CRITICAL CARE

SECRETS

CRITICAL CARE

F

P
E.l
Co
Bu

Je
He
Ha
Bo

ELSEVIER

MOSBY

3251 Riverport Lane
St. Louis, Missouri 63043

Critical Care Secrets
Fifth Edition

ISBN: 978-0-323-08500-7

Notice

Knowledge and best practice in this field are constantly changing. As new research and experience broaden our knowledge, changes in practice, treatment, and drug therapy may become necessary or appropriate. Readers are advised to check the most current information provided (i) on procedures featured or (ii) by the manufacturer of each product to be administered, to verify the recommended dose or formula, the method and duration of administration, and contraindications. It is the responsibility of the practitioner, relying on his or her own experience and knowledge of the patient, to make diagnoses, to determine dosages and the best treatment for each individual patient, and to take all appropriate safety precautions. To the fullest extent of the law, neither the Publisher nor the editors assume any liability for any injury and/or damage to persons or property arising out of or related to any use of the material contained in this book.

Library of Congress Cataloging-in-Publication Data
Critical care secrets / [edited by] Polly E. Parsons, Jeanine P. Wiener-Kronish. – 5th ed.
    p. ; cm. – (Secrets series)
Includes bibliographical references and index.
ISBN 978-0-323-08500-7 (pbk. : alk. paper)
I. Parsons, Polly E., 1954- II. Wiener-Kronish, Jeanine P., 1951- III. Series: Secrets series.
[DNLM: 1. Critical Care–Examination Questions. WX 18.2]
616.02'8–dc23

2012017925

Executive Content Strategist: James Merritt
Content Development Specialist: Barbara Cicalese
Publishing Services Manager: Anne Altepeter
Project Manager: Louise King
Design Manager: Steven Stave

Working together to grow
libraries in developing countries

www.elsevier.com | www.bookaid.org | www.sabre.org

ELSEVIER | BOOK AID International | Sabre Foundation

Printed in China

Last digit is the print number: 9 8 7 6 5 4 3 2 1

To our husbands, Jim and Daniel, and our children, Alec, Chandler, Jessica, and Samuel, for their patience and support, and for allowing us to take the time to complete this edition

CONTRIBUTORS

Neil Agrawal, MD
Cardiology Specialist, Oklahoma Heart Institute, Tulsa, Oklahoma

Ali Al-Alwan, MD
Clinical Instructor, Pulmonary and Critical Care Medicine, University of Vermont College of Medicine; Fellow, Pulmonary and Critical Care Medicine, Fletcher Allen Health Care, Burlington, Vermont

Hasan B. Alam, MD, FACS
Professor of Surgery, Harvard Medical School; Director of Surgical Critical Care/Acute Care Surgery Fellowship Program, Division of Trauma, Emergency Surgery, and Surgical Critical Care, Massachusetts General Hospital, Boston, Massachusetts

Rae M. Allain, MD
Assistant Professor of Anesthesia, Harvard Medical School; Division Chief, Thoracic, Vascular, Radiology, and Neuroanesthesia, Department of Anesthesia, Critical Care, and Pain Medicine, Massachusetts General Hospital, Boston, Massachusetts

Gilman B. Allen, MD
Associate Professor of Medicine, Director of Medical Intensive Care Unit, Pulmonary and Critical Care Medicine, University of Vermont College of Medicine; Attending Physician, Pulmonary and Critical Care Medicine, Fletcher Allen Health Care, Burlington, Vermont

Michael N. Andrawes, MD
Instructor, Department of Anesthesia, Critical Care, and Pain Medicine, Massachusetts General Hospital/Harvard Medical School, Boston, Massachusetts

Abbas Ardehali, MD, FACS
Professor of Surgery and Medicine, Division of Cardiothoracic Surgery, UCLA; Director of Heart, Lung, and Heart/Lung Transplant Programs, Division of Cardiothoracic Surgery, Ronald Reagan UCLA Medical Center; Chief, Division of Cardiac Surgery, Veterans Affairs Greater Los Angeles Healthcare System, Los Angeles, California

Aranya Bagchi, MBBS
Clinical Fellow in Anesthesia, Department of Anesthesia, Critical Care and Pain Medicine, Massachusetts General Hospital/Harvard Medical School, Boston, Massachusetts

Keith Baker, MD, PhD
Assistant Professor of Anesthesia, Harvard Medical School; Assistant Anesthetist, Department of Anesthesia, Critical Care, and Pain Medicine, Massachusetts General Hospital, Boston, Massachusetts

Arna Banerjee, MD
Assistant Professor of Anesthesiology and Surgery, Department of Anesthesiology and Critical Care, Vanderbilt University Medical Center, Nashville, Tennessee

Carolyn E. Bekes, MD, MHA, FCCM
Professor of Medicine, Cooper Medical School of Rowan University; Chief Medical Officer, Cooper University Hospital, Camden, New Jersey

William J. Benedetto, MD
Anesthesia Instructor, Department of Anesthesia, Critical Care, and Pain Management, Massachusetts General Hospital, Boston, Massachusetts

Pavan K. Bendapudi, MD
Clinical Fellow, Pathology Department, Harvard Medical School; Clinical Fellow, Blood Transfusion Service, Brigham and Women's Hospital, Boston, Massachusetts

John R. Benjamin, MD, MSc
Fellow in Critical Care Medicine, Department of Anesthesia, Critical Care, and Pain Management, Massachusetts General Hospital, Boston, Massachusetts; Commander, Medical Corps, United States Navy, Walter Reed Memorial Military Medical Center, Bethesda, Maryland

Philip E. Bickler, MD, PhD
Professor, Department of Anesthesia and Perioperative Care, UCSF, San Francisco, California

Luca M. Bigatello, MD
Adjunct Professor of Anesthesiology, Tufts University School of Medicine, Boston; Director, Surgical Critical Care, Department of Anesthesiology and Pain Medicine, St. Elizabeth's Medical Center, Brighton, Massachusetts

Edward A. Bittner, MD, PhD
Assistant Professor of Anesthesia, Harvard Medical School; Associate Director, Surgical Intensive Care Unit, Program Director, Critical Care-Anesthesiology Fellowship, Department of Anesthesia, Critical Care, and Pain Medicine, Massachusetts General Hospital, Boston, Massachusetts

Brad W. Butcher, MD
Fellow, Department of Internal Medicine, Division of Nephrology, UCSF Medical Center, San Francisco, California

Michael E. Canham, MD
Associate Professor of Medicine, National Jewish Medical and Research Center, University of Colorado Health Sciences Center, Denver, Colorado

William E. Charash, MD, PhD
Associate Professor, Surgery, Chief, Division of Trauma, Burns, and Surgical Critical Care, University of Vermont College of Medicine, Burlington, Vermont

Jonathan E. Charnin, MD
Instructor, Harvard Medical School; Assistant Residency Program Director, Department of Anesthesia, Critical Care, and Pain Medicine, Massachusetts General Hospital, Boston, Massachusetts

Hovig V. Chitilian, MD
Instructor in Anesthesia, Harvard Medical School; Staff Anesthesiologist, Department of Anesthesia, Critical Care, and Pain Medicine, Massachusetts General Hospital, Boston, Massachusetts

Alexandra F.M. Cist, MD
Instructor in Medicine, Harvard Medical School; Assistant in Medicine, Pulmonary and Critical Care Unit, Massachusetts General Hospital, Boston, Massachusetts

Jaina Clough, MD
Assistant Professor, Primary Care Internal Medicine, University of Vermont College of Medicine/
Fletcher Allen Health Care, Burlington, Vermont

J. Perren Cobb, MD
Associate Professor, Departments of Anesthesia and Surgery, Harvard University; Director,
Critical Care Center, Vice-Chair for Critical Care, Department of Anesthesia, Critical Care, and
Pain Medicine, Massachusetts General Hospital, Boston, Massachusetts

Elizabeth Cox, MD
Anesthesia Resident, Department of Anesthesia, Critical Care, and Pain Medicine, Massachusetts
General Hospital, Boston, Massachusetts

Bruce A. Crookes, MD, FACS
Associate Professor of Surgery, Department of Surgery, Medical University of South Carolina,
Charleston, South Carolina

Harold L. Dauerman, MD
Professor of Medicine, University of Vermont College of Medicine; Director, Cardiovascular
Catheterization Laboratories, Fletcher Allen Health Care, Burlington, Vermont

Marc A. DeMoya, MD
Assistant Professor of Surgery, Division of Trauma, Emergency Surgery, and Surgical
Critical Care, Massachusetts General Hospital/Harvard Medical School, Boston,
Massachusetts

Anne E. Dixon, MA, BM, BCh
Associate Professor, Department of Medicine, University of Vermont College of Medicine,
Burlington, Vermont

Cameron Donaldson, MD
Clinical Instructor, University of Vermont College of Medicine; Fellow, Cardiology, Fletcher Allen
Health Care, Burlington, Vermont

Shawn P. Fagan, MD
Medical Director, Division of Burns, Massachusetts General Hospital and Shriners Hospital for
Children, Boston, Massachusetts

Peter J. Fagenholz, MD
Attending Surgeon, Department of Surgery, Division of Trauma, Emergency Surgery, and Critical
Care, Massachusetts General Hospital; Instructor in Surgery, Harvard Medical School, Boston,
Massachusetts

Corey R. Fehnel, MD
Clinical Fellow, Neurology, Harvard Medical School; Neurocritical Care Fellow, Massachusetts
General Hospital, Boston, Massachusetts

Michael G. Fitzsimons, MD, FCCP
Director, Division of Cardiac Anesthesia, Assistant Professor, Department of Anesthesia, Critical
Care, and Pain Medicine, Massachusetts General Hospital, Boston, Massachusetts

Zechariah S. Gardner, MD
Assistant Professor, Primary Care Internal Medicine, University of Vermont College of Medicine;
Attending Physician, Hospitalist Medicine, Primary Care Internal Medicine, Fletcher Allen Health
Care, Burlington, Vermont

Edward E. George, MD, PhD
Medical Director, Post Anesthesia Care Units, Assistant Anesthetist, Department of Anesthesia, Critical Care, and Pain Management, Massachusetts General Hospital, Boston, Massachusetts; Assistant Professor in Anesthesia, Harvard Medical School, Boston, Massachusetts; Commander, Medical Corps, United States Navy, Walter Reed Memorial Military Medical Center, Bethesda, Maryland

Matthew P. Gilbert, DO, MPH
Assistant Professor of Medicine, Endocrinology, Diabetes, and Metabolism, University of Vermont College of Medicine, Burlington, Vermont

Jeremy Goverman, MD, FACS
Instructor, Department of Surgery, Harvard Medical School; Assistant in Surgery, Division of Burns, Massachusetts General Hospital; Medical Staff, Burns, Shriners Hospital for Children, Boston, Massachusetts

Christopher Grace, MD, FACP
Director, Infectious Diseases Unit, Fletcher Allen Health Care; Professor of Medicine, Department of Medicine, University of Vermont College of Medicine, Burlington, Vermont

Michael A. Gropper, MD, PhD
Professor and Executive Vice Chairperson, Department of Anesthesia and Perioperative Care, Director, Critical Care Medicine, Investigator, Cardiovascular Research Institute, UCSF, San Francisco, California

Jennifer M. Hall, DO
Fellow, Geriatric Psychiatry, Duke University Hospital, Durham, North Carolina

Michael E. Hanley, MD
Professor of Medicine, Division of Pulmonary and Critical Care Medicine, University of Colorado Denver Health Sciences Center; Associate Director of Medicine, Denver Health Medical Center, Denver, Colorado

C. William Hanson, III, MD
Professor of Anesthesiology and Critical Care, University of Pennsylvania, Philadelphia, Pennsylvania

John E. Heffner, MD
Professor of Medicine, Oregon Health and Science University; William M. Garnjobst Chair, Department of Medicine, Providence Portland Medical Center, Attending Physician, The Oregon Clinic, Portland, Oregon

David C. Hooper, MD
Professor of Medicine, Harvard Medical School; Associate Chief, Division of Infectious Diseases, Chief, Infection Control Unit, Massachusetts General Hospital, Boston, Massachusetts

Christopher D. Huston, MD
Associate Professor, Infectious Diseases, Departments of Medicine, and Microbiology and Molecular Genetics, University of Vermont College of Medicine, Burlington, Vermont

James L. Jacobson, MD
Associate Professor, Psychiatry, University of Vermont College of Medicine; Director, Outpatient Psychiatry Department and Psychopharmacology Clinic, Fletcher Allen Health Care, Burlington, Vermont

Daniel W. Johnson, MD
Instructor, Harvard Medical School; Department of Anesthesia, Critical Care, and Pain Medicine, Massachusetts General Hospital, Boston, Massachusetts

Christine Haas Jones, MD
Assistant Professor of Medicine, University of Vermont College of Medicine, Burlington, Vermont

David A. Kaminsky, MD
Associate Professor, Pulmonary and Critical Care Medicine, University of Vermont College of Medicine; Attending Physician, Pulmonary and Critical Care Medicine, Fletcher Allen Health Care, Burlington, Vermont

George Kasotakis, MD
Instructor in Surgery, Harvard Medical School; Acute Care Surgery Fellow, Division of Trauma, Emergency Surgery, and Surgical Critical Care, Massachusetts General Hospital, Boston, Massachusetts

Dinkar Kaw, MD
Associate Professor of Medicine, Division of Nephrology, Department of Medicine, University of Toledo College of Medicine, Toledo, Ohio

David R. King, MD, FACS
Instructor, Department of Surgery, Harvard Medical School; Attending Surgeon, Division of Trauma, Emergency Surgery, and Surgical Critical Care, Massachusetts General Hospital, Boston, Massachusetts

Themistoklis Kourkoumpetis, MD
Postdoctoral Research Fellow, Division of Infectious Diseases, Massachusetts General Hospital/ Harvard Medical School, Boston, Massachusetts

Asheesh Kumar, MD
Assistant Professor, Department of Anesthesiology, Uniformed Health Sciences University, Bethesda, Maryland

David J. Kuter, MD, DPhil
Professor of Medicine, Harvard Medical School; Chief of Hematology, Department of Medicine, Massachusetts General Hospital, Boston, Massachusetts

Stephen E. Lapinsky, MBBCh, MSc, FRCPC
Professor, Department of Medicine, University of Toronto; Site Director, Intensive Care Unit, Mount Sinai Hospital, Toronto, Ontario, Canada

Jack L. Leahy, MD
Professor of Medicine and Chief of Endocrinology, Diabetes, and Metabolism, University of Vermont College of Medicine, Burlington, Vermont

Kay B. Leissner, MD, PhD
Instructor, Department of Anesthesia, Harvard Medical School; Adjunct Assistant Professor of Anesthesiology, Boston University School of Medicine; Adjunct Assistant Professor of Anesthesiology, Tufts University School of Medicine, Boston; Chief, Anesthesiology Service, Veterans Affairs Boston Healthcare System, West Roxbury, Massachusetts

Martin M. LeWinter, MD
Professor, Medicine and Molecular Physiology and Biophysics, University of Vermont College of Medicine; Attending Physician, Cardiology, Fletcher Allen Health Care, Burlington, Vermont

Stuart L. Linas, MD
Rocky Mountain Kidney Professor of Renal Research and Professor of Medicine, University of Colorado School of Medicine; Chief of Nephrology, Denver Health Sciences Center, Denver, Colorado

Kathleen D. Liu, MD, PhD, MAS
Assistant Professor, Departments of Medicine and Anesthesia, UCSF, San Francisco, California

Madison Macht, MD
Fellow, Pulmonary Sciences and Critical Care Medicine, University of Colorado Denver, Aurora, Colorado

Theodore W. Marcy, MD, MPH
Professor Emeritus of Medicine, Pulmonary Disease and Critical Care Medicine, University of Vermont College of Medicine, Burlington, Vermont

Annis Marney, MD, MSCI
Assistant Professor of Medicine, Division of Diabetes, Endocrinology, and Metabolism, University of Vermont College of Medicine; Attending Physician, Fletcher Allen Health Care, Burlington, Vermont

Jenny L. Martino, MD, MSPH
Attending Physician, Pulmonary and Critical Care Medicine, PeaceHealth Medical Group, PeaceHealth Southwest Medical Center, Vancouver, Washington

Philip McArdle, MB, BCh, BAO, FFARCSI
Associate Professor, Department of Anesthesiology, University of Alabama at Birmingham, Birmingham, Alabama

David W. McFadden, MD, FACS
Professor and Chair, Department of Surgery, University of Connecticut School of Medicine, Farmington, Connecticut

Ursula McVeigh, MD
Assistant Professor, Department of Family Medicine, University of Vermont College of Medicine; Interim Director, Palliative Care Service, Fletcher Allen Health Care, Burlington, Vermont

Ali Y. Mejaddam, MD
Trauma Research Fellow, Division of Trauma, Emergency Surgery, and Surgical Critical Care, Massachusetts General Hospital/Harvard Medical School, Boston, Massachusetts

Prema R. Menon, MD
Clinical Instructor, Pulmonary/Critical Care, University of Vermont College of Medicine/Fletcher Allen Health Care, Burlington, Vermont

David W. Miller, MD
Assistant Professor, Department of Anesthesiology, Division of Critical Care and Perioperative Medicine, Co-Director, Neurosciences Intensive Care Unit, University of Alabama at Birmingham, Birmingham, Alabama

Benoit Misset, MD
Professor of Intensive Care Medicine, Paris Descartes University; Head of Medical Surgical Intensive Care Unit, Paris Saint-Joseph Hospital Network, Paris, France

Sarah Mooney, MBBCh, MRCP
Fellow, Infectious Diseases, University of Vermont College of Medicine/Fletcher Allen Health Care, Burlington, Vermont

Amy E. Morris, MD
Assistant Professor, Division of Pulmonary and Critical Care Medicine, University of Washington, Seattle, Washington

Marc Moss, MD
Roger S. Mitchell Professor of Medicine, Division of Pulmonary Sciences and Critical Care Medicine, University of Colorado Denver, Aurora, Colorado

Eleftherios E. Mylonakis, MD, PhD, FIDSA
Associate Professor of Medicine, Division of Infectious Diseases, Massachusetts General Hospital/Harvard Medical School, Boston, Massachusetts

Claus U. Niemann, MD
Professor of Anesthesia and Surgery, Department of Anesthesia and Perioperative Care, and Department of Surgery, Division of Transplantation, UCSF, San Francisco, California

Cindy Noyes, MD
Assistant Professor of Medicine, Infectious Disease, Fletcher Allen Health Care/University of Vermont College of Medicine, Burlington, Vermont

Ala Nozari, MD, PhD
Assistant Professor of Anesthesia, Harvard Medical School; Assistant Anesthetist, Department of Anesthesia, Critical Care, and Pain Medicine, Massachusetts General Hospital, Boston, Massachusetts

Islem Ouanes, MD
Assistant Professor of Intensive Care Medicine, Intensive Care Unit, University Hospital Fattouma Bourguiba, University of Monastir, Monastir, Tunisia

Pratik Pandharipande, MBBS, MSCI
Associate Professor of Anesthesiology, Department of Anesthesiology and Critical Care, Vanderbilt University Medical Center and Tennessee Valley Healthcare System, Nashville, Tennessee

Manuel Pardo, Jr., MD
Professor and Vice Chair for Education, Department of Anesthesia and Perioperative Care, UCSF, San Francisco, California

Kapil Patel, MD
Clinical Assistant Professor of Medicine, Pulmonary and Critical Care Medicine, University of Maryland Medical Center, Baltimore, Maryland; Attending Physician, Pulmonary and Critical Care Medicine, Upper Chesapeake Medical Center, Bel-Air, Maryland

William Peery, MD
Assistant Professor of Surgery, Department of Surgery, West Virginia University, Charleston, West Virginia

Sarah Pesek, MD
Clinical Instructor, Surgery, University of Vermont College of Medicine; Surgical Resident, Fletcher Allen Health Care, Burlington, Vermont

Kristen K. Pierce, MD
Assistant Professor of Medicine, Infectious Disease, University of Vermont College of Medicine/Fletcher Allen Health Care, Burlington, Vermont

Jean-François Pittet, MD
Director, Division of Critical Care and Perioperative Medicine, Professor and Vice-Chair, Department of Anesthesiology, University of Alabama at Birmingham, Birmingham, Alabama

Louis B. Polish, MD
Associate Professor of Medicine, Division of Infectious Diseases, Director, Internal Medicine Clerkship, University of Vermont College of Medicine, Burlington, Vermont

Nitin Puri, MD, FACP
Medical Intensivist, Pulmonary/Critical Care, Inova Fairfax Hospital, Falls Church, Virginia

Allan Ramsay, MD
Professor Emeritus, Department of Family Medicine, University of Vermont College of Medicine, Burlington, Vermont; Interim Medical Director, Hospice of the Champlain Valley, Colchester, Vermont

Daniel Saddawi-Konefka, MD, MBA
Clinical Fellow, Department of Anesthesia, Harvard Medical School; Resident, Department of Anesthesia, Critical Care, and Pain Medicine, Massachusetts General Hospital, Boston, Massachusetts

Neeraj K. Sardana, MD
Fellow, Department of Gastroenterology and Hepatology, University of Vermont College of Medicine/Fletcher Allen Health Care, Burlington, Vermont

Richard H. Savel, MD, FCCM
Associate Professor of Clinical Medicine and Neurology, Albert Einstein College of Medicine; Medical Co-Director, Surgical Intensive Care Unit, Montefiore Medical Center, Bronx, New York

Ulrich H. Schmidt, MD, PhD
Associate Professor, Department of Anesthesia, Critical Care, and Pain Medicine, Harvard Medical School; Medical Director, Surgical Intensive Care Unit and Respiratory Care Services, Massachusetts General Hospital, Boston, Massachusetts

Lynn M. Schnapp, MD
Professor, Pulmonary and Critical Care Medicine and Center for Lung Biology, University of Washington; Attending Physician, Medical and Trauma Intensive Care Unit, Harborview Medical Center, Seattle, Washington

Alison Schneider, MD
Clinical Instructor and Fellow, Endocrinology, Diabetes, and Metabolism, University of Vermont College of Medicine, Burlington, Vermont

Joel J. Schnure, MD
Associate Professor, University of Vermont College of Medicine; Co-Director, Division of Endocrinology, Diabetes, and Metabolism, Fletcher Allen Health Care; Burlington, Vermont

Lee H. Schwamm, MD, FAHA
Vice Chairman, Department of Neurology, C. Miller Fisher Endowed Chair and Director, TeleStroke and Acute Stroke Services, Massachusetts General Hospital; Professor of Neurology, Harvard Medical School, Boston, Massachusetts

Joseph I. Shapiro, MD
Dean, Marshall University Joan C. Edwards School of Medicine, Huntington, West Virginia

Shailendra Sharma, MD
Academic Hospitalist, Denver Hospital and Health Authority; Nephrology Fellow, University of Colorado School of Medicine, Denver, Colorado

Kenneth Shelton, MD
Clinical Fellow in Anesthesia, Department of Anesthesia, Critical Care, and Pain Medicine, Massachusetts General Hospital/Harvard Medical School, Boston, Massachusetts

Erica S. Shenoy, MD, PhD
Research Fellow in Medicine, Harvard Medical School; Clinical and Research Fellow, Division of Infectious Diseases, Infection Control Unit, Massachusetts General Hospital, Boston, Massachusetts

David Shimabukuro, MDCM
Medical Director, Department of Anesthesia and Perioperative Care, UCSF, San Francisco, California

Stuart F. Sidlow, MD
Attending Anesthesiologist, Department of Anesthesiology, Pennsylvania Hospital, Philadelphia, Pennsylvania

Aaron B. Skolnik, MD
Clinical Fellow, Department of Medical Toxicology, Banner Good Samaritan Medical Center, Phoenix, Arizona

Peter S. Spector, MD
Professor of Medicine, Department of Medicine, University of Vermont College of Medicine; Director, Cardiac Electrophysiology, Attending Physician, Cardiology, Fletcher Allen Health Care, Burlington, Vermont

Antoinette Spevetz, MD, FCCM, FACP
Associate Professor of Medicine, Cooper Medical School of Rowan University; Associate Director, MSICU for Operations, Director, Intermediate Care Unit, Section of Critical Care Medicine, Cooper University Hospital, Camden, New Jersey

Renee D. Stapleton, MD, PhD
Assistant Professor, Medicine, Pulmonary, and Critical Care Medicine, University of Vermont College of Medicine, Burlington, Vermont

Scott C. Streckenbach, MD
Assistant Professor, Anesthesia, Massachusetts General Hospital/Harvard Medical School, Boston, Massachusetts

Benjamin T. Suratt, MD
Associate Professor of Medicine and Associate Chief, Division of Pulmonary and Critical Care Medicine, University of Vermont College of Medicine; Attending Physician, Department of Medicine, Fletcher Allen Health Care, Burlington, Vermont

Lynda S. Tilluckdharry, MB, BCh, BAO, LRCP&SI
Consultant, Rheumatology and Immunology, Cross Crossing Medical Center, San Fernando, Trinidad and Tobago, West Indies

Gwendolyn M. van der Wilden, MSc
Clinical Research Fellow, Surgery, Division of Trauma, Emergency Surgery, and Surgical Critical Care, Massachusetts General Hospital, Boston, Massachusetts

Susan A. Vassallo, MD
Assistant Professor of Anesthesia, Harvard Medical School; Anesthetist, Department of Anesthesia, Critical Care, and Pain Management, Massachusetts General Hospital, Boston, Massachusetts

George C. Velmahos, MD, PhD, MSEd
John Francis Burke Professor of Surgery, Harvard Medical School; Chief, Division of Trauma, Emergency Surgery, and Surgical Critical Care, Massachusetts General Hospital, Boston, Massachusetts

Joseph L. Weidman, MD
Anesthesiology Resident, Department of Anesthesiology, Critical Care, and Pain Medicine, Massachusetts General Hospital, Boston, Massachusetts

Jeanine P. Wiener-Kronish, MD
Henry Isaiah Dorr Professor of Research and Teaching in Anesthetics and Anesthesia, Harvard Medical School; Anesthetist-in-Chief, Massachusetts General Hospital, Boston, Massachusetts

Susan R. Wilcox, MD
Staff Physician, Department of Anesthesia, Critical Care, and Pain Medicine, and Department of Emergency Medicine, Massachusetts General Hospital, Boston, Massachusetts

Chad Wilson, MD, MPH
Assistant Professor of Surgery, New York University School of Medicine, New York, New York

Marie E. Wood, MD
Professor of Medicine, University of Vermont College of Medicine, Burlington, Vermont

Daniel Yagoda, MPH
Health Engineer, Critical Care Center, Massachusetts General Hospital, Boston, Massachusetts

Jon (Kai) Yamaguchi, MD, FACS
Assistant Professor of Surgery, University of Vermont College of Medicine; Chief, Division of Transplant Surgery, Fletcher Allen Health Care, Burlington, Vermont

Michael Young, MD
Professor of Medicine, Pulmonary and Critical Care, Wake Forest University; Medical Director and Attending Physician, Intermediate Care and Medical Intensive Care Unit, Wake Forest/Baptist Medical Center, Winston-Salem, North Carolina

Pierre Znojkiewicz, MD
Clinical Instructor and Fellow, Cardiology, University of Vermont College of Medicine, Burlington, Vermont

PREFACE

Over the course of the past five editions of *Critical Care Secrets*, critical care medicine has become increasingly complex. The fundamentals and clinical skills required to care for critically ill patients continue to transcend subspecialties, so in this edition we have again included chapters from a wide range of specialists, including pulmonologists, surgeons, anesthesiologists, psychiatrists, pharmacists, and infectious disease experts. We have asked these experts to pose the key questions in critical care and formulate the answers so practitioners can identify effective solutions to their patients' medical and ethical problems.

A broad understanding of anatomy, physiology, immunology, and inflammation is fundamentally important to effectively care for critically ill patients. For example, it is hard to imagine understanding the principles of mechanical ventilation without being aware of the principles of gas and fluid flow, pulmonary mechanics, and electronic circuitry. Accordingly, the authors have incorporated these key elements into this edition. In addition, critical care medicine requires knowledge of protocols and guidelines that are continuously evolving and that increasingly dictate best practices.

In this fifth edition of *Critical Care Secrets*, we have again been fortunate to have many of the leaders in critical care contribute chapters in their areas of expertise. In addition to substantially revising and updating chapters from the previous edition, we have included new chapters on timely topics such as intensive care unit ultrasound, extracorporeal membrane oxygenation, influenza, disaster medicine, arterial and central venous catheters, the immunocompromised host, toxic alcohol and cardiovascular drug poisoning, palliative care, and organ donation.

We sincerely thank all of the authors who contributed their time and expertise to this endeavor. We believe they have captured the essence of critical care medicine and have presented it in a format that will be useful to everyone, from students to experienced clinicians.

Polly E. Parsons, MD
Jeanine P. Wiener-Kronish, MD

CONTENTS

Top 100 Secrets 1

I. BASIC LIFE SUPPORT

1. General Approach to the Critically Ill Patient...........................9
   Manuel Pardo, Jr., MD, and Michael A. Gropper, MD, PhD

2. General Approach to Trauma Patients............................... 13
   Peter J. Fagenholz, MD, and Hasan B. Alam, MD, FACS

3. Cardiopulmonary Resuscitation.................................... 20
   David Shimabukuro, MDCM

4. Assessments of Oxygenation 28
   Asheesh Kumar, MD, Michael E. Canham, MD, and Ulrich H. Schmidt, MD, PhD

5. Pulse Oximetry, Capnography, and Blood Gas Analysis 33
   Philip E. Bickler, MD, PhD

6. Hemodynamic Monitoring 39
   Daniel Saddawi-Konefka, MD, MBA, and Jonathan E. Charnin, MD

7. Fluid Therapy... 47
   Elizabeth Cox, MD, and Keith Baker, MD, PhD

8. Nutrition in Critically Ill Patients.................................... 50
   Renee D. Stapleton, MD, PhD

9. Mechanical and Noninvasive Ventilation............................ 58
   Manuel Pardo, Jr., MD

10. Discontinuation of Mechanical Ventilation 63
    Theodore W. Marcy, MD, MPH, and Jenny L. Martino, MD, MSPH

II. PROCEDURES

11. Arterial and Central Venous Catheters............................... 69
    Hovig V. Chitilian, MD

12. Ultrasound in the Intensive Care Unit 74
    Daniel W. Johnson, MD

13. Extracorporeal Membrane Oxygenation............................. 79
    Michael G. Fitzsimons, MD, FCCP, and Michael N. Andrawes, MD

14. Tracheal Intubation and Airway Management 87
   Manuel Pardo, Jr., MD

15. Tracheotomy and Upper Airway Obstruction 93
   John E. Heffner, MD

16. Chest Tubes 100
   Gwendolyn M. van der Wilden, MSc, and David R. King, MD, FACS

17. Bronchoscopy 106
   Amy E. Morris, MD, and Lynn M. Schnapp, MD

18. Pacemakers and Defibrillators 113
   Scott C. Streckenbach, MD, and Kenneth Shelton, MD

19. Circulatory Assist Devices 121
   Joseph L. Weidman, MD, Michael N. Andrawes, MD, and Michael G. Fitzsimons, MD, FCCP

III. PULMONARY MEDICINE

20. Acute Bacterial Pneumonia 131
   Kenneth Shelton, MD, Jeanine P. Wiener-Kronish, MD, and Aranya Bagchi, MBBS

21. Asthma 142
   Ali Al-Alwan, MD, Gilman B. Allen, MD, and David A. Kaminsky, MD

22. Chronic Obstructive Pulmonary Disease 151
   Anne E. Dixon, MA, BM, BCh

23. Cor Pulmonale 157
   Luca M. Bigatello, MD, and Kay B. Leissner, MD, PhD

24. Acute Respiratory Failure, Acute Lung Injury/Acute Respiratory
   Distress Syndrome, and Acute Chest Syndrome 166
   Prema R. Menon, MD, and Gilman B. Allen, MD

25. Hemoptysis 171
   Michael E. Hanley, MD

26. Venous Thromboembolism and Fat Embolism 177
   Madison Macht, MD, and Marc Moss, MD

IV. CARDIOLOGY

27. Heart Failure and Valvular Heart Disease 185
   Martin M. LeWinter, MD, and Neil Agrawal, MD

28. Acute Myocardial Infarction 192
   Cameron Donaldson, MD, and Harold L. Dauerman, MD

29. Dysrhythmias and Tachyarrhythmias 197
   Pierre Znojkiewicz, MD, and Peter S. Spector, MD

30. Aortic Dissection 204
   Asheesh Kumar, MD, and Rae M. Allain, MD

31. Pericardial Disease (Pericarditis and Pericardial Tamponade) 212
   Stuart F. Sidlow, MD, and C. William Hanson, III, MD

V. INFECTIOUS DISEASE

32. Sepsis, Severe Sepsis, and Septic Shock............................ 217
   David Shimabukuro, MDCM, Richard H. Savel, MD, FCCM, and Michael A. Gropper, MD, PhD

33. Endocarditis.. 223
   Louis B. Polish, MD

34. Meningitis and Encephalitis in the Intensive Care Unit................ 232
   Cindy Noyes, MD, and Christopher D. Huston, MD

35. Disseminated Fungal Infections 240
   Themistoklis Kourkoumpetis, MD, and Eleftherios E. Mylonakis, MD, PhD, FIDSA

36. Multidrug-Resistant Bacteria 246
   Christopher Grace, MD, FACP

37. Bioterrorism... 252
   Sarah Mooney, MBBCh, MRCP, and Christopher Grace, MD, FACP

38. Skin and Soft Tissue Infections 262
   Erica S. Shenoy, MD, PhD, and David C. Hooper, MD

39. Influenza.. 271
   Christopher Grace, MD, FACP

40. Immunocompromised Host 277
   Kristen K. Pierce, MD

VI. RENAL DISEASE

41. Hypertension 293
   Stuart L. Linas, MD, and Shailendra Sharma, MD

42. Acute Renal Failure 299
   Dinkar Kaw, MD, and Joseph I. Shapiro, MD

43. Renal Replacement Therapy and Rhabdomyolysis.................... 306
   Brad W. Butcher, MD, and Kathleen D. Liu, MD, PhD, MAS

44. Hypokalemia and Hyperkalemia 315
   Stuart L. Linas, MD, and Shailendra Sharma, MD

45. Hyponatremia and Hypernatremia 322
   Brad W. Butcher, MD, and Kathleen D. Liu, MD, PhD, MAS

VII. GASTROENTEROLOGY

46. Gastrointestinal Bleeding in the Critically Ill Patient.................. 329
   George Kasotakis, MD, and George C. Velmahos, MD, PhD, MSEd

47. Acute Pancreatitis.. 336
   *Neeraj K. Sardana, MD, Jon (Kai) Yamaguchi, MD, FACS,
   and David W. McFadden, MD, FACS*

48. Hepatitis and Cirrhosis 343
   Zechariah S. Gardner, MD, and Jaina Clough, MD

49. Acute Abdomen and Peritonitis.................................... 352
William E. Charash, MD, PhD, and Sarah Pesek, MD

VIII. ENDOCRINOLOGY

50. Diabetic Ketoacidosis and Hyperosmolar Hyperglycemic State......... 359
Joel J. Schnure, MD, and Jack L. Leahy, MD

51. Management of Hyperglycemia in the Critically Ill.................... 369
Matthew P. Gilbert, DO, MPH, and Alison Schneider, MD

52. Adrenal Insufficiency in the Intensive Care Unit...................... 374
Michael Young, MD

53. Thyroid Disease in the Intensive Care Unit 379
Annis Marney, MD, MSCI

IX. HEMATOLOGY/ONCOLOGY

54. Blood Products and Coagulation 385
George Kasotakis, MD, and Hasan B. Alam, MD, FACS

55. Thrombocytopenia and Platelets................................... 392
Chad T. Wilson, MD, MPH, and Hasan B. Alam, MD, FACS

56. Disseminated Intravascular Coagulation 397
Pavan K. Bendapudi, MD, and David J. Kuter, MD, DPhil

57. Oncologic Emergencies (Including Hypercalcemia) 404
Marie E. Wood, MD

X. RHEUMATOLOGY

58. Rheumatologic Disease in the Intensive Care Unit.................... 411
Lynda S. Tilluckdharry, MB, BCh, BAO, LRCP&SI, and Christine Haas Jones, MD

XI. NEUROLOGY

59. Coma... 423
Ala Nozari, MD, PhD, Corey R. Fehnel, MD, and Lee H. Schwamm, MD, FAHA

60. Brain Death 428
Corey R. Fehnel, MD, Ala Nozari, MD, PhD, and Lee H. Schwamm, MD, FAHA

61. Status Epilepticus... 434
Ala Nozari, MD, PhD, Corey R. Fehnel, MD, and Lee H. Schwamm, MD, FAHA

62. Stroke 441
Corey R. Fehnel, MD, Ala Nozari, MD, PhD, and Lee H. Schwamm, MD, FAHA

63. Guillain-Barré Syndrome.. 448
Ala Nozari, MD, PhD, Corey R. Fehnel, MD, and Lee H. Schwamm, MD, FAHA

64. Myasthenia Gravis 452
Corey R. Fehnel, MD, Ala Nozari, MD, PhD, and Lee H. Schwamm, MD, FAHA

65. Alcohol Withdrawal 456
     Bruce A. Crookes, MD, FACS, and William Peery, MD

XII. SURGERY AND TRAUMA

66. Burns and Frostbite 461
     Shawn P. Fagan, MD, and Jeremy Goverman, MD, FACS

67. Pneumothorax 468
     Madison Macht, MD, and Michael E. Hanley, MD

68. Flail Chest and Pulmonary Contusion 475
     Susan R. Wilcox, MD, and Edward A. Bittner, MD, PhD

69. Cardiac Trauma 482
     Ali Y. Mejaddam, MD, and Marc A. DeMoya, MD

XIII. PERIOPERATIVE CARE

70. Liver and Heart Transplantation 489
     Claus U. Niemann, MD, and Abbas Ardehali, MD, FACS

XIV. SEDATION AND PAIN MANAGEMENT

71. Use of Paralytic Agents in the Intensive Care Unit 497
     David W. Miller, MD, and Jean-François Pittet, MD

72. Pain Management in the Intensive Care Unit 504
     Philip McArdle, MB, BCh, BAO, FFARCSI, and Jean-François Pittet, MD

73. Sedation and Delirium 512
     Pratik Pandharipande, MBBS, MSCI, and Arna Banerjee, MD

XV. EMERGENCY MEDICINE

74. Disaster Medicine: Impact on Critical Care Operations 521
     John R. Benjamin, MD, MSc, and Edward E. George, MD, PhD

75. Allergy and Anaphylaxis 527
     Susan A. Vassallo, MD

76. Hypothermia 534
     Peter J. Fagenholz, MD, and Edward A. Bittner, MD, PhD

77. Heat Stroke 541
     William J. Benedetto, MD

XVI. TOXICOLOGY

78. General Toxicology and Toxidromes 545
     Aaron B. Skolnik, MD, and Susan R. Wilcox, MD

79. Analgesics and Antidepressants 552
     Aaron B. Skolnik, MD, and Susan R. Wilcox, MD

80. Toxic Alcohol Poisoning 558
   Aaron B. Skolnik, MD, and Susan R. Wilcox, MD

81. Poisoning by Cardiovascular Drugs 562
   Aaron B. Skolnik, MD, and Susan R. Wilcox, MD

82. Neuroleptic Malignant Syndrome 565
   Jennifer M. Hall, DO, and James L. Jacobson, MD

XVII. OBSTETRICS

83. Care of the Critically Ill Pregnant Patient 571
   Stephen E. Lapinsky, MBBCh, MSc, FRCPC

XVIII. ETHICS

84. Ethics 577
   Alexandra F.M. Cist, MD

85. Palliative Care 582
   Ursula McVeigh, MD, and Allan Ramsay, MD

86. Organ Donation 588
   Benjamin T. Suratt, MD, and Kapil Patel, MD

XIX. ADMINISTRATION

87. Intensive Care Unit Organization, Management, and Value 593
   Daniel Yagoda, MPH, Ulrich H. Schmidt, MD, PhD, and J. Perren Cobb, MD

88. Quality Assurance and Patient Safety in the Intensive Care Unit 598
   Nitin Puri, MD, FACP, Antoinette Spevetz, MD, FCCM, FACP, and Carolyn E. Bekes, MD, MHA, FCCM

89. Scoring Systems for Comparison of Disease Severity in Intensive Care Unit Patients 603
   Benoit Misset, MD, and Islem Ouanes, MD

TOP 100 SECRETS

These secrets are 100 of the top board alerts. They summarize the concepts, principles, and most salient details of critical care medicine.

1. Elevated lactate levels suggest tissue hypoperfusion, and normal lactate clearance is suggestive of adequate fluid resuscitation.

2. Always assume that even a single episode of hypotension in a trauma patient is due to bleeding, and proceed accordingly.

3. Good cardiopulmonary resuscitation can make a difference for a successful resuscitation from cardiac arrest. Know and perform it well.

4. Time to defibrillation is the most important factor in a return of spontaneous circulation from ventricular tachycardia and/or ventricular fibrillation.

5. Pulse oximetry is good for continuous monitoring, but arterial blood gases (ABGs) are best for diagnosis and acute management. If oximetry does not fit the clinical picture, obtain an ABG.

6. Use the alveolar gas equation to help understand mechanisms of hypoxemia.

7. Hemodynamic monitoring assesses whether the circulatory system has adequate performance to supply oxygen and sustain the "fire of life." Monitoring provides data to guide therapy but is not therapeutic.

8. There is no proved benefit to colloid over crystalloid in acute resuscitation.

9. Starting enteral nutrition early in critically ill patients increased survival.

10. Enteral feeding in patients with shock is acceptable after the patient is resuscitated and hemodynamically stable, even if the patient is receiving stable lower doses of vasopressors.

11. The primary indications for mechanical ventilation are inadequate oxygenation, inadequate ventilation, and elevated work of breathing.

12. Low tidal volume mechanical ventilation can lead to improved outcomes in the patient with acute respiratory distress syndrome.

13. Daily weaning assessments improve patient outcomes.

14. The rate of central venous catheter–related bloodstream infections can be reduced through a combination of the use of maximal sterile barrier precautions, 2% chlorhexidine-based antiseptic, centralization of line insertion supplies, and daily evaluation of the need for continued central access.

15. Subclavian venous catheters have the lowest risk of bloodstream infection.

16. *Lung sliding* on ultrasound examination effectively rules out pneumothorax at the site of the transducer.

17. Extracorporeal membrane oxygenation can be used successfully in patients with respiratory failure in whom low tidal volume ventilation is failing.

18. Nonrecognition of an esophageal intubation leads to death; direct visual confirmation or detection of carbon dioxide must be done to confirm the proper location of an endotracheal tube.

19. If a tracheostomy tube falls out of its stoma within the first 1 to 5 days of placement, do not attempt to reinsert it blindly. Perform translaryngeal intubation instead because blind attempts at reinsertion misplace the tube into a paratracheal track, compress the trachea, and cause asphyxia.

20. Any airway or stomal bleeding that develops more than 48 hours after tracheotomy should suggest the possibility of a tracheoarterial fistula, which develops as a communication between the trachea and a major intrathoracic artery.

21. A retrospective study showed that positive pressure ventilation (PPV) does not influence the rate of recurrent pneumothorax or chest tube placements after removal. Consequently, presence of mechanical PPV is not an indication to leave a chest tube in place.

22. Chest physiotherapy appears to be as effective as bronchoscopy in treating atelectasis, although bronchoscopy has a role in retained, inspissated secretions or foreign bodies.

23. Pulmonary artery line placement in patients with a newly implanted (less than 3 months) implantable cardioverter defibrillator or pacemaker is associated with high risk of lead dislodgment, especially if there is a coronary sinus lead.

24. Intraaortic balloon pumps should be considered in patients who may benefit from increased diastolic pressures (persistent refractory angina, cardiovascular compromise from myocardial ischemia/infarction) or decreased afterload (acute mitral regurgitation, cardiogenic shock).

25. Clinical judgment should supplement severity of illness scores in defining patients with severe community-acquired pneumonia.

26. The use of clinical criteria alone will lead to the overdiagnosis of ventilator-associated pneumonia.

27. A normal PCO_2 in acute asthma is a warning sign of impending respiratory failure.

28. Noninvasive mechanical ventilation reduces the need for intubation in patients with a chronic obstructive pulmonary disease exacerbation and impending respiratory failure.

29. Chronic hypoxemia is the most common cause of pulmonary hypertension.

30. Patients with acute lung injury and acute respiratory distress syndrome die of multiorgan dysfunction far more frequently than they do of refractory hypoxemia.

31. For most patients, bronchial artery embolization is the treatment of choice to stop hemorrhaging in massive hemoptysis.

32. Because death from massive hemoptysis is more commonly caused by asphyxiation than exsanguination, it is important to emergently maintain airway patency and protect the nonbleeding lung.

33. Deep venous thrombosis and pulmonary embolism are common and often underdiagnosed in critically ill patients.

34. The key to treating heart failure is determining the cause, that is, reduced ejection fraction, normal/preserved ejection fraction, restrictive cardiomyopathy, hypertrophic cardiomyopathy, or right ventricular failure.

35. The best clinical guide to help in choosing which treatment is appropriate for the critically ill patient with heart failure is to assess volume and perfusion status.

36. Acute myocardial infarction, complicated by out-of-hospital cardiac arrest, has a very high mortality, and hypothermia may improve chances for survival and neurologic recovery.

37. It is important to distinguish hemodynamically unstable arrhythmias that need immediate cardioversion/defibrillation from other more stable rhythms.

38. When managing acute aortic dissection, adequate beta blockade must be established *before* the initiation of nitroprusside to prevent propagation of the dissection from a reflex increase in cardiac output.

39. Pulsus paradoxus is when there is respiratory variation on arterial waveform seen during pericardial tamponade of >10 mm Hg.

40. Severe sepsis = sepsis plus acute organ dysfunction.

41. Early diagnosis and therapeutic interventions in patients with severe sepsis or septic shock are associated with better outcomes.

42. Between 60% and 80% of cases of endocarditis result from streptococcal infection. *Staphylococcus aureus* tends to be the most common etiologic agent of infective endocarditis in intravenous (IV) drug users.

43. *Streptococcus pneumoniae* remains the most common cause of community-acquired bacterial meningitis, and treatment directed to this should be included in the initial empiric regimen.

44. Most patients do not require computed tomographic scan before lumbar puncture; however, signs and symptoms that suggest elevated intracranial pressure should prompt imaging. These include new-onset neurologic deficits, new-onset seizure, and papilledema. Severe cognitive impairment and immune compromise are also conditions that warrant consideration for imaging.

45. If you suspect disseminated fungal infection, do not wait for cultures to treat.

46. Reducing multidrug-resistant bacteria can only be accomplished by using fewer antibiotics, not more.

47. Clinical or laboratory identification of an unusual pathogen (i.e., anthrax, smallpox, plague) should raise suspicion for a biologic attack.

48. Pain disproportionate to physical findings; skin changes including hemorrhage, sloughing, or anesthesia; rapid progression; crepitus; edema beyond the margin of erythema; and systemic involvement should prompt intense investigation for deep infection and involvement of surgical consultants as needed in the case of necrotizing fasciitis or gas gangrene.

49. During influenza season all persons admitted to the intensive care unit (ICU) with respiratory illness should be presumed to have influenza and be tested and treated.

50. Asplenic individuals are at risk for infection with encapsulated organism.

51. The greatest degree of immunosuppression in solid organ transplant recipients is in the 1 to 6 months after transplantation.

52. Severe hypertension in absence of end organ damage can be safely treated outside the setting of intensive care and reduction in blood pressure be achieved gently over hours to days.

53. The serum creatinine level may not change much during acute renal failure in patients with decreased muscle mass.

54. In the analysis of acid-base disorders, a normal serum pH does not imply that there is not an acid-base disorder; rather it points to mixed disorder.

55. Serum magnesium level should be checked and corrected, if low, in patients with refractory hypokalemia.

56. Overly rapid correction of hyponatremia or hypernatremia can result in devastating long-term neurologic sequelae.

57. If a patient has neurologic symptoms associated with hyponatremia, one of the immediate goals of therapy should be correction of serum sodium to a *safe* level.

58. Be systematic in your workup of gastrointestinal tract bleeding. Follow an algorithm.

59. In a patient with acute pancreatitis, make sure the patient's fluid is replenished with an adequate amount of IV fluid. This is as important as, if not more important than, the other facets of treatment, including pain control, nutritional support, correcting electrolyte abnormalities, treating infection (if present), and treating the underlying cause.

60. Steroids should be considered for the treatment of severe alcoholic hepatitis as defined by a Maddrey's discriminate score ≥ 32.

61. Abdominal compartment syndrome is an underappreciated diagnosis.

62. This is no secret—we all share the responsibility for reducing nosocomial infections.

63. Worsening confusion or a new impairment in mental state during treatment of diabetic ketoacidosis or hyperosmolar hyperglycemic state is life-threatening cerebral edema until proved otherwise.

64. Administering insulin without adequate fluid replacement during treatment of diabetic ketoacidosis or hyperosmolar hyperglycemic state can lead to profound hypotension, shock, or cardiovascular collapse.

65. An IV insulin infusion is the safest and most effective way to treat hyperglycemia in critically ill patients.

66. If the blood pressure of an ICU patient with septic shock responds poorly to repeated fluid boluses and vasopressors, hydrocortisone should be given regardless of cortisol levels.

67. In most cases you do not need to treat nonthyroidal illness syndrome with levothyroxine despite low thyroxine, triiodothyronine, and thyroid-stimulating hormone levels; instead follow expectantly, and recheck laboratory values in 4 to 6 weeks.

68. Stable anemia is well tolerated in critically ill patients. Transfuse blood products only when necessary or if hemoglobin level drops below 7 gm/dL.

69. Although disseminated intravascular coagulation typically presents with bleeding or laboratory abnormalities suggesting deficient hemostasis, *hyper*coagulability and accelerated thrombin generation actually underlie the process.

70. Surgery for cord compression can keep people ambulatory longer than radiation alone.

71. For a neutropenic fever, draw cultures, give broad-spectrum antibiotics, then complete the workup.

72. In a patient in the ICU who is seen with multiorgan failure or a clinical picture resembling fulminant sepsis, consider the diagnosis of systemic lupus erythematosus or vasculitis.

73. Respiratory pattern, autonomic functions, and brain stem reflexes are critical in identifying the cause of coma and should be recorded in all patients.

74. No ancillary test can replace an experienced clinical examination for determination of brain death.

75. The mainstay of treatment for status epilepticus includes stabilizing the patient, controlling the seizures, and treating the underlying cause.

76. ICU admission, invasive hemodynamic monitoring, and respiratory support with frequent vital capacity measurements are keys to following patients with Guillain-Barré syndrome.

77. Tachypnea is often the first sign of respiratory muscle weakness. Respiratory muscle strength is ideally measured by maximum inspiratory flow and vital capacity (VC) in patients with myasthenia gravis. A quick surrogate for forced VC is to ask the patient to count to the highest number possible during one expiration.

78. Benzodiazepines are the preferred agents for the treatment of alcohol withdrawal.

79. Time should not be wasted pursuing radiographic confirmation when a tension pneumothorax is suspected in a hemodynamically unstable patient. Either formal tube thoracostomy should be immediately performed or an Angiocath inserted into the second intercostal space along the midclavicular line.

80. The condition of a significant number of patients with flail chest and/or pulmonary contusion can be safely and effectively managed without intubation by using aggressive pulmonary care, including face-mask oxygen, continuous positive airway pressure, chest physiotherapy, and pain control.

81. The model for end-stage liver disease (MELD) calculates the severity of liver disease.

82. Delirium is a disturbance of consciousness with inattention, accompanied by a change in cognition or perceptual disturbances that develop over a short period of time, fluctuate over days, and remain underdiagnosed.

83. Therapeutic hypothermia (temperature 30°-34° C) improves neurologic outcomes in comatose survivors of cardiac arrest.

84. Heat stroke is a true medical emergency requiring immediate action: Delay in cooling increases mortality.

85. When caring for a critically ill poisoned patient, the diagnostic and therapeutic interventions should be started on the basis of the clinical presentation, with use of the history, the physical examination, and recognition of toxidromes.

86. Syrup of ipecac and gastric lavage have no role in the routine management of the poisoned patient.

87. Oral or IV *N*-acetylcysteine should be administered promptly to any patient with suspected or confirmed acetaminophen toxicity.

88. Patients with methanol and ethylene glycol ingestions present with an osmolal gap, which closes with metabolism and develops an anion gap acidosis. Isopropanol toxicity begins with an osmolal gap but is not metabolized to an anion gap.

89. Patients with toxic alcohol ingestion and any vision disturbance, severe metabolic acidosis, or renal failure should undergo urgent hemodialysis.

90. The treatment of choice for calcium channel blocker toxicity is hyperinsulinemia-euglycemia therapy to maximize glucose uptake into cardiac myocytes.

91. Neuroleptic malignant syndrome can occur at any age in either sex with exposure to any antipsychotic medication.

92. Although radiologic investigations and drug treatment may carry some risk of harm to the fetus, necessary tests and treatment should not be avoided in the critically ill mother.

93. Patients and their families are the experts on the patient's goals and values, and clinicians are the experts on determining which clinical interventions are indicated to try to achieve reasonable clinical goals.

94. Timely ethics consultation in the ICU may mitigate conflict and reduce ICU length of stay, hospital length of stay, ventilator days, and costs.

95. Only discuss treatment choices after the patient or family has been updated on medical condition, prognosis, and possible outcomes and once overall goals of medical care are agreed on.

96. Family conferences are more successful when providers listen more and talk less. Encourage the family to discuss their understanding of illness, their emotions, and who the patient is as a person. Then respond with statements of support and understanding.

97. All patients with impending brain death or withdrawal of care should be screened for the possibility of organ donation.

98. The gap between those patients awaiting a transplant and those donating organs is widening exponentially—the vast majority of those on the transplant list will die waiting.

99. The hospital systems investing today in advanced informatics, automated decision analysis, telemedicine, and/or regionalized care will be the leading systems tomorrow.

100. Patient safety remains a concern in critically ill patients, and a primary barrier to improving patient safety is physicians' inability to change their practice patterns.

I. BASIC LIFE SUPPORT

GENERAL APPROACH TO THE CRITICALLY ILL PATIENT

Manuel Pardo, Jr., MD, and Michael A. Gropper, MD, PhD

This book deals with many different aspects of critical care. Each disorder has specific diagnostic and management issues. However, when initially evaluating a patient, one must have a conceptual framework for the patterns of organ system dysfunction that are common to many types of critical illness. Furthermore, in the patient with multiple organ failure, resuscitation or stabilization is often more important than establishing an immediate, specific diagnosis.

1. **Which organ systems are most commonly dysfunctional in critically ill patients?**
   The respiratory system, the cardiovascular system, the internal or metabolic environment, the central nervous system (CNS), and the gastrointestinal tract.

2. **What system should be evaluated first?**
   The first few minutes of evaluation should address life-threatening physiologic abnormalities, usually involving the airway, the respiratory system, and the cardiovascular system. The evaluation should then expand to include all organ systems.

3. **Which should be performed first—diagnostic maneuvers or therapeutic maneuvers?**
   The management of a critically ill patient differs from the typical sequence of history and physical examination followed by diagnostic tests and therapeutic plans. The pace of assessment and therapy is quicker, and simultaneous evaluation and treatment are necessary to prevent further physiologic deterioration. For example, if a patient has a tension pneumothorax, the immediate placement of a chest tube may be lifesaving. Extra time should not be taken to transport the patient to a monitored setting. If there are no obvious life-threatening abnormalities, it may be appropriate to transfer the patient to the intensive care unit (ICU) for further evaluation. Many patients are admitted to the ICU solely for continuous electrocardiogram monitoring and more frequent nursing care.

4. **How do you evaluate the respiratory system?**
   The most important function of the lungs is to facilitate oxygenation and ventilation. Physical examination may reveal evidence of airway obstruction or respiratory failure. These signs include cyanosis, tachypnea, apnea, accessory muscle use, gasping respirations, and paradoxic respirations. Auscultation may reveal rales, rhonchi, wheezing, or asymmetric breath sounds.

5. **Define *paradoxic respirations* and *accessory muscle use.* What is their significance?**
   Normal breathing involves simultaneous rise and fall of the abdomen and chest wall.
   - A patient with *paradoxic respirations* has asynchrony of abdominal and chest wall movement. With inspiration, the chest wall rises as the abdomen falls. The opposite occurs with exhalation.
   - *Accessory muscle use* refers to the contraction of the sternocleidomastoid and scalene muscles with inspiration. These patients have increased work of breathing, which is the

amount of energy the body consumes for the work of the respiratory muscles. Most patients use accessory muscles before they have development of paradoxic respirations. Without support from a mechanical ventilator, patients with paradoxic respirations or increased work of breathing will eventually have respiratory muscle fatigue, hypoxemia, and hypoventilation.

6. **What supplemental tests are useful in evaluating the respiratory system?**
   Although all tests should be individualized to the particular clinical situation, arterial blood gas (ABG) analysis, pulse oximetry, and chest radiography rapidly provide useful information at a relatively low cost-benefit ratio.

7. **What therapy should be considered immediately in a patient with obvious respiratory failure?**
   Mechanical ventilation may be an immediate life-sustaining therapy in a patient with obvious or impending respiratory failure. Mechanical ventilation can be carried out *invasively* or *noninvasively*. Invasive ventilation is carried out via endotracheal intubation or tracheotomy. Noninvasive ventilation is instituted with a nasal mask or a full face mask. Even if the patient does not have obvious respiratory distress, supplemental oxygen should be administered until the oxygen saturation is measured. The risk of development of oxygen-induced hypercarbia is rare in any patient, including those with an acute exacerbation of chronic obstructive pulmonary disease.

8. **How do you evaluate the cardiovascular system?**
   The most important function of the cardiovascular system is the delivery of oxygen to the body's vital organs. The determinants of oxygen delivery are cardiac output and arterial blood oxygen content. The blood oxygen content, in turn, is determined primarily by the hemoglobin concentration and the oxygen saturation. It is difficult to determine the hemoglobin concentration and the oxygen saturation by physical examination alone. Therefore the initial evaluation of the cardiovascular system focuses on evidence of vital organ perfusion. New technology may allow rapid assessment of hemoglobin with use of a noninvasive spectrophotometric sensor.

9. **How is vital organ perfusion assessed?**
   The measurement of heart rate and blood pressure is the first step. If the systolic blood pressure is below 80 mm Hg or the mean blood pressure is below 50 mm Hg, the chances of inadequate vital organ perfusion are greater. However, because blood pressure is determined by cardiac output and peripheral vascular resistance, it is not possible to estimate cardiac output from blood pressure alone. The vital organs and their method of initial evaluation are as follows:
   - **Lungs** (see Questions 4-7)
   - **Skin:** Assess warmth and capillary refill in all extremities.
   - **CNS:** Assess level of consciousness and orientation.
   - **Heart:** Measure blood pressure and heart rate, and ask for symptoms of myocardial ischemia (e.g., chest pain).
   - **Kidneys:** Measure urine output and creatinine level.

10. **What supplemental tests are useful in the initial evaluation of the cardiovascular system?**
    Electrocardiography is a potentially useful diagnostic test with a low cost-benefit ratio. Cardiac enzyme tests, such as troponin measurement, are generally available within hours and can suggest myocardial injury. Other tests, which may entail more risk and cost, should be determined after the initial evaluation. These may include echocardiography, right-sided heart catheterization, central venous pressure measurement, or coronary angiography.

11. **What therapies should be considered immediately in a patient with hypotension and evidence of inadequate vital organ function?**
Fluid and vasopressor therapy can rapidly restore vital organ perfusion, depending on the cause of the deterioration. In most patients, a fluid challenge is well tolerated, although it is possible to precipitate heart failure and pulmonary edema in a volume-overloaded patient. Other therapies that may be immediately lifesaving include thrombolysis or coronary angioplasty for an acute myocardial infarction. Patients with hypotension from sepsis may benefit from early therapy involving defined goals for blood pressure, central venous pressure, central venous oxygen saturation, and hematocrit.

12. **How do you evaluate the metabolic environment?**
The clinical laboratory is required for most metabolic tests. It is difficult to evaluate the metabolic environment by physical examination alone.

13. **Why are metabolic changes important to detect in a critically ill patient?**
Metabolic abnormalities such as acid-base, fluid, and electrolyte disturbances are common in critical illness. These disorders may compound the underlying illness and require specific treatment themselves. They may also reflect the severity of the underlying disease. Metabolic disorders such as hyperkalemia and hypoglycemia can be life threatening. Prompt testing and treatment may reduce morbidity and improve patient outcome.

14. **Which laboratory tests should be performed in the initial evaluation of the metabolic environment?**
The selected tests should have a rapid reporting time, be widely available, and be likely to produce a change in management. Tests that fit these criteria include measurements of glucose, white blood cell count, hemoglobin, hematocrit, electrolytes, anion gap, blood urea nitrogen, creatinine, and pH. Elevated lactate levels suggest tissue hypoperfusion, and normal lactate clearance is suggestive of adequate fluid resuscitation. Some of these tests may be unnecessary in a particular patient, and supplemental testing may be useful in others.

15. **How do you evaluate the CNS?**
A neurologic examination is the first step in evaluating the CNS. The examination should include assessment of mental status (i.e., level of consciousness, orientation, attention, and higher cortical function). CNS disturbances in critical illness can be subtle. Common changes include fluctuations in mental status, changes in the sleep-wake cycle, or abnormal behavior. The remainder of the neurologic examination includes assessment of respiratory pattern, cranial nerves, sensation, motor function, and reflexes. Delirium, which is common in ICU patients, can be evaluated with the confusion assessment method (CAM-ICU).

16. **What diagnostic tests and therapies should be immediately considered in a patient with altered mental status?**
Oxygen therapy may be useful in patients with altered mental status from hypoxemia. Pulse oximetry or ABG analysis should be done to evaluate this. Intravenous dextrose may be lifesaving in patients with hypoglycemia. Additional diagnostic tests may be indicated depending on the clinical situation. Lumbar puncture, head computed tomographic (CT) or magnetic resonance imaging scan, electroencephalography, and metabolic testing may be useful in directing specific therapies. Patients with acute ischemic stroke may benefit from tissue plasminogen activator therapy, which is most effective when administered within 90 minutes of symptom onset.

17. **How do you evaluate the gastrointestinal tract?**
History and abdominal and rectal examination are the first steps in an initial evaluation of the gastrointestinal tract. Abdominal catastrophes such as bowel obstruction and bowel perforation are common inciting events leading to multiple organ failure. In addition, abdominal distention can reduce the compliance of the respiratory system, leading to progressive atelectasis and hypoxemia. Further diagnostic tests such as chest radiography, abdominal

ultrasonography, plain radiography of the abdomen, or abdominal CT scan may be useful in certain patients. For example, the finding of free air in the abdomen may lead to surgery for correction of bowel perforation.

18. **Besides the information about current organ system function, what else should one learn about a patient in the initial evaluation?**
After assessing current medical status, one should develop a sense for the physiologic reserve of the patient, as well as the potential for further deterioration. This information may often be gained by observing the patient's response to initial therapeutic maneuvers. It is also important to realize that patients may not desire cardiopulmonary resuscitation or other life-support therapies. If the patient has completed an advance directive, such as a durable power of attorney for health care, these guidelines should be followed or discussed further with the patient.

19. **What measures can be taken to reduce patient morbidity in the ICU?**
The prevention of complications in the ICU is an important patient safety issue. Each ICU should develop strategies to prevent complications such as venous thromboembolism, nosocomial pneumonia, and central line infections. In the last several years, a number of clinical trials have focused on reducing morbidity and mortality among critically ill patients. Many of these studies have evaluated common ICU problems such as acute respiratory distress syndrome, sepsis, and postoperative hyperglycemia. Practices such as hand washing can have a major impact on the incidence of complications.

KEY POINTS: GENERAL APPROACH TO CRITICALLY ILL PATIENTS

1. In the first few minutes, try to identify any life-threatening problems that require immediate treatment.

2. In patients with respiratory distress, consider whether immediate mechanical ventilation is necessary to prevent respiratory arrest.

3. Administer a fluid challenge for hypotensive patients without evidence of pulmonary edema.

4. When possible, use treatment strategies that have demonstrated benefit in clinical trials of critically ill patients.

BIBLIOGRAPHY

1. Dellinger RP, Levy MM, Carlet JM, et al: Surviving Sepsis Campaign: international guidelines for management of severe sepsis and septic shock: 2008. Crit Care Med 36:296-327, 2008.

2. Ely EW, Margolin R, Francis J, et al: Evaluation of delirium in critically ill patients: validation of the Confusion Assessment Method for the Intensive Care Unit (CAM-ICU). Crit Care Med 29:1370-1379, 2001.

3. Fonarow GC, Smith EE, Saver JL, et al: Timeliness of tissue-type plasminogen activator therapy in acute ischemic stroke: patient characteristics, hospital factors, and outcomes associated with door-to-needle times within 60 minutes. Circulation 123:750-758, 2011.

4. Luce JM: End-of-life decision making in the intensive care unit. Am J Respir Crit Care Med 182:6-11, 2010.

5. Miller RD, Ward TA, Shiboski SC, et al: A comparison of three methods of hemoglobin monitoring in patients undergoing spine surgery. Anesth Analg 112:858-863, 2011.

6. Pronovost P, Needham D, Berenholtz S, et al: An intervention to decrease catheter-related bloodstream infections in the ICU. N Engl J Med 355:2725-2732, 2006.

CHAPTER 2

GENERAL APPROACH TO TRAUMA PATIENTS

Peter J. Fagenholz, MD, and Hasan B. Alam, MD, FACS

1. **Which trauma patients need to be admitted to the intensive care unit (ICU)?**
   Patients who are receiving mechanical ventilation or require vasopressor support will obviously be admitted to the ICU. As care has shifted to nonoperative management of many injuries, the ability to closely monitor patients is critical. For example, a patient with a grade 4 splenic laceration who undergoes splenectomy may be able to be managed after surgery on a regular ward, whereas that same patient, if managed without surgery, would likely require closer observation in an ICU.

   Examples of trauma patients who may not meet clear-cut "critical care" criteria but who demand close serial observation that is often best carried out in an ICU include those with potential extremity compartment syndrome, nonoperative high-grade solid-organ injuries, significant closed-head injuries, and nonoperative penetrating abdominal trauma. Depending on local capacity a highly monitored observation or "step-down" unit may also be appropriate for these types of patients. If in doubt, admit them to a more-monitored rather than less-monitored setting.

2. **What is the top priority when a trauma patient first presents?**
   Airway evaluation and management are the critical starting point for the evaluation of any trauma patient. Airway compromise is the most important cause of early preventable death in trauma patients. The airway must be secured before further evaluation or treatment is undertaken.

3. **How is the airway managed in trauma patients?**
   Airway management is discussed thoroughly in Chapter 14, but trauma patients can pose a unique set of airway management challenges. Maxillofacial, laryngotracheal, and neck injury; intracranial hypertension; hemodynamic instability; thermal injury to the airway; and the need for maintaining in-line cervical spine stabilization are common conditions that can complicate airway management in trauma.

   All trauma care providers should have experience with airway evaluation and management from manual airway maneuvers (e.g., jaw thrust, chin lift), to the use of mechanical airway devices (oropharyngeal and nasopharyngeal airways), to bag-mask ventilation, to rapid-sequence endotracheal intubation, to the use of airway adjuncts such as the bougie or laryngeal mask airway, to establishing a surgical airway. A general algorithm for trauma airway management is shown in Figure 2-1.

4. **What are the most important causes of hypotension in the trauma patient?**
   Hemorrhagic shock—bleeding—is the most common cause of hypotension in the trauma patient. A vigorous search for bleeding is the key to the initial evaluation of any trauma patient with hypotension. Even a single episode of hypotension (systolic blood pressure [SBP] < 100-110 mm Hg) should be considered a potential harbinger of serious injury requiring interventional hemorrhage control. Methods for rapid localization of hemorrhage are discussed in Question 5.

   Obstructive shock is that caused by tension pneumothorax or pericardial tamponade. Pericardial tamponade is usually diagnosed with the help of ultrasound examination. Tension pneumothorax is usually diagnosed clinically by mechanism and physical examination.

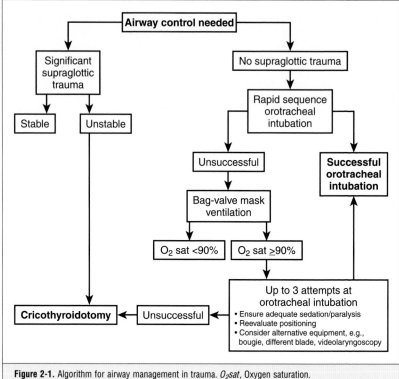

Figure 2-1. Algorithm for airway management in trauma. O_2sat, Oxygen saturation.

Occasionally ultrasound or chest radiographic examination may be of assistance, but one should never wait to obtain these studies when the diagnosis is suspected.

Spinal shock is a form of neurogenic shock that occurs because of the loss of sympathetic tone and peripheral vasodilation that occurs with high (typically T4 level or above) spinal cord injuries. It should be suspected when the patient has had a compatible mechanism of injury, the hypotension is accompanied by bradycardia, and results of the neurologic examination are consistent (lower extremity paralysis, loss of rectal tone, and a compatible sensory level).

Cardiogenic shock may result from traumatic cardiac contusion or occasionally from preexisting cardiac pathologic condition (coronary disease, valvular lesions, congestive heart failure) in patients with other, noncardiac trauma.

5. **How can I rapidly identify the source of bleeding in hemorrhagic shock?**
    Delayed control of bleeding ranks with airway compromise as a major preventable cause of trauma death. To be controlled, the source of bleeding must be rapidly identified. Hypotension due to hemorrhage typically does not occur until a trauma patient has lost 30% to 40% of his or her blood volume. This quantity of blood can be lost only into a limited number of places. The most important of these places are, externally, the chest, the abdomen, the retroperitoneum, and occasionally the thighs. Patients with hypotension should not undergo prolonged imaging such as computed tomography (CT), and all these potential areas of bleeding must usually be evaluated in the emergency department in a matter of minutes. This is possible with

reasonable sensitivity for major hemorrhage with use of a combination of physical examination, ultrasound scan, and plain radiography, all modalities that are widely and quickly available.

Physical examination is the most important tool for identifying external sources of bleeding. External bleeding is often missed or underappreciated when it is due to scalp wounds (which can result in significant blood loss); wounds in the back or axillae, which may be missed by a cursory examination; or mangled extremities, which may be diffusely oozing.

Physical examination and chest radiographic examination are the keys to identifying thoracic bleeding. Both can be done quickly. Ultrasound may be a useful adjunct (see extended focused abdominal sonography for trauma [E-FAST] later). If reasonable suspicion exists for intrathoracic bleeding, tube thoracostomy may be both diagnostic and therapeutic.

The abdomen is usually evaluated by FAST. If it cannot be performed, or is technically limited, diagnostic peritoneal aspiration or lavage is an alternative.

The retroperitoneum cannot be directly evaluated without CT, but most hemodynamically significant retroperitoneal bleeding is the result of pelvic fractures, which can be detected on a plain radiograph of the pelvis. Although retroperitoneal bleeding due to pelvic fractures generally correlates with the severity of the fracture, even relatively minor fractures may occasionally produce major hemorrhage. Similarly, femur fractures, especially if bilateral, suggest the possibility of significant hemorrhage into the thighs.

6. **What is the role of the FAST examination in evaluating the trauma patient with hemodynamic instability?**

The FAST examination has become a standard part of the evaluation of the trauma patient. It involves an ultrasound examination of four locations: the right and left upper quadrants of the abdomen, the pelvis, and the pericardium. The primary role of FAST is to evaluate for hemoperitoneum in patients with blunt trauma who are hemodynamically unstable. In these patients, when no other explanation for hypotension exists, positive FAST examination results can quickly identify the need for laparotomy, saving the time that might otherwise be spent obtaining more involved imaging such as CT. Patients with blunt trauma who are hemodynamically stable but have intraabdominal fluid identified on FAST should not be rushed to the operating room but should undergo CT imaging. Many common injuries, such as splenic and liver lacerations, which can result in positive FAST examination results, do not require surgical exploration and can be better defined on CT, which is safe to perform if the patient is hemodynamically stable. FAST can also identify pericardial tamponade. E-FAST includes sonography of the thorax to assess for hemothorax or pneumothorax. In many centers, FAST is routinely performed even in stable patients to establish a baseline for comparison if the patient's condition later deteriorates.

7. **What is *damage control resuscitation*?**

Damage control resuscitation refers to the practice of administering blood products early in the course of resuscitation of patients with massive hemorrhage (anticipated need for > 10 U packed red blood cell [PRBC] transfusion) to limit the coagulopathy associated with crystalloid administration or isolated PRBC transfusion. Observational data from the battlefield and civilian trauma centers suggest that early administration of fresh frozen plasma (FFP) and platelets reduces mortality and postoperative transfusion after major hemorrhage. The optimal ratio of PRBC/FFP/platelets that should be administered in the setting of massive bleeding is a matter of debate, and no controlling evidence is available. The U.S. Army has adopted a policy of administering these products in a 1:1:1 ratio for battlefield casualties requiring massive transfusion. Other investigators have achieved reductions in mortality by instituting a 4:2:1 ratio in place of unstructured transfusion. Whatever the exact ratio chosen, it is ideal to have in place a massive transfusion protocol that allows the blood bank to deliver blood products rapidly in a fixed ratio. This allows the desired ratio to be achieved and simplifies the process of care when caring for these critically ill patients. Massive transfusion protocols using the different product ratios described earlier have been shown to reduce mortality in case-controlled studies.

Whenever this quantity of transfusion is required, the use of a combination rapid transfuser–fluid warmer is highly recommended to prevent hypothermia. It should be reemphasized that these guidelines apply only to the massively transfused patient and that excessive blood products in patients with minimal hemorrhage may even be harmful.

8. **What is *hypotensive resuscitation*?**
   Hypotensive resuscitation, also known as permissive hypotension, refers to the principle of gaining hemorrhage control before restoration of euvolemia and normal blood pressure. The most important steps in treatment of the bleeding trauma patient are identifying the source of bleeding and stopping it. If vigorous fluid resuscitation proceeds before these goals have been met, hemodilution, hypothermia, and increased blood pressure may actually work to increase bleeding by causing coagulopathy and by *popping the clot*. Hypotensive resuscitation, in which a minimal blood pressure to provide end-organ perfusion is maintained until definite hemorrhage control (whether surgical, endovascular, or otherwise), has been associated with improved survival in patients with penetrating torso trauma.

9. **When fluid resuscitation of the bleeding trauma patient is begun, how should it be carried out?**
   Adequate intravenous access is a prerequisite for large-volume resuscitation. Large-bore (14 gauge or 16 gauge) peripheral intravenous cannulas are ideal because they can be placed quickly and have a large diameter and short length, which allows rapid infusion. Even larger-bore peripheral and central lines (7.5 F to 8.5 F) allow still more rapid infusion though may be more time-consuming to place. Multiport central lines are not appropriate for significant volume resuscitation, because their small diameter and length result in slow rates of infusion. When large-volume transfusion is anticipated, all effort should be made to use a rapid infuser–fluid warmer system to reduce coagulopathy due to hypothermia. If bleeding patients are taken to the operating room, a cell saver suction system can reduce transfusion requirements.

10. **What is damage control surgery?**
    The term *damage control* comes from the U.S. Navy, in which it refers to the ability of a ship to sustain damage but be adequately repaired in the field to allow completion of its mission, with definitive repair deferred until return to port. Damage control surgery refers to operations performed in patients whose condition is unstable to control hemorrhage and limit contamination, without completing definitive repair of all injuries. This commonly includes maneuvers such as resecting bowel without performing an anastomosis, placing temporary vascular shunts without performing definitive vessel repair, packing for control of hemorrhage, and the use of rapid temporary closure techniques. Damage control operations are followed by a period of resuscitation in the ICU, during which physiologic homeostasis is restored by the correction of coagulopathy, hypothermia, electrolyte abnormalities, and other derangements. Finally, reoperation for definitive repair of injuries is the final step.

11. **What are the signs of abdominal compartment syndrome, and how is it managed?**
    Abdominal compartment syndrome occurs when high intraabdominal pressure causes end-organ compromise. Abdominal compartment syndrome in trauma usually occurs because of massive fluid resuscitation, which causes visceral edema, occasionally compounded by an intraabdominal hematoma, or packs placed for hemostasis. A tense distended abdomen, respiratory distress (or high peak inspiratory pressures if mechanically ventilation is used), and oliguria constitute the classic clinical triad of abdominal compartment syndrome. This triad is often accompanied by hypotension. Respiratory distress and high peak inspiratory pressures result from the abdominal pressure pushing up on the diaphragm, oliguria results from compression of the renal vein disturbing perfusion to the kidney and causing acute kidney injury, and hypotension is caused by decreased venous return via the inferior vena cava.

When abdominal compartment syndrome is suspected, intraabdominal pressure can be measured by transducing the pressure measured via a bladder catheter. An intraabdominal pressure >20 mm Hg in the proper clinical setting is highly suggestive of abdominal compartment syndrome. Although medical management with diuresis (which may reduce visceral edema) and paralysis (which increases abdominal wall compliance) may occasionally be sufficient, definitive therapy requires surgical decompression of the abdomen.

12. **How can I clear the cervical spine?**
The cervical spine should be immobilized in blunt trauma patients who have had significant force to the head or neck. In awake patients with an intact sensorium who can focus on the examination, the cervical spine can be cleared by physical examination alone. The midline bony structures of the neck from C1 to C7 should be carefully palpated. Next, the examiner should push down on the top of the patient's head, axially loading the cervical spine. Finally, the patient should be asked to flex and extend the neck and turn the head from side to side. If all these maneuvers can be completed without eliciting pain or tenderness, cervical spinal immobilization is not necessary. If pain or tenderness is identified at any point, a cervical collar should be reapplied immediately, and a CT scan of the cervical spine performed.

In patients who are not clinically examinable, radiographic evaluation should begin with a CT scan of the cervical spine. Our practice is to discontinue cervical immobilization if the attending radiologist and trauma surgeon agree that the CT scan is completely normal, meaning not only is there no fracture but there is no abnormality of any kind, including no prevertebral soft tissue swelling, and no loss of normal lordosis. This is an area of some debate, and other practitioners recommend routine magnetic resonance imaging before discontinuing cervical immobilization in unexaminable patients.

13. **Should patients with spinal cord injury receive steroids?**
Patients with acute blunt spinal cord injury may derive slight functional benefit from early administration of high-dose steroids, though their use is debated. If the decision is made to treat with steroids, methylprednisolone should be administered with a bolus of 30 mg/kg and an infusion started at 5.4 mg/kg per hour. If the first dose is administered within 3 hours of injury, the infusion should be continued for 24 hours. If the first dose is administered between 3 and 8 hours after injury, the infusion should be continued for 48 hours, and if the first dose cannot be administered within 8 hours of injury it should not be administered at all.

14. **How is closed-head injury managed?**
The following are the key management principles for patients with closed-head injury:
- Maintain normal blood pressure (SBP >90 mm Hg).
- Maintain normal oxygenation (O_2 saturation >90%, PaO_2 >60 mm Hg).
- Hyperosmolar therapy (mannitol 0.25-1 g/kg or hypertonic saline solution) should be used when lateralizing signs or signs of herniation are present.
- Steroids are contraindicated and increase mortality.

Although it is difficult to demonstrate benefit for each of these interventions individually, when instituted as a bundle they can result in a decrease in mortality for patients with brain injury.

When discrete traumatic mass lesions such as acute subdural or epidural hemorrhage occur, these should be surgically evacuated. No benefit is proved for decompressive craniotomy for patients with persistently elevated intracranial pressure without a surgically amenable mass lesion.

15. **What are the options for treating massive bleeding from pelvic fractures?**
Pelvic fractures can often be appreciated on physical examination when instability of the pelvic ring is detected. A plain anteroposterior radiographic film of the pelvis, easily obtained in the trauma bay, confirms the diagnosis. Pelvic fractures may be associated with massive bleeding from the rich pelvic plexus of veins and occasionally from associated pelvic arterial structures.

Because the bleeding typically occurs diffusely from multiple sources, it is not possible to identify and ligate the bleeding vessels. Arrest of hemorrhage relies on three primary modalities:

Pelvic immobilization, which can be temporarily obtained in the trauma bay by wrapping the pelvis with a sheet, but is definitively achieved by surgical internal or external fixation.

Preperitoneal pelvic packing, a damage control technique in which the extraperitoneal pelvis is packed with laparotomy pads to compress bleeding vessels. These are removed at a second operation when bleeding is controlled.

Angiographic embolization, which can directly address pelvic arterial bleeding and may help to stop venous bleeding by reducing pelvic vascular inflow.

These techniques are best performed simultaneously in an operating room capable of accommodating endovascular intervention.

16. **When is chemical deep venous thrombosis (DVT) prophylaxis safe in traumatically injured patients?**

Trauma patients in general are at high risk for the development of venous thrombosis and thromboembolism, and so prompt initiation of prophylaxis against DVT is important. The American College of Chest Physicians recommends immediate initiation of thromboprophylaxis with low-molecular-weight heparin in all trauma patients except those with a contraindication because of active bleeding or a high risk of clinically important bleeding. What exactly comprises a contraindication in trauma remains subjective. Retrospective data suggest that chemical prophylaxis is safe in patients whose condition is stable, even with closed-head and solid-organ injuries, and that chemical DVT prophylaxis can be safely initiated 24 to 72 hours after injury in these patients. Large randomized trials are still needed to better define the best thromboprophylaxis regimen and the optimal timing for initiation of thromboprophylaxis in patients with major trauma.

KEY POINTS: GENERAL APPROACH TO TRAUMA PATIENTS

1. Untreated airway compromise is a major cause of preventable death in trauma. Secure the airway early.

2. Bleeding is the most common cause of hypotension in the trauma patient.

3. Sources of major bleeding can be identified within minutes in the emergency department by using a combination of physical examination, bedside ultrasound scan, and radiographs.

4. In the bleeding patient, fluid infusion should be minimized until control of hemorrhage is obtained.

5. Massively bleeding patients should undergo transfusion by use of a protocol with a fixed ratio of FFP to PRBC to platelets.

BIBLIOGRAPHY

1. Alam HB: Advances in resuscitation strategies. Int J Surg 9:5-12, 2011.

2. American College of Surgeons Committee on Trauma : Advanced Trauma Life Support Course Manual, 8th ed. Chicago, American College of Surgeons, 2008.

3. An G, West MA: Abdominal compartment syndrome: a concise clinical review. Crit Care Med 36:1304-1310, 2008.

4. Bickell WH, Wall MJ Jr., Pepe PE, et al: Immediate versus delayed fluid resuscitation for hypotensive patients with penetrating torso injuries. N Engl J Med 331:1105-1109, 1994.

5. Bracken MB, Shepard MJ, Holford TR, et al: Administration of methylprednisolone for 24 or 48 hours or tirilazad mesylate for 48 hours in the treatment of acute spinal cord injury. Results of the Third National Acute Spinal Cord Injury Randomized Controlled Trial. National Acute Spinal Cord Injury Study. JAMA 277:1597-1604, 1997.

6. Brain Trauma Foundation; American Association of Neurological Surgeons; Congress of Neurological Surgeons: Guidelines for the management of severe traumatic brain injury. J Neurotrauma 24(1 Suppl):S1-106, 2007.

7. Burlew CC, Moore EE, Smith WR, et al: Preperitoneal pelvic packing/external fixation with secondary angioembolization: optimal care for life-threatening hemorrhage from unstable pelvic fractures. J Am Coll Surg 212:628-635, discussion 635-637, 2011.

8. Cooper DJ, Rosenfeld JV, Murray L, et al: DECRA Trial Investigators. Australian and New Zealand Intensive Care Society Clinical Trials Group: Decompressive craniectomy in diffuse traumatic brain injury. N Engl J Med 364:1493-1502, 2011.

9. Geerts WH, Bergqvist D, Pineo GF, et al: American College of Chest Physicians: Prevention of venous thromboembolism: American College of Chest Physicians Evidence-Based Clinical Practice Guidelines (8th ed). Chest 133(6 Suppl):381S-453S, 2008.

10. Gruen RL, Jurkovich GJ, McIntyre LK, et al: Patterns of errors contributing to trauma mortality: lessons learned from 2,594 deaths. Ann Surg 244:371-380, 2006.

11. Langeron O, Birenbaum A, Amour J: Airway management in trauma. Minerva Anestesiol 75:307-331, 2009.

12. Lee JC, Peitzman AB: Damage-control laparotomy. Curr Opin Crit Care 12:346-350, 2006.

13. Patel NY, Riherd JM: Focused assessment with sonography for trauma: methods, accuracy, and indications. Surg Clin North Am 91:195-207, 2011.

14. Sanddal TL, Esposito TJ, Whitney JR, et al: Analysis of preventable trauma deaths and opportunities for trauma care improvement in Utah. J Trauma 70:970-977, 2011.

15. Schoenfeld AJ, Bono CM, McGuire KJ, et al: Computed tomography alone versus computed tomography and magnetic resonance imaging in the identification of occult injuries to the cervical spine: a meta-analysis. J Trauma 68:109-113, 2010.

16. Seamon MJ, Feather C, Smith BP, et al: Just one drop: the significance of a single hypotensive blood pressure reading during trauma resuscitations. J Trauma 68:1289-1294, 2010.

CHAPTER 3

CARDIOPULMONARY RESUSCITATION

David Shimabukuro, MDCM

Most of the information provided in this chapter can be reviewed in greater detail by referring to specific guidelines published by the American Heart Association (AHA), in conjunction with the International Liaison Committee on Resuscitation. Please visit the AHA's website at http://www.heart.org and follow the links to Cardiopulmonary Resuscitation and Emergency Cardiovascular Care (CPR & ECC). Also see the Bibliography at the end of this chapter. This chapter focuses on basic life support (BLS) and the management of pulseless arrest (a part of advanced cardiovascular life support [ACLS]).

1. **What is meant by cardiopulmonary resuscitation (CPR)?**
   To most people, *CPR* refers to BLS, which encompasses closed-chest compressions and rescue breathing. For health care providers, the term can be much broader and can include
   - ACLS
   - Pediatric advanced life support (PALS)
   - Advanced trauma life support (ATLS)
   Thus it is very important for the physician to be specific whenever discussing resuscitation with patients and their families.

2. **Is iatrogenic cardiopulmonary arrest very common?**
   It probably occurs much more often than it really should. Without a doubt, errors of omission and commission contribute to the incidence and poor outcome of in-hospital cardiopulmonary arrests. In a study of 562 in-hospital arrests, a major unsuspected diagnosis was present (and proved by autopsy) in 14% of cases. The two most common missed diagnoses were pulmonary embolus and bowel infarction, which together accounted for 89% of all missed conditions. Retrospective reviews indicate that as many as 15% of in-hospital arrests are probably avoidable. These cases can be attributed to respiratory insufficiency and hemorrhage that are often undetected or diagnosed too late, because aberrations in patients' vital signs and their complaints (especially dyspnea) are frequently ignored.

   Direct iatrogenesis also contributes to in-hospital cardiopulmonary arrests. Almost every procedure, including esophagogastroduodenoscopy, bronchoscopy, central venous line placement, and an abdominal computed tomography scan with contrast, has, on occasion, been associated with an arrest. The injudicious use of lidocaine, sedative-hypnotics, and opiates is primarily responsible for these types of arrests throughout the hospital. Careful hemodynamic monitoring, especially pulse oximetry, by a dedicated practitioner can decrease the occurrence of this easily avoidable complication.

3. **What are the four major components of BLS?**
   - Recognition of an unresponsive patient who is not breathing or not breathing in a normal manner
   - Activation of the emergency medical system with acquisition of an automated external defibrillator (AED)
   - Closed-chest cardiac compressions with ventilations
   - Actual defibrillation

4. **What is the *CAB* of resuscitation?**

   According to all published guidelines, the *CAB* of resuscitation is compressions, airway, and breathing. This has replaced the old mnemonic of *ABCD* because initial resuscitation now begins with closed-chest compressions once it has been established that the patient is unresponsive, is not breathing, and has no pulse. After 30 chest compressions, the airway is opened and two breaths are delivered. Thus the sequence is compressions, airway, and breathing (CAB).

5. **How is BLS performed?**

   For any patient in cardiac arrest, the most important steps are to
   1. Immediately recognize unresponsiveness
   2. Check for lack of breathing or lack of normal breathing
   3. Activate emergency response system and retrieve an AED
   4. Check for a pulse (no more than 10 seconds)
   5. Start cycles of 30 chest compressions followed by two breaths
   This applies to all patients, regardless of location (in hospital or out of hospital).

   - **Responsiveness:** A quick check for the presence of breathing or lack of normal breathing should be performed when assessing a patient who may be in cardiac arrest. If the patient is unresponsive, then the emergency response system should be activated and an AED or defibrillator should be quickly retrieved (i.e., call 911 or call a *code*).

   - **Compressions:** Because a pulse can be very difficult to assess, it may be necessary to use other clues, such as whether the patient is breathing spontaneously or moving. Regardless, the health care provider should take no more than 10 seconds to check for a definitive pulse at either the carotid or femoral artery. If the patient has no pulse or no signs of life, or the rescuer is unsure, chest compressions should be started immediately. The heel of the hand should be placed longitudinally on the lower half of the sternum, between the nipples. The sternum should be depressed at least 5 cm (2 inches) at a rate of at least 100 compressions per minute. Complete chest recoil is necessary to allow for venous return and is important for effective CPR. The pattern should be 30 compressions to two breaths (30:2 equals one cycle of CPR) regardless of whether one or two rescuers are present. Pulse checks and signs of life should be assessed after every five cycles (equivalent to 2 minutes) of CPR. Once the AED or defibrillator arrives, it should be attached without delay so that an electrical shock can be immediately delivered to improve the likelihood of a return of spontaneous circulation (ROSC).

   - **Airway:** With the new 2010 BLS guidelines, the importance of airway management has taken more of a secondary role. The old mnemonic ABCD (airway, breathing, circulation, and defibrillation) with "look, listen, and feel" has been changed to CAB (compressions, airway, and breathing). This change is due to evidence proving the importance of chest compressions and the need to quickly restore blood flow to improve the likelihood of ROSC. Airway maneuvers should still be attempted, but they should occur quickly and efficiently and minimize interruptions in chest compressions. Opening of the airway can be achieved by a simple head tilt–chin lift technique. A jaw thrust maneuver can be used in patients with suspected cervical spine injury. Simple airway devices, such as nasal or oral airways, can be inserted to displace the tongue from the posterior oropharynx. Definitive airway management, such as placement of an endotracheal tube, is an aspect of ACLS and should never be a part of BLS.

   - **Breathing:** Although several large out-of-hospital studies have demonstrated that chest compression–alone CPR is not inferior to traditional compression-ventilation CPR, health care providers are still expected to provide assisted ventilation. A lone rescuer, outside the hospital setting, should not use a bag-mask for ventilation, but should use mouth-to-mouth or mouth-to-mask. Care should be taken to avoid rapid or forceful breaths. Delivered tidal volumes are given over a 1-minute period and should be just enough to produce visible chest rise. Large tidal volumes should be avoided because they would promote hyperventilation and decrease preload. Hyperventilation in the patient with cardiac arrest receiving closed-chest compressions has been proved to be detrimental for neurologic recovery.

- **Defibrillation:** An AED or defibrillator should be attached to the patient as soon as possible. Proper electrode pad or paddle placement on the chest wall should be to the right of the upper sternal border below the clavicle and to the left of the nipple with the center in the midaxillary line. If using a portable out-of-hospital AED device, turn the AED on first and then follow the voice commands. If the defibrillator's electrical output is adjustable, then the initial voltage delivered should be the manufacturer's recommendation. When this is unknown, 200 J should be used. Immediately after the shock, closed-chest compressions are resumed.

  Of note, BLS should ideally be performed only by those persons who have been certified by the AHA, or other similar organization. However, it is not uncommon for 911 operators to provide instruction over the phone when no other qualified individual is nearby. Certification is easily obtained by attending one or two classes taught by qualified instructors. Most communities offer these classes to the general public.

6. **How does blood flow during closed-chest compressions?**
Two basic models derived from animal studies explain the movement of blood during closed-chest compressions:
- In the **cardiac pump** model, the heart is squeezed between the sternum and spine. Systole occurs when the heart is compressed; the atrioventricular valves close and the pulmonary and aortic valves open, ensuring ejection of blood with unidirectional, antegrade flow. Diastole occurs with the release of the squeezed heart resulting in a fall in intracardiac pressures; the atrioventricular valves open while the pulmonary and aortic valves close. Blood is subsequently drawn into the heart from the venae cavae and lungs.
- In the **thoracic pump** model, the heart is considered a passive conduit. Closed-chest compression results in uniformly increased pressures throughout the thoracic cavity. Forward flow of blood occurs with each squeeze of the heart and thorax because of the relative noncompliance of the arterial system (i.e., they resist collapse) and the one-way valves preventing retrograde flow in the venous system. Both of these models probably contribute to blood flow during CPR.

7. **What is the main determinant of a successful resuscitation?**
Two principal factors can highly influence the outcome of resuscitation.
- The first factor is access to defibrillation. For most adults, the primary cause of sudden, nontraumatic cardiac arrest is ventricular tachycardia (VT) or ventricular fibrillation (VF), for which the recommended treatment is electrical defibrillation.
- The second factor is time—or more specifically, time to defibrillation. Survival from a VF arrest decreases by 7% to 10% for each minute of delay. Defibrillation at the earliest possible moment is vital in facilitating a successful resuscitation.

  Of interest, only 15% to 20% of patients who have an out-of-hospital arrest survive to discharge; the percentage is even lower for those who have an in-hospital event.

8. **What is the role of pharmacologic therapy during ACLS?**
The immediate goals of pharmacologic therapy are to improve myocardial blood flow, increase ventricular inotropy, and terminate life-threatening arrhythmias, thereby restoring and/or maintaining spontaneous circulation. Combined α/β-adrenergic agonists, such as epinephrine, and smooth-muscle V_1 agonists, such as vasopressin, augment the mean aortic-to-ventricular end-diastolic pressure gradient (coronary perfusion pressure) by increasing arterial vascular tone. Phenylephrine and norepinephrine also increase arterial pressure and myocardial blood flow, but neither has been shown to be superior to epinephrine. Of note, recent data have shown that vasopressin plus epinephrine may be advantageous over epinephrine alone when comparing patients' survival rates to hospital discharge and residual neurologic deficits. None of the studies reached statistical significance.

In addition to improving or maintaining myocardial blood flow, pharmacologic therapy during ACLS is also aimed at terminating or preventing arrhythmias, which can further damage an already severely ischemic heart. VT and VF markedly increase myocardial oxygen consumption at a time when oxygen supply is tenuous because of poor delivery. Intracellular acidosis only causes the myocardium to be more dysfunctional and irritable, which makes the heart more vulnerable to arrhythmias. Amiodarone, a class III antiarrhythmic agent, has become the drug of choice for the treatment of the majority of life-threatening arrhythmias.

9. **Is sodium bicarbonate indicated in the routine management of cardiopulmonary arrest?**
   No! The primary treatment of metabolic acidosis from tissue hypoperfusion and hypoxia during a cardiac arrest is adequate chest compressions and ventilations. The metabolic acidosis is usually unimportant in the first 15 to 18 minutes of resuscitation. If appropriate ventilation can be maintained, the arterial pH usually remains above 7.2. Some argue that, during CPR, ventilation is at best suboptimal, leading to a combined metabolic and respiratory acidosis, dropping the pH well below 7.2. Studies have shown that severe acidosis leads to depression of myocardial contractile function, ventricular irritability, and a lowered threshold for VF. In addition, a markedly low pH interferes with the vascular and myocardial responses to adrenergic drugs and endogenous catecholamines, reducing cardiac chronotropy and inotropy. Although it is appealing to administer sodium bicarbonate in this situation, the clinician must keep in mind that the bicarbonate ion, after combining with a hydrogen ion, generates new carbon dioxide. Cell membranes are highly permeable to carbon dioxide (more so than bicarbonate), and therefore administration of sodium bicarbonate causes a paradoxic intracellular acidosis. The resultant intramyocardial hypercapnia leads to a profound decline in cardiac contractile function and failure of resuscitation. The generated carbon dioxide also needs to be eliminated to prevent worsening of an already present respiratory acidosis. Given the poor cardiac output during CPR and probable suboptimal ventilation, this may be quite difficult.
   Because the optimal acid-base status for resuscitation has not been established and no buffer therapy is needed in the first 15 minutes, the routine administration of sodium bicarbonate for acidosis resulting from a cardiac arrest is not recommended. Only restoration of the spontaneous circulation with adequate tissue perfusion and oxygen delivery can reverse this ongoing process.

10. **What are the arrhythmias associated with most cardiopulmonary arrests?**
    Most sudden nontraumatic cardiopulmonary arrests in adults are caused by VF or VT from myocardial ischemia or infarct from coronary artery disease. Electrolyte disturbances (hypokalemia or hypomagnesemia), prolonged hypoxia, and drug toxicity can also be important inciting factors in patients with multiple medical problems. Also not uncommon are bradyasystolic arrests (as many as 50% of in-hospital arrests). One cause of this arrhythmia could be unrecognized hypoxemia or acidemia. Other causes include heightened vagal tone precipitated by medications, an inferoposterior myocardial infarction (Bezold-Jarisch reflex), or invasive procedures. A third common arrest rhythm seen is pulseless electrical activity (PEA). A common etiology is prolonged arrest itself. Typically, after 8 minutes or more of VF, electrical defibrillation induces a slow, wide-complex PEA that tends to be terminal and is known as a pulseless idioventricular rhythm. On most occasions of an unsuccessful resuscitation, VF degrades to pulseless idioventricular rhythm before the patient becomes asystolic. The rhythm of PEA can also be narrow and fast, which accompanies other reversible life-threatening conditions, rather than just representing a terminal rhythm. Examples are cardiac tamponade, hypovolemia, pulmonary embolus, or tension pneumothorax. These are discussed later in some detail.

11. **What are the most common, immediately reversible causes of cardiopulmonary arrest?**

An alert clinician should recognize, at the patient's bedside, the following treatable causes of cardiopulmonary arrest:

- **Hypovolemia:** This should be suspected in all cases of arrest associated with rapid blood loss. This *absolute* hypovolemia occurs in settings such as trauma (pelvic fractures), gastrointestinal hemorrhage, or rupture of an abdominal aortic aneurysm. A *relative* hypovolemia can occur with sepsis or anaphylaxis resulting from extensive capillary leak. Regardless of the type, a large amount of fluid (crystalloid, colloid, blood) should be rapidly administered and the cause of the hypovolemia corrected (e.g., by taking the patient to the operating room or administering antibiotics).

- **Hypoxia:** Hypoxia from a variety of causes can lead to a cardiac arrest. Tracheal intubation with the delivery of a high concentration of oxygen is the treatment of choice while the cause of the hypoxia is determined and definitive management instituted.

- **Hydrogen ions (acidosis):** These can lead to myocardial failure resulting in cardiogenic shock and arrest. The high hydrogen ion concentration also increases myocardial irritability and arrhythmia formation. A known preexisting severe acidosis can be partially compensated for by hyperventilation, but sodium bicarbonate may still need to be administered. The underlying cause of the acidosis should be diagnosed and corrected.

- **Hyperkalemia:** This condition is encountered in patients with renal insufficiency, diabetes, and profound acidosis. Peaked T waves and a widening of the QRS complex, with the electrical activity eventually deteriorating to a sinus-wave pattern, herald hyperkalemia. Treatment includes the administration of calcium chloride, sodium bicarbonate, insulin, and glucose. *Hypokalemia* and other electrolyte disturbances leading to a cardiac arrest are much less common. Treating the abnormality should help restore spontaneous circulation.

- **Hypothermia:** This condition should be easily detected on examination of the patient. The electrocardiogram (ECG) may reveal Osborne waves that are pathognomonic. All resuscitation efforts should be continued until the patient is euthermic.

- **Tablets or toxins:** Ingestion of these items should be considered in those patients with an out-of-hospital cardiac arrest. Some of the more common intoxications include carbon monoxide poisoning after prolonged exposure to smoke or exhaust fumes from incomplete combustion, cyanide poisoning during fires involving synthetic materials, and drug overdoses (intentional or unintentional). High-flow, high-concentration, and, if possible, hyperbaric oxygen, along with the management of acidosis, are the cornerstones of treatment for carbon monoxide and cyanide poisonings. In addition, intravenous (IV) sodium nitrite and sodium thiosulfate can be used to help remove cyanide from the circulation. Tricyclic antidepressant drugs act as a type Ia antiarrhythmic agent and cause slowing of cardiac conduction, ventricular arrhythmias, hypotension, and seizures. Aggressive alkalinization of blood and urine, in addition to seizure control, should aid in controlling toxicity. An opiate overdose causes hypoxia from hypoventilation, whereas an overdose of cocaine can lead to myocardial ischemia. Naloxone reverses the effects of opioids and should be administered immediately if an opioid overdose is suspected.

- **Cardiac tamponade:** Cardiac tamponade presents with hypotension, a narrowed pulse pressure, elevated jugular venous pressure, distant and muffled heart sounds, and low-voltage QRS complexes on the ECG. Trauma patients and patients with malignancies are at greatest risk. Pericardiocentesis or subxiphoid pericardiorrhaphy can be lifesaving.

- **Tension pneumothorax:** This condition must be recognized immediately. Most often it occurs in patients who have had trauma or in patients receiving positive-pressure ventilation. The signs of a tension pneumothorax are rapid-onset hypotension, hypoxia, and an increase in airway pressures. Subcutaneous emphysema and reduced breath sounds on the affected side with tracheal deviation toward the unaffected side are commonly noted. The placement of a 14- or 16-gauge IV catheter into the second intercostal space at the midclavicular line or into the fifth intercostal space at the anterior axillary line for immediate decompression is imperative for restoration of circulation. A chest tube can be placed after the tension pneumothorax is converted to a simple pneumothorax.

- **Thrombosis of a coronary artery:** This condition can lead to myocardial ischemia and infarct. Reperfusion is a vital determinant for eventual outcome. Cardiac catheterization is the primary choice if it is immediately available; thrombolysis is a good alternative.
- **Thrombosis of the pulmonary artery:** Thrombosis of the pulmonary artery can be devastating. Some patients may be seen initially with dyspnea and chest pain, similar to acute coronary syndromes, but those who are seen in cardiac arrest have a minimal chance of survival. Therapy would include immediate thrombolysis to unload the right ventricle while restoring pulmonary blood flow.

12. How should VF be treated?

Early defibrillation with a single nonsynchronized electrical shock at an energy level of 360 J for a monophasic waveform defibrillator or the manufacturer's recommendation (see later) for a biphasic waveform defibrillator is recommended to minimize myocardial damage. A single subsequent shock, after five cycles (2 minutes) of CPR, should continue if the patient remains in pulseless VT or VF. If using a biphasic waveform defibrillator, the energy level equivalent to a 360-J monophasic waveform shock, as determined by the manufacturer, should be used. If this energy level is not known and it is firmly established that one is using a biphasic waveform defibrillator, it is recommended that a single shock of 200 J be administered.

If the initial single shock is not successful at terminating the VF, according to ACLS guidelines, epinephrine or vasopressin should be given while CPR continues. After five cycles, or 2 minutes of CPR, the rhythm should be reevaluated. If the patient remains in VF or pulseless VT, the defibrillator should be charged while CPR continues (if the charge time is more than 5-10 seconds; most standard hospital defibrillators charge within 5 seconds). When ready, the patient should be cleared and the shock delivered; CPR should be immediately reinstituted and rhythm analysis delayed for 2 minutes. After five cycles, or 2 minutes of CPR, the patient should once again be reevaluated by a pulse check and a rhythm check. If this process continues to be unsuccessful, an antiarrhythmic agent, amiodarone, should be administered. Venous access and a definitive airway should be obtained during periods of patient reevaluation. CPR is not to be interrupted unless absolutely necessary. The sequence should always be five cycles of CPR, patient evaluation, charge of defibrillator with CPR in progress (if long charge time), defibrillation, immediate resumption of five cycles of CPR with drug administration and patient evaluation.

13. Is pulseless idioventricular rhythm treatable?

Delayed electrical defibrillation or prolonged VF frequently results in a pulseless idioventricular rhythm or asystole. In the majority of cases, the idioventricular rhythm is not amenable to treatment and results in death. In animal experiments, high-dose epinephrine (0.1-0.2 mg/kg) has helped to restore cardiac contractility and pacemaker activity; however, several clinical studies have shown no benefit in long-term survival or neurologic outcome. It is not recommended.

14. How is asystole treated?

Asystole is treated identically to PEA. These two rhythms do not require defibrillation (asystole has no electrical activity whereas PEA is an organized electrical rhythm). However, given the grim prognosis for successful resuscitation, the clinician should rapidly determine whether any evidence exists that resuscitation should not be attempted when approaching a patient in asystole. If resuscitation is appropriate, perform CPR for 2 minutes and then reconfirm the absence of electrical cardiac activity (a flatline in an ECG may be due to technical mistakes). Rotate the monitoring leads 90 degrees (if using paddles), and maximize the amplitude to detect fine VF (if present, defibrillation should be performed immediately). If using the pads and ECG leads, cycle through the various leads (I, III, III). Verify the absence of pulses at the carotid or femoral artery. Epinephrine 1 mg is administered every 5 minutes; vasopressin 40 U can replace the first or second dose. The use of atropine is not recommended. Throughout the resuscitation, the clinician should always consider stopping resuscitative efforts.

Contrary to asystole, PEA has a more favorable outcome. However, the underlying cause needs to be addressed for the resuscitation to be successful. Reversible causes of cardiopulmonary arrest were reviewed earlier (see Question 11).

15. **What are the appropriate routes of administration of drugs during resuscitation?**
The preferred choice is by the IV route. If a central venous catheter is in place, this should be used over a peripheral venous line. Administration of drugs through a peripheral venous line will result in a slightly delayed onset of action, although the peak drug effect is similar to that achieved via the central route. Drugs administered peripherally should be followed with at least 20 mL of normal saline solution to ensure central delivery. Intracardiac administration should not be performed.

Virtually every resuscitation drug can be administered in conventional doses via the intraosseous (IO) route. Because of the ease of insertion via readily available kits, this method is preferred in all patients when an IV line cannot be readily obtained.

The *NAVEL* drugs (i.e., naloxone, atropine, vasopressin, epinephrine, lidocaine) are absorbed systemically after endotracheal administration. Although pulmonary blood flow, and hence systemic absorption, is minimal during CPR, recent animal studies suggest that comparable hemodynamic responses can occur. At this time, two to three times the standard IV doses are recommended for the endotracheal route. Of note, the endotracheal administration of drugs should only be considered when attempts on obtaining an IV or IO line have failed.

16. **What is the usual outcome of in-hospital CPR?**
Most patients who receive CPR in the hospital do not survive. In fact, only 5% to 20% of patients live to be discharged home. Furthermore, many patients who do survive have severe impairments of independence and cognition. Unfortunately, it is not yet possible to confidently predict the outcome of in-hospital resuscitation.

KEY POINTS: CARDIOPULMONARY RESUSCITATION

1. Iatrogenic cardiopulmonary arrests can occur during procedures; extra care needs to be taken to monitor patients during procedures.

2. Compressions, Airway, and Breathing (C-A-B); NOT airway, breathing, and circulation (A-B-C).

3. Remember the reversible causes of cardiac arrest: hypovolemia, hypoxia, hydrogen ions (acidosis), hyperkalemia, toxins, tamponade, tension pneumothorax, coronary thrombosis, pulmonary thrombosis.

4. If IV access is not readily available, then move to the IO route.

5. Only 5% to 20% of inpatients will undergo CPR and survive their hospitalization.

BIBLIOGRAPHY

1. Bedell SE, Fulton EJ: Unexpected findings and complications at autopsy after cardiopulmonary resuscitation (CPR). Arch Intern Med 146:1725-1728, 1986.

2. Brown CG, Martin DR, Pepe PE, et al: A comparison of standard-dose and high-dose epinephrine in cardiac arrest outside the hospital. N Engl J Med 327:1051-1055, 1992.

3. Dorian P, Cass D, Schwartz B, et al: Amiodarone as compared with lidocaine for shock-resistant ventricular fibrillation. N Engl J Med 346:884-890, 2002.

4. Field JM, Hazinski MF, Sayre MR, et al: Part 1: executive summary: 2010 American Heart Association Guidelines for Cardiopulmonary Resuscitation and Emergency Cardiovascular Care. Circulation 122(3 Suppl):S640-S656, 2010.

5. Gueugniaud PY, David JS, Chanzy E, et al: Vasopressin and epinephrine vs. epinephrine alone in cardiopulmonary resuscitation. N Engl J Med 359:21-30, 2008.

6. McGrath RB: In-house cardiopulmonary resuscitation—after a quarter of a century. Ann Emerg Med 16:1365-1368, 1987.

7. Paradis NA, Martin GB, Rivers EP, et al: Coronary perfusion pressure and the return of spontaneous circulation in human cardiopulmonary resuscitation. JAMA 263:1106-1113, 1990.

8. Shimabukuro DS, Liu LL: Cardiopulmonary resuscitation. In Miller RD, Pardo M, Jr (eds): Basics of Anesthesia, 6th ed. Philadelphia, Saunders, 2011, pp 715-728.

9. SOS-KANTO Study Group: Cardiopulmonary resuscitation by bystanders with chest compression only (SOS-KANTO): an observational study. Lancet 369:920-926, 2007.

CHAPTER 4

ASSESSMENTS OF OXYGENATION

Asheesh Kumar, MD, Michael E. Canham, MD, and Ulrich H. Schmidt, MD, PhD

1. **What do arterial blood gas (ABG) instruments measure?**

   The current ABG instruments measure pH, PCO_2, and PO_2 using three separate electrodes. The blood gas samples are placed through an inlet into a temperature-controlled chamber (usually 37° C) where the blood is exposed to these three electrode tips. Newer ABG machines have simultaneous CO-oximeter measurements as well. Consequently, with use of an absorption spectrophotometer, measurements of reduced hemoglobin, oxyhemoglobin, carboxyhemoglobin, and methemoglobin can also be made. Often, hemoglobin and basic electrolytes can be measured simultaneously.

2. **When should ABGs be used?**

   Analysis of ABGs is used extensively in the critical care setting to evaluate both acid-base status and oxygen and carbon dioxide gas exchange. Analysis of ABGs can be useful in virtually any critical care situation, especially with regard to the acid-base status, adequacy of perfusion, and adequacy of gas exchange.

3. **What alternatives exist to measure respiratory gases and gas exchange?**

   ABGs, specifically acid-base status, are useful for evaluation of systemic pH, especially in the setting of significant metabolic acidoses. However, alternative mechanisms are clinically available to measure systemic oxygen and carbon dioxide levels.

   - **Pulse oximetry:** Pulse oximetry is a noninvasive, continuous method of measuring the saturation of hemoglobin by using the differential absorption of different wavelengths of light depending on the loading conditions of oxygen that can significantly reduce the number of ABGs measured in critically ill patients. Further, recent studies have validated the use of respiratory variation in pulse oximetry to detect fluid responsiveness in critically ill patients.
   - **End-tidal carbon dioxide:** In patients without significant pulmonary pathologic conditions, an end-tidal carbon dioxide monitor can approximate the plasma levels of carbon dioxide, indicating ongoing metabolic production and adequacy of ventilation.
   - **Bicarbonate:** Levels of serum bicarbonate can provide guidance about serum levels of carbon dioxide and pH, especially in the chronic setting. Elevations of serum bicarbonate can indicate chronic retention of carbon dioxide.
   - **Exhaled carbon dioxide:** The content of exhaled carbon dioxide over a given period of time can be measured by several commercially available devices. This can provide information regarding total body carbon dioxide production, as well as the adequacy of carbon dioxide elimination. Specifically, with use of the Bohr equation, the dead-space fraction can be calculated to assess the adequacy of ventilation and underlying degrees of pulmonary pathologic conditions.
   - **Calculated minute ventilation:** The overall minute ventilation can be calculated by multiplying the tidal volume by respiratory rate. Again, the minute ventilation can provide information about metabolic demands and production.

4. **What is the alveolar gas equation?**

   The alveolar gas equation is a formula used to approximate the partial pressure of oxygen in the alveolus (PAO_2).

$$PAO_2 = (PB - PH_2O)FiO_2 - (PaCO_2/R)$$

where PB is the barometric pressure, PH_2O is the water vapor pressure (usually 47 mm Hg), FiO_2 is the fractional concentration of inspired oxygen, and R is the gas exchange ratio. (The rate of CO_2 production to O_2 utilization is usually approximately 0.8 at rest). For example, at sea level:

$$PAO_2 = (760 - 47)0.21 - (40/0.8) = 100 \text{ mm Hg}$$

As demonstrated by the alveolar gas equation, significant alterations of other values can affect the alveolar oxygen level. For example, significant elevation of plasma carbon dioxide can lead to a decrease in the partial pressure of alveolar oxygen. Further, changes in the respiratory quotient (e.g., supplemental nutrition with high carbohydrate content) can further decrease alveolar oxygenation because of a high CO_2 production–to–O_2 utilization ratio.

5. **What is the alveolar-arterial PO$_2$ difference, or *A – a gradient* (A – aO$_2$ gradient)?**
After calculation of the PAO_2 from the alveolar gas equation, the A – aO_2 gradient can be obtained by subtracting the PaO_2 measured from the ABG. The alveolar-to-arterial (A – aO_2) oxygen gradient is the difference between the amount of the oxygen in the alveoli (PAO_2) and the amount of oxygen dissolved in the plasma (PaO_2), as measured by ABG. For example, at sea level (with $PCO_2 - 40$, $PO_2 - 92$):

$$PAO_2 - PaO_2 = A - aO_2 \text{ gradient}$$

$$100 \text{ mm Hg} - 92 \text{ mm Hg} = 8 \text{ mm Hg}$$

The normal A – aO_2 gradient is dependent on age, body position, and nutritional status. A normal A – a gradient for a young adult nonsmoker breathing air is between 5 and 10 mm Hg. Normally, the A – a gradient increases with age. For every decade a person has lived, his or her A – a gradient is expected to increase by 1 mm Hg. The A – aO_2 gradient is widened under normal conditions by age, obesity, fasting, supine position, and heavy exercise. One predictive equation for estimating PO_2 (at PB = 760 mm Hg) in relation to age is as follows: $PO_2 = 109 - 0.43 \times$ Age (in years).

6. **How is the A – aO$_2$ gradient useful? What can cause significant elevations of the A – aO$_2$ gradient?**
The A – aO_2 gradient may be affected by significant cardiopulmonary conditions that result in hypoxemia and/or hypocarbia. However, it must be noted that the A – a gradient normally increases with higher FiO_2, resulting in an elevated gradient without clinical hypoxemia. When receiving a high FiO_2, both PAO_2 and PaO_2 can increase. However, the PAO_2 increases disproportionately, causing the A – a gradient to increase. In one series, the A – a gradient in men breathing air and 100% oxygen varied from 8 to 82 mm Hg in patients younger than 40 years of age and from 3 to 120 mm Hg in patients older than 40 years of age.
Clinically significant hypoxemia associated with a widened A – aO_2 gradient is commonly due to:

- **V/Q mismatch:** The normal heterogeneity of V/Q matching in the lung can be significantly altered by many disease states, resulting in a widened A – aO_2 gradient and clinical hypoxemia. Commonly, this can be seen with atelectasis, pneumonia, aspiration, pulmonary edema, and/or acute lung injury or adult respiratory distress syndrome (ARDS).
- **Right-to-left shunt:** A right-to-left shunt exists when blood passes from the right to the left side of the heart without being oxygenated. Numerous anatomic shunts exist physiologically that contribute to the normal A – aO_2 gradient, such as the bronchial and thebesian circulation. Pathologic shunts can develop when nonventilated alveoli are perfused (atelectasis, pneumonia, edema, ARDS, pulmonary fibrosis).

- **Diffusion impairment:** Diffusion impairment occurs when a limitation exists to the movement of oxygen from the alveoli into the pulmonary vasculature. This can be due to overall destruction of lung parenchyma, such as severe emphysema, or pathologic changes in the air-blood interface in the lung, such as fibrosis.

7. **What clinical conditions can present with a normal $A - aO_2$ gradient?**
   Conditions that purely lower the alveolar concentration of oxygen without concomitant pulmonary pathologic conditions can result in clinically significant hypoxemia with a normal $A - aO_2$ gradient. Because many can result in complicating factors that cause significant elevations of the $A - aO_2$ gradient, such as atelectasis, consolidation, or aspiration events, these conditions are clinically rarely seen in isolation. Clinical hypoxemia with a normal $A - aO_2$ gradient occurs in the setting of low inspired partial pressure of oxygen (PiO_2). On the basis of the alveolar gas equation, this results from multiple factors.
   - **Low FiO_2:** This can be seen in a variety of clinical situations, such as hypoxic mixtures of inhaled gases. These are also readily correctable by administration of higher concentrations of oxygen; failure to respond to such therapy should prompt investigation of other causes of hypoxemia.
   - **Low PB:** Atmospheric pressure at sea level is approximately 760 mm Hg. As altitude increases, PB decreases; with significant elevations of altitude, low alveolar oxygen levels can develop. The mean measured PAO_2 measured at 8400 m (descent from summit of Mount Everest) above sea level was 30 mm Hg with an $A - aO_2$ gradient of 5.41 mm Hg.
   - **Significant hypercarbia (elevated $PaCO_2$):** Elevations of arterial carbon dioxide levels can result in decreases in alveolar oxygen levels. Pure hypercarbia is often the result of hypoventilation syndromes. These can be related to multiple factors:
     - Central nervous system (CNS) depression, such as drug overdose, structural CNS lesions, or ischemic CNS lesions that affect the respiratory center
     - Obesity hypoventilation (Pickwickian) syndrome
     - Impaired neural conduction, such as amyotrophic lateral sclerosis, Guillain-Barré syndrome, high cervical spine injury, or phrenic nerve paralysis
     - Muscular weakness, such as myasthenia gravis, muscular dystrophy, or residual neuromuscular blockade
     - Poor chest wall elasticity, such as a flail chest or kyphoscoliosis

8. **What are point-of-care (POC) ABGs?**
   Current technology allows measurement of ABGs at the bedside with handheld blood gas analysis devices that use disposable cartridges. Several commercially available devices provide different test options to measure in addition to routine ABG values. Consequently, the reliability of each measured parameter may differ from one device to another.

9. **How do POC ABGs work? What are their advantages and disadvantages?**
   The heparinized ABG specimen is placed into the POC cartridge, where the blood flows to different sites-sensors for analysis. The pH and PCO_2 are measured by direct potentiometry, and the PO_2 is measured amperometrically. The values for HCO_3, total CO_2, base excess, and oxygen saturation are calculated. POC testing can be performed by nurses, physicians, and respiratory therapists, and the ABG results are obtained more rapidly and may influence critical decisions. The major disadvantages include cost per cartridge, lack of preanalysis calibrations to ensure accuracy, and a lack of CO-oximetry measurements.

10. **Given that oximetry is so readily available, painless, and accurate, why is ABG analysis necessary?**
    Oximetry and the newer technology that made it more accessible, affordable, and accurate have decreased the need for ABG analysis in monitoring oxygen saturation. In fact, the number of ABGs done has decreased with the influx of oximeters into virtually every department in a

hospital. However, relying on oximetry alone can lead to misdiagnosis, increased cost, and potentially fatal respiratory arrest. Common clinical scenarios include

- **Hypercarbia:** An increased PCO_2 from hypoventilation (e.g., in a patient receiving narcotics) can often be missed by a reassuring oxygen saturation. Although the pulse oximeter provides information regarding systemic oxygenation, it cannot provide data regarding systemic conditions of carbon dioxide. An ABG or venous blood gas measurement is necessary for further evaluation, because oxygenation can be maintained despite rising PCO_2 and impending respiratory failure.

- **Carbon monoxide (CO):** CO diffuses rapidly across the pulmonary capillary membrane and binds to hemoglobin with approximately 240 times the affinity of oxygen. Standard pulse oximetry cannot screen for CO exposure, because it cannot differentiate carboxyhemoglobin from oxyhemoglobin, inasmuch as they absorb the same emitted light wavelength. Arterial blood gas measurements tend to be normal because PO_2 reflects oxygen dissolved in blood, and this process is not affected by CO. Acute CO poisoning must be clinically suspected on the basis of a suggestive history and associated physical examination findings (e.g., singed nasal hair, soot); specialized eight-wavelength pulse oximeters and ABG analysis with CO-oximetry are required to detect systemic CO.

- **Abnormal hemoglobin or hemoglobin variants:** Methemoglobin is an altered state of hemoglobin in which the ferrous (Fe^{2+}) irons of heme are oxidized to the ferric (Fe^{3+}) state, which are unable to bind oxygen. In addition, the oxygen affinity of any remaining ferrous hemes is increased, resulting in a leftward shift of the oxygen dissociation curve. Large amounts of methemoglobin production can be induced by various drugs, including antibiotics and local anesthetics, such as benzocaine (commonly used for oropharyngeal topicalization). Methemoglobinemia may be clinically suspected by the presence of clinical cyanosis in the presence of a normal arterial PO_2 as obtained by ABGs. Classically, oxygen saturation as measured by pulse oximetry drops to 85%, as methemoglobin absorbs both wavelengths of light (660 and 940 nm) emitted by pulse oximetry resulting in an average value regardless of the true percentage of oxyhemoglobin.

KEY POINTS: ASSESSMENTS OF OXYGENATION

1. Multiple reliable methods are available for monitoring the adequacy of gas exchange in the critical care setting.

2. The ABG and the alveolar gas equation can be used to evaluate the mechanisms of hypoxemia in critically ill patients.

BIBLIOGRAPHY

1. Barton CW: Correlation of end-tidal CO_2 measurements to arterial $PaCO_2$ in non-intubated patients. Ann Emerg Med 23:562-563, 1994.

2. Durbin CG, Rostow SK: More reliable oximetry reduces the frequency of arterial blood gas analyses and hastens weaning after cardiac surgery: a prospective, randomized trial of the clinical impact of a new technology. Crit Care Med 30:1735-1740, 2002.

3. Feissel M, Teboul JL, Merlani P, et al: Plethysmographic dynamic indices predict fluid responsiveness in septic ventilated patients. Intensive Care Med 33:993-999, 2007.

4. Fu ES, Downs JB, Schweiger JW, et al: Supplemental oxygen impairs detection of hypoventilation by pulse oximetry. Chest 126:1552-1558, 2004.

5. Hampson NB: Pulse oximetry in severe carbon monoxide poisoning. Chest 114:1036-1041, 1998.

6. Hess D, Schlottag A, Levin B, et al: An evaluation of the usefulness of end-tidal PCO_2 to aid weaning from mechanical ventilation following cardiac surgery. Respir Care 36:837-843, 1991.

7. Michael PW, Grocott MB, Martin DS, et al: Arterial blood gases and oxygen content in climbers on Mount Everest. N Engl J Med 360:140-149, 2009.

8. Mithoefer JC, Bossman OG, Thibeault DW, et al: The clinical estimation of alveolar ventilation. Am Rev Respir Dis 98:868-871, 1968.

9. Nuckton TJ, Alonso JA, Kallet RH, et al: Pulmonary dead-space fraction as a risk factor for death in the acute respiratory distress syndrome. N Engl J Med 346:1281-1286, 2002.

10. Perkins GD, McAuley DF, Giles S, et al: Do changes in pulse oximeter oxygen saturation predict equivalent changes in arterial oxygen saturation? Crit Care 7:R67, 2003.

11. Rodríguez-Roisin R, Roca J: Mechanisms of hypoxemia. Intensive Care Med 31:1017-1019, 2005.

12. Severinghaus JW, Astraup P, Murray JF: Blood gas analysis and critical care medicine. Am J Respir Crit Care Med 157:S114-S122, 1998.

13. Siddiki H, Kojicic M, Li G, et al: Bedside quantification of dead-space fraction using routine clinical data in patients with acute lung injury: secondary analysis of two prospective trials. Crit Care 14:R141, 2010.

14. Story DA: Alveolar oxygen partial pressure, alveolar carbon dioxide partial pressure, and the alveolar gas equation. Anesthesiology 84:101, 1996.

15. Tobin MJ: Respiratory monitoring in the intensive care unit. Am Rev Respir Dis 138:1625-1642, 1988.

PULSE OXIMETRY, CAPNOGRAPHY, AND BLOOD GAS ANALYSIS

Philip E. Bickler, MD, PhD

CHAPTER 5

PULSE OXIMETRY

1. What is pulse oximetry and how does it work?

Pulse oximetry is the continuous noninvasive estimation of arterial hemoglobin-oxygen saturation. It is used routinely to monitor oxygenation in diverse clinical settings, including the operating room, emergency department, and intensive care unit. Clinical use of pulse oximetry falls into two main categories:

1. It is used as a screening or warning for arterial hemoglobin-oxygen desaturation.
2. It is used as an end point for titration of therapeutic interventions. Because pulse oximeters detect pulsatile blood flow, they also monitor heart rate and can provide a relative perfusion index.

Pulse oximeters function by transmitting red light (660 nm, absorbed by oxyhemoglobin [O_2Hb]) and infrared light (940 nm, absorbed by deoxyhemoglobin [deoxyHb]) from two light-emitting diodes (LEDs) through tissue containing pulsatile blood. The saturation of hemoglobin with oxygen is a function of the ratio of red to infrared light absorption from the pulsatile and nonpulsatile components of the signals. Thus the saturation (SpO_2) is a function of the *ratio of two ratios*, cancelling out most differences caused by finger thickness, pigmentation, and other factors. A microprocessor algorithm is used to calculate the arterial saturation on the basis of calibration studies done by comparing true saturation measured on arterial blood with a CO-oximeter with the pulse oximeter reading. This calibration is factory set and is not adjustable.

Pulse oximeter probes can be applied to any site that allows orientation of the LED and photodetector opposite one another across a vascular bed. If the tissue is too thick, the signal is attenuated before reaching the detector and the oximeter cannot function. Oximeters can be applied to fingers, toes, earlobes, lips, cheeks, and the bridge of the nose. Esophageal and oral probes are also in development. Several manufacturers offer reflectance oximeter probes that can be applied to flat tissue surfaces such as the forehead or chest. Recently introduced earlobe-mounted sensors combine a pulse oximeter and a transcutaneous CO_2 electrode. Many pulse oximeters now include noise and artifact rejection software. This refinement aids the determination of SpO_2 in patients with low perfusion or motion (e.g., tremor).

2. How accurate are pulse oximeters?

Pulse oximetry is accurate within 2% to 3% of the true O_2Hb levels as measured in vitro with multiwavelength oximeters. The U.S. Food and Drug Administration requires manufacturers to demonstrate that their instruments confirm to this degree of accuracy in human subjects at between 70% and 100% oxygen saturation. Because the principle of measurement is based on a ratio of absorbance ratios, no calibration of the instrument by the user is needed or possible.

3. What factors interfere with pulse oximetry?

Most errors in oximetry measurement are the result of poor signal quality (i.e., hypoperfusion, vasoconstriction) or excessive noise (i.e., motion artifact). Optical interference may be introduced by extraneous light from fluorescent sources or infrared surgical navigation systems.

Intravenous dyes (methylene blue, indocyanine green) and nail polishes (especially green, blue, or black) absorb at the wavelengths used by the oximeter and can produce artificially low measurements. Contamination from venous pulsations caused by dependent venous pooling or valvular insufficiency may also cause low readings. For a similar reason, the simultaneous arterial and venous pulsation during cardiopulmonary resuscitation (CPR) make oximeter data unreliable. Extreme hyperbilirubinemia has been reported to have variable effects on SpO_2 values. The presence of dysfunctional hemoglobin species can alter the ability of oximetry to reflect the true oxygen saturation. Studies show that darkly pigmented skin can falsely increase saturation estimates derived by some widely used pulse oximeters by up to 7% in the range of 70% to 80% saturation.

4. **What effects does dyshemoglobinemia have on pulse oximetry?**
Because pulse oximeters use two wavelengths of light, they are capable of differentiating only two species of hemoglobin: Hb and O_2Hb. Given that abnormal hemoglobin species such as carboxyhemoglobin (CoHb) or methemoglobin (MetHb) also absorb red and infrared light, their presence affects the SpO_2 measurement, and their quantitative contribution cannot be determined. The pulse oximeter assumes that only functional hemoglobin is present (O_2Hb or Hb), and the oxygen saturation is calculated on the basis of these amounts.

For example, CoHb is read by the limited wavelength analysis of a pulse oximeter as O_2Hb (CoHb is scarlet red), which will falsely elevate the SpO_2 reading. The absorption pattern of MetHb is interpreted by the pulse oximeter as 85% saturation; thus, progressively higher levels of MetHb cause the SpO_2 value to converge on 85% regardless of the actual SaO_2. When the presence of significant amounts of dysfunctional hemoglobin is suspected, a CO-oximeter should be used to determine O_2Hb saturation. A multiwavelength laboratory CO-oximeter determines SaO_2 more accurately in the presence of dysfunctional hemoglobins because it possesses wavelengths of light that can be used to detect the presence of CoHb and MetHb.

The presence of fetal hemoglobin has not been shown to significantly affect the accuracy of SpO_2 measurements because its light absorption properties are similar to those of adult hemoglobin.

CAPNOGRAPHY

5. **What is capnography, and how does it work?**
Capnography is the continuous measurement and graphic display of exhaled carbon dioxide. It is a noninvasive method to assess both ventilation and cardiac output. Most commonly, infrared light absorption by CO_2 is the method used to determine the CO_2 concentration. Sampling usually occurs in one of two ways. In a mainstream capnograph, CO_2 levels are measured with a sensor (light source and detector) placed directly in the patient's breathing circuit. With sidestream capnography, a continuous sample of airway gas is diverted from the patient's breathing circuit or airway to the capnograph for analysis and display. The mainstream method has a very rapid response time, but, because the sensor must be placed near the patient, long-term monitoring may be cumbersome. The sidestream method, because it uses a thin plastic sampling tube, is lighter and allows for greater flexibility, but, because transit time is unavoidable, a slower response time (approximately 3-5 seconds) results. Because of mixing of gases in the sample stream, the absolute values of the plateau and baseline may also be attenuated. The sidestream device can also be used with a modified nasal cannula or face mask to monitor CO_2 concentrations in the breath of patients who do not have endotracheal tubes in place.

The most commonly used method for measuring carbon dioxide in expired gases is infrared light absorbance. In addition, technologies such as Raman spectrometry and mass spectrometry are reliable, accurate, and responsive but generally more expensive. However, these options also offer detection of a variety of other gases and anesthetic vapors. Colorimetric detectors that attach to endotracheal tubes are available to help assess endotracheal tube placement. The colorimetric detector uses a pH-sensitive indicator strip to semiquantitatively detect exhaled CO_2. Although portable and convenient, these devices yield results that are often more difficult to interpret than conventional capnographs, and they do not provide continuous measurement of CO_2.

6. **What does the capnogram reveal about a patient's condition?**
A capnograph provides a continuous display of the CO_2 concentration of gases in the airways. A normal capnogram is shown in Figure 5-1. The CO_2 partial pressure at the end of normal exhalation (phase III in the figure, end-tidal CO_2 [$PETCO_2$]) is a reflection of gas leaving alveoli and is an estimate of the alveolar CO_2 partial pressure ($PACO_2$). When ventilation and perfusion are well matched, the $PACO_2$ approximates the arterial PCO_2 ($PaCO_2$), and thus $PaCO_2$ equals $PACO_2$ plus $PETCO_2$. The presence of cyclical exhaled CO_2 is useful in confirming airway patency, verifying endotracheal tube placement, and verifying the adequacy of pulmonary ventilation. In addition, decreases in cardiac output caused by hypovolemia or cardiac dysfunction result in decreased pulmonary perfusion. This causes an increased alveolar dead space, which dilutes $PETCO_2$. Animal studies show that a 20% decrease in cardiac output causes a 15% decrease in $PETCO_2$.

Alterations in the shape of the capnogram in a patient with an endotracheal tube and mechanical ventilation often provide clues to alterations in pulmonary pathologic condition and malfunction of ventilation equipment. For example, a staircase pattern in phase II may indicate sequential emptying of the lung, which may occur in main stem partial bronchial obstruction. An upward sloping plateau during expiration is a classic indication of late emptying of poorly ventilated alveolar spaces with elevated PCO_2, which may occur with expiratory obstruction at the level of smaller airways, as seen in chronic obstructive pulmonary disease (COPD), bronchospasm, and other forms of ventilation-perfusion mismatching. A pulmonary embolus is another cause of a decrease in end-tidal CO_2.

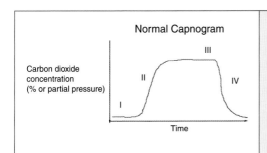

Normal Capnogram

Carbon dioxide concentration (% or partial pressure)

I II III IV

Time

Figure 5-1. A capnogram is a plot of airway CO_2 versus time. Phase I (inspiratory baseline) refers to inspired gas devoid of CO_2. Phase II (beginning expiration) represents expiration of anatomic dead space followed by gas from respiratory bronchioles and alveoli. Phase III (alveolar plateau) corresponds with exhalation of alveolar gases. The last portion of the plateau is termed *end-tidal* ($PETCO_2$). Phase IV (inspiratory downslope) is the beginning of the next inspiration.

7. **What factors affect the arterial–end-tidal CO_2 gradient?**
The normal gradient between $PaCO_2$ and $PETCO_2$, $P(a - ET)CO_2$, is <6 mm Hg. The gradient between $PaCO_2$ and $PETCO_2$ increases when pulmonary perfusion is reduced or ventilation is maldistributed. This occurs with the development of high ventilation-perfusion alveolar units (increased dead space ventilation). The result is an increased $P(a - ET)CO_2$ and decreased $PETCO_2$. Examples of this state are COPD, pulmonary hypoperfusion, and pulmonary emboli. Technical failures such as accidental extubation and endotracheal tube cuff leak can also cause a decrease in $PETCO_2$.

8. **Can capnography assist in CPR efforts?**
   In the course of CPR, capnography not only can help verify tracheal intubation, it can also monitor the adequacy of circulatory assistance. The presence of exhaled CO_2 during CPR is useful in that it provides evidence of enough circulation to produce CO_2 transport from tissues to the lungs. Thus, assuming constant minute ventilation and CO_2 production, changes in $PETCO_2$ reflect the status of overall circulation. Some investigators have suggested that if the $PETCO_2$ is >15 mm Hg at the beginning of CPR, it may predict successful resuscitation. Failure to achieve any recovery of $PETCO_2$ should prompt consideration of a diagnosis of inadequate cardiac filling. This may be caused by hypovolemia, tamponade, pneumothorax, or pulmonary embolism. Low $PETCO_2$ also may be caused by alveolar hyperventilation, or it may indicate ineffective CPR. The return of spontaneous circulation is heralded with a substantial increase in $PETCO_2$, primarily because of increased flow of hypercarbic blood to the lungs.

ARTERIAL BLOOD GASES

9. **What do arterial blood gas (ABG) instruments measure?**
   ABG instruments measure pH, PCO_2, and PO_2 using three separate electrodes. The blood gas samples are placed through an inlet into a temperature-controlled chamber (usually 37° C) where the blood is exposed to these three electrodes. The information from an ABG is essential in evaluating gas transport in blood, because the shape of the O_2Hb dissociation curve depends on blood pH (Fig. 5-2).

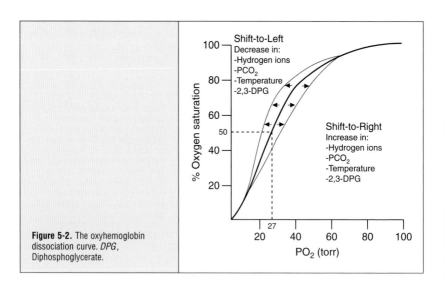

Figure 5-2. The oxyhemoglobin dissociation curve. *DPG*, Diphosphoglycerate.

10. **When should ABGs be obtained?**
    Analysis of ABGs is used extensively in critical care to evaluate both acid-base status and oxygen and carbon dioxide gas exchange. Analysis of ABGs is indicated in virtually all cardiopulmonary conditions.

11. **How is an ABG used to calculate the $A - a$ gradient?**
    The alveolar gas equation is a formula used to approximate the partial pressure of oxygen in the alveolus (PAO_2).

$$PAO_2 = (PB - PH_2O)FiO_2 - (PaCO_2/R)$$

where PB is the barometric pressure, PH_2O is the water vapor pressure (usually 47 mm Hg), FiO_2 is the fractional concentration of inspired oxygen, and R is the gas exchange ratio. (The rate of CO_2 production to O_2 utilization is usually approximately 0.8 at rest). For example, at sea level:

$$PAO_2 = (760 - 47)0.21 - (40/0.8) = 100 \text{ mm Hg}$$

After calculation of the PAO_2 from the alveolar gas equation, the $A - aO_2$ gradient can be obtained by subtracting the PaO_2 measured from the ABGs. For example, at sea level (with $PCO_2 = 40$, $PO_2 = 92$):

$$PAO_2 - PaO_2 = A - aO_2 \text{ gradient}$$

$$100 \text{ mm Hg} - 92 \text{ mm Hg} = 8 \text{ mm Hg}$$

The normal $A - aO_2$ gradient is dependent on age, body position, and nutritional status. The $A - aO_2$ gradient is widened under normal conditions by age, obesity, fasting, supine position, and heavy exercise. One predictive equation for estimating PO_2 (at PB = 760 mm Hg) in relation to age is as follows: $PO_2 = 109 - 0.43 \times$ Age (in years). The $A - aO_2$ gradient may be increased by any significant cardiopulmonary condition that results in hypoxemia and/or hypocarbia. Hypoxemia caused by simple alveolar hypoventilation will not widen the $A - aO_2$ gradient. Most pulmonary emboli, on the other hand, will widen the $A - aO_2$ gradient, because, even if hypoxemia does not occur, hypocarbia is very common.

12. **Given that pulse oximetry is painless and accurate, why is ABG analysis even necessary?**
Oximetry and the newer technology that made it more accessible, affordable, and accurate have decreased the need for ABG analysis in monitoring oxygen saturation. In fact, in many hospitals the number of ABGs done has decreased with the influx of oximeters into virtually every department in a hospital. However, relying on oximetry alone can lead to misdiagnosis, increased cost, and potentially fatal respiratory arrest. Consider the following examples of pitfalls of using oximetry alone that have been observed in practice.
   1. A patient was noted to have oxygen desaturation via oximetry during a routine check after minor orthopedic surgery. The physicians evaluated this by ordering a chest radiograph, pulmonary function tests, and a ventilation-perfusion lung scan, the results of all of which were normal. Finally, ABG analysis was done and revealed alveolar hypoventilation alone with a normal $A - aO_2$ gradient. The oxygen desaturation was simply the result of an increased PCO_2 from hypoventilation in a patient receiving narcotics.
   2. After an episode of smoke inhalation, a patient came to the emergency department because of headache and nausea. The oxygen saturation by oximetry was normal, and the patient was nearly dismissed after symptomatic treatment alone. Fortunately, recognizing the limitation of oximetry in differentiating oxygenated hemoglobin from CoHb, the physician drew an ABG sample, which revealed profound carbon monoxide poisoning. The patient was treated appropriately with 100% oxygen and close monitoring.
   3. A patient with fever and sepsis had a respiratory rate of 40/min, and a chest radiograph revealed bilateral alveolar infiltrates. Oxygen was initiated, and with the use of pulse oximetry, the oxygen saturation was 90% after breathing 100% O_2 by nonrebreathing mask. Unfortunately, the house officer did not draw an ABG sample and failed to realize that, with marked hyperventilation and respiratory alkalosis, the O_2Hb dissociation curve is shifted to the left, thereby causing a much higher oxygen saturation for a given PaO_2. Had ABG analysis been done at that time, it would have revealed pH 7.58, $PACO_2$ 22 mm Hg, PAO_2 50 mm Hg, and O_2 saturation 90%, all clearly indicating intubation and assisted ventilation with positive end-expiratory pressure.

KEY POINTS: PULSE OXIMETRY, CAPNOGRAPHY, AND BLOOD GAS ANALYSIS

1. Pulse oximeter accuracy is strongly degraded by low perfusion states; accept only numeric estimates of saturation that are associated with clean perfusion signals.

2. Pulse oximeters may interpret dyes, skin pigment, and dyshemoglobinemia as alterations in hemoglobin-oxygen saturation.

3. The capnogram contains important information concerning airways disease and cardiopulmonary pathology.

BIBLIOGRAPHY

1. Aoyagi T, Miyasaka K: The theory and applications of pulse spectrophotometry. Anesth Analg 94(1 Suppl): S93-S95, 2002.

2. Bickler PE, Feiner JR, Severinghaus JW: Effects of skin pigmentation on pulse oximeter accuracy at low saturation. Anesthesiology 102:715-719, 2005.

3. Callaham M, Barton C: Prediction of outcome of cardiopulmonary resuscitation from end-tidal carbon dioxide concentration. Crit Care Med 18:358-362, 1990.

4. Feiner JR, Bickler PE: Improved accuracy of methemoglobin detection by pulse CO-oximetry during hypoxia. Anesth Analg 111:1160-1167, 2010.

5. Gravenstein JS, Jaffe MB, Paulus DA, (eds): Capnography: Clinical Aspects. Cambridge, United Kingdom, Cambridge University Press, 2004.

6. Kugelman A, Wasserman Y, Mor F, et al: Reflectance pulse oximetry from core body in neonates and infants: comparison to arterial blood oxygen saturation and to transmission pulse oximetry. J Perinatol 24:366-371, 2004.

7. Robertson FA, Hoffman GM: Clinical evaluation of the effects of signal integrity and saturation on data availability and accuracy of Masimo SE and Nellcor N-395 oximeters in children. Anesth Analg 98:617-622, 2004.

8. Severinghaus JW, Astraup P, Murray JF: Blood gas analysis and critical care medicine. Am J Respir Crit Care Med 157:S114-S122, 1998.

9. Sorbini CA, Grassi V, Solinas E, et al: Arterial oxygen tension in relation to age in healthy subjects. Respiration 25:3-13, 1968.

CHAPTER 6

HEMODYNAMIC MONITORING

Daniel Saddawi-Konefka, MD, MBA, and Jonathan E. Charnin, MD

1. **What is the purpose of hemodynamic monitoring?**

   Oxygen and fuels are brought to the tissues and waste products are removed by the flow of blood. The goal of hemodynamic monitoring is to assess whether the circulatory system has adequate performance in this regard to sustain organ function and life. Notably, hemodynamic monitoring provides data to guide therapy but is not by itself therapeutic.

2. **How do manual blood pressure cuffs differ from automatic blood pressure cuffs?**

   Manual auscultation of the blood pressure assigns systolic value to the pressure measured when the first Korotkoff sound is heard and diastolic value to the pressure measured when the fourth Korotkoff sound disappears. Automatic blood pressure cuffs measure oscillations in pressure, caused by blood flow across a range of blood pressures; they determine only the mean blood pressure, which is determined by the point of greatest oscillation. With use of proprietary algorithms, the systolic and diastolic blood pressures are calculated. Both methods are susceptible to error with poor cuff size (which should cover two thirds of the limb segment), motion artifact, arrhythmia, and extremes of blood pressure.

3. **How are arterial lines calibrated, and what factors affect readings?**

   Arterial lines generate blood pressure readings using pressure transducers. To yield useful information, the transducers must first be zeroed and leveled (positioned appropriately). Second, the system should be monitored for damping and resonance.

   Zeroing and leveling eliminate the effects of atmospheric pressure and hydrostatic pressure, respectively, on blood pressure readings. Atmospheric pressures are set to zero so that reported values are relative pressures. If the system is not zeroed appropriately, measurements will continuously offset by a fixed amount. Errors can also occur if the transducer is physically lowered so that it will read a higher pressure and vice versa (potential energy is replaced by pressure to maintain energy in the fluid; read about Bernoulli's equation for more). Therefore it is crucial to position the transducer at the height of interest (e.g., external acoustic meatus to approximate pressure at the circle of Willis).

   Damping is the tendency of an oscillating system to decrease oscillation amplitude. In the case of an arterial line, the systolic and diastolic readings tend to converge around the mean pressure. Damping results from medium or large air bubbles in the circuit, compliant tubing between the transducer and cannulation site, loose connections, or kinks. Resonance or *whip* causes falsely increased systolic readings and falsely decreased diastolic readings. It occurs when the system's frequency of oscillation (i.e., heart rate) matches the system's natural frequency of vibration causing whip in the signal. The classic example of this (though not easy to accomplish) is breaking a wine glass by singing a note of the same frequency as the wine glass's resonant frequency.

4. **In what situations should arterial line placement be considered?**

   - Inability to obtain noninvasive blood pressures.
   - Hemodynamic instability. Patients who need monitoring because of extremely high blood pressure, extremely low blood pressure, or extremely volatile blood pressure.

- Need for rigorous blood pressure control. Patients who need blood pressure kept within a tight range (e.g., status post aortic aneurysm repair).
- Need for frequent arterial blood sampling. Patients with severe ventilation compromise, oxygenation compromise, or other condition where it is useful to follow serial laboratory values with an arterial line.

Choice of cannulation site is important because each site has unique benefits and risks. The radial artery is often chosen given the convenient location and good collateral supply to the hand. In patients with severe vasoconstriction, however, a femoral line may be preferable because the radial pressure may underestimate central arterial pressure.

5. **How do arterial tracings differ between proximal and distal cannulation sites?**
Arterial tracings become more peaked with higher systolic pressures but similar mean pressures as one transduces sites progressively distal from the aorta. The dicrotic notch representing aortic valve closure is seen in the aorta and its largest branches but becomes lost in peripheral arteries. A smaller second wave of pressure during diastole represents pressure waves reflecting off the peripheral resistance arterioles. This phenomenon can sometimes cause a pulse-oximeter to *double count* the pulse.

6. **List indications for central line placement.**
Central lines are indicated for monitoring the central venous pressure, infusing concentrated vasopressors, delivering total parenteral nutrition, sampling central venous blood for analysis, and obtaining venous access when peripheral access cannot be obtained.

7. **Describe the central venous waveform components. Which part of the waveform cycle should be reported as the central venous pressure?**
Central venous pressures have predictable waveforms. These waveforms have upward deflections representing atrial contraction ("a" wave), ventricular contraction that causes the tricuspid valve to bulge into the atrium ("c" wave), and passive venous return of blood during diastole ("v" wave). (Note the somewhat counterintuitive fact that ventricular contraction coincides with the "c" wave, not the "v" wave.) The downslope after the "c" wave is called the "x" descent, and the downslope after the "v" wave is called the "y" descent. See Figure 6-1.

Central venous pressure should reflect the end-diastolic distention of the ventricle. Therefore the pressure measured should be immediately before systole. This corresponds to the valley immediately before the "c" wave and immediately after the "a" wave. In addition, because intrathoracic pressure (which is transmitted to the central veins) varies with respiration, pressures should be measured at end-expiration to minimize this effect on measurements.

8. **List the indications for pulmonary artery catheter (PAC) placement.**
Indications to place a PAC include monitoring pulmonary artery pressures, measuring cardiac output by using thermodilution, assessing left ventricular filling pressures, and allowing sampling of true mixed-venous blood.

9. **Describe complications of central line or PAC placement.**
Central line complications include pneumothorax, arterial puncture, line infection, arrhythmia, hematoma, and deep venous thrombosis. Rarer complications include thoracic duct injury and cardiac tamponade.

All the aforementioned central line complications can also arise during PAC placement. In addition, PAC placement can result in transient right bundle branch block through direct mechanical irritation of the right ventricle; therefore, PACs are relatively contraindicated in patients with left bundle branch blocks because of the potential for complete heart block. Lastly, pulmonary arterial rupture, which is usually fatal, can occur if care with the balloon tip is not taken.

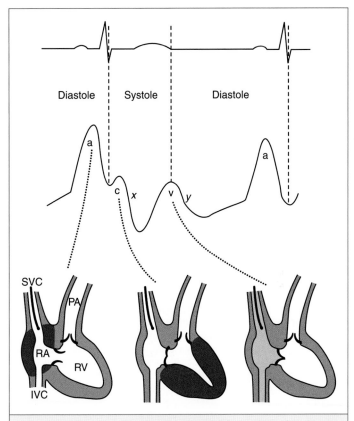

Figure 6-1. Central venous waveform components. *IVC*, Inferior vena cava; *PA*, pulmonary artery; *RA*, right atrium; *RV*, right ventricle; *SVC*, superior vena cava.

10. **Describe normal pressures and waveforms encountered as a PAC is advanced.**
The inflated balloon on the distal tip will advance with the flow of blood through the superior vena cava, right atrium, right ventricle, and ultimately the pulmonary artery. Different waveforms are obtained at each position as illustrated below.

The right atrial pressures are similar to central venous pressures described in question 7. Right ventricular pressures will have systolic components that are in phase with (i.e., occur synchronously with) systemic arterial systolic pressures and have low diastolic pressures that increase during diastole. Systolic pulmonary arterial pressures will also be in phase with systemic arterial systolic pressures and have similar waveforms that gradually decrease during diastole. The pulmonary artery occlusion pressure (PAOP)—or wedge pressure if no balloon is used—reflects the left atrial pressure and thereby left ventricular filling. Because the wedge pressure reflects the left atrial pressures, it may have "a," "c," and "v" waves, although in practice these may difficult to identify. Large "v" waves due to mitral regurgitation can occur on the PAOP trace, but these large "v" waves will occur during late systole and early diastole. See Figure 6-2.

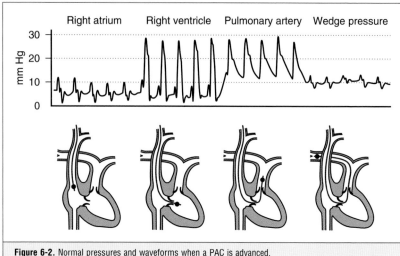

Figure 6-2. Normal pressures and waveforms when a PAC is advanced.

11. **Normally, central venous pressures gauge right ventricular end-diastolic volume and pulmonary arterial occlusion pressures gauge left ventricular end-diastolic volume. What factors alter these relationships?**
    Physiologic or pathologic conditions that affect the relationship between measured pressures and ventricular volumes can be understood by appreciating the following concepts:
    - Transducers measure atrial pressures as surrogates for ventricular end-diastolic volumes. In patients with severely stenotic valves, pressures will be elevated and therefore overestimate the volumes.

    - $Volume_{ventricle} = Compliance_{ventricle} \cdot (P_{inside\ ventricle} - P_{outside\ ventricle})$

    From this it becomes clear that:
    - A less compliant ventricle will have less volume for the same pressure (e.g., left ventricular hypertrophy).
    - Volume depends on the relationship between pressure inside and pressure outside the ventricle. In cases where the pressures externally compressing the ventricle are high (e.g., high positive end-expiratory pressure [PEEP], increased intraabdominal pressures), the pressures inside the ventricles will overestimate the volumes. This is also the case with intraventricular dependence where a severely dilated right ventricle could compress the left ventricle.

12. **Describe how thermodilution with a PAC can be used to determine cardiac output.**
    The principle of thermodilution cardiac output is that a bolus of cold injectate will lower the temperature of the blood as it flows through the right side of the heart. Cold saline solution is bolused proximal to the right side of the heart, and the temperature is measured by the distal tip of the catheter in the pulmonary artery. Higher blood flow (i.e., cardiac output) means the cold is diluted in a larger volume of blood, and smaller temperature changes will be measured. Conversely, low cardiac output shows high temperature change with the bolus, because the cold bolus comprises a much higher portion of the flow that passes the temperature probe.

The modified Stewart-Hamilton equation describes this:

$$CO = \frac{(T_{body} - T_{injectate}) \cdot V_1 \cdot K_1}{AUC}$$

where CO is cardiac output, T_{body} is the temperature of the body, $T_{injectate}$ is the temperature of the injectate, V_1 is the volume of the injectate, K_1 represents properties specific to the catheter and measuring system, and AUC is the area under the curve of the temperature change. In simple terms, the equation relates that flow (a volume per time) is equal to quantity (of *cold*) per time divided by concentration (in this case a temperature *concentration*). Again, even more simply:

$$Flow\ (L/min) = \frac{Quantity\ per\ time("temperature"/min)}{Concentration("temperature"/L)}$$

13. **How is a fluid challenge useful in the intensive care unit (ICU) setting?**
Determining volume status (i.e., which side of the Frank-Starling curve a patient is on) in the ICU can be very difficult but remains important to thoughtfully optimize hemodynamics. A time-honored test is to give a fluid bolus and look for a change in hemodynamics. If a bolus has a salutary effect (increase in blood pressure or cardiac output), then the patient is likely on the ascending portion of the Frank-Starling curve, and another fluid bolus may be indicated to improve hemodynamics. If a fluid bolus produces minimal effect, then it is likely that the patient is near the top of the Frank-Starling curve. If a fluid bolus causes deterioration in the blood pressure or cardiac output, then the patient may be volume overloaded on the descending portion of the curve.
A similar test of volume status is the *passive leg raise*. To perform this test, blood pressure or cardiac output is measured with the patient supine. The patient's legs are then passively elevated, delivering a reversible *autotransfusion* of approximately 500 mL of blood (i.e., blood rushes to the central veins from the legs because of hydrostatic pressure). If the passive leg raise improves hemodynamics, additional volume may be indicated. If the effect is negative, it can be quickly reversed by lowering the legs, which is an advantage over the fluid bolus technique where the bolus cannot be quickly removed.

14. **Can arterial lines tell us anything more than pressure?**
Arterial lines can be used to assess both fluid responsiveness and cardiac output. With the ubiquity of arterial lines in ICUs, these techniques can be very useful.
- **Fluid responsiveness:** If central veins are not adequately filled (i.e., with a patient with hypovolemia), changes in intrathoracic pressure during positive-pressure variation can result in highly significant effects on cardiac output and blood pressure. Variation in pulse pressure or systolic pressure of greater than 10% to 12% is predictive of positive fluid responsiveness. Note that this technique holds only for sedated patients (with no spontaneous respirations) receiving positive-pressure ventilation with regular cardiac rhythm.
- **Cardiac output:** As the arterial pulse pressure waveform reflects the stroke volume, algorithms have been developed to continuously monitor cardiac output through waveform analysis. These techniques are challenged by nonlinearity of pressure to volume translation, damping and resonance issues, and flow-independent systemic vascular resistance changes.

15. **What are transpulmonary thermodilution and transpulmonary lithium dilution?**
Similar to thermodilution with PACs (see question 12), these techniques use the Stewart-Hamilton equation to approximate cardiac output using temperature (in the case of thermodilution) or lithium concentration (in the case of lithium dilution). Boluses (of either cold injectate or lithium) are injected in central veins, and temperatures or lithium concentrations are

measured in arterial lines. Commercial applications typically use these techniques to calibrate some form of arterial waveform analysis to provide a continuous determination of cardiac output (e.g., the PiCCO and LiDCO devices).

16. What is impedance cardiac output?

With impedance cardiac output, current is applied across the chest and the impedance (resistance) is calculated. With each heartbeat, the impedance decreases (as the low-resistance blood-filled aorta expands). Combining the impedance change and heart rate allows estimation of the cardiac output. Limitations of this technique in the critically ill have resulted in lack of widespread adoption.

17. How is Fick's principle used to measure cardiac output?

Fick's principle allows highly accurate calculation of cardiac output. Total oxygen consumption, VO_2, in the tissues must equal the delivered oxygen less the returned oxygen. Delivered oxygen is equal to cardiac output multiplied by arterial oxygen content (C_a, determined in a systemic artery). Returned oxygen is equal to cardiac output multiplied by mixed venous oxygen content (C_v, determined in the pulmonary artery). Oxygen consumption can also be measured directly with a closed-loop spirometer. Setting these two equal to each other allows us to generate the following equation:

$$VO_2 = (CO \cdot C_a) - (CO \cdot C_v)$$

Rearranging, cardiac output is calculated as

$$CO = \frac{VO_2}{C_a - C_v}$$

In this equation, oxygen content of blood, C, is calculated as

$$C = Hgb \cdot 1.34 \; SpO_2 + 0.003 \cdot PO_2$$

where Hgb is hemoglobin (measured in grams per deciliter), SpO_2 is hemoglobin saturation with oxygen (measured as a percentage), and PO_2 is the partial pressure of oxygen in blood (measured in millimeters of mercury).

18. How is cardiac output measured with transesophageal aortic Doppler?

Doppler technology relies on frequency change of sound waves as they reflect off moving objects. With transesophageal aortic Doppler, the Doppler probe lies in the esophagus and reflects sound from the blood pumping through the aorta, and the velocity of blood in the aorta is determined. By assuming an aortic diameter (based on height, weight, age, sex) or measuring the diameter directly, a flow can be calculated (flow = area × velocity time integral × heart rate). Because this calculates flow only in the descending aorta, a certain percentage (typically around 30%) is added to determine total cardiac output.

19. Describe some of the general applications of bedside ultrasound examination to monitor hemodynamics in the ICU.

Ultrasound scan provides real-time noninvasive data, and its utility in critical care is tremendous and growing. To cover ICU ultrasound applications in detail is beyond the scope of this chapter, but certain key points bear mentioning. Ultrasound can be used to directly assess cardiac output and function (stroke volume, contractility/ventricular function, valvular function) with transthoracic or transesophageal echocardiography. Fluid responsiveness can be gauged by measuring the change in inferior vena cava diameter during a respiratory cycle, similar to assessing systolic pressure variation, in a patient receiving mechanical ventilation. The presence of pulmonary edema can be seen, but not quantified, by ultrasound examination of the lung. Technical limitations make the usefulness of ultrasound quite variable. Also, it is a very operator-dependent technology, and specific training coupled with frequent practice is required.

20. **Is it possible to look more directly at tissue perfusion?**
    Many methods to assess tissue perfusion (the ultimate gauge of adequate hemodynamics) have been and are being developed. Although many more exist than are covered in this chapter, some include

    - **Gastric tonometry:** Carbon dioxide accumulation in gut mucosa typically results from decreased perfusion. Therefore measurement of gastric carbon dioxide via nasogastric or orogastric tube can provide a gauge for whether tissue perfusion is adequate.
    - **Tissue oxygenation (StO$_2$):** Tissue oxygenation is a measure of the ratio of oxygenated to nonoxygenated hemoglobin in a sample of tissue. It differs from arterial oxygenation (SpO$_2$), which represents systemic arterial oxygenation, in that tissue oxygenation is a local measurement at the microcirculation level. Think of this as a pulse oximeter for muscle or deeper tissues.
    - **Confocal microscopy:** With use of confocal techniques, these microscopes can look under the skin or mucosa of the tongue. Confocal microscopes can actually watch red blood cells moving through capillaries. This technology is not currently being used for bedside monitoring, but it is often cited as a research tool when studying perfusion.

KEY POINTS: HEMODYNAMIC MONITORING

1. Hemodynamic monitoring is our way of attempting to determine whether tissue perfusion is adequate; it provides data to guide therapy but is not by itself therapeutic.

2. Arterial transducers must first be zeroed and leveled to eliminate the effects of atmospheric pressure and hydrostatic pressure on readings. In addition, system readings should be monitored for damping (where readings erroneously converge to the mean pressure) and resonance (where readings erroneously diverge from the mean pressure).

3. Central lines have predictable waveforms with upward deflections during atrial contraction (the "a" wave), ventricular contraction (the "c" wave), and passive venous return (the "v" wave). To gauge end-diastolic volume, the pressure reported should be at the valley immediately preceding the "c" wave.

4. Fluid responsiveness in critically ill patients can be assessed with fluid challenge, the passive leg raise test, systolic pressure variation, pulse pressure variation, ultrasound examination of the inferior vena cava, and several other methods.

BIBLIOGRAPHY

1. Brennan J, Blair J, Goonewardena S, et al: Reappraisal of the use of inferior vena cava for estimating right atrial pressure. J Am Soc Echocardiogr 20:857-861, 2007.

2. Chatterjee K: The Swan-Ganz catheters: past, present and future: a viewpoint. Circulation 119:147-152, 2009.

3. Cholley B, Payen D: Noninvasive techniques for measurements of cardiac output. Curr Opin Crit Care 11:424-429, 2005.

4. Isakow W, Shuster D: Extravascular lung water measurements and hemodynamic monitoring in the critically ill: bedside alternatives to the pulmonary artery catheter. Am J Physiol Lung Cell Mol Physiol 291:1118-1131, 2006.

5. Jensen M, Sloth E, Larsen K, et al: Transthoracic echocardiography for cardiopulmonary monitoring in intensive care. Eur J Anaesthesiol 21:700-707, 2004.

6. Karamanoglu M, O'Rourke M, Avolio A, et al: An analysis of the relationship between central aortic and peripheral upper limb pressure waves in man. Eur Heart J 14:160-167, 1993.

7. Monnet X, Rienzo M, Osman D: Passive leg raising predicts fluid responsiveness in the critically ill. Crit Care Med 34:1402-1407, 2006.

8. Munis J, Lozada L: Giraffes, siphons and starling resistors: cerebral perfusion pressure revisited. J Neurosurg Anesthesiol 12:290-296, 2000.

9. Pittman J, Ping J, Mark J: Arterial and central venous pressure monitoring. Int Anesthesiol Clin 42:13-30, 2004.

10. Seneff M: Arterial line placement and care. In Irwin RS, Rippe JM (eds): Irwin and Rippe's Intensive Care Medicine, 6th ed. Philadelphia, Lippincott Williams & Wilkins, 2008, pp 36-45.

CHAPTER 7

FLUID THERAPY

Elizabeth Cox, MD, and Keith Baker, MD, PhD

1. **How is water distributed throughout the body?**
   Total body water comprises 60% of body weight in males and 50% of body weight in females. The distribution of this water is 40% in intracellular space (30% in females because of larger amounts of subcutaneous tissue and smaller muscle mass) and 20% in extracellular space. The extracellular fluid is broken down into 15% interstitial and 5% plasma. Total body water decreases with age; 75% to 80% of a newborn infant's weight is water.

2. **What are sensible and insensible fluid losses? How are maintenance fluid requirements calculated?**
   - Insensible losses (nonmeasurable)
     □ Skin: 600 mL
     □ Lungs: 200 mL
   - Sensible losses (measurable)
     □ Fecal: 200 mL
     □ Urine: 800-1500 mL
     □ Sweat: Variable
   These losses account for 2000 to 2500 mL/day, giving a 24-hour fluid requirement of 30 to 35 mL/kg to maintain normal fluid balance.

3. **What are fluid maintenance requirements for children?**
   Twenty-four–hour fluid requirements for children have been formulated on the basis of weight:
   - **4:2:1** rule: **4** mL/kg per hour for the first 10 kg
   - Then add additional **2** mL/kg per hour for the next 10 kg to 20 kg
   - Then add **1** mL/kg per hour for every kilogram after that
     EXAMPLE: 30-kg child
     40 + 20 + 10 = 70 mL/hr maintenance

4. **Describe the clinical features of volume deficit and volume excess.**
   - Deficits (low volume)
     □ Central nervous system: decreased mentation in severe cases
     □ Cardiovascular: tachycardia, hypotension (in later stages)
     □ Skin: decreased turgor in subacute volume loss
     □ Renal: decreased urine output
   - Excesses (volume overload)
     □ Distended neck veins
     □ Pulmonary edema
     □ Peripheral edema

5. **What are the classes of hemorrhagic shock, and what fluid should be administered in each class?**
   See Table 7-1.

TABLE 7-1. SEVERITY OF HEMORRHAGIC SHOCK				
	I	II	III	IV
Blood loss (mL)	<750	750-1500	1500-2000	>2000
Blood loss (% BV)	<15	15-30	30-40	>40
Pulse rate (beats/min)	<100	>100	>120	>140
Blood pressure	Normal	Normal	Decreased	Decreased
Respiratory rate (respirations/min)	14-20	20-30	30-40	>35
Urine output (mL/hr)	>30	20-30	5-15	Negligible
CNS symptoms	Normal	Anxious	Confused	Lethargic
Resuscitation fluid	LR	LR	LR + blood	LR + blood

BV, Blood volume; *CNS*, central nervous system; *LR*, lactated Ringer's solution.

6. **What is the 3:1 rule in fluid therapy after acute blood loss?**
   Three milliliters of crystalloid is given for each milliliter of blood loss to compensate for administered fluid that is lost into the interstitial and intracellular spaces. This is a starting dose. Most patients need more than this and will need 5:1 to restore normovolemia. Please see Chapter 54 for description of blood replacement in patients who require massive transfusions (greater than 10 U of packed red blood cells).

7. **What empiric replacement fluids can be used for fluid losses?**
   - **Sweat:** 5% dextrose (D_5) ¼ normal saline solution with 5 KCl/L
   - **Gastric, colon:** D_5 ½ normal saline solution with 30 KCl/L
   - **Bile, pancreas, small bowel:** lactated Ringer's solution
   - **Third space (interstitial loss):** lactated Ringer's solution

8. **What is the difference between crystalloids and colloids? Give examples of each.**
   - **Crystalloids:** Crystalloids are mixtures of sodium chloride and other physiologically active solutes. The distribution of sodium will determine the distribution of the infused crystalloid. Examples are normal saline solution, lactated Ringer's solution, and hypertonic saline solution.
   - **Colloids:** High-molecular-weight substances that stay in the vascular space and exert an osmotic force are colloids. Examples are albumin, hetastarch, dextran, and blood.

9. **Describe the composition of normal saline and lactated Ringer's solution. Which should be used for acute resuscitation?**
   Table 7-2 summarizes the composition of normal saline and lactated Ringer's solution. Lactated Ringer's solution is preferable for acute volume replacement because normal saline solution can result in hyperchloremic metabolic acidosis.

TABLE 7-2. COMPOSITION OF CRYSTALLOIDS

FLUID	NA (mmol/L)	CL (mmol/L)	K (mmol/L)	CA (mg/dL)	LACTATE (mmol/L)	PH
Normal saline solution	154	154	—	—	—	6.0
Lactated Ringer's solution	130	109	4	3	28	6.5

10. **What evidence-based data exist to support the use of various resuscitation fluids?**
    - **Lactated Ringer's solution:** This remains the least expensive and best fluid for trauma resuscitation.
    - **Albumin, hetastarch and other colloids:** No evidence from randomized controlled trials exists to demonstrate that resuscitation with colloids reduces the risk of death, pulmonary edema, or hospital stay compared with resuscitation with crystalloids in patients with trauma or burns, or after surgery. Because colloids are more expensive, it is difficult to justify their continued use in this setting.
    - **Hypertonic saline solution:** The only benefit is shown in patients with head trauma–cerebral edema.

Acknowledgement

The editors gratefully acknowledge the contributions of James E. Wiedeman, MD, and Mark W. Bowyer, MD, DMCC, COL, USAF, MC, authors of this chapter in the previous edition.

KEY POINTS: FLUID THERAPY

1. Total body water is 60% of body weight (40% intracellular and 20% extracellular). Plasma (blood) volume is 5% of body weight.

2. Diagnose volume deficit or excess by clinical examination, not laboratory study results.

3. Avoid fluid and electrolyte abnormalities by measuring and replacing ongoing gastrointestinal losses with appropriate fluids.

4. Use lactated Ringer's solution for acute volume resuscitation.

5. There is no proved benefit to colloid over crystalloid in acute resuscitation.

BIBLIOGRAPHY

1. Alderson P, Bunn F, Lefebvre C, et al: Albumin Reviewers: Human albumin solution for resuscitation and volume expansion in critically ill patients. Cochrane Database System Rev 4:CD001208, 2004.

2. Fan E, Stewart TE: Albumin in critical care: SAFE but worth the salt? Crit Care 8:297-299, 2004.

3. Perel P, Roberts I: Colloids versus crystalloids for fluid resuscitation in critically ill patients. Cochrane Database System Rev 3:CD000567, 2011.

CHAPTER 8

NUTRITION IN CRITICALLY ILL PATIENTS

Renee D. Stapleton, MD, PhD

1. **Why is nutrition therapy in critical illness important?**

   Critical illness is most often accompanied by a catabolic stress state in which patients demonstrate a systemic inflammatory response, hypermetabolism, multiple organ dysfunction, infectious complications, and malnutrition. Malnutrition is associated with impaired immunologic function and increased morbidity and mortality in acutely ill patients. Therefore nutrition therapy is important to attempt to improve patient outcomes.

2. **What are the goals of nutritional therapy in critically ill patients?**

   Over the past decade, there has been a shift away from the concept of nutrition *support*, where nutrition was provided as a fuel to support patients during a time of critical illness, toward the concept of nutrition *therapy*, where nutritional interventions are focused on modulating the immunologic and inflammatory response of critical illness. Therefore the generally accepted goals of nutritional delivery in critically ill patients are to
   - Provide nutritional therapy consistent with the patient's condition
   - Prevent nutrient deficiencies
   - Avoid complications related to delivering nutrition
   - Improve patient outcomes

3. **How should the nutritional status of critically ill patients be assessed?**

   Nutritional status assessment in critically ill patients is difficult. Traditionally, albumin, prealbumin, and anthropometric measurements have been used to assess nutritional status. However, these are inaccurate in critical illness because of fluid resuscitation and the acute phase response. Therefore one must rely on information such as recent weight loss, comorbid illnesses, and recent gastrointestinal (GI) dysfunction.

4. **What mode of feeding (enteral or parenteral) should be initiated in critically ill patients?**

   Unless an absolute contraindication to enteral nutrition (EN) exists (such as ischemic bowel or bowel obstruction), EN should be initiated preferentially over parenteral nutrition (PN). Several randomized controlled trials (RCTs) have compared EN with PN in critically ill patients with an intact GI tract. When these studies were aggregated in a meta-analysis, no difference in survival was seen. However, EN is associated with a significant reduction in infectious complications, and it is less expensive than PN. Evidence also suggests that lack of use of the GI tract rapidly results in atrophy of gut luminal mucosa, which may lead to bacterial translocation across the gut wall and into the systemic circulation. Even small amounts of, or trophic, EN increase blood flow to the gut, preserve GI epithelial structures, and maintain villous height. EN also improves immune function by supporting gut-associated lymphoid tissue. EN is therefore recommended over PN unless the patient has an absolute contraindication to enteral feeding (discussed later).

5. **When should EN be initiated in critically ill patients?**
Early EN is usually defined as initiating enteral feedings within 48 hours of intensive care unit (ICU) admission. Many RCTs have compared early EN versus delayed nutrient intake in critically ill patients receiving mechanical ventilation, and, when these results were aggregated, early EN was associated with a trend toward mortality reduction and a significant reduction in infectious complications. Starting EN early does not seem to affect the duration of mechanical ventilation or ICU length of stay. The presence of bowel sounds and the passage of flatus are not necessary before the institution of EN.

6. **How many calories should critically ill patients receive?**
Energy expenditure varies with age, sex, body mass, and type and severity of illness. During critical illness, total energy expenditure (TEE) can be measured with indirect calorimetry. However, in clinical practice, resting energy expenditure (REE) is usually estimated by using a variety of available equations and is then multiplied by a *stress factor* of 1.0 to 2.0 to estimate TEE (and therefore caloric requirements). Roughly 25 kcal/kg ideal body weight is often the standard practice, and other equations, such as Harris-Benedict, Ireton-Jones, and Weir, are commonly used (Table 8-1). Unfortunately, predictive equations tend to be inaccurate. The optimal amount of calories to provide critically ill patients is unclear given the paucity of existing data, but studies do suggest that providing an amount of calories closer to goal calories is associated with improved clinical outcomes.

TABLE 8-1. EXAMPLES OF PREDICTIVE EQUATIONS FOR REE IN CRITICAL ILLNESS

Harris-Benedict	Men: $[66.5 + (13.8 \times AdjBW) + (5 \times Ht) - (6.8 \times Age)] \times 1.3$ Women: $[655 + (9.6 \times AdjBW) + (1.8 \times Ht) - 4.7 \times Age)] \times 1.3$
Owen	Men: $879 + (10.2 \times ActBW)$ Women: $795 + (7.2 \times ActBW)$
Mifflin	Men: $5 + (10 \times ActBW) + (6.25 \times Ht) - (5 \times Age)$ Women: $161 + (10 \times ActBW) + (6.25 \times Ht) - (5 \times Age)$
Ireton-Jones equation for obesity	Men: $606 + (9 \times ActBW) - (12 \times Age) + 400$ (if ventilated) $+ 1400$ Women: $ActBW - (12 \times Age) + 400$ (if ventilated) $+ 1444$
Ireton-Jones for patients with mechanical ventilation	Men $= 2206 - (10 \times Age) + (5 \times ActBW) + 292$ (if trauma) $+ 851$ (if burn) Women $= 1925 - (10 \times Age) + (5 \times ActBW) + 292$ (if trauma) $+ 851$ (if burn)
25 kcal/kg	BMI <25: $ActBW \times 25$ BMI ≥ 25: $IBW \times 25$

ActBW, Actual body weight = weight on admission (kilograms); *AdjBW*, adjusted body weight = ideal body weight + 0.4 (actual body weight − ideal body weight); *BMI*, body mass index; *Ht*, height (centimeters); *IBW*, ideal body weight = 50 + 2.3 per inch >60 inches (men), 45.5 + 2.3 per inch >60 inches (women).

7. **What should be the composition of EN in critically ill patients?**

Few data are available to inform the macronutrient composition of enteral feedings. In general, critically ill patients should receive an amount of protein daily between 1.5 and 2.0 g/kg of ideal body weight. The use of whole protein, or polymeric, formulas is recommended because insufficient data exist to support the routine use of peptide-based formulas in most patients. In most enteral formulas, approximately 25% to 30% of calories are from fat. Similar to the situation with protein, evidence in the literature is insufficient to support the routine use of high-fat or low-fat enteral formulas. In some ICU populations, specific enteral formulas are recommended (discussed later). For example, formulas containing arginine are often considered in patients who have had elective surgery, trauma, or burns but should generally not be used in patients with sepsis. Specific formulas designed for patients with renal failure are also available.

8. **Should critically ill patients in shock and/or receiving vasopressors receive EN?**

Ischemic bowel is a very rare complication of EN but has been reported in critically ill patients and can be fatal. Therefore the general recommendation is that EN be avoided in patients who are in shock and in those patients in whom resuscitation is active, vasopressors are being initiated, or vasopressor doses are increasing. Once patients are resuscitated and hemodynamically stable, EN may be initiated, even if they are receiving stable lower doses of vasopressors. However, special attention should be paid to signs of enteral feeding intolerance such as abdominal distention or increasing gastric residual volumes (GRVs).

9. **Should gastric or small-bowel EN be used?**

EN can be delivered through an intragastric gastric (nasogastric or orogastric) or postpyloric (either in the duodenum or jejunum) feeding tube. Enteral tubes may also be surgically placed. Each option has risks and benefits. In patients who have endotracheal tubes in place, nasal tubes can increase the risk of sinusitis. Intragastric feeding tubes can be placed at the bedside, and their position can be immediately confirmed radiographically (it is not sufficient to assess placement with auscultation alone). However, successful placement of a small-bowel feeding tube at the bedside varies from 11% to 93% depending on technique and operator experience. The use of endoscopy or fluoroscopy for postpyloric feeding tube placement can cause delays in initiating enteral feeding. In a meta-analysis of gastric versus small-bowel feeding in ICU patients, small-bowel feeding was not found to be associated with any improvement in survival but was associated with a reduction in infections, particularly pneumonia. Therefore the routine use of small-bowel enteral feeding is recommended when possible. However, in many ICUs, obtaining access to the small bowel may be logistically difficult and expensive if fluoroscopy or endoscopy is needed. In ICUs where obtaining small-bowel access is less feasible, small-bowel feedings should be considered for patients showing signs of intolerance to intragastric feeding (see later) or at high risk for aspiration (e.g., must remain in supine position).

10. **Should EN be delivered continuously or in boluses?**

Continuous feeding delivers a small amount of feeding formula continuously over a 24-hour period, whereas bolus feeding delivers a large volume of formula over a short period of time. Because one pseudorandomized study found that aggressive early EN via bolus feeding was harmful, it is generally thought that bolus feeding is less safe than continuous feeding. However, a paucity of evidence is available on this topic.

11. **How should enteral feeding tolerance be monitored?**

Patients should be monitored frequently (e.g., every 4 to 6 hours) for tolerance of EN, especially in the first few days after initiating enteral feedings. This monitoring should include an assessment of pain (often difficult in critically ill patients), abdominal distention, and stooling. GRVs should also be measured frequently. However, evidence suggests that higher GRVs as high as 250 to 500 mL are not associated with an increased risk for pneumonia or aspiration. Thus the recently published American Society for Parenteral and Enteral Nutrition (A.S.P.E.N.) and Society of Critical Care Medicine (SCCM) *Guidelines for the Provision and Assessment of Nutrition Support Therapy in the Adult Critically Ill Patient* recommend that GRVs between 250 and 500 mL should prompt clinicians to take measures to reduce the risk of aspiration (e.g., elevate the head of the patient's bed) but that automatic cessation of enteral feeding should not occur for GRVs <500 mL unless other signs of intolerance are present.

McClave SA, Martindale RG, Vanek VW, et al: Guidelines for the Provision and Assessment of Nutrition Support Therapy in the Adult Critically Ill Patient: Society of Critical Care Medicine (SCCM) and American Society for Parenteral and Enteral Nutrition (A.S.P.E.N.). JPEN J Parenter Enteral Nutr 33:277-316, 2009.

12. **How should critically ill patients be positioned during enteral feeding?**
Two prior randomized trials have compared semirecumbent with supine positioning in ICU patients. In one study (Drakulovic, 1999), the incidence of pneumonia was significantly reduced in patients in the semirecumbent position. The other study (van Nieuwenhoven, 2006) did not achieve the target positioning and did not find a reduction in infections. On the basis of these limited data, it is recommended that critically ill patients have the head of their beds raised to as close to 45 degrees as possible.

Drakulovic MB, Torres A, Bauer TT, et al: Supine body position as a risk factor for nosocomial pneumonia in mechanically ventilated patients: a randomised trial. Lancet 354:1851-1858, 1999.

van Nieuwenhoven CA, Vandenbroucke-Grauls C, van Tiel FH, et al: Feasibility and effects of the semirecumbent position to prevent ventilator-associated pneumonia: a randomized study. Crit Care Med 34:396-402, 2006.

13. **Should motility agents be used in critically ill patients?**
The use of motility agents is recommended when clinically feasible, especially in patients with signs of enteral feeding intolerance. Motility agents including erythromycin or metoclopramide have been found to improve gastric emptying and tolerance of EN but do not seem to change outcomes in critically ill patients. In one study, administration of enteral naloxone (to reverse the side effects of opioid narcotics on the GI tract) resulted in an increased volume of EN infused, decreased GRVs, and decreased incidence of ventilator-associated pneumonia.

14. **Should feeding protocols be used in ICUs?**
Nurse-driven feeding protocols that include rapid startup of enteral feeding, goal infusion rate, orders for GRVs, and directions for when to stop and start feedings increase the percentage of goal calories administered. In an effort both to start enteral feedings in the critically ill patient early and to provide an amount of calories close to goal, feeding protocols should be implemented.

15. **When is EN contraindicated?**
Contraindications to EN include conditions that lead to a nonfunctioning GI tract such as ischemic bowel, intestinal obstruction, severe malabsorption, and severe short gut syndrome. In general, pancreatitis, enterocutaneous fistulae, and recent GI surgery are not contraindications to enteral feeding.

16. **What are some complications of enteral feeding, and how can they be minimized?**
EN is not without risks, and complications can be categorized as GI, mechanical, or metabolic.
- **GI complications** include diarrhea, nausea, vomiting, constipation, aspiration, and ischemic bowel. Decreased gastric motility occurs in a majority of critically ill patients, and therefore nausea and vomiting with resultant aspiration are not uncommon. These can be minimized with semirecumbent positioning, placement of a small-bowel feeding tube, and continuous rather than bolus enteral feeding (discussed earlier). Ileus also commonly occurs

in a critical care setting, often as a result of opioid administration, and can be treated with small doses of oral naloxone that do not affect the analgesia of opioids. Diarrhea is common in the ICU and may be due to antibiotics or other medications. If diarrhea develops in a patient receiving EN, infectious causes (i.e., *Clostridium difficile*) should first be ruled out. If those tests are negative, stool-bulking agents such as banana flakes can be administered. Alternative strategies to decrease diarrhea include increasing soluble fiber intake or changing to another enteral formula.

- **Mechanical complications** include obstruction of the feeding tube with medications; erosion of the feeding tube into nasal or gastric mucosa with risk of bleeding, infection, or perforation; accidental insertion of the feeding tube into the pulmonary tree with risk of injury; displacement of the tube with risk of aspiration; and sinusitis. To minimize these complications, tubes should be soft and well lubricated for insertion, and tube position should always be verified radiographically before use (auscultation over the stomach alone is not adequate).
- **Metabolic complications** include hyperglycemia, electrolyte derangements, and overfeeding. Monitoring of blood glucose and electrolytes can detect these and lead to appropriate changes in feedings. If overfeeding is a concern, a metabolic cart (indirect calorimetry) can be performed to measure TEE.

17. **When should PN be used in critically ill patients?**
    EN is the preferred method of delivering nutrition therapy in critically ill patients, and measures such as placing a small-bowel feeding tube and starting motility agents should be used in patients who have signs of intolerance to enteral feedings before considering initiating PN. However, PN is appropriate in some ICU patients, including those in whom EN is not feasible (e.g., ongoing intolerance or contraindication to enteral feeding) and those who are obviously malnourished at admission. Data answering this question are sparse, but the recent A.S.P.E.N.-SCCM Guidelines recommend that PN be considered in the following three circumstances:
    - After 7 days of hospitalization in critically ill patients who are not malnourished but in whom enteral feeding has not been feasible or who have only received a fraction of goal calories
    - On admission in critically ill patients who are malnourished and in whom enteral feeding is not feasible
    - During the perioperative period in a patient undergoing major GI surgery who is either malnourished or when the period of time during which EN is not feasible is expected to be longer than 5 to 7 days

    Given these recommendations, very few patients in a medical ICU should need PN.

18. **What are some complications of PN?**
    - **Mechanical complications** in patients receiving PN include those related to the catheter used for delivery of PN, such as pneumothorax and venous thromboembolism.
    - **Metabolic complications** from PN include hyperglycemia and electrolyte abnormalities. Hyperglycemia can be treated with an appropriate insulin protocol for hyperglycemia associated with critical illness.
    - **Infectious complications** from parenteral feeding include central line–associated bloodstream infection and sepsis.
    - **Hepatobiliary complications.** PN can occasionally cause elevated hepatic transaminase, alkaline phosphatase, and bilirubin levels, as well as steatosis (i.e., fatty liver), and acalculous cholecystitis may result.

19. **Which pharmaconutrients or specialized formulas should critically ill patients receive?**
    - **Glutamine.** Although data are limited, supplemental enteral glutamine (when using a feeding formula that is not already supplemented with glutamine) decreases hospital length of stay, ICU length of stay, and mortality in burn and mixed ICU patients and therefore

should be added to enteral regimens when feasible. This effect is likely explained by glutamine's role in maintaining the integrity of the GI lumen. It can be administered as a powder mixed with water and infused through the feeding tube, and the dose should be 0.3 to 0.5 g/kg per day.

- **Parenteral glutamine** potentially has an even larger benefit than enteral glutamine and has been shown to reduce mortality and infections in patients receiving PN. Outside of North America, the dipeptide formulation of intravenous glutamine is available and should be used. In North America, however, intravenous glutamine is available only in a formulation that has limited solubility and requires excess fluid administration.

- **Antioxidants:** A prior meta-analysis found that antioxidants and minerals reduced mortality in critically ill patients. On the basis of these results, critically ill patients (particularly those with burns or trauma and receiving mechanical ventilation) should receive antioxidant vitamins (vitamins E and C) and minerals (selenium, zinc, and copper). Very few data are currently available on individual nutrients.

- **Arginine:** Enteral feeding formulas containing arginine should be used in patients undergoing major elective surgery and in those with trauma, burns, and head and neck cancer. On the basis of results from prior studies, however, patients with sepsis should not receive arginine because it has been suggested that it may increase mortality.

- **Omega-3 fatty acids:** The use of feeding formulas containing omega-3 fatty acids (fish oil) in patients with acute lung injury and sepsis is currently quite controversial. Three prior trials comparing an enteral formula containing omega-3 fatty acids, borage oil (γ-linolenic acid [GLA]), and antioxidants with placebo found benefit. However, two additional recent randomized trials (one used a liquid fish oil supplement and another used a twice-daily supplement containing fish oil, GLA, and antioxidants) found no benefit.

20. **What nutrition therapy should patients with acute kidney injury (AKI) receive?**
Like most other critically ill patients, patients with AKI should receive early EN with standard amounts of protein and calories. Protein restriction should not be used to delay the initiation of dialysis. Specific enteral formulas designed for renal failure that have varying electrolyte compositions (e.g., lower phosphate or potassium) or are calorie dense (i.e., fluid restricted) can be used if needed.

21. **What nutrition therapy should patients with acute pancreatitis receive?**
Early EN is now standard of care in patients with acute pancreatitis. In past decades, patients with acute pancreatitis were not allowed any enteral intake and were fed parenterally. In recent times, however, research has found that these patients have improved outcomes if they receive early EN started within 48 hours of admission, even in cases of severe acute pancreatitis. Two trials have also found that outcomes in these patients are not different when they are fed gastrically versus jejunally.

22. **How might propofol influence the nutritional support provided to critically ill patients?**
Propofol is a sedative commonly used in an ICU setting that is delivered as a 10% lipid emulsion and provides 1.1 kcal/mL. When patients are receiving propofol for longer periods of time (i.e., more than 3-4 days) or in large doses, the calories received from propofol should be taken into account in relation to the overall caloric prescription to avoid excess delivery of calories. Because propofol can also cause hypertriglyceridemia, which can lead to acute pancreatitis, serum triglyceride levels should be measured in patients receiving larger doses of propofol.

KEY POINTS: NUTRITION IN CRITICALLY ILL PATIENTS

1. EN should be used in the vast majority of ICU patients rather than PN.

2. EN should be started within 24 to 48 hours of ICU admission.

3. After patients with shock are resuscitated and hemodynamically stable, they can safely receive EN even if they are receiving stable lower doses of vasopressors.

4. In patients intolerant of EN, measures such as semirecumbent positioning and motility agents should be attempted before starting PN.

5. Patients with acute pancreatitis, even if it is severe, should receive EN, which can be delivered either gastrically or jejunally.

BIBLIOGRAPHY

1. Canadian critical care nutrition clinical practice guidelines: topics. http://criticalcarenutrition.com/docs/cpg/1.0envspn_07_FINAL.pdf. Accessed August 1, 2011.

2. Canadian critical care nutrition clinical practice guidelines: topics. http://criticalcarenutrition.com/docs/cpg/2.0early_FINAL.pdf. Accessed August 1, 2011.

3. Cerra FB, Benitez MR, Blackburn GL, et al: Applied nutrition in ICU patients. A consensus statement of the American College of Chest Physicians. Chest 111:769-778, 1997.

4. Drakulovic MB, Torres A, Bauer TT, et al: Supine body position as a risk factor for nosocomial pneumonia in mechanically ventilated patients: a randomised trial. Lancet 354:1851-1858, 1999.

5. Gadek JE, DeMichele SJ, Karlstad MD, et al: Effect of enteral feeding with eicosapentaenoic acid, gamma-linolenic acid, and antioxidants in patients with acute respiratory distress syndrome. Crit Care Med 27:1409-1420, 1999.

6. Heyland DK, Dhaliwal R, Suchner U, et al: Antioxidant nutrients: a systematic review of trace elements and vitamins in the critically ill patient. Intensive Care Med 31:327-337, 2005.

7. Heyland DK, Drover JW, Dhaliwal R, et al: Optimizing the benefits and minimizing the risks of enteral nutrition in the critically ill: role of small bowel feeding. JPEN J Parenter Enteral Nutr 26(6 Suppl):S51-S55, 2002.

8. Ibrahim EH, Mehringer L, Prentice D, et al: Early versus late enteral feeding of mechanically ventilated patients: results of a clinical trial. JPEN J Parenter Enteral Nutr 26:174-181, 2002.

9. Khalid I, Doshi P, DiGiovine B: Early enteral nutrition and outcomes of critically ill patients treated with vasopressors and mechanical ventilation. Am J Crit Care 19:261-268, 2010.

10. McClave SA, Chang WK, Dhaliwal R, et al: Nutrition support in acute pancreatitis: a systematic review of the literature. JPEN J Parenter Enteral Nutr 30:143-156, 2006.

11. McClave SA, Martindale RG, Vanek VW, et al: Guidelines for the Provision and Assessment of Nutrition Support Therapy in the Adult Critically Ill Patient: Society of Critical Care Medicine (SCCM) and American Society for Parenteral and Enteral Nutrition (A.S.P.E.N.). JPEN J Parenter Enteral Nutr 33:277-316, 2009.

12. Meissner W, Dohrn B, Reinhart K: Enteral naloxone reduces gastric tube reflux and frequency of pneumonia in critical care patients during opioid analgesia. Crit Care Med 31:776-780, 2003.

13. Pontes-Arruda A, Aragão AM, Albuquerque JD: Effects of enteral feeding with eicosapentaenoic acid, gamma-linolenic acid, and antioxidants in mechanically ventilated patients with severe sepsis and septic shock. Crit Care Med 34:2325-2333, 2006.

14. Rice TW, Wheeler AP, Thompson BT, et al, for the NHLBI ARDS Clinical Trials Network: Enteral omega-3 fatty acid, gamma-linolenic acid, and antioxidant supplementation in acute lung injury. JAMA 306:1574-1581, 2011.

15. Singer P, Theilla M, Fisher H, et al: Benefit of an enteral diet enriched with eicosapentaenoic acid and gamma-linolenic acid in ventilated patients with acute lung injury. Crit Care Med 34:1033-1038, 2006. Erratum in: Crit Care Med 34:1861, 2006.

16. Stapleton RD, Martin TR, Weiss NS, et al: A phase II randomized placebo-controlled trial of omega-3 fatty acids for the treatment of acute lung injury. Crit Care Med 39:1655-1662, 2011.

17. Suchner U, Heyland DK, Peter K: Immune-modulatory actions of arginine in the critically ill. Br J Nutr 87 (1 Suppl):S121-S132, 2002.

18. van Nieuwenhoven CA, Vandenbroucke-Grauls C, van Tiel FH, et al: Feasibility and effects of the semirecumbent position to prevent ventilator-associated pneumonia: a randomized study. Crit Care Med 34:396-402, 2006.

CHAPTER 9

MECHANICAL AND NONINVASIVE VENTILATION

Manuel Pardo, Jr., MD

1. **What are the primary indications for mechanical ventilation?**
   The primary indications for mechanical ventilation are inadequate oxygenation, inadequate ventilation, and elevated work of breathing.

2. **What is the difference between conventional and noninvasive ventilation?**
   - The conventional approach to mechanical ventilation involves use of an airway device inserted directly into a patient's trachea.
   - Noninvasive ventilation is mechanical ventilation without the use of an endotracheal tube or tracheotomy. See Figure 9-1.

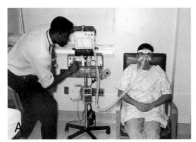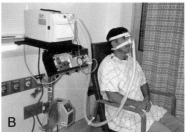

Figure 9-1. A demonstration of noninvasive positive-pressure ventilation with a nasal mask. **A,** The respiratory therapist is adjusting the inspiratory pressure support level and checking for proper mask fit. **B,** The mask must be fitted properly to minimize air leak but avoid excessive pressure on the skin.

3. **What are the main types of mechanical ventilation?**
   The two main types are positive-pressure and negative-pressure ventilation. With positive-pressure ventilation, positive pressure is applied to the airway to inflate the lungs directly. This can be accomplished with an artificial airway (e.g., endotracheal tube) or with a nasal or face mask (noninvasive ventilation). With negative-pressure ventilation, negative pressure is applied to the abdomen and thorax to draw air into the lungs through the upper airway. This form of ventilation is typified by the *iron lung* negative pressure ventilators used after the polio epidemics in the first half of the 20th century. For the remainder of this chapter, noninvasive ventilation will refer to noninvasive positive-pressure ventilation.

4. **What are the advantages of noninvasive ventilation compared with conventional mechanical ventilation with an endotracheal tube?**
   In most studies of noninvasive ventilation in the intensive care unit (ICU) setting, the main outcome measure has been reduced need for tracheal intubation. For those patients who avoid

intubation, the main advantage is the avoidance of artificial airway complications. Several studies document a lower infection rate (e.g., nosocomial pneumonia and sinusitis) with noninvasive ventilation, which may be related to the maintenance of the protective glottic barrier. Other advantages include reduced need for sedative medications. Some noninvasive ventilation trials have demonstrated reductions in ICU length of stay, ICU mortality, or in-hospital mortality.

5. **What are the disadvantages and contraindications of noninvasive ventilation?**
   Patient selection is crucial to ensuring success with noninvasive ventilation. Patients who are uncooperative, need immediate intubation, have upper airway pathologic conditions, are hemodynamically unstable, or have excessive secretions are not likely to have successful ventilation. Noninvasive ventilation should be contraindicated in these patients. In practical terms, noninvasive ventilation can initially require significant attention by the respiratory therapist and/or ICU nurse.

6. **Which patients with acute respiratory failure are most likely to benefit from noninvasive ventilation?**
   Patients with acute exacerbations of chronic obstructive pulmonary disease are most likely to benefit, in terms of reduction in need for tracheal intubation and decreased mortality. Other populations likely to have a decreased intubation rate with noninvasive ventilation include patients with immune compromise from solid organ transplants or hematologic malignancies, cardiogenic pulmonary edema, respiratory failure after lung resection, and respiratory failure immediately after elective abdominal surgery. If noninvasive ventilation is used for patients that do not fit in these categories, consider limiting the time to 2 hours unless clear improvement is evident.

7. **What are the most commonly used modes of mechanical ventilation?**
   For noninvasive ventilation, the most common mode is pressure support ventilation. For conventional ventilation, the three most commonly used modes are assist control ventilation, synchronized intermittent mandatory ventilation (SIMV), and pressure support ventilation.

8. **How does pressure support ventilation work?**
   Pressure support ventilation requires the patient to trigger each breath. When a patient inhales and generates inspiratory gas flow, the ventilator rapidly delivers a preset inspiratory pressure, typically 5 to 20 cm H_2O. The ventilator's inspiratory flow stops when a certain threshold flow has been reached, typically 25% of the peak flow rate. During the expiratory phase of the respiratory cycle, positive end-expiratory pressure (PEEP) is often applied, typically between 5 and 10 cm H_2O. The patient's work of breathing is reduced, proportional to the amount of inspiratory pressure that is set. This is usually judged by the patient's tidal volume, which can vary with each breath on the basis of patient effort and lung mechanics. Because minute ventilation is not guaranteed during pressure support ventilation, the patient may have hypoventilation if the pulmonary process is severe enough or if respiratory depressant sedatives are administered.

9. **How do the assist control and SIMV modes differ?**
   Assist control and SIMV share some common features. Both deliver a preset tidal volume and respiratory rate. Thus a minimum minute ventilation is guaranteed, unlike pressure support ventilation, which requires the patient to have an intact respiratory drive.
   Assist control and SIMV differ in how they manage patient-initiated inspirations above the preset respiratory rate. With assist control, every additional patient-initiated breath receives the preset tidal volume. During SIMV, the additional breaths depend on the patient's respiratory muscles to generate the tidal volume.

10. **Why is pressure support commonly combined with SIMV?**
    Because additional breaths above the preset respiratory rate depend on the patient's effort and lung mechanics, the addition of pressure support can provide a reduction in the work of breathing. This may be desirable if added respiratory workload is imposed on the patient, for example, from a small-diameter endotracheal tube.

11. **How does the clinician choose the initial ventilator settings?**
    The ventilator settings initially chosen depend on the reason for mechanical ventilation. Most patients with respiratory failure have some combination of hypoxemia, hypoventilation, or elevated work of breathing. The clinician has some choices to make, including:
    - Mode of ventilation: assist control, SIMV, pressure support
    - Tidal volume
    - FiO_2
    - PEEP

    For a patient who must have guaranteed minute ventilation and the greatest reduction in work of breathing, the assist control mode is most commonly chosen. Tidal volume and respiratory rate are selected to maintain arterial pH in the normal range. The inspired oxygen is initially set to 100%, and PEEP is set to at least 5 cm H_2O. Both FiO_2 and PEEP are adjusted to prevent hypoxemia, as judged by arterial PO_2 or pulse oximetry.

12. **What factors are used to select tidal volume?**
    For many years, clinicians selected tidal volumes of 10 to 12 mL/kg and adjusted respiratory rate to achieve normocarbia. The rationale for selecting larger than normal tidal volumes included prevention of atelectasis and ease of normalizing PCO_2. However, the growing recognition of ventilator-associated lung injury led to alternate mechanical ventilation strategies, especially in the patient with acute respiratory distress syndrome (ARDS). A ventilation strategy using tidal volumes in the normal range of 6 mL/kg (based on ideal body weight) was shown to offer better clinical outcomes, including mortality, than ventilation using a higher tidal volume of 12 mL/kg. For patients without ARDS or lung injury, it is not clear whether the use of 6 mL/kg tidal volume is associated with improved outcomes, but a general trend has been to avoid use of high tidal volumes.

13. **How is the optimal PEEP setting determined?**
    The determination of optimal PEEP in the patient with mechanical ventilation has been a source of controversy for decades. The goal of PEEP use is partly determined by the cause of respiratory failure. A patient with normal oxygenation who has mechanical ventilation may receive a *low* level of PEEP, 5 cm H_2O, to help prevent atelectasis. A patient with pulmonary edema and hypoxemia may benefit from higher levels of PEEP (10 cm H_2O or higher) to recruit alveoli that are collapsed; in such a patient there may be a reduced FiO_2 requirement and improved lung compliance. Because high inspired oxygen concentration can itself cause lung injury, the use of PEEP may allow use of a lower FiO_2.

14. **What is auto-PEEP?**
    Auto-PEEP, also called intrinsic PEEP, is the development of PEEP because of incomplete exhalation before delivery of a positive-pressure breath. Auto-PEEP can be seen in patients with high minute ventilation requirement (e.g., ARDS) or diseases of airflow limitation (e.g., asthma). Physiologically, auto-PEEP behaves similarly to applied PEEP. Detection of auto-PEEP can be difficult, although modern ventilators often incorporate an expiratory hold (occlusion of expiratory valve before inspiration) to measure this otherwise-hidden pressure.

15. **How can auto-PEEP be reduced?**
    Reduction of auto-PEEP involves treatment of the underlying disorder. Adjustment of the mechanical ventilator to maximize expiratory time may also provide some benefit. The approach may include increasing inspiratory flow rate and lowering minute ventilation by decreasing respiratory rate and/or tidal volume.

16. **How does mechanical ventilation affect the cardiovascular system?**
    Positive-pressure ventilation results in positive intrathoracic pressure, which decreases venous return. The resulting decrease in cardiac output may lead to hypotension. The reduction in preload may be most dangerous in a patient with right-sided heart failure. In addition, the inflation of the lungs with positive pressure increases the right ventricular afterload, which is also potentially hazardous for the failing right ventricle. On the other hand, positive intrathoracic pressure increases the pressure gradient for aortic blood flow out of the thorax, thus facilitating some degree of left ventricular afterload reduction.

17. **How are ventilator settings adjusted after the initial settings have been instituted?**
    Evaluation includes subjective assessment of the patient's work of breathing and degree of respiratory distress. A patient who is dyssynchronous with mechanical ventilation may need adjustment of the ventilator mode, tidal volume, or intravenous sedation. PEEP and FiO_2 are adjusted to avoid hypoxemia and hyperoxia (see question 13). Tidal volume and respiratory rate may also be adjusted on the basis of measured arterial pH and PCO_2 (see question 12). pH is also affected by the presence of metabolic acidosis or alkalosis. Peak and plateau airway pressures are assessed to determine respiratory compliance. The peak pressure is measured at the end of inspiration, whereas the plateau pressure is measured after a brief inspiratory pause.

18. **How can peak and plateau airway pressure be used to evaluate the patient's respiratory system?**
    The peak airway pressure reflects respiratory resistance and compliance, whereas plateau airway pressure reflects only compliance. Therefore a large difference between peak and plateau pressure suggests a source of increased resistance (e.g., secretions, narrowed endotracheal tube, bronchospasm). An elevated peak and plateau pressure (with less than 5 cm difference between the two) implies reduced compliance (e.g., pulmonary edema, chest wall restriction).

19. **What is permissive hypercarbia?**
    Traditionally, mechanical ventilation parameters were adjusted to normalize blood gases, including normal PCO_2. For patients with severe bronchospasm (e.g., acute asthma exacerbation), the strategy of normalizing the PCO_2 can lead to auto-PEEP, air trapping, and even life-threatening barotrauma. Similarly, a patient with severe ARDS has markedly elevated dead space, requiring extremely high minute ventilation to achieve normal PCO_2. Ventilator-associated lung injury can result from repeated stretching of alveoli, with accompanying release of inflammatory mediators. A ventilation strategy that allows the PCO_2 to become elevated *(permissively)* minimizes the risk of barotrauma in both types of patients and is a cornerstone of management, in addition to treating the underlying disease processes.

20. **What are the complications of mechanical ventilation?**
    Major complications include ventilator-associated lung injury, barotrauma (including pneumomediastinum and pneumothorax), hemodynamic compromise, and pneumonia. Ventilator-associated pneumonia is now recognized as one of the most severe health care–associated infections in the critically ill patient. Other complications of mechanical ventilation can stem from the use of sedation, which is almost always needed in the patient with respiratory failure.

21. **What are the complications unique to noninvasive ventilation?**
    Complications of noninvasive ventilation include pressure necrosis of the skin, aerophagia, and intolerance of the mask. The incidence of mask intolerance can be as high as 25%. In addition, the presence of the face mask may complicate nutrition because oral feeding requires mask removal and the presence of a nasoenteric tube may interfere with mask seal. Pulmonary toilet measures such as tracheal suctioning are also more difficult compared with those in the patient with a tracheal tube in place.

KEY POINTS: MECHANICAL VENTILATION

1. The primary indications for mechanical ventilation are inadequate oxygenation, inadequate ventilation, and elevated work of breathing.

2. The patient populations most likely to benefit from noninvasive ventilation are those with acute exacerbations of chronic obstructive pulmonary disorder, cardiogenic pulmonary edema, and immune compromise.

3. The assist control mode provides a guaranteed minute ventilation and full support of all patient-initiated breaths.

4. Pressure support ventilation requires intact respiratory drive from the patient; tidal volume and minute ventilation are variable and depend on patient effort.

5. Low tidal volume mechanical ventilation can lead to improved outcomes in the patient with acute respiratory distress syndrome.

BIBLIOGRAPHY

1. Acute Respiratory Distress Syndrome Network: Ventilation with lower tidal volumes as compared with traditional tidal volumes for acute lung injury and the acute respiratory distress syndrome. N Engl J Med 342:1301-1308, 2000.
2. Calfee CS, Matthay MA: Recent advances in mechanical ventilation. Am J Med 118:584-591, 2005.
3. Squadrone V, Coha M, Cerutti E, et al: Continuous positive airway pressure for treatment of postoperative hypoxemia: a randomized controlled trial. JAMA 293:589-595, 2005.

CHAPTER 10

DISCONTINUATION OF MECHANICAL VENTILATION

Theodore W. Marcy, MD, MPH, and Jenny L. Martino, MD, MSPH

1. **What proportion of patients can be readily removed from mechanical ventilation?**

   The majority of patients (75%) supported with mechanical ventilation are able to resume unsupported breathing within 7 days of intubation if the illness that resulted in respiratory failure resolves or improves. One of the clinician's challenging tasks is to determine when the patient is ready for ventilator discontinuation. Continuing mechanical ventilation beyond the time that is necessary exposes the patient to risks for nosocomial infection and ventilator-induced lung injury. Conversely, removing ventilatory support from a patient prematurely can lead to severe stress from respiratory and cardiovascular decompensation and exposes the patient to the risks associated with reintubation including increased mortality rate, increased time in the intensive care unit (ICU), and need for long-term care in a rehabilitation facility.

2. **When should patients receiving mechanical ventilation be assessed for ventilator discontinuation?**

   Every patient receiving mechanical ventilation should be assessed for ventilator discontinuation on a *daily* basis as long as his or her medical status meets the following criteria:
   - Lung injury stable or resolving
   - Adequate gas exchange with low positive end-expiratory pressure (PEEP) and fraction of inspired oxygen (FiO_2) requirements (e.g., PEEP <5-8 cm H_2O, FiO_2 <0.4-0.5)
   - Hemodynamic stability (e.g., not requiring pressors, no serious arrhythmias)
   - Patient capable of initiating inspiratory efforts

   Evidence indicates that systematic daily weaning assessments improve patient outcomes, reduce the number of days patients are dependent on the ventilator, and reduce the number of patients who require tracheostomies.

3. **How, exactly, should this assessment be done?**

   As of yet, no systematic weaning protocol has been agreed on. However, most protocols have a stepwise assessment that varies in the details. The above criteria should be assessed daily as a *wean screen*. For the patients who pass the daily wean screen, there is first an initial brief trial or *readiness assessment* during which patients are closely observed for 1 to 5 minutes while receiving minimal or no support (continuous positive airway pressure [CPAP] ≤5 cm H_2O, T-piece trial, 5 to 7 cm H_2O pressure support from the ventilator, or automatic tube compensation) to assess their ability to undergo a formal spontaneous breathing trial (SBT). If the patient does well during the readiness assessment, an SBT is performed for between 30 and 120 minutes. During this time patients are closely monitored for signs of respiratory insufficiency, hemodynamic deterioration, problems with gas exchange, or patient discomfort. Full ventilatory support is promptly reinitiated if problems develop. Successfully completing an SBT is highly predictive of successful ventilator discontinuation. These steps are illustrated in Figure 10-1.

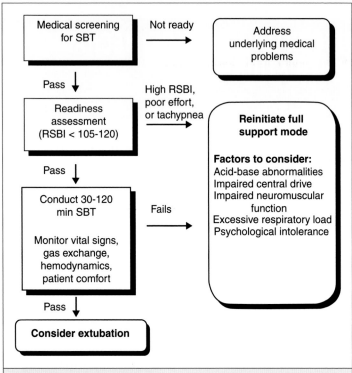

Figure 10-1. A protocol for daily assessment for extubation. *RSBI,* Rapid shallow breathing index calculated by frequency of breaths per minute divided by tidal volume in liters; *SBT,* spontaneous breathing trial.

4. **What is the rapid shallow breathing index (RSBI)? What does it predict?**
   The RSBI is calculated by using the following formula:

$$\frac{\text{Respiratory rate(breaths/min)}}{\text{Tidal volume(L)}}$$

   Higher values for the RSBI signify a pattern of breathing often seen in patients with respiratory muscle fatigue who tend to have weak inspiratory efforts and consequently higher respiratory rates. Values greater than 105 to 120 predict patients who may not tolerate an SBT. However, the observed RSBI value can be increased by recent suctioning, anxiety, fever, and the size of the endotracheal tube. Clinicians should be aware that the RSBI will generally be lower during use of minimal support modes (pressure support, CPAP) in comparison with when patients are just using a T-piece. The RSBI is most often measured during the readiness assessment to identify patients who may go forward with an SBT. The RSBI does not predict the ability for the patient to have the endotracheal tube removed on its own.

5. **To which mode should the ventilator be set during the SBT?**
   The specific ventilatory mode during the SBT is not critical. The choices usually include one of the following:
   - T-piece circuit that provides a constant flow of oxygen past the endotracheal tube with an extension downstream to prevent entrainment of room air

- Low levels of pressure support ventilation of 5 to 8 cm H_2O
- CPAP

A disadvantage of T-piece trials is that the patient is not connected to the ventilator's alarm systems that supplement clinician monitoring for apnea or tachypnea. The choice among these options will depend on each provider's experience and preferences.

6. **What are the traditional weaning parameters, and how are they used?**

Traditional weaning parameters include maximal inspiratory pressure, minute volume, vital capacity, maximum voluntary ventilation, thoracic compliance, and respiratory resistance. In the past, they were used to predict the likelihood of success with weaning trials. It is now known that they do not discriminate well between patients who will have success and those who will have failure after extubation. Assessment during a carefully monitored SBT appears to provide the most clinically useful information regarding ventilator discontinuation. Measurement of traditional weaning parameters is generally not necessary.

7. **Describe what to do about sedation and analgesia with such a patient.**

Patients are often medicated with sedatives and analgesics while receiving mechanical ventilation to reduce patient pain and discomfort and to limit patient movements that could lead to accidental extubation or other injuries. Continuous sedation may provide a more constant level of sedation, but this has been associated with a longer duration of mechanical ventilation, days spent in the ICU, and hospitalization compared with intermittent sedation protocols. Patients randomly assigned to undergo a planned interruption of continuous sedation on a daily basis had reduced days of mechanical ventilation and days in the ICU compared with those who were randomly assigned to receive continuous sedation. No adverse effects of interruption of sedation were apparent. The optimal method of providing sedation and analgesia for these patients is not known. However, minimizing sedatives to the level that achieves a specified sedation target and attempting to awaken the patient daily appear to be important aspects of patient management during mechanical ventilation. It is also important to have the daily sedation vacation correspond with the weaning trial to ensure an accurate assessment of the patient's ability to breathe. Systematic improvements in sedation practice are associated with improvements in outcomes including shorter ICU and hospital length of stay, duration of mechanical ventilation, and costs.

8. **What do you do with patients who have failure during the SBT?**

Two actions are necessary:

- Return the patient to a full ventilatory support mode (e.g., assist/control).
- Perform a comprehensive review of potential contributing factors to the failure.

To sustain spontaneous ventilation successfully, patients must have an intact respiratory center drive and adequate neuromuscular function and not have excessive loads on the respiratory muscles. Box 10-1 provides one method of systematically reviewing possible causes of failure during an SBT. Patients often have more than one cause for failure to wean, and correction of these factors may require multiple interventions. In general, it is recommended to wait 24 hours before attempting another SBT.

9. **What criteria are important when considering removal of an artificial airway?**

Successful completion of an SBT does not necessarily indicate that the patient is ready for extubation. Reintubation for respiratory failure occurs in approximately 10% to 15% of patients in most well-run ICUs. This rate is higher among those who have had endotracheal tubes in place for longer than 48 hours, who are older, or who have increased severity of illness, anemia, or cardiac failure. Unfortunately, reintubation is associated with a significantly increased mortality compared with patients not requiring reintubation, even when controlling for the severity of illness among these patients. Patients should be able to protect their airway, should demonstrate good cough effort, and should not have copious secretions. Patients should be responsive and able to follow commands. The difficulty of reintubating the patient's airway should be taken into account; the threshold for extubation in someone with a difficult airway should be higher. A cuff

---

BOX 10-1. FACTORS TO CONSIDER WHEN TESTS OF INSPIRATORY EFFORTS OR SPONTANEOUS BREATHING TRIALS FAIL IN PATIENTS

1. The patient has an increasing $PaCO_2$ without increases in respiratory effort or rate.
   (a) Inadequate respiratory center drive because of excessive narcotics, sedatives, hypothyroidism, or brain injury
   (b) Appropriate compensation for metabolic alkalosis because of excessive diuresis or nasogastric suctioning
   (c) Return to a chronic hypercapnic state after inappropriate overventilation in patients with COPD or sleep apnea
2. The patient has tachypnea, tachycardia, or distress.
   (a) Impaired neuromuscular function
      - Fatigue due to prolonged high loads, inadequate rest, or ventilator dyssynchrony
      - Hypothyroidism
      - Electrolyte deficiencies (e.g., hypokalemia, hypophosphatemia, hypomagnesemia)
      - Critical illness myopathy or polyneuropathy
      - Steroid myopathy
      - Effects of drugs (e.g., aminoglycosides, neuromuscular antagonists)
      - Sepsis
      - Diaphragmatic paresis or paralysis due to phrenic nerve injury resulting from cold cardioplegia or thoracic or neck surgery
      - Prolonged malnutrition
   (b) Excessive respiratory load
      - Increased airway resistance (e.g., asthma, COPD, excessive secretions, small endotracheal tube)
      - Air trapping and increased threshold load due to positive residual pressures (particularly in patients with COPD)
      - Decreased respiratory system compliance (e.g., pulmonary edema, fibrosis, pneumonia, abdominal distention, thoracic cage abnormalities, pleural effusions)
      - High minute ventilation requirements (e.g., fever, sepsis, metabolic acidosis, high physiologic dead space, excessive caloric intake, pulmonary embolism)
   (c) Impaired left ventricular function
   (d) Psychological dependence: a diagnosis of exclusion but not rare in patients in ICUs

---

COPD, Chronic obstructive pulmonary disease.

leak test can be performed if there is concern about postextubation upper airway obstruction. Though the presence of a leak is reassuring, the absence of a leak does not necessarily predict stridor after extubation.

10. **What about using noninvasive ventilation (NIV) for patients who have respiratory failure after extubation?**
   The initial use of NIV—ventilators that interface with the patient through a full face or nasal mask rather than an endotracheal tube—has improved outcomes in subsets of patients who are seen with acute respiratory failure, particularly patients with chronic obstructive pulmonary disease (COPD) and cardiogenic pulmonary edema. However, the situation may be different in patients who have respiratory failure after extubation.
   A recent Cochrane review found that in patients with COPD in whom extubation failed, NIV may be a reasonable option. NIV had a positive effect on mortality and ventilator-associated pneumonia, length of stay in the ICU and hospital, and total duration of ventilation in COPD patients in whom extubation failed. Patients need close monitoring if this approach is tried. NIV may also be useful as a prophylactic measure in patients who are thought to be high reintubation risks. The full utility of NIV after failure of extubation needs to be further elucidated. The majority of positive trials enrolled exclusively or predominately patients with COPD.

11. **Define prolonged mechanical ventilatory support (PMV).**

    A recent consensus conference defined patients receiving PMV as those who need at least 6 hours/day of ventilatory support for ≥ 21 days. These patients generally require a tracheostomy for optimal care. It is estimated that approximately 3% to 7% of patients receiving mechanical ventilatory support meet this definition. One-year survival rates among these patients range from 23% to 76%, with older age and poor functional status before the acute illness predicting a worse prognosis. In patients receiving PMV, the criteria used in the weaning protocols previously described for acutely ill patients do not apply. Many of these patients are managed in long-term care units outside the ICU.

12. **Should these patients be managed with different modes of ventilation?**

    Patients who are ventilator dependent after 14 to 21 days despite improvement in disease state may require different management strategies. Multidisciplinary rehabilitation with focus on ventilatory support, nutrition, physical therapy, and psychosocial support are all important aspects. Gradual reduction in ventilatory support may be used in PMV patients. Many clinicians wean patients to approximately 50% of their maximal support levels without using SBTs. Once at the 50% level, daily SBTs are started. Ventilatory support should be withdrawn gradually during the day, with progressively longer SBTs, allowing rest and sleep on full support modes at night. Once the patient tolerates spontaneous ventilation throughout the day, withdrawal of nocturnal ventilation may proceed relatively quickly. The success rate of ventilator discontinuation is only 50% to 60%. As in acutely ill patients, a therapist-driven protocol approach to weaning appears to improve outcomes in comparison with clinical judgment alone. Clinicians should continue efforts to identify and correct physiologic reasons for the patient's inability to resume spontaneous ventilation (see Box 10-1).

13. **Why is there such an emphasis on protocols?**

    In most recent studies, systematic weaning protocols, protocols to minimize or interrupt sedation, and raising the head of the bed have been associated with improved patient outcomes and reductions in the cost of care. Protocols run by nonphysicians produce faster liberation from the ventilator unless the physician-run usual care aggressively follows guidelines, in which case there is no difference. A recent Cochrane review found that protocolized weaning in critically ill adults resulted in a reduced shorter duration of mechanical ventilation by 25%, weaning duration was reduced by 78%, and ICU length of stay was reduced by 10%.

KEY POINTS: DISCONTINUATION OF MECHANICAL VENTILATION

1. Daily systematic assessments of patients receiving mechanical ventilation for the ability to breathe spontaneously are important in achieving timely discontinuation of ventilator support and reducing complications related to artificial airways and mechanical ventilation.

2. A respiratory therapist–driven or nurse-driven protocol for this daily assessment can safely reduce the duration of mechanical ventilation and performs better than standard physician assessments.

3. Sedation and analgesia should be minimized or interrupted on a daily basis.

4. Before removing the artificial airway, patients should be able to protect their airway, should demonstrate good cough effort, and should not have copious secretions.

5. Systematic attention to medical conditions that impair spontaneous breathing, such as left ventricular dysfunction, muscle fatigue, and metabolic abnormalities, should be part of this daily assessment. This can guide the medical care for those patients in whom a spontaneous breathing trial fails or who require prolonged ventilatory support.

WEBSITE

Institute for Healthcare Improvement (IHI) Knowledge Center: Implement the IHI Ventilator Bundle
http://www.ihi.org/knowledge/Pages/Changes/ImplementtheVentilatorBundle.aspx

BIBLIOGRAPHY

1. Blackwood B, Alderdice F, Burns KE, et al: Protocolized versus non-protocolized weaning for reducing the duration of mechanical ventilation in critically ill adult patients. Cochrane Database Syst Rev 5;CD006904, 2010.

2. Burns KE, Adhikari NK, Keenan SP, et al: Noninvasive positive pressure ventilation as a weaning strategy for intubated adults with respiratory failure. Cochrane Database Syst Rev 8;CD004127, 2010.

3. El-Khatib MF, Bou-Khalil P: Clinical review: liberation from mechanical ventilation. Crit Care 12:221, 2008.

4. Ely E, Meade M, Haponik E, et al: Mechanical ventilator weaning protocols driven by nonphysician health-care professionals: evidence-based clinical practice guidelines. Chest 120(6 Suppl):454S-463S, 2001.

5. Epstein SK, Ciubotaru RL, Wong JB: Effect of failed extubation on the outcome of mechanical ventilation. Chest 112:186-192, 1997.

6. Esteban A, Anzueto A, Frutos F, et al: Characteristics and outcomes in adult patients receiving mechanical ventilation: a 28-day international study. JAMA 287:345-355, 2002.

7. Jackson DL, Proudfoot CW, Cann KF, et al: A systematic review of the impact of sedation practice in the ICU on resource use, costs and patient safety. Crit Care 14:R59, 2010. Available online at http://ccforum.com/content/14/2/R59. Accessed February 4, 2012.

8. Kress J, Pohlman A, O'Connor M, et al: Daily interruption of sedative infusions in critically ill patients undergoing mechanical ventilation. N Engl J Med 342:1471-1477, 2000.

9. Krishan J, Moore D, Robeson C, et al: A prospective, controlled trial of a protocol-based strategy to discontinue mechanical ventilation. Am J Respir Crit Care Med 169:673-678, 2004.

10. MacIntyre N: Discontinuing mechanical ventilatory support. Chest 132:1049-1056, 2007.

11. MacIntyre N, Epstein S, Carson S, et al: Management of patients requiring prolonged mechanical ventilation: report of a NAMDRC consensus conference. Chest 128:3937-3954, 2005.

12. MacIntyre NR, Cook DJ, Ely EW, et al: Evidence based guidelines for weaning and discontinuing mechanical ventilation: a collective task force facilitated by the American College of Chest Physicians; the American Association for Respiratory Care; and the American College of Critical Care Medicine. Chest 120(6 Suppl):375S-395S, 2001.

13. Patel KN, Ganatra KD, Bates JH, et al: Variation in the rapid shallow breathing index associated with common measurement techniques and conditions. Respir Care 54:1462-1466, 2009.

14. Tobin M: Advances in mechanical ventilation. N Engl J Med 344:1986-1996, 2001.

15. Yang KL, Tobin MJ: A prospective study of indexes predicting the outcome of trials of weaning from mechanical ventilation. N Engl J Med 324:1445-1450, 1991.

ARTERIAL AND CENTRAL VENOUS CATHETERS

Hovig V. Chitilian, MD

CHAPTER 11

1. **What are the indications for intraarterial blood pressure monitoring?**
   - Inability to obtain noninvasive blood pressure measurements (i.e., burn or multitrauma patient with all extremities affected; during cardiopulmonary bypass; in patients with left ventricular assist devices)
   - Need for beat-to-beat monitoring of blood pressure because of patient's underlying condition
   - Need for multiple blood drawings for laboratory testing

2. **Which are the common sites for intraarterial catheter placement? What is the effect of the catheter site on the measured blood pressure?**
   The common sites are the radial, brachial, axillary, femoral, and dorsalis pedis arteries. As the monitoring site is moved further distally in the arterial tree, systolic pressures increase and diastolic pressures decrease when compared with central arterial pressure. The mean arterial pressure, however, remains the same between peripheral and central arterial waveforms.

3. **What additional data can be determined from the intraarterial pressure waveform?**
   In addition to direct pressure measurements, the arterial pressure waveform can be used to determine a patient's fluid responsiveness, as well as cardiac output. Changes in the arterial pressure waveform with mechanical ventilation have been shown to predict fluid responsiveness (a measurable increase in stroke volume with the administration of fluid). Goal-directed intraoperative fluid management based on arterial waveform changes has been shown to improve outcome in patients undergoing high-risk surgery. In addition, a number of commercially available devices exist that allow the continuous measurement of cardiac output with use of arterial pressure waveform analysis.

4. **What are the most common complications of arterial catheterization?**
   Vascular insufficiency (3%-5%), bleeding (1.5%-2.5%), and infection (<1%)

5. **What are the risk factors for vascular complications in patients with intraarterial catheters?**
   Concomitant use of vasopressors, prior arterial injury, duration of cannulation longer than 48 or 72 hours, hematoma formation, presence of disseminated intravascular coagulation, reduced cardiac output, and female sex

6. **What is the risk of permanent distal ischemic damage?**
   Studies have suggested that the rate of arterial occlusion is lower in axillary and femoral catheters compared with radial artery catheters; however, the rate of permanent distal ischemic damage is comparable at 0.1% to 0.2%. The incidence of permanent ischemic damage to the hand after radial artery catheterization has been reported to be 0.09%.

7. **Is the modified Allen's test useful?**
   There is no evidence that the modified Allen's test (a test of circulatory supply to the hand based on alternating occlusion of the radial and ulnar arteries) can predict hand ischemia with radial artery cannulation.

8. **What is the risk of arterial catheter–related bloodstream infection (BSI)?**
   The incidence of BSIs associated with arterial catheters is 0.8% or 1.7 per 1000 catheter days. Data are conflicting regarding the association of the site of catheterization with risk of infection with some studies suggesting that radial or dorsalis pedis arterial sites are associated with a decreased incidence of BSI when compared with the femoral artery.

9. **What measures can be taken to reduce the risk of BSI associated with intraarterial catheters?**
   The Centers for Disease Control and Prevention do not recommend routine replacement of peripheral arterial catheters at fixed time intervals as a method for preventing catheter-related BSIs. The use of full-barrier sterile precautions (chlorhexidine skin preparation, mask, hat, sterile gloves, gown, and sheet) has not been shown to reduce the risk of bacterial colonization or BSI when compared with the use of hand washing, chlorhexidine preparation, and sterile gloves for the placement of radial or dorsalis pedis arterial catheters.

10. **What are the indications for central venous cannulation?**
    - Monitoring cardiac filling pressures
    - Rapid administration of fluid
    - Intravenous administration of drugs or fluids that are potentially damaging to peripheral veins or tissues (vasoactive medications, parenteral nutrition)
    - Insertion of pulmonary artery catheter or transvenous pacing wires
    - Aspiration of air embolus
    - Access for hemodialysis or hemofiltration
    - Venous access in the instance of difficult peripheral venous access

11. **Which veins are commonly used, and how are they accessed?**
    The most commonly accessed central veins are the internal jugular, the subclavian, and the femoral veins. With use of either anatomic landmarks or ultrasound guidance, the vein is accessed percutaneously with a *finder* needle of a gauge smaller than the catheter. A guidewire is then passed through the needle and into the vein. The needle is removed, and a dilator is passed over the wire and into the vein to dilate the tissues and venous entry point. The dilator is removed, and the catheter is then passed over the wire and into the vein.

12. **What are the complications associated with central venous catheterization?**
    It is estimated that more than 15% of patients who receive central venous catheters have complications. Significant complications include arterial puncture, hematoma, pneumothorax, hemothorax, air embolus, and bloodstream infections. The risk of each complication varies with the location of the vein that is cannulated. The most common mechanical complications are arterial puncture, hematoma, and pneumothorax. Internal jugular venous catheterization and subclavian venous catheterization carry similar risks of mechanical complications. Subclavian venous cannulation carries the highest risk of pneumothorax (1.5%-3%). Femoral venous cannulation carries the highest risk of arterial puncture (9%-15%) followed by internal jugular venous cannulation (6%-9.5%).

13. **Is there any benefit to the use of ultrasound guidance?**
    The use of ultrasound guidance for central venous catheterization has been shown to reduce the number of cannulation attempts, as well as the incidence of a number of mechanical complications, including arterial puncture, hematoma, pneumothorax, brachial plexus injury, and

infection. The data showing the benefit of ultrasound guidance of central venous catheterization has prompted regulatory agencies in both the United States and Europe to recommend the routine use of ultrasound guidance for establishing central venous access.

14. How can ultrasound be used to establish central venous access?

Ultrasound-guided vascular access should be conducted with a linear probe using a 7- to 12-MHz frequency range. In general, imaging with higher ultrasound frequencies yields greater resolution but lower penetration. The use of lower ultrasound frequencies yields greater penetration but reduced resolution. Blood vessels can be visualized in the long axis (ultrasound beam parallel to the vessel) or in the short axis (ultrasound beam perpendicular to the vessel). Likewise, the needle can be visualized in the plane of the ultrasound beam and parallel to it (*in-plane* visualization) or perpendicular to the plane of the ultrasound beam *(out of plane)*. During imaging, the ultrasound probe should always be held perpendicular to the skin. The relevant ultrasound anatomy should be identified in the short axis, and the vein of interest should be examined for evidence of thrombosis or aberrant anatomy. The vessel of interest should be centered on the screen, and its depth should be noted. Veins should be distinguished from arteries on the basis of their thinner walls, compressibility, and nonpulsatile flow.

15. What is the risk of central venous catheter–related bloodstream infection (CRBSI)?

It is estimated that approximately 80,000 central venous CRBSIs occur in intensive care units in the United States each year. The total associated cost has been estimated to be $0.67 to $2.7 billion.

16. What are the risk factors for CRBSI in patients with central venous catheters?

- Prolonged hospitalization before catheterization
- Prolonged duration of catheterization
- Heavy microbial colonization at the insertion site
- Heavy microbial colonization of the catheter hub
- Internal jugular venous catheterization
- Neutropenia
- Total parenteral nutrition through the catheter
- Substandard care of the catheter

    The subclavian site of insertion is associated with the lowest risk of CRBSI.

17. What is the pathogenesis of CRBSI?

CRBSI arises from bacterial colonization of the central venous catheter. The two methods of colonization are:

- Migration of bacteria along the skin-catheter interface
- Contamination of a catheter access port

    Common bacterial pathogens in hospital-acquired CRBSI include coagulase-negative *Staphylococcus aureus*, *S. aureus*, *Enterococcus* species, *Candida* species, *Escherichia coli*, and *Klebsiella* species.

18. How is a CRBSI diagnosed?

CRBSI should be suspected in patients who have evidence of a BSI (such as fever) and an indwelling central venous catheter. The Infectious Diseases Society of America (IDSA) guidelines recommend that the diagnosis be confirmed with simultaneous quantitative blood cultures drawn through the central venous catheter and a peripheral vein with at least a threefold greater colony count from the central line sample. Alternatively, the diagnosis can be made if the blood culture drawn from the catheter becomes positive over a 2-hour period before the simultaneously drawn peripheral culture.

19. **How is a CRBSI treated?**

Once cultures are obtained, treatment of CRBSI involves removal of the catheter and initiation of systemic antibiotics. Because gram-positive cocci are the most common pathogens, empiric therapy with vancomycin is recommended until culture results and sensitivities are obtained. In patients who receive total parenteral nutrition, are taking a prolonged course of broad-spectrum antibiotics, have a hematologic malignancy, have had stem cell or solid organ transplantation, or have femoral catheterization, empiric coverage should include antibiotics with activity against gram-negative bacilli and *Candida* species.

20. **What steps are recommended to prevent CRBSI?**

Recommendations by the IDSA to prevent CRBSI include
- Performance of hand hygiene before catheter insertion
- Centralization of central line insertion supplies in a line cart or kit
- Use of maximal sterile barrier precautions
- Skin preparation with 2% chlorhexidine-based antiseptic
- Preferential use of the subclavian vein and avoidance of the femoral vein
- Disinfection of catheter ports before access
- Evaluation of the need for continued central catheter use on a daily basis

The use of ultrasound guidance for central venous catheter insertion has also been shown to reduce the risk of CRBSI.

KEY POINTS: ARTERIAL AND CENTRAL VENOUS CATHETERS

1. Indications for intraarterial blood pressure monitoring: inability to obtain noninvasive blood pressure measurements, need for beat-to-beat monitoring of blood pressure, need for multiple blood drawings for laboratory testing.

2. Common complications of intraarterial catheter placement: vascular insufficiency, hematoma, and infection.

3. Common indications for central venous cannulation: monitoring of cardiac filling pressures, central administration of drugs, rapid administration of fluid, and insertion of pulmonary artery catheter.

4. Prevention of central venous CRBSIs includes performance of hand hygiene before catheter insertion, use of maximal sterile barrier precautions, preferential use of the subclavian vein, and skin preparation with 2% chlorhexidine-based antiseptic.

BIBLIOGRAPHY

1. Brzezinski M, Luisetti T, London MJ: Radial artery cannulation: a comprehensive review of recent anatomic and physiologic investigations. Anesth Analg 109:1763-1781, 2009.
2. de Waal EEC, Wappler F, Buhre WF: Cardiac output monitoring. Curr Opin Anaesthesiol 22:71-77, 2009.
3. Fragou M, Grawanis A, Dimitriou V, et al: Real-time ultrasound-guided subclavian vein cannulation versus the landmark method in critical care patients: a prospective randomized study. Crit Care Med 39:1607-1612, 2011.
4. Frezza EE, Mezghebe H: Indications and complications of arterial catheter use in surgical or medical intensive care units: analysis of 4932 patients. Am Surg 64:127-131, 1998.
5. Karakitsos D, Labropoulos N, De Groot E, et al: Real-time ultrasound-guided catheterisation of the internal jugular vein: a prospective comparison with the landmark technique in critical care patients. Crit Care 10:R162, 2006.
6. Lipira AB, Mackinnon SE, Fox IK: Axillary arterial catheter use associated with hand ischemia in a multi-trauma patient: case report and literature review. J Clin Anesth 23:325-328, 2011.

7. Maki DG, Kluger DM, Crnich CJ: The risk of bloodstream infection in adults with different intravascular devices: a systematic review of 200 published prospective studies. Mayo Clin Proc 81:1159-1171, 2006.

8. Making health care safer: a critical analysis of patient safety practices. Agency for Healthcare Research and Quality publication 01-E058; Rockville, Maryland; Jul 20, 2001.

9. Mark JB, Barbeito A: Arterial and central venous pressure monitoring. Anesthesiol Clin 24:717-735, 2006.

10. McGee DC, Gould MK: Preventing complications of central venous catheterization. N Engl J Med 348:1123-1133, 2003.

11. Michard F: Stroke volume variation: from applied physiology to improved outcomes. Crit Care Med 39:402-403, 2011.

12. O'Grady NP, Alexander M, Dellinger EP, et al: Guidelines for the prevention of intravascular catheter–related infections. Am J Infect Control 30:476-489, 2002.

13. Rijnders BJA, Wijngaerden EV, Wilmer A, et al: Use of full sterile barrier precautions during insertion of arterial catheters: a randomized trial. Clin Infect Dis 36:743-748, 2003.

14. Scheer B, Perel A, Pfeiffer UJ: Clinical review: complications and risk factors of peripheral arterial catheters used for hemodynamic monitoring in anaesthesia and intensive care medicine. Crit Care 6:199-204, 2002.

15. Weber DJ, Rutala WA: Central line–associated bloodstream infections: prevention and management. Infect Dis Clin North Am 25:77-102, 2011.

CHAPTER 12

ULTRASOUND IN THE INTENSIVE CARE UNIT

Daniel W. Johnson, MD

1. **What is point-of-care ultrasound, and how is it used in the intensive care unit (ICU)?**

   Point-of-care ultrasound is the application of ultrasound by the bedside clinician for the purpose of answering diagnostic questions or guiding procedures. Traditionally, after consultation was requested by the bedside clinician, ultrasound examination was performed and interpreted by radiologists, cardiologists, and their sonographers. With the advent of point-of-care ultrasonography, the clinician can apply the ultrasound device himself or herself to answer specific questions without the inherent inefficiencies of consulting imaging services.

   Point-of-care ultrasound is of particular value in the ICU, where the patient's status changes rapidly and diagnostic and therapeutic applications of ultrasound are necessary immediately.

2. **What are the main variables that determine ultrasound image quality?**

   The most important variables are frequency, depth, and gain. Ultrasound frequency is largely determined by transducer selection. High-frequency transducers provide excellent resolution but limit the depth at which structures can be viewed. When viewing structures close to the body's surface, a high-frequency transducer should be used. When viewing deep structures, a low-frequency transducer must be used. Increasing the depth allows the user to view more structures, but with increased depth comes a reduction in resolution. Increasing the gain increases the intensity, or brightness, of the image.

3. **How can the ultrasound transducer be manipulated to optimize image quality?**

   The transducer can be moved to a different location on the body, it can be tilted, or it can be rotated about an axis. When manipulating an ultrasound transducer, the user must take care to alter only the location *or* the tilt *or* the rotation at one time. Novice users frequently attempt to alter two or three of these at the same time, which makes image acquisition more difficult.

4. **Where is the ultrasound transducer placed for cardiac imaging?**

   Because bone effectively blocks the transmission of ultrasound waves and creates an acoustic shadow on the ultrasound image display, the sonographer must use *windows* that allow ultrasound waves to avoid the sternum and ribs. The main echocardiographic windows are depicted in Figure 12-1.

5. **What questions can be answered by focused transthoracic echocardiography?**

   Focused transthoracic echocardiography is used to answer specific clinical questions, the answers to which impact immediate medical decision making. Examples of such questions:
   - Is the left ventricular systolic function hyperdynamic, normal, depressed, or severely depressed?
   - Is the right ventricle dilated?
   - Is right ventricular systolic function normal or depressed?
   - Is a pericardial effusion present, and, if so, is there evidence of tamponade?
   - Do any of the valves appear grossly abnormal on two-dimensional imaging?
   - Does the inferior vena cava (IVC) appear underfilled, normal, or overloaded?

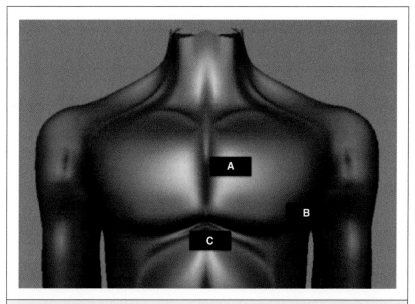

Figure 12-1. Main echocardiographic windows. *A*, Parasternal; *B*, apical; *C*, subcostal. (Modified from Ferrada P, Murthi S, Anand RJ, et al: Transthoracic focused rapid echocardiographic examination: real-time evaluation of fluid status in critically ill trauma patients. J Trauma 70:56-62, 2011.)

With advanced training, the intensivist can perform comprehensive transthoracic and/or transesophageal examinations. Figure 12-2 is an example of a normal subcostal four-chamber view obtained in the ICU.

6. **What does severe hypovolemia look like on echocardiography?**
   In the setting of severe hypovolemia, the left ventricle appears hyperdynamic with near or complete effacement of the small left ventricular cavity (in other words, the ejection fraction approaches 100%). In the setting of shock, subcostal imaging of the IVC is also useful for determining a patient's volume status. A large IVC with minimal respiratory variation suggests that the patient will not be fluid responsive. A small IVC with marked respiratory variation suggests that the patient will likely be fluid responsive.

7. **How can pneumothorax be ruled out with pleural ultrasound?**
   The presence of *lung sliding* effectively rules out pneumothorax at the site of the ultrasound transducer. The transducer is applied to the chest in the sagittal plane. The user identifies rib shadows with a bright pleural line in between the ribs. In the normal subject, movement of the visceral pleura against the parietal pleura creates a characteristic pattern known as "lung sliding" on the ultrasound display. By applying the probe in multiple locations on the right and left chest, the user can detect lung sliding and rule out pneumothorax. Because a variety of lung and pleural pathologies can cause a lack of lung sliding, it is important to know that, although lung sliding can rule out pneumothorax, a lack of lung sliding requires the user to work through a differential diagnosis that includes pneumothorax, acute respiratory distress syndrome, atelectasis, pleural disease, and contralateral main-stem intubation.

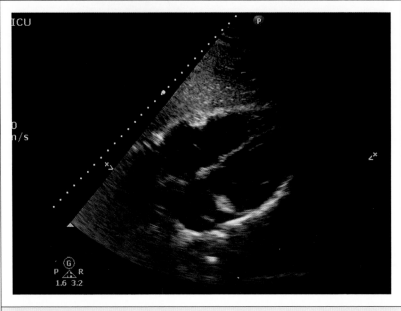

Figure 12-2. Normal subcostal four-chamber view.

8. **If "air is the enemy of ultrasound," how can ultrasound examination of the lung be useful?**

A number of normal and pathologic states can be detected by lung ultrasound examination, often by interpretation of stereotypical patterns of artifact. Normal aerated lung exhibits a reverberation artifact with horizontal lines known as *A lines* across the ultrasound display. When fluid accumulates in the lung interstitium or alveoli, artifacts known as *B lines* appear on the ultrasound display. B lines are bright vertical lines that extend from the most superficial aspect of the display to the edge of the display. In general, the number of B lines correlates with the quantity of fluid accumulation in the lung.

9. **How does fluid in the pleural space appear on ultrasound?**

Pleural effusion and hemothorax, like all free fluid, appear black on the ultrasound display.

Although it is impossible to determine the nature of free fluid by imaging alone, the history and physical examination provide the context that allows the clinician to narrow the differential diagnosis.

When sufficient pleural fluid has accumulated to collapse nearby lung, the atelectatic lung can be seen *floating* in pleural fluid. Ultrasound imaging of pleural fluid can help the intensivist to determine whether thoracentesis or thoracostomy tube placement would be possible and can be used for procedural guidance.

10. **What is the FAST examination?**

FAST stands for "focused abdominal sonography for trauma." It is performed to evaluate for free fluid (blood) and cardiac activity in trauma patients, particularly those with shock. The FAST examination consists of:

- Low-frequency ultrasound examination of the right upper quadrant (for blood between the diaphragm and liver, between liver and kidney, or around the kidney)
- Left upper quadrant (for blood between diaphragm and spleen, between spleen and kidney, or around the kidney)
- Heart and pericardial space (for evidence of cardiac activity and pericardial fluid)
- Pelvis

The trauma surgeon uses the positive (free fluid present) or negative (free fluid not present) result of the FAST examination to aid in decision making regarding need for immediate surgery versus ongoing diagnostic evaluation.

11. **What is the smallest amount of abdominal free fluid detectable by the FAST examination?**
The sensitivity of the FAST examination depends on the location of the free fluid, position of the patient, and quality of imaging and interpretation. In general, the FAST examination is capable of detecting free fluid in quantities greater than 250 mL.

12. **Which ultrasound transducer is appropriate for vascular access?**
A high-frequency transducer is essential for ultrasound-guided vascular access. High-frequency imaging results in excellent resolution and a high-quality image with limited depth. Low frequency results in less resolution with greater depth.

13. **What are some of the ways ultrasound can be used for central venous access?**
The most common application involves imaging of the internal jugular vein in short axis (in cross section). Ultrasound examination allows the operator to view the relationship between the internal jugular vein and the carotid artery and thus optimize needle placement and trajectory during the procedure. When used properly, ultrasound reduces the risk of carotid artery puncture and reduces the number of attempts necessary for successful cannulation of the internal jugular vein. A similar technique can be applied to the femoral vein. Increasingly, intensivists are using ultrasound to visualize the subclavian-axillary vein before placement of central lines at this site.

14. **Are there other applications of ultrasound for vascular access?**
Ultrasound can facilitate placement of arterial catheters in both superficial (e.g., radial) and deep (e.g., femoral, axillary, brachial) vessels. Placement of arterial catheters by landmark and palpation alone is sometimes impossible, and in some of these cases ultrasound guidance leads to successful placement. Ultrasound can also be used to facilitate placement of peripheral intravenous lines. Critically ill patients' peripheral veins are frequently difficult to access by traditional techniques because of prior lines, repeated phlebotomy, and soft-tissue edema. Ultrasound allows the intensivist to visualize and access veins that would be undetectable by inspection and palpation alone.

15. **How can ultrasound be used to screen for deep venous thrombosis (DVT)?**
Because most lower-extremity DVTs are located at the branch points of the venous system, ultrasound examination of these sites is useful in ruling out DVT. The venous system is viewed with a high-frequency transducer in cross section at the proximal thigh (where the common femoral vein joins with the greater saphenous vein) and in the popliteal fossa. A distance of 5 to 10 cm of vein should be examined in both the femoral and popliteal regions. If the common femoral vein and popliteal vein are fully compressible and no thrombus is visualized, the patient is unlikely to have a significant DVT.

16. **Where can I learn critical care ultrasound techniques?**
The best way to learn these techniques is to train with someone who is already an expert in point-of-care ultrasound. Local, regional, and national courses in critical care ultrasound are available throughout the year and are open to all health care professionals and trainees.

Several high-quality texts and articles describe these ultrasound techniques in detail. Online resources including full curricula in critical care ultrasound are also available. Many critical care fellowships currently include training in point-of-care ultrasound. After training in point-of-care ultrasound, the clinician must use ultrasound examination regularly to continue to improve in imaging and interpretation.

KEY POINTS: ULTRASOUND IN THE INTENSIVE CARE UNIT

1. High frequency provides excellent image resolution with poor depth. Low frequency allows deep imaging at the expense of image resolution.

2. Free fluid appears black on the ultrasound display.

3. Left ventricular systolic function can be accurately estimated by focused echocardiography.

4. Pneumothorax can be ruled out by ultrasound detection of lung sliding in multiple sites over the chest.

5. Ultrasound imaging of full compression of the common femoral vein and popliteal vein can be used to screen for lower-extremity DVT.

BIBLIOGRAPHY

1. Blaivas M: Ultrasound in the detection of venous thromboembolism. Crit Care Med 35(5 Suppl):S224-S234, 2007.

2. Feissel M, Michard F, Faller JP, et al: The respiratory variation in inferior vena cava diameter as a guide to fluid therapy. Intensive Care Med 30:1834-1837, 2004.

3. Lichtenstein DA, Menu Y: A bedside ultrasound sign ruling out pneumothorax in the critically ill: lung sliding. Chest 108:1345-1348, 1995.

4. Mayo PH, Beaulieu Y, Doelken P, et al: American College of Chest Physicians/La Société de Réanimation de Langue Française statement on competence in critical care ultrasonography. Chest 135:1050-1060, 2009.

5. Moore CL, Copel JA: Point-of-care ultrasonography. N Engl J Med 364:749-757, 2011.

6. Noble VE, Nelson B: Manual of Emergency and Critical Care Ultrasound, 2nd ed. New York, Cambridge University Press, 2011.

CHAPTER 13

EXTRACORPOREAL MEMBRANE OXYGENATION

Michael G. Fitzsimons, MD, FCCP, and Michael N. Andrawes, MD

1. **What is extracorporeal membrane oxygenation (ECMO)?**

   ECMO is a means to provide peripheral oxygenation, ventilation, and circulation to a variety of patients with diseases of the heart and/or lungs for periods of days or weeks. The lungs of patients with severe respiratory failure have an impaired ability to perform the necessary functions of the thoracic cavity, primarily oxygenation and ventilation. Data show that patients with respiratory failure who cannot receive oxygenation or ventilation adequately with use of low tidal volumes without high plateau pressures can be treated with ECMO successfully. Certain patients with hemodynamic failure who lack the ability to meet the metabolic demands of the organs of the body despite pharmacologic support may also benefit from ECMO.

2. **What is the history of ECMO?**

   ECMO was developed as an extension of cardiopulmonary bypass. The first reported use of ECMO for respiratory failure in an adult patient was reported in 1972 in a young man with adult respiratory distress syndrome after a motor vehicle accident. This was followed in 1976 by the first use of ECMO in neonatal patients. Since its development ECMO has been shown to improve survival in neonates with respiratory failure from a variety of causes compared with more traditional therapy. The benefits in adult patients are more controversial.

3. **How is ECMO different from cardiopulmonary bypass?**

   Cardiopulmonary bypass was developed as a means to provide short-term support to patients undergoing cardiac surgery. The setup necessary for cardiopulmonary bypass is also designed to accomplish several other tasks including suction and venting of the field and cardiac chambers and administration of cardioplegia (Table 13-1).

TABLE 13-1. DIFFERENCES AND SIMILARITIES BETWEEN ECMO AND CARDIOPULMONARY BYPASS

PARAMETER	ECMO	CARDIOPULMONARY BYPASS
Oxygenation	Yes	Yes
Ventilation	Yes	Yes
Circulatory support	Yes	Yes
Venous reservoir	No	Yes
Ability to deliver cardioplegia	No	Yes
Ability to administer medications into circuit	No	Yes
Supplemental pumps (e.g., suction, vent)	No	Yes
Heating and cooling	Yes	Yes
Ability to adjust oxygenation	Yes	Yes
Ability to add fluids directly to circuit	No	Yes
Ability to administer anesthetics in line	No	Yes

4. What are clinical situations where ECMO may be beneficial?

ECMO has been used for the short-term hemodynamic and respiratory support for numerous conditions (Box 13-1).

BOX 13-1. POTENTIAL CLINICAL USES OF ECMO

- Adult respiratory distress syndrome
- Acute respiratory failure associated with viral infection
- Bridge to heart transplantation
- Bridge to lung transplantation
- Acute massive pulmonary emboli
- Primary graft failure after heart transplantation
- Right ventricular failure after heart transplantation
- Severe refractory status asthmaticus
- Low cardiac output syndrome after cardiopulmonary bypass
- Support during liver transplantation
- Hemodynamics and respiratory support during surgery for mediastinal mass excision
- Support during carinal resection
- Support during high-risk percutaneous coronary interventions
- Support during high-risk electrophysiology procedures
- Burn-associated respiratory failure
- Respiratory failure due to near drowning
- Respiratory support for congenital diaphragmatic hernia
- Rewarming after accidental hypothermia
- Reexpansion pulmonary edema
- Severe myocarditis
- Post obstructive pulmonary edema
- Pancreatitis
- Fat emboli syndrome
- Amniotic fluid embolism
- Drug overdose

---

5. Are there any diagnostic modalities that may indicate when emergent ECMO is indicated?

Transesophageal echocardiography (TEE) allows real-time assessment of cardiac function. Acute pulmonary thromboemboli, amniotic fluid embolism, and air emboli cause an acute pressure overload on the right ventricle. Acute right ventricular pressure overload results in ventricular dilatation, tricuspid regurgitation, and a shift of the interventricular septum toward the left, further impairing filling of the left ventricle and a reduction in cardiac output. TEE may also be used to guide proper placement of the venous return cannula into the right atrium when ECMO is initiated.

6. What does the literature show regarding ECMO?

Dr. Warren Zapol performed the first randomized study to evaluate the effectiveness of ECMO in adult patients with severe acute respiratory failure. This study, published in 1979, determined that ECMO could support respiratory gas exchange but did not increase long-term survival. Subsequent studies have generally demonstrated survival rates of approximately 50% for patients with primary respiratory failure. Older patients, those having complications while receiving ECMO, and those having prolonged ventilation before ECMO were predictors of higher mortality. Survival for patients with primary cardiac failure also tends to be less.

7. **Are there any contraindications to ECMO?**

   Few absolute contraindications to ECMO exist. Patient or proxy refusal is an absolute contraindication. Patients with "do not resuscitate" orders should not be subject to ECMO. Irreversible respiratory failure in patients who are not candidates for lung transplantation should preclude the use of ECMO. Severe bleeding and peripheral vascular disease increase the risk of complications with ECMO. Some have argued against the use in elderly patients, although one study demonstrated that 41.7% of patients older than 75 years with cardiogenic shock treated with ECMO survived to discharge.

8. **What are the components of an ECMO circuit?**

   An ECMO circuit contains several key components including the vascular access, tubing, driving force (pump), gas exchange unit (oxygenator-ventilator), and interface or console. Vascular access is most commonly established in the femoral artery and veins. The cannulas are sized between 21F and 28F for adults and smaller for newborns and children. The venous or *drainage* cannula may be positioned into the right atrium under echocardiography or fluoroscopic guidance. The arterial or *return* cannula is placed in the other femoral vein (venovenous [VV] ECMO) or femoral artery (venoarterial [VA] ECMO).

   Most ECMO circuits have a membrane gas exchange unit. This gas exchange unit consists of a series of hollow fibers through which the blood passes. Gas is passed in a countercurrent manner allowing exchange across the membranes. The pump system may be either a roller system or a centrifugal system. A roller pump system consists of flexible tubing in a track. The *roller* compresses the tubing and forces the blood forward with each turn. Such flow is independent of systemic vascular resistance, and high pressures can develop. Centrifugal pumps have been popular in Europe and are becoming more popular in the United States. Centrifugal pumps contain a magnetically driven impeller, which cycles at several thousand rotations

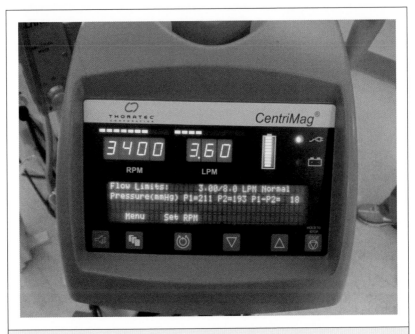

Figure 13-1. CentriMag ECMO console.

per minute generating a pressure gradient across the pump head and propelling blood forward. It is preload and afterload dependent. If flow into the pump is decreased, then flow and pressure will be decreased. The CentriMag blood pump is a magnetically levitated centrifugal device that produces unidirectional flow and may generate flows up to 10 L/min (Figs. 13-1 and 13-2).

9. **How is vascular access established for ECMO?**
   Several potential sites exist for both venous and arterial cannulation for patients requiring ECMO. The decision as to which cannulation strategy is necessary depends on the goals (Table 13-2). The venous or *drainage* cannula for adult patients should be 23F to 25F and the return cannula 17F to 21F.

10. **What does one monitor while using ECMO?**
    Monitoring patients subject to ECMO is a multidisciplinary task. Surgeons, intensivists, perfusionists, anesthesiologists, respiratory therapists, and nurses may all be involved in the care of these patients. Maintenance of normal physiologic parameters is the goal (Table 13-3). Flow rates, sweep speed, and FiO_2 are adjusted to attain such measure.

11. **How is ventilation managed while a patient is receiving ECMO?**
    The avoidance of barotrauma is a prime benefit of ECMO. Most patients will be given *rest* settings to avoid complications associated with high volume and high pressure ventilation. Inspiratory pressures are often limited to 20 to 25 cm H_2O with a positive end-expiratory pressure of 10 to 15 cm H_2O and a low respiratory rate. Terragni demonstrated that ECMO allows tidal

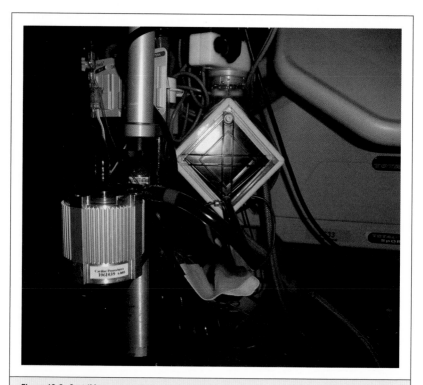

Figure 13-2. CentriMag pump and gas exchange system.

TABLE 13-2. CANNULATION SITES FOR ECMO

CANNULATION TECHNIQUE	SITE OF VENOUS DRAINAGE	SITE OF BLOOD RETURN	BENEFITS	DOWNSIDE
VV	Drainage from IVC via femoral vein	Return via right atrium or SVC	No arterial cannulation, easy to establish	No hemodynamic support, susceptible to shunt
VA	Drainage from the IVC via femoral vein	Femoral artery or axillary artery; the carotid artery has been used in neonates.	Hemodynamic support, decreased pulmonary blood flow, ability to relax lungs	Requires arterial cannulation; lower flows will not distribute blood above diaphragm
Mixed venous and VA	Drainage from IVC via femoral vein	Femoral artery or aorta and SVC		

IVC, Inferior vena cava; *SVC,* superior vena cava.

TABLE 13-3. GOALS FOR MANAGEMENT DURING ECMO

PARAMETER	GOAL
Flow rates (mL/kg/min)	50-80
Mean arterial pressure (adult) (mm Hg)	65-95
Sweep speed (gas flow) (mL/kg/min)	50-80
FiO_2 (%)	100
pH	7.35-7.45
$PaCO_2$ (mm Hg)	35-45
SpO_2 (arterial or return cannula) (%)	100
SpO_2 (VA ECMO) (%)	>95
SpO_2 (VV ECMO) (%)	85-92

volumes less than 6 mL/kg to be used. An improvement in morphologic markers of lung protection and a reduction in pulmonary cytokines are observed.

12. **What problems are commonly encountered during the clinical management of ECMO?**
Acute problems tend to fall into three categories:
1. Inadequate flow, commonly due to either hypovolemia or malposition of the drainage cannula

2. Poor oxygenation, maybe due to an inadequate FiO_2 or shunt of blood through the lungs
3. Inadequate ventilation, due to malfunction of the gas exchange assembly or low *sweep speed*

13. **How does one wean a patient from ECMO?**
    The technique of weaning a patient from ECMO support depends on the type of ECMO (VV or VA) and the purpose of the support. In general the lungs and heart assume more responsibility for oxygenation, ventilation, and circulation. Sidebotham et al. describe their technique for weaning ECMO (Table 13-4).

14. **What are complications of ECMO?**
    Most adult ECMO is established with peripheral cannulation of the femoral artery. Lower limb ischemia may occur because of occlusion of arterial inflow and may be treated with decannulation or supplemental cannulation of the superficial femoral artery. Neither body mass index, body surface area, nor cannula size predicts limb ischemia. Abdominal compartment syndrome may occur in both adult and pediatric patients receiving ECMO and is likely due to massive fluid resuscitation in an effort to achieve adequate ECMO flows. Other complications include bleeding, clot formation, stroke, renal failure, and nosocomial infection. Mechanical mishaps such as failure of the pump and oxygenator must be considered in planning support.

TABLE 13-4. WEANING A PATIENT FROM ECMO SUPPORT		
MEASURE	**VV ECMO**	**VA ECMO**
Purpose of support	Oxygenation-ventilation	Hemodynamic support
Measure of improvement	Increased SpO_2 and PaO_2 Decreased $PaCO_2$ Improved CXR Increased lung compliance	Return of pulsatile arterial waveform Improved cardiac function by echocardiography
Technique	Provide full ventilatory support Reduce gas "sweep" Reduce flows to 1-2 L/min	Adjust inotropic support to provide acceptable hemodynamics Reduce flows to 1-2 L/min
Monitoring during weaning	Maintenance of SpO_2/PaO_2	Echocardiography (cardiac function) Blood pressure Cardiac output Central venous pressure Pulmonary artery pressure
When to discontinue	Acceptable ABG 2-3 hr after weaning and tolerance of flow reduction to zero	Acceptable hemodynamics after 1-2 hr of minimal or no hemodynamics support.

Modified from Sidebotham D, McGeorge A, McGuinness S, et al: Extracorporeal membrane oxygenation for treating severe cardiac and respiratory failure in adults: part 2—technical considerations. J Cardiothorac Vasc Anesth 24:164-172, 2010.
ABG, Arterial blood gases; *CXR,* chest radiograph.

15. **How does one transfer a patient receiving ECMO?**
    The transfer of patients with severe respiratory failure and hemodynamic failure to large medical centers is increasingly common. The University of Michigan reviewed all patients transferred between 1990 and 1999 while receiving ECMO. Patients were transferred over a range of 2 to 790 miles. No patients died during transport. Complications noted included power failure, circuit tubing leakages, circuit rupture, membrane lung thrombosis, membrane lung leakage, and hyperventilation.

KEY POINTS: EXTRACORPOREAL MEMBRANE OXYGENATION

ECMO may provide temporary support to patients with failure of the cardiopulmonary system by:

1. Providing primary oxygenation and circulation for patients with primary cardiac failure (VA ECMO)

2. Providing extracorporal oxygenation and carbon dioxide removal for patients with respiratory failure (VV ECMO)

ECMO is different from cardiopulmonary bypass in several ways:

1. ECMO circuits cannot deliver cardioplegia.
2. ECMO circuits do not have supplemental pumps.
3. ECMO circuits do not have a venous reservoir.

The primary components of an ECMO circuit are:

1. Vascular access
2. Tubing
3. Pump
4. Gas exchange mechanism

Common potential complications of ECMO are:

1. Lower limb ischemia
2. Bleeding
3. Clot formation
4. Stroke
5. Renal failure
6. Infection

BIBLIOGRAPHY

1. Augustin P, Lasocki S, Dufour G, et al: Abdominal compartment syndrome due to extracorporeal membrane oxygenation in adults. Ann Thorac Surg 90:e40-e41, 2010.

2. Aziz TA, Singh G, Popjes E, et al: Initial experience with CentriMag extracorporeal membrane oxygenation for support of critically ill patients with refractory cardiogenic shock. J Heart Lung Transplant 29:66-71, 2010.

3. Brogan TV, Thiagarajan RR, Rycos PT, et al: Extracorporeal membrane oxygenation in adults with severe respiratory failure: a multi-center database. Intensive Care Med 35:2105-2114, 2009.

4. Foley DS, Pranikoff T, Younger JG, et al: A review of 100 patients transported on extracorporeal life support. ASAIO J 48:612-619, 2002.

5. Hill JD, O'Brien TG, Murray JJ, et al: Prolonged extracorporeal oxygenation in severe acute respiratory failure (shock lung syndrome). Use of the Bramson membrane lung. N Engl J Med 286:629-634, 1972.

6. Meilck F, Quintel M: Extracorporeal membrane oxygenation. Curr Opin Crit Care 11:87-93, 2005.

7. Peek GJ, Mugford M, Tiruvoipai R, et al: CESAR trial collaboration. Efficacy and economic assessment of conventional ventilator support versus extracorporeal membrane oxygenation for severe adult respiratory failure [CESAR]; a multicenter randomized controlled trial. Lancet 374:1351-1363, 2009.

8. Saito S, Nakatani T, Kobayashi J, et al: Is extracorporeal life support contraindicated in elderly patients? Ann Thorac Surg 83:140-145, 2007.

9. Sidebotham D, McGeorge A, McGuinness S, et al: Extracorporeal membrane oxygenation for treating severe cardiac and respiratory failure in adults: part 2—technical considerations. J Cardiothorac Vasc Anesth 24:164-172, 2010.

10. Terragni PP, Del Sorbo L, Mascia L, et al: Tidal volume lower than 6 ml/kg enhances lung protection. Role of extracorporeal carbon dioxide removal. Anesthesiology 111:826-835, 2009.

11. Zapol WM, Snider MT, Hill JD, et al: Extracorporeal membrane oxygenation in severe acute respiratory failure. A randomized prospective study. JAMA 242:2193-2196, 1979.

12. Zapol WM, Snider MT, Schneider RC: Extracorporeal membrane oxygenation for acute respiratory failure. Anesthesiology 46:272-285, 1977.

TRACHEAL INTUBATION AND AIRWAY MANAGEMENT

CHAPTER 14

Manuel Pardo, Jr., MD

1. **What is the airway?**

   The airway is the conduit through which air and oxygen must pass before reaching the lungs. It includes the anatomic structures extending from the nose and mouth to the larynx and trachea.

2. **What is airway management?**

   Airway management is the procedure for ensuring that the airway remains patent. It is the first step in the ABCs of basic resuscitation (B = breathing, C = circulation).

3. **Why does airway management generally precede management of breathing and circulation?**

   If the airway is completely obstructed, no oxygen can reach the lungs, and the heart and circulation will have no oxygen to distribute to the body's vital organs. However, the 2010 American Heart Association (AHA) *Guidelines for Cardiopulmonary Resuscitation and Emergency Cardiovascular Care* now recommend beginning cardiopulmonary resuscitation with 30 chest compressions before delivering two rescue breaths. Although there is no proven mortality benefit to managing the airway after the circulation, the AHA rationale is that blood flow to vital organs depends on chest compressions.

   Note: In addition, the AHA recommends "hands-only" chest compressions (i.e., no rescue breathing at all) for the untrained lay rescuer of a victim in cardiac arrest.

4. **Describe the ways to manage the airway.**

   The airway may remain patent without any intervention and can be managed with or without tracheal intubation. Airway management without intubation can involve a variety of maneuvers. In unconscious patients, the tongue commonly obstructs the airway. Techniques to open the airway include the head tilt–chin lift maneuver and the jaw thrust maneuver. Placement of oral or nasal airways may also help to maintain a patent airway. The use of a face mask with a bag-valve device (e.g., Ambu bag) is the usual next step in airway management. In the majority of patients, it is possible to maintain a patent airway without tracheal intubation. If tracheal intubation is required, it can be accomplished through surgical or nonsurgical techniques.

5. **What are the indications for tracheal intubation?**

   There are five main indications:
   - Upper airway obstruction
   - Inadequate oxygenation
   - Inadequate ventilation
   - Elevated work of breathing
   - Airway protection

6. **Explain why upper airway obstruction is an indication for tracheal intubation.**

   If the upper airway is obstructed and cannot be opened with the previously described maneuvers, the trachea must be intubated to avoid life-threatening hypoxemia. Although intubation will bypass the anatomic area of obstruction, the cause should be determined to evaluate appropriate timing of extubation or need for further treatment.

7. **Explain how to evaluate hypoxemia as an indication for tracheal intubation.**
If the patient's oxygen saturation is consistently less than 90% despite the use of high-flow oxygen delivered through a face mask, tracheal intubation should be considered. One hundred percent oxygen can be delivered reliably only with an endotracheal tube. Other factors to consider are the adequacy of cardiac output, blood hemoglobin concentration, presence of chronic hypoxemia, and reason for the hypoxemia. For example, patients with hypoxemia due to intracardiac right-to-left shunts may have chronic hypoxemia. In these patients, the administration of 100% oxygen with an endotracheal tube may not be effective in raising the oxygen saturation level.

8. **Explain how to evaluate hypoventilation as an indication for tracheal intubation.**
With hypoventilation, the blood PCO_2 progressively rises, which also lowers the blood pH level (respiratory acidosis). With increasing CO_2 levels, patients eventually become unconscious (CO_2 narcosis). Low systemic pH may be associated with abnormal myocardial irritability and contractility. The exact level of pH or PCO_2 that requires assisted ventilation must be determined for each patient. Chronic respiratory acidosis (e.g., in a patient with severe chronic obstructive pulmonary disease) is usually better tolerated than acute respiratory acidosis.

9. **Explain how to evaluate elevated work of breathing as an indication for tracheal intubation.**
Normally, the respiratory muscles account for less than 5% of the total body oxygen consumption. In patients with respiratory failure, this can increase to as much as 40%. It can be difficult to assess the work of breathing by clinical examination. However, patients who have rapid shallow breathing, use of accessory respiratory muscles, or paradoxic respirations have a predictably high work of breathing. The results of an arterial blood gas analysis (i.e., pH, PCO_2, and PO_2) may be initially normal in such patients. Eventually, the respiratory muscles fatigue and fail, causing inadequate oxygenation and ventilation. Mechanical ventilation can sometimes be done without tracheal intubation (see Chapter 9) but is more reliably accomplished with intubation.

10. **Explain airway protection as an indication for tracheal intubation.**
In an awake patient, protective airway reflexes normally prevent the pulmonary aspiration of gastric contents. Patients with altered mental status from a variety of causes may lose these protective reflexes, increasing the risk of aspiration pneumonia. Tracheal intubation with a cuffed tube can decrease the risk of aspiration. However, liquids can still leak around the endotracheal tube cuff, and the glottic barrier is bypassed, which plays a role in bacterial colonization of the lower airways.

11. **What are the surgical techniques for tracheal intubation?**
Surgical techniques include cricothyroidotomy or tracheotomy, which involves placing an endotracheal tube directly into the trachea through the cricothyroid membrane or between two tracheal rings.

12. **What are the commonly used nonsurgical techniques for tracheal intubation?**
Nonsurgical techniques can be divided into techniques that incorporate direct vision and *blind* techniques. The most commonly used direct vision intubation technique is direct laryngoscopy. The laryngoscope is placed in the mouth and manipulated to expose the larynx. An endotracheal tube is then placed through the larynx into the trachea. Another direct vision technique uses the flexible fiberoptic bronchoscope. An endotracheal tube is loaded onto the bronchoscope, which is advanced through the larynx via the nose or mouth. Once the bronchoscope is in the trachea, the endotracheal tube is advanced into position. Blind intubation is generally performed through the nose because the nasopharynx guides the endotracheal tube toward the larynx. Some laryngoscopes incorporate a video screen to allow improved vision of glottic structures via a small camera at the tip of the laryngoscope blade.

13. **Which drugs can be given to facilitate tracheal intubation?**
Sedative or analgesic agents are given to reduce the discomfort of laryngoscopy and to blunt the hemodynamic response. Muscle relaxants can make direct laryngoscopy easier to perform. The main risks of sedative or analgesic drugs in this setting are hypotension and respiratory depression. The muscle relaxants cause paralysis of all skeletal muscle, including the respiratory muscles. If the trachea cannot be intubated, the patient may not resume spontaneous breathing if sedatives, analgesics, or muscle relaxants have been given.

14. **What equipment should be prepared before direct laryngoscopy is attempted?**
Before laryngoscopy is attempted, all equipment should be checked for proper function. This includes laryngoscope blades, laryngoscope handle, suction source, suction catheter, oxygen source, self-inflating bag or breathing circuit, face mask, oral airways, nasal airways, sedative agents, muscle relaxants, intravenous line, and patient monitors.

15. **How is direct laryngoscopy accomplished?**
The technique varies slightly depending on the type of blade used (Figs. 14-1 and 14-2). First, the head is placed in the *sniffing* position with cervical spine in flexion and atlantooccipital joint in extension. The blade is inserted into the right side of the mouth. Then the tongue is moved to the left. With a curved (Macintosh) blade, the tip is inserted between the base of the tongue and the superior

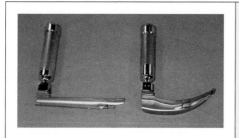

Figure 14-1. Two types of commonly used laryngoscope blades. The straight blade *(left)* is a size 3 Wisconsin blade. The curved blade *(right)* is a size 3 Macintosh blade.

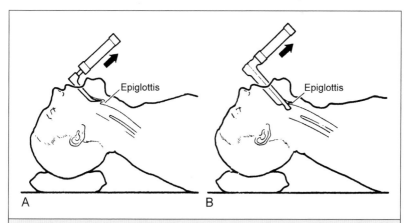

Figure 14-2. Procedure for direct laryngoscopy. *A,* A curved laryngoscope blade is placed in the vallecula. Lifting the blade forward and upward exposes the larynx. *B,* A straight blade is used to lift the epiglottis directly and expose the larynx. (From Gal TJ: Airway management. In Miller RD [ed]: Miller's Anesthesia, 6th ed. New York, 2005, Churchill Livingstone, p 1634.)

surface of the epiglottis, an area called the *vallecula*. If a straight (Miller or Wisconsin) blade is used, the tip is manipulated to lift the epiglottis. With both blade types, once the tip is in position, the blade is moved forward and upward to expose the larynx. An endotracheal tube is then inserted into the trachea. Gentle downward pressure on the thyroid cartilage may help to improve the view of the larynx.

16. **What maneuver can be performed to minimize the risk of aspiration during direct laryngoscopy?**
Cricoid pressure consists of firm manual pressure on the cricoid cartilage. This maneuver can occlude the esophagus and reduce the chance of gastric distention from mask ventilation. It can also prevent regurgitation of gastric contents into the pharynx. However, controversy exists about the effectiveness of this maneuver.

17. **What is a difficult airway? What is a difficult intubation?**
A difficult airway is a clinical situation in which an anesthesiologist or other specially trained clinician has difficulty with mask ventilation or tracheal intubation. Difficult intubation can be defined as one requiring more than three attempts at laryngoscopy or more than 10 minutes of laryngoscopy. Although the definitions are arbitrary, the inability to maintain a patent airway (with or without intubation) may be associated with anoxic brain injury and death.

18. **How do you evaluate the airway for potential difficulty?**
The history should address the ease of prior tracheal intubations. Patients who have general anesthesia for surgery frequently undergo tracheal intubation. The anesthetic record for the procedure should document the ease of intubation and the equipment used. On examination, one must evaluate four anatomic features: mouth opening, pharyngeal space, neck extension, and submandibular compliance.

19. **How do you evaluate mouth opening and pharyngeal space to predict difficult intubation?**
In the adult, a mouth opening of two to three fingerbreadths is usually adequate. One measure of pharyngeal space is the Mallampati class (Fig. 14-3). The patient is asked to sit upright with the head in a neutral position. Then he or she is asked to open the mouth as widely as possible and protrude the tongue as far as possible. The classification is based on the pharyngeal structures seen.
- **Class I:** The soft palate, fauces, entire uvula, and tonsillar pillars are visible.
- **Class II:** The soft palate, fauces, and part of the uvula are visible.
- **Class III:** The soft palate and base of the uvula are visible.
- **Class IV:** The soft palate is not visible at all.

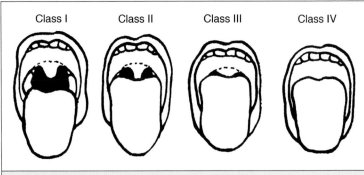

Figure 14-3. The Mallampati classification to evaluate pharyngeal space.

Intubation is generally easier in patients with class I airways than in patients with class IV airways. However, this test addresses only one of the four anatomic features required for easy direct laryngoscopy.

20. **How do you evaluate neck extension and submandibular compliance to predict difficult intubation?**
A normal adult has approximately 35 degrees of extension at the atlantooccipital joint. A decrease in extension may make it impossible to view the larynx with direct laryngoscopy. It can be difficult to assess the submandibular compliance by physical examination. Assessment of the mandibular space can be attempted by measuring the distance from the chin to the thyroid cartilage, the *thyromental distance*. An adult with less than 6.5 cm of thyromental distance may have a greater chance of difficult intubation than one with greater than 6.5 cm. Combining the various physical examination tests improves the ability to predict a difficult intubation, but no combination is foolproof.

21. **How do you manage a potentially difficult intubation?**
Three types of plans must be made when managing a difficult airway. The first is the primary approach to the intubation. The second is the plan for an emergency nonsurgical airway. Finally, a plan should exist for an emergency surgical airway (cricothyroidotomy or tracheotomy).
Many factors affect the management plan for a potentially difficult airway. These factors include the indication for intubation, the urgency of the intubation, the availability of skilled personnel, and the availability of special equipment. Because an awake, cooperative, spontaneously breathing patient normally has a patent airway, an awake intubation may be the safest. Topical or local anesthetics can be used to decrease airway sensation and patient discomfort.

22. **What are the ways to provide an emergency nonsurgical airway?**
If tracheal intubation and mask ventilation are not possible and the airway is not patent, an emergency airway must be provided. The options for providing an emergency nonsurgical airway include laryngeal mask ventilation, transtracheal jet ventilation, or esophageal-tracheal Combitube ventilation. The laryngeal mask is the most widely available of the three options. It is inserted into the posterior pharynx and lies opposite the larynx. In elective situations, it has a success rate of more than 90%. It is less successful in emergencies, but its widespread availability makes it a valuable option in managing the difficult airway. Special versions of the laryngeal mask incorporate features designed to facilitate blind passage of an endotracheal tube into the trachea.
Note: Emergency intubations are associated with up to a 2% mortality because of the underlying conditions of the patient and the difficulties associated with the intubations. The risks are increased by performing direct laryngoscopy more than twice.

23. **How is tracheal intubation confirmed?**
Auscultation for bilateral breath sounds and absence of stomach inflation should be done after each intubation attempt. However, these signs may still be present with an esophageal intubation. Carbon dioxide capnography is one of the most reliable methods to confirm placement. The laryngoscopic view may be useful. If an experienced clinician clearly sees the tube between the vocal cords, this is definitive confirmation. The endotracheal tube itself commonly blocks sight of the vocal cords, and inexperienced clinicians may insert the tube in the esophagus despite having a good view of the larynx. Other confirmation methods include fiberoptic bronchoscopy or an esophageal detector device.

24. **What are the immediate, short-term complications of tracheal intubation?**
Immediate complications of intubation include dental injury, cervical spine injury, pharyngeal trauma, laryngeal injury, aspiration of gastric contents, and tracheal rupture. Nosebleed is a risk with nasal intubations. The most common injuries are minor lip trauma and dental injury.

KEY POINTS: AIRWAY MANAGEMENT IN PATIENTS IN THE INTENSIVE CARE UNIT

1. In most patients, it is possible to maintain a patent airway without tracheal intubation.

2. Before managing a patient's airway, confirm the availability and function of all equipment that may be used.

3. The five main indications for tracheal intubation are upper airway obstruction, inadequate oxygenation, inadequate ventilation, elevated work of breathing, and airway protection.

4. To predict a difficult intubation, evaluate four anatomic features on physical examination: mouth opening, pharyngeal space, neck extension, and submandibular compliance.

5. Confirm endotracheal tube placement immediately with a reliable method such as carbon dioxide capnography.

BIBLIOGRAPHY

1. American Society of Anesthesiologists: Practice guidelines for management of the difficult airway: http://ecommerce.asahq.org/p-177-practice-guidelines-for-management-of-the-difficult-airway.aspx. Accessed October 13, 2011.

2. Berg RA, Hemphill R, Abella BS, et al: Part 5: adult basic life support: 2010 American Heart Association guidelines for cardiopulmonary resuscitation and emergency cardiovascular care. Circulation 122:S685-S705, 2010.

3. El-Orbany M, Connolly LA: Rapid sequence induction and intubation: current controversy. Anesth Analg 110:1318-1325, 2010.

4. Henderson J: Airway management in the adult. In Miller RD (ed): Miller's Anesthesia, 7th ed. New York, Churchill Livingstone, 2010, pp 1573-1610.

TRACHEOTOMY AND UPPER AIRWAY OBSTRUCTION

John E. Heffner, MD

CHAPTER 15

1. **What are the different techniques for a surgical airway?**
   - A *standard surgical tracheotomy* is an open surgical procedure that allows insertion of a tracheostomy tube into the trachea between cartilaginous rings.
   - A *percutaneous dilatational tracheotomy* refers to various procedures that have in common either a modified Seldinger technique for placing a modified tracheostomy tube or a forceps technique to cannulate and dilate tracheal tissue between cartilaginous rings.
   - A *cricothyroidotomy* is a technique for placement of an airway into the trachea through the cricothyroid space. A cricothyroidotomy can be performed as a surgical procedure through an incision, as a percutaneous procedure by a Seldinger technique, or as a needle cricothyroidotomy for emergency airway access.
   - A *minitracheotomy* allows percutaneous placement of a 7 F cannula through the tracheal rings to allow suctioning for patients with difficulty clearing airway secretions.

2. **How is a percutaneous tracheotomy performed?**
   Most intensivists perform a percutaneous tracheotomy by the Ciaglia technique, which inserts a needle into the trachea under bronchoscopic guidance. A guidewire placed through the needle allows insertion of a Teflon introducer dilator followed by a single curved dilator that increases in caliber from the tip to base where it matches the dimensions of a tracheostomy tube. After stomal dilatation, a tracheostomy tube loaded onto an introducer is inserted over the guidewire. Percutaneous tracheotomy can also be performed with insertion of a balloon catheter between tracheal rings that dilates a stoma tract after balloon inflation. Also, a specialized guidewire dilating forceps (called a GWDF technique) has a groove that allows loading of a guidewire onto forceps and dilates the trachea, threads the wire, and inserts a tracheostomy tube over the wire by a Seldinger technique. In the United States the Ciaglia technique with a curved, graduated dilator is the most commonly performed percutaneous procedure for tracheotomy.

3. **What are the indications for a tracheotomy?**
   The four indications for tracheotomy are as follows:
   - Maintenance of an airway for patients with upper airway obstruction
   - Airway access for suctioning retained secretions
   - Prevention of aspiration for patients with glottic dysfunction
   - Airway support for patients who require long-term mechanical ventilation

4. **What are the relative advantages of percutaneous versus surgical tracheotomy?**
   Both techniques provide effective and safe access to the trachea for critically ill patients. No high-quality prospective randomized trials have provided evidence that one procedure is better than the other. However, many studies suggest that percutaneous tracheotomy has advantages of shorter procedure time, ease of performing the procedure in the intensive care unit (ICU), decreased cost by avoiding use of an operating room (OR), provision of a tighter stoma that decreases stomal bleeding and improves tube stability, and lower risk of stomal infections. Performance of the procedure in the patient's ICU room also expedites an earlier tracheostomy by avoiding the need to schedule OR time. Some surgeons, however, perform standard surgical tracheotomies in the ICU, thereby diminishing the cost benefits of percutaneous tracheotomy by

avoiding use of the OR. When a standard surgical tracheotomy is done in the ICU, the ICU room must have adequate lighting and otherwise simulate the OR environment and resources.

5. **Is emergency tracheotomy the surgical procedure of choice in patients with apnea and acute upper airway obstruction when intubation fails?**
   No. Tracheotomy is acceptably safe when performed electively in an OR environment under controlled clinical conditions. Risks of surgical complications increase fivefold, however, when tracheotomy is applied in an emergency situation. An emergency cricothyroidotomy provides the greatest likelihood of successful airway placement with the lowest risks for complications in patients with acute upper airway obstruction who cannot undergo translaryngeal intubation. Advantages of a cricothyroidotomy in this setting derive from the superficial location of the cricothyroid membrane that allows rapid and reliable insertion of an airway.

6. **Can a percutaneous tracheotomy be safely performed in a patient receiving mechanical ventilation who requires positive end-expiratory pressure (PEEP)?**
   Percutaneous tracheotomy can be performed successfully in patients with severe respiratory failure who require high levels of PEEP. In one reported series the procedure was performed under bronchoscopic guidance for patients with mean PEEP levels of 16.6 cm H_2O (range, 12-20 cm H_2O), and no deterioration of arterial oxygen was found at 1 and 24 hours after the procedure compared with patients with lower PEEP levels (mean, 7.6 cm H_2O; range, 5.4-9.8 cm H_2O).

7. **How is a cricothyroidotomy performed?**
   The cricothyroid membrane is located approximately 2 to 3 cm below the thyroid notch. The membrane, which is typically 1 cm in height, lies below the vocal cords but within the subglottic larynx. For a surgical cricothyroidotomy, a scalpel is used to incise the overlying skin and stab the membrane. The resultant opening into the airway is enlarged with a spreader, allowing placement of a tracheostomy tube. For a percutaneous cricothyroidotomy, commercially available instruments designed for emergency situations allow puncture of the membrane and introduction of an airway cannula in one maneuver.

8. **Why do all patients not undergo a cricothyroidotomy rather than a tracheotomy?**
   For long-term airway access, cricothyroidotomy has a higher incidence of delayed airway damage; therefore most intensivists limit its use to 3 to 7 days after emergency insertion. If a patient remains ventilator dependent after this time, recommendations exist to convert a patient with a cricothyroidotomy to a tracheotomy. No studies exist to support this recommendation, however, with some studies reporting more airway injury in patients who undergo conversion.

9. **What are the complications of tracheotomy?**
   Tracheotomy complications are categorized as intraoperative, early postoperative, and late postoperative. The most common complications during each of these periods are listed in Box 15-1.

10. **What is the most lethal complication of tracheotomy in the perioperative period?**
    Inadvertent decannulation of a tracheostomy tube during the first 1 to 5 days after its placement represents a potentially lethal clinical event. It may take several days for a tracheostomy incision to form a stomal tract that allows blind replacement of a decannulated tracheostomy tube. Before this time, attempts to reinsert a tracheostomy tube will most likely create a false tissue tract in the pretracheal space. Subsequent attempts to provide ventilation to the patient with positive pressure through a misplaced tube result in profound cervical emphysema and external compression of the trachea, leading to asphyxia.

BOX 15-1. COMPLICATIONS OF TRACHEOTOMY

Intraoperative Complications	**Early Postoperative Complications**
Cardiopulmonary arrest	Hemorrhage
Hemorrhage	Subcutaneous emphysema
Pneumothorax and pneumomediastinum	Inadvertent decannulation
Recurrent laryngeal nerve injury	Wound infection
Tracheoesophageal fistula	Pneumonia
Tracheal ring fracture and herniation	Tube obstruction

Late Complications
Tracheal stenosis
Subglottic stenosis
Tracheoesophageal fistula
Tracheoinnominate fistula
Tracheocutaneous fistula

---

11. **Can patients with mechanical ventilation and a tracheostomy speak?**

Several techniques promote speech in patients with mechanical ventilation and a tracheostomy tube in place. Patients with low to moderate minute ventilation requirements can whisper intelligibly if the tracheostomy tube cuff is deflated to allow a small *cuff leak* during the ventilatory inspiratory cycle. Addition of a small amount of PEEP creates a leak throughout inspiration and expiration and promotes more continuous and spontaneous speech. A *speaking tracheostomy tube* provides an external cannula that directs compressed gas to exit the tube below the vocal cords, allowing some patients to communicate in whispered tones. An *electrolarynx* placed against the neck near the laryngeal cartilage generates a vibratory tone that can be articulated with practice into intelligible speech. If patients have limited or no mechanical ventilatory requirements, a one-way valve can be placed in-line between a fenestrated tracheostomy tube with a deflated cuff and the ventilator tubing, allowing expiration through the native airway and promoting intelligible speech.

12. **What is the ideal size of a tracheostomy tube for a patient?**

No one size is best for all patients because tracheal caliber and clinical situations vary. Small-caliber tubes may decrease the incidence of tracheal stenosis at the stoma site because of the smaller tracheal incision required. Unfortunately, small tubes present difficulties in airway suctioning, spontaneous ventilation, and fiberoptic bronchoscopy. Furthermore, small tubes have small cuffs that may damage the tracheal mucosa because they require high intracuff pressures to overdistend to seal the airway. Overly large tubes require wide stomas and prohibit adequate cuff inflation to cushion the rigid tube from the tracheal mucosa and to effectively prevent aspiration. The best approximation of ideal size requires the surgeon to select a tube with an outer diameter two thirds the inner caliber of the patient's trachea at the point of insertion.

13. **Why is it important to monitor intracuff pressures?**

Cuff pressures in excess of mucosal capillary perfusion pressures (usually 25 mm Hg) can rapidly cause mucosal ischemia and resultant tracheal stenosis. If a tracheostomy tube is underinflated (< 18 mm Hg) in a patient undergoing mechanical ventilation, the risks for aspiration and nosocomial pneumonia increase. Therefore most experts recommend maintaining cuff pressure between 18 and 25 mm Hg. Clinicians should notice the units of measurement of cuff pressures and make the appropriate conversion from centimeters of water to millimeters of mercury to allow adherence to cuff pressure standards (Cuff pressure in millimeters of mercury = [Measured cuff pressure in centimeters of water]/1.36).

14. **Should tracheostomy tube cuff pressures be directly measured periodically in patients undergoing mechanical ventilation?**
Frequent monitoring of cuff pressure with a pressure gauge provides the only measure to prevent tracheal injury at the cuff site. Other techniques, such as finger palpation of the external inflation bulb, minimal occlusive volume, and the tension felt by the operator on an inflating syringe, do not substitute for direct measurements of intracuff pressure.

KEY POINTS: MAINTAINING APPROPRIATE INTRACUFF ✓ PRESSURES

1. Maintain intracuff pressures between 18 mm Hg and 25 mm Hg.

2. Measure pressures routinely with a pressure gauge.

3. Check intracuff pressures when patients go for anesthesia.

4. Intracuff pressures can increase markedly when patients travel by air during helicopter transport.

15. **What precautions should be exercised in patients with a cuffed tracheostomy tube who undergo general anesthesia?**
Some volatile anesthetics, such as nitrous oxide, diffuse more rapidly into a tracheostomy tube cuff than oxygen or nitrogen can diffuse out and thereby increase intracuff pressures. During a 2-hour operation, cuff pressures may increase from 15 mm Hg to over 80 mm Hg, which can cause ischemic injury to the tracheal mucosa. Appropriate precautions include frequent monitoring of cuff pressures in the OR or inflation of the tube cuff at the outset of the surgical procedure with the anesthetic gas mixture administered to the airway. Similarly, cuff pressures should undergo frequent monitoring while patients with tracheotomies are transported by helicopter or planes between facilities because increased altitude and lower barometric pressures will also cause cuff overinflation.

16. **What should the clinician consider in any patient with airway hemorrhage after the first 48 hours of insertion of a tracheostomy tube?**
Bleeding within the first 48 hours of tracheotomy is usually a result of hemorrhage from the incisional wound. Any bleeding that develops more than 48 hours after surgery should suggest the possibility of a tracheoarterial fistula, which develops as a communication between the trachea and a major intrathoracic artery. The innominate artery is most commonly involved because it lies nine to 12 tracheal rings below the cricoid cartilage within reach of a tracheostomy tube. A tube cuff or tip can erode the anterior tracheal wall as a result of pressure necrosis and penetrate the artery. This life-threatening complication requires immediate evaluation by a thoracic surgeon capable of performing an emergency sternotomy for ligation of the innominate artery because massive hemorrhage often develops after an initial *herald* episode of mild to moderate bleeding.

17. **How should you evaluate a patient who continues to have cough and shortness of breath 2 months after removal of a tracheostomy tube?**
Although these symptoms often accompany underlying lung disease, they also occasionally represent the only clinical manifestations of a tracheoesophageal fistula. Patients undergoing positive-pressure mechanical ventilation may experience gastric distention or frequent belching. Recurrent aspiration of esophageal secretions may manifest as nosocomial

pneumonia. A tracheoesophageal fistula related to pressure necrosis by the tube cuff or catheter tip occurs as a complication of tracheostomy in fewer than 1% of patients. Risk factors include excessive tube movement, high ventilator inflation pressures, overinflated cuffs, prolonged intubation, diabetes mellitus, and the presence of a nasogastric tube.

Suspicion of a tracheoesophageal fistula should be pursued by endoscopic evaluation by either tracheoscopy or bronchoscopy, which can establish the location and extent of the fistula.

18. **Do ventilator-dependent patients wean faster from the ventilator if an *early* tracheotomy is performed?**
No high-quality studies have definitively answered the question whether routine, early tracheotomy within the first 4 to 7 days of mechanical ventilation improves clinical outcomes in general populations of critically ill patients. These studies are difficult to design because physicians demonstrate tremendous inaccuracies during the first 4 to 7 days of mechanical ventilation in identifying which patients may undergo successful extubation within the next few days, thereby avoiding an unnecessary tracheotomy. Accumulated evidence and expert opinion, however, conclude that tracheotomy versus continued endotracheal intubation does not improve survival or even shorten hospital stay. However, tracheotomy may improve patient comfort, decrease sedation needs, and allow earlier mobilization. There is no clear evidence that early tracheotomy decreases risk for ventilator-associated pneumonia.

19. **When should a tracheotomy be performed in a ventilator-dependent patient?**
Because clinical studies have not determined the ideal time to perform a tracheotomy in patients who require long-term mechanical ventilation, clinicians must individualize the decision. A tracheotomy should be considered when a patient appears likely to benefit from the procedure and when a need for prolonged ventilation becomes apparent. The potential benefits of tracheotomy over prolonged translaryngeal intubation include improved comfort, enhanced ability to communicate, and greater mobility. The *anticipatory* approach of estimating likely duration of ventilator dependency and likelihood of benefiting from tracheotomy is preferred over the routine selection of patients for tracheotomy after an obligate duration of intubation, which has been termed *calendar watching*.

20. **Describe the role of a fenestrated tracheostomy tube in the ICU.**
Newer fenestrated tracheostomy tubes with multiple small holes in their greater curvature assist speech and weaning from tracheostomy in spontaneously breathing patients without stimulating growth of granulation tissue. After removal of an inner cannula (if present) and deflation of the cuff, patients can breathe around the cuff and through the fenestrations in addition to the stoma to decrease airway resistance. Placement of a one-way valve, such as the Passy-Muir valve, on the tracheostomy tube allows patients to inhale through the tube and exhale out their native upper airways, thereby promoting speech.

Some physicians recommend placement of a fenestrated tracheostomy tube to facilitate gradual weaning toward decannulation. Others prefer to use a tracheal button, arguing that placement of a fenestrated tube interferes with spontaneous clearing of secretions through the native airway and delays decannulation.

21. **What is a tracheal button?**
Tracheal buttons, such as the Olympic tracheal button and the Montgomery tracheal button, assist weaning from a tracheostomy tube (Fig. 15-1). Designed as a straight, rigid, or flexible plastic or Silastic tube, tracheal buttons fit through the stoma to maintain its patency in case patients need suctioning or reinsertion of a tracheostomy tube through the tract. The button is ideal for patients with borderline ventilatory status because the distal end abuts the anterior tracheal wall and does not protrude into the airway to impede respiration or clearance of secretions by coughing.

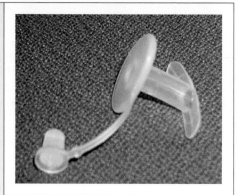

Figure 15-1. A tracheotomy stoma button. The silicone distal flange deforms to allow placement into the trachea through the stoma tract.

22. **Why do patients aspirate after removal of a tracheostomy tube?**
Scarring at the stoma site may interfere with the rostrocaudal excursion of the larynx during swallowing, which is necessary for glottic closure. In addition, prolonged diversion of ventilation away from the glottis causes attenuation of the vocal cord adductor response that is important in aspiration prevention.

23. **When should you suspect upper airway obstruction after decannulation of a tracheostomy tube?**
Patients may have upper airway obstruction immediately after decannulation, or obstruction may develop up to 6 months later. Causes of delayed upper airway obstruction after decannulation include subglottic or tracheal stenosis and tracheomalacia. These complications may progress slowly with a gradual narrowing of the airway causing exercise-induced dyspnea, which may be ascribed to the patient's underlying respiratory condition or recovery from critical illness. Stridor and other classic manifestations of upper airway obstruction may be later findings after the airway is narrowed more than 90%. Late presentations with sudden onset of stridor may result from acute illnesses, such as bronchitis or pneumonia that unveils the underlying airway narrowing.

BIBLIOGRAPHY

1. Allan JS, Wright CD: Tracheoinnominate fistula: diagnosis and management. Chest Surg Clin North Am 13:331-341, 2003.
2. Clec'h C, Alberti C, Vincent F, et al: Tracheostomy does not improve the outcome of patients requiring prolonged mechanical ventilation: a propensity analysis. Crit Care Med 35:132-138, 2007.
3. deBoisblanc BP: Percutaneous dilational tracheostomy techniques. Clin Chest Med 24:399-407, 2003.
4. Diaz-Reganon G, Minambres E, Ruiz A, et al: Safety and complications of percutaneous tracheostomy in a cohort of 800 mixed ICU patients. Anaesthesia 63:1198-1203, 2008.
5. Durbin CGJ: Tracheostomy: why, when, and how? Respir Care 55:1056-1068, 2010.
6. Francois B, Clavel M, Desachy A, et al: Complications of tracheostomy performed in the ICU: subthyroid tracheostomy vs surgical cricothyroidotomy. Chest 123:151-158, 2003.
7. Heffner JE: Toward leaner tracheostomy care: first observe, then improve. Respir Care 54:1635-1637, 2009.
8. Helm M, Gries A, Mutzbauer T: Surgical approach in difficult airway management. Best Pract Res Clin Anaesthesiol 19:623-640, 2005.
9. Hess DR: Tracheostomy tubes and related appliances. Respir Care 50:497-510, 2005.

10. Higgins KM, Punthakee X: Meta-analysis comparison of open versus percutaneous tracheostomy. Laryngoscope 117:447-454, 2007.

11. Mooty RC, Rath P, Self M, et al: Review of tracheo-esophageal fistula associated with endotracheal intubation. J Surg Educ 64:237-240, 2007.

12. O'Connor HH, White AC: Tracheostomy decannulation. Respir Care 55:1076-1081, 2010.

13. Scales DC, Ferguson ND: Early vs late tracheotomy in ICU patients. JAMA 303:1537-1538, 2010.

14. Scales DC, Thiruchelvam D, Kiss A, et al: The effect of tracheostomy timing during critical illness on long-term survival. Crit Care Med 36:2547-2557, 2008.

15. Silvester W, Goldsmith D, Uchino S, et al: Percutaneous versus surgical tracheostomy: a randomized controlled study with long-term follow-up. Crit Care Med 34:2145-2152, 2006.

16. Talving P, DuBose J, Inaba K, et al: Conversion of emergent cricothyrotomy to tracheotomy in trauma patients. Arch Surg 145:87-91, 2010.

17. Terragni PP, Antonelli M, Fumagalli R, et al: Early vs late tracheotomy for prevention of pneumonia in mechanically ventilated adult ICU patients: a randomized controlled trial. JAMA 303:1483-1489, 2010.

18. Wain JCJ: Postintubation tracheal stenosis. Semin Thorac Cardiovasc Surg 21:284-289, 2009.

19. Zias N, Chroneou A, Tabba MK, et al: Post tracheostomy and post intubation tracheal stenosis: report of 31 cases and review of the literature. BMC Pulm Med 8:18, 2008.

CHAPTER 16

CHEST TUBES

Gwendolyn M. van der Wilden, MSc, and David R. King, MD, FACS

1. **What is a chest tube?**
   A chest tube is properly called a tube thoracostomy and is generally used to evacuate the pleural space of air, blood, serous effusion, bile, chyle, pus, or other fluid. This allows reexpansion of the lung and reapposition of the visceral and parietal pleura.

2. **Define occult *pneumothorax*.**
   An occult pneumothorax occurs when air is trapped within the pleural space but is only identified on a computed tomography scan after a normal chest radiograph. It can be spontaneous or caused by blunt and/or penetrating trauma. Approximately 2% to 10% of trauma patients will be seen with an occult pneumothorax. There are generally no associated clinical findings.
   An occult pneumothorax requires reimaging to evaluate progression but usually does not require treatment. The need for positive-pressure ventilation (PPV) (i.e., a trip to the operating room for nonchest or nonlung injury) is *not* an indication for pleural space decompression of an occult pneumothorax.

3. **What is a hemothorax and how to treat it?**
   When blood accumulates in the pleural cavity because of blunt or penetrating injuries, it is called a hemothorax. Before a hemothorax can be detected on a standard chest radiograph, 200 to 300 mL of blood must be present within the pleural space. It takes up to 1 L before systemic signs of shock and hypoperfusion will manifest.
   Normally, large chest tubes (32 F-40 F) will be used to evacuate a large-volume hemothorax, and in 85% the bleeding will spontaneously cease and the lung will reexpand. Large amounts of undrained clotted blood (loculated hemothorax) will be evacuated via operative drainage (video-assisted thoracoscopic surgery). Thoracotomy is required only rarely (Box 16-1).

BOX 16-1. INDICATIONS FOR THORACOTOMY AFTER TRAUMA

1. Initial chest tube output of 1500 mL of blood (massive hemothorax)
2. Persistent drainage of 200 to 300 mL/hr

---

4. **What are the indications to place a chest tube?**
   See Table 16-1.

5. **What can go wrong? What are some possible complications?**
   See Box 16-2.

6. **How do you choose between a pigtail and a chest tube?**
   See Table 16-2.

TABLE 16-1. INDICATIONS TO PLACE A CHEST TUBE

IN ACUTE SETTING	NONACUTE

PTX
  ■ Spontaneous (when PTX is large or progressive and if the patient is clinically unstable)
  ■ Iatrogenic (when PTX is large or progressive or the patient is clinically unstable)
  ■ Tension PTX
  ■ Caused by penetrating chest trauma
Hemothorax
Esophageal rupture with leak into pleural space
	Drainage of pleural effusions
	Chylothorax
	Parapneumonic effusion or empyema
	Postoperative care (e.g., after coronary bypass, thoracotomy, or lobectomy)

PTX, Pneumothorax.

BOX 16-2. COMPLICATIONS OF CHEST TUBE PLACEMENT

Insertional
- Intercostal vessel laceration
- Lung parenchyma perforation
- Perforation of visceral organs (lung, heart, diaphragm, and intraabdominal organs)

Positional
- Postremoval pneumothorax
- Drain dislodgment
- Nonfunctional
  - Kinked
  - Clotted

Infective
- Empyema
- Insertion site wound infection

Intercostal Neuralgia

Reexpansion Pulmonary Edema

---

7. **What does the triangle of safety mean?**

A chest tube is placed in the anterior axillary or midaxillary line in the fifth to sixth intercostal space. This is between the anterior border of the latissimus dorsi, the lateral border of the pectoralis major muscle, the apex just below the axilla, and a line above the horizontal level of the nipple: the triangle of safety. It is a safe place because of its location above the diaphragm and a very thin chest wall musculature, allowing rapid and minimally painful insertion.

TABLE 16-2. CHOOSING BETWEEN A PIGTAIL AND A CHEST TUBE

INDICATION	SIZE (F)
Pneumothorax	
■ Large but stable	16-24
■ Large and unstable	Pigtail (14 or smaller)
■ With mechanical ventilation	24-28
■ Traumatic (blood in addition to air)	28-40
Hemothorax	32-40
Malignant pleural effusion	Pigtail (14 or smaller)
Parapneumonic effusion or empyema	10-14 or 16-24 (when fluid is viscous)

8. **Describe the consecutive steps of a tube thoracostomy.**
   - Prepare and drape the skin around the area of insertion.
   - Administer local anesthesia (1% lidocaine) if the patient is conscious.
   - Make a 2-cm incision over the rib, below the site chosen for insertion.
   - Create a subcutaneous tunnel, using blunt dissection, and spread the muscle using a Kelly clamp.
   - Gently enter the pleural space. Explore the space digitally to make sure you are in the pleural cavity and that no adhesions exist between the visceral and parietal pleura.
   - Insert the tube (clamped at the insertion end with the Kelly clamp), and place apically and anteriorly for a pneumothorax or superiorly and posteriorly for a hemothorax or pleural effusion.
   - After placement, secure the tube to the skin of the chest wall, and connect to an underwater seal with controlled negative pressure suction.

9. **How is a pigtail placed?**
   A pigtail is placed by using the Seldinger technique.
   - Prepare and drape the skin around the area of insertion.
   - Administer local anesthesia (1% lidocaine) if the patient is conscious.
   - Make a very small incision parallel to the intercostal space, just above the rib, and insert an introducer needle into the pleural space and aspirate for air or fluid.
   - Insert a guidewire through the introducer needle into the pleural space, again apical for a pneumothorax or inferiorly for a fluid collection.
   - Dilate the tract for the chest tube by passing a dilator(s) over the guidewire. Pass the chest drain with dilator over the guidewire into the pleural space, and finally remove guidewire and dilator, leaving the chest drain in place.
   - Make sure to suture the chest tube into place, and connect it to the drainage system.
   - The entire process may be facilitated by ultrasonographic guidance at the bedside.

10. **When can you remove a chest tube?**
    Before you remove the chest tube, there needs to be compliance with the following criteria:
    1. The lung must be fully expanded again (a final chest radiograph can be helpful here).
    2. During Valsalva maneuver or coughing, there must be no air leak in the water seal chamber.
    3. The daily amount of fluid drainage should be less than 100 to 200 mL.
    4. The fluid should be serous.
    5. The patient's clinical status has improved.

11. **How long does a trial of water seal need to be before chest tube removal?**
    For chest tubes placed for a traumatic pneumothorax, a prospective randomized trial demonstrated that a short 6-hour trial of water seal is adequate to allow occult air leaks to become clinically or radiographically apparent. Therefore chest tubes placed for a traumatic pneumothorax may safely be removed after 6 hours on water seal.

12. **Do you need to give the patient antibiotics before placing a chest tube?**
Much controversy exists as to whether prophylactic antibiotics should be administered before placing a chest tube. Some trials show a reduction in infections (especially in patients with penetrating chest trauma), but most trials showed no benefit. Generally, a single dose of gram-positive coverage should be given before chest tube placement if the tube is being placed for trauma. Otherwise, no antibiotics are indicated.

13. **What is a tension pneumothorax or hemothorax?**
See Box 16-3.

BOX 16-3. TENSION PNEUMOTHORAX OR HEMOTHORAX

What Happens:
- Complete lung collapse
- Tracheal deviation
- Mediastinal shift

All Leading to the Following:
- Decreased venous return to the heart
- Hypotension
- Respiratory distress

Clinical Signs:
- Dyspnea
- Tachypnea
- Hypotension
- Diaphoresis
- Distended neck veins

---

14. **Needle decompression or tube thoracostomy?**
Needle decompression is the standard of care, first-line treatment for a tension pneumothorax by rapidly decompressing the pleural space. A large-bore needle is inserted in the second intercostal space in the midclavicular line. Subsequently, a regular chest tube will be placed.
  In every other pneumothorax or hemothorax, a chest tube is generally recommended.
  For spontaneous pneumothoraces, two recent studies, however, showed that needle aspiration alone in the emergency department is at least as safe and effective as a regular chest tube. It also shortened the hospital length of stay.

15. **Why avoid rapid pulmonary reexpansion?**
Rapid reexpansion can lead to reexpansion pulmonary edema, which has a mortality rate as high as 20%. It occurs during rapid evacuation of a chronic pleural effusion or rapid reexpansion of the lung in case of a chronic pneumothorax.
  Treatment of this reexpansion pulmonary edema is supportive, because the disease is usually self-limited. Supplemental oxygen and sometimes mechanical ventilation are necessary.
  Asking the patient to breathe deeply and cough to expand the lung before applying suction can prevent rapid reexpansion from occurring.

16. **How do you place a chest tube in a patient who is either morbidly obese or has anorexia nervosa?**
- Morbidly obese: Because of enormous amounts of subcutaneous tissue, safe placement of a chest tube sometimes is not feasible. A recent case report describes the use of a minimally invasive trocar with laparoscope to visualize the intercostal musculature, parietal pleura, and lung parenchyma. The laparoscope was then withdrawn, and the tube was placed through the trocar and into the chest. Finally, the trocar was withdrawn, keeping the tube in place.

- Anorexia nervosa: Because of starvation, the total lung protein content, connective tissue, hydroxyproline, and elastin levels decrease. This makes the lung much more vulnerable to iatrogenic injury at the time of chest tube insertion. A review of the literature suggests that these patients may require higher levels of suction, promoting lung expansion, or switching from suction or water seal drainage to a Heimlich valve earlier in the patient's course.

17. **Do you place chest tubes in a population with high prevalence of human immunodeficiency virus (HIV) and tuberculosis?**
A high rate of complications is related to chest tube placement in patients with HIV, such as pneumonia, empyema, sepsis, and necrotizing fasciitis. A recent review of the literature suggested that conservative management of small pneumothoraces may be appropriate.

18. **What is the influence of PPV on chest tube removal?**
A retrospective study showed that PPV does not influence the rate of recurrent pneumothorax or chest tube placements after removal. Consequently presence of mechanical PPV is not an indication to leave a chest tube in place.

KEY POINTS: CHEST TUBES

1. All patients in unstable condition with hemothorax or pneumothorax should have a tube thoracostomy.

2. Large tubes are chosen for hemothorax, and smaller tube (or pigtails) are selected for pneumothorax or serous effusions.

3. Tube thoracostomy is not required for occult pneumothoraces.

4. Chest tubes placed for a traumatic pneumothorax may safely be removed after 6 hours on water seal.

5. Presence of mechanical PPV is not an indication to leave a chest tube in place.

BIBLIOGRAPHY

1. Ali HA, Lippmann M, Mundathaje U, et al: Spontaneous hemothorax: a comprehensive review. Chest 134:1056, 2008.

2. Baumann MH, Strange C, Heffner JE, et al: Management of spontaneous pneumothorax: an American College of Chest Physicians Delphi consensus statement. Chest 119:590, 2001.

3. Biffl WL, Narayanan V, Gaudiani JL, et al: The management of pneumothorax in patients with anorexia nervosa: a case report and review of the literature. Patient Safety in Surgery 4(1):1, 2010.

4. Dev SP, Nascimiento B Jr, Simone C, et al: Videos in clinical medicine. Chest-tube insertion. N Engl J Med 357: e15, 2007.

5. Ho KK, Ong ME, Koh MS, et al: A randomized controlled trial comparing minichest tube and needle aspiration in outpatient management of primary spontaneous pneumothorax. Am J Emerg Med 29:1152-1157, 2011.

6. Kim YK, Kim H, Lee CC, et al: New classification and clinical characteristics of reexpansion pulmonary edema after treatment of spontaneous pneumothorax. Am J Emerg Med 27:961-967, 2009.

7. Martino K, Merrit S, Boyakye K, et al: Prospective randomized trial of thoracostomy removal algorithms. J Trauma 46:369-371, discussion 372-373, 1999.

8. Maxwell RA, Campbell DJ, Fabian TC, et al: Use of presumptive antibiotics following tube thoracostomy for traumatic hemopneumothorax in the prevention of empyema and pneumonia—a multi-center trial. J Trauma 57:742, 2004.

9. Moore FO, Goslar PW, Coimbra R, et al: Blunt traumatic occult pneumothorax: is observation safe? Results of a prospective. AAST multicenter study. J Trauma 70:1019-1025, 2011.

10. Schaefer GP, Pender J, Toschlog EA, et al: Endoscopically-assisted tube thoracostomy placement in a super-morbidly obese patient with penetrating thoracoabdominal trauma. Am Surg 77:119-120, 2011.

11. Schulman CI, Cohn SM, Blackbourne L, et al: How long should you wait for a chest radiograph after placing a chest tube on water seal? A prospective study. J Trauma 59:92-95, 2005.

12. Sethuraman KN, Duong D, Mehta S, et al: Complications of tube thoracostomy placement in the emergency department. J Emerg Med 40:14-20, 2011.

13. Tawil I, Gonda JM, King RD, et al: Impact of positive pressure ventilation on thoracostomy tube removal. J Trauma 68:818-821, 2010.

14. Tebb ZD, Talley B, Macht M, et al: An argument for the conservative management of small traumatic pneumathoraces in populations with high prevalence of HIV and tuberculosis: an evidence-based review of the literature. Int J Emerg Med 3:391-397, 2010.

15. Zehtabchi S, Rios CL: Management of emergency department patients with primary spontaneous pneumothorax: needle aspiration or tube thoracostomy? Ann Emerg Med 51:91-100, 2008.

CHAPTER 17

BRONCHOSCOPY

Amy E. Morris, MD, and Lynn M. Schnapp, MD

1. **What is flexible bronchoscopy?**

   Bronchoscopy literally means "to see the airways." This procedure allows visualization of the upper airways, trachea, and bronchi. Flexible bronchoscopy uses a small-caliber fiberoptic scope, which is passed through the nose or mouth or through a tracheostomy or endotracheal tube (Fig. 17-1). The bronchoscope is then directed down the trachea to the main carina (Fig. 17-2) and beyond to the regions of interest. In most patients, the airways can be visualized at least to the segmental bronchi.

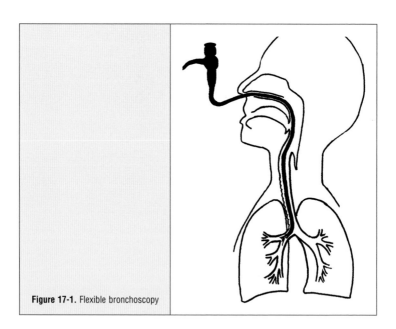

Figure 17-1. Flexible bronchoscopy

2. **How is flexible bronchoscopy performed?**

   Flexible bronchoscopy can be performed at the bedside or in a specialized suite with the assistance of a nurse and a respiratory therapist. Preparation includes the following steps:

   1. Set up suction equipment and monitoring for cardiac rhythm, blood pressure, and oxygenation saturation. Supplemental oxygen should be provided via nasal cannula or face mask.
   2. Numb the patient's nose and pharynx with topical lidocaine.
   3. Control cough and gag with small doses of short-acting narcotic and benzodiazepines.
   4. Lubricate the bronchoscope with topical lidocaine jelly. Anesthesia of the posterior pharynx, vocal cords, and carinas is particularly important because advancing the bronchoscope past these areas is most likely to cause the patient to cough.

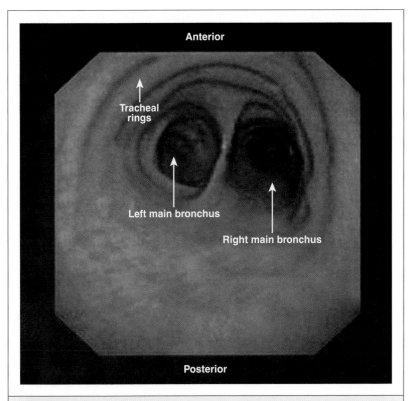

Figure 17-2. Bronchoscopic view of the distal trachea, main carina, and right and left main stem bronchi.

3. **How is rigid bronchoscopy different from flexible bronchoscopy?**
   Rigid bronchoscopy is performed while the patient is receiving mechanical ventilation under general anesthesia, with use of a rigid hollow tube that provides a large working channel and direct illumination. This technique is preferable to flexible bronchoscopy when more suction is required (as in the work-up of hemoptysis), during removal of some foreign bodies, during surgical or laser removal of endobronchial lesions, or in the placement of endobronchial stents. Rigid bronchoscopy requires a stable cervical spine and the ability to manipulate the mandible.

4. **When should intubation be considered before bronchoscopy?**
   A spontaneously breathing patient scheduled to undergo flexible bronchoscopy without an artificial airway or mechanical ventilation should be cooperative, without violent coughing, and without risk for upper airway obstruction or hypoxic or hypercarbic respiratory failure. Patients who do not fit these criteria, but in whom bronchoscopy is considered a necessary procedure, may require intubation before the procedure. In all cases, equipment for endotracheal intubation should be easily accessible.

5. **How is bronchoscopy different for patients receiving mechanical ventilation?**
   Fiberoptic bronchoscopy can be performed through an endotracheal tube at least 7.0 mm in diameter. Topical anesthesia is achieved with 1 to 2 mL of 2% lidocaine through the

endotracheal tube, followed by additional boluses as needed during the procedure. A silicone-based lubricant is applied to the bronchoscope to facilitate passage through the endotracheal tube. The bronchoscope will partially obstruct the tube, causing increased airway pressure and potentially increased air trapping. The respiratory therapist should set the ventilator on a volume mode with increased peak airway pressure limits to ensure that the patient receives adequate minute ventilation. The fractional concentration of oxygen in inspired gas (FiO_2) should be increased (usually to 1.0) because bronchoscopy and lavage may cause transient hypoxia.

6. **What are the indications for bronchoscopy in the intensive care unit (ICU)?**
   Bronchoscopy allows inspection of the airways, collection of samples from the lower airways, and performance of various interventions (Table 17-1). In the ICU, it is most commonly used to diagnose infection via bronchoalveolar lavage (BAL) or protected specimen brush. In BAL, the tip of the bronchoscope is wedged into a subsegmental bronchus while aliquots of saline solution (typically 30 mL each) are injected and aspirated into sterile traps. Alveolar contents are collected while the bronchoscope position prevents flooding of other regions of the lung. The protected specimen brush is a sterile brush with a gelatin cap that is inserted into a potentially infected area, agitated, then withdrawn and sent for culture.

TABLE 17-1.   INDICATIONS FOR BRONCHOSCOPY

STEP	INDICATION	GOAL
Inspection	Hemoptysis	Localize bleeding
		Search for endobronchial lesion
	Infection	Identify evidence of inflammation or pus
	Aspiration	Look for foreign bodies
	Mass	Look for endobronchial masses
	Chest trauma	Find evidence of airway injury
	Inhalational injury	Find evidence of airway injury
Sample collection	Pulmonary infiltrates (infectious)	Obtain samples for Gram stain, silver stain, bacterial cultures, and viral and fungal studies
	Pulmonary infiltrates (noninfectious)	Identify alveolar hemorrhage
		Check for eosinophilia (analyze cell count and differential)
	Mass or adenopathy	Perform transbronchial biopsy for cytologic or pathologic analysis
Interventions	Hemoptysis	Control bleeding
	Bronchial obstruction	Remove mucus or foreign bodies
		Perform laser removal of masses
		Place stent
	Alveolar proteinosis	Perform lavage
	Intubation	Visualize anatomy for tube placement

7. **What other kinds of samples can be collected by bronchoscopy?**
   - **Cytology brush:** An abrasive brush is agitated against potentially malignant tissue and then sent for cytologic analysis.
   - **Transbronchial biopsy:** The bronchoscope is advanced into subsegmental bronchi; then biopsy forceps are pushed past distal airways into the pulmonary parenchyma to obtain lung tissue. This technique may be used to diagnose infection (i.e., fungal disease), granulomatous diseases (i.e., sarcoidosis), or malignancy.
   - **Transbronchial needle aspiration:** A technique used in diagnosis and staging of cancer. A short, rigid needle is thrust through the airway wall, usually near the main carina, into subcarinal or paratracheal lymph nodes. Suction is then applied to aspirate cells, which are sent for cytologic evaluation.

8. **What is endobronchial ultrasound examination (EBU)?**
   EBU uses a specialized bronchoscope with a small ultrasound transducer at its tip. In addition to direct visualization of the airways, the operator is able to see ultrasound images of the tissue structures deep to the airway mucosa, such as lymph nodes and blood vessels. EBU allows more precise sampling of lymph nodes or other submucosal masses than blind needle aspiration. It is most often used in the staging of lung cancer, often in conjunction with transesophageal ultrasound examination. The sensitivity of these ultrasound-assisted biopsy techniques rivals surgical mediastinoscopy while incurring less morbidity, and they are increasingly used in this setting. It is not commonly performed in the ICU.

9. **List the absolute and relative contraindications for bronchoscopy.**
   - **Absolute contraindications:** These include an inability to maintain a patent airway during the procedure, such as in upper airway obstruction, laryngospasm, or intubation with a small endotracheal tube; an inability to oxygenate or ventilate adequately during bronchoscopy; active cardiac ischemia; malignant arrhythmias; and severe hemodynamic instability.
   - **Relative contraindications:** These include poor patient cooperation, elevated intracranial pressure, and severe coagulopathy. Patients with impending respiratory failure or laryngeal edema may undergo bronchoscopy more safely if the airway is secured by elective endotracheal intubation before the procedure.

10. **What are the potential complications of bronchoscopy?**
    Flexible bronchoscopy is generally a safe procedure. However, complications do occur, with an incidence in observational studies of 0.1% for death and 2% to 5% for major complications (Table 17-2). Sources of complication include the bronchoscopic procedure itself and anesthetic or sedative medications.

11. **What is the role of bronchoscopy in the diagnosis of community-acquired pneumonia (CAP)?**
    CAP in an immunocompetent host does not require microbiologic confirmation by bronchoscopy and is typically treated with empiric antibiotics. However, bronchoscopy may be indicated in patients with preexisting lung disease, immunosuppression, or critical illness because the microbiologic flora involved are less predictable. In patients whose conditions fail to respond to initial treatment for CAP, bronchoscopic sampling may provide information about bacterial resistance or atypical organisms or may reveal noninfectious etiologies.

12. **Discuss the role of bronchoscopy in a patient with immunosuppression and pulmonary infiltrates.**
    The differential diagnosis of pulmonary infiltrates in an immunocompromised host is broad and includes infectious and noninfectious etiologies. Bronchoscopy is particularly useful in these patients to guide therapy by collecting samples that are analyzed by culture, special stains, and serologies. These methods are useful in the diagnosis of infections with *Pneumocystis jiroveci*,

TABLE 17-2.   POTENTIAL COMPLICATIONS OF BRONCHOSCOPY

INTERVENTION	POTENTIAL COMPLICATION	PREVENTION
Passing bronchoscope through nose	Epistaxis, nasal discomfort	Topical anesthesia and vasoconstriction
Passing bronchoscope through pharynx	Gagging, emesis, aspiration	Topical anesthesia, benzodiazepines
Passing bronchoscope into trachea	Laryngospasm, cough, laryngeal trauma	Topical anesthesia
	Bronchospasm	Pretreatment with beta agonists
Bronchoalveolar lavage	Postprocedure fever	Minimize lung contamination by oral secretions
	Hypoxemia	Supplemental oxygen; good wedge technique
Cytology brush	Endobronchial hemorrhage	Avoid vascular lesions
Transbronchial biopsy	Hemorrhage	Avoid vascular lesions
	Pneumothorax	Avoid distal biopsies; consider fluoroscopy
Topical lidocaine administration	Arrhythmias, seizures	Use <7 mg/kg (<25 mL) of 2% lidocaine
Conscious sedation	Hypotension	Intravenous access, prehydration in patients with hypovolemia
	Respiratory depression	Avoid oversedation, stimulate patient

atypical bacteria, viruses (e.g., cytomegalovirus, respiratory syncytial virus, adenovirus), fungal pathogens, and mycobacteria. In addition, bronchoscopy and cytology may reveal alveolar hemorrhage, malignancy, or other noninfectious sources that are more common in this population than in immunocompetent hosts.

13. **What is the role of bronchoscopy in the diagnosis of ventilator-associated pneumonia (VAP)?**
The clinical diagnosis of VAP is made when a patient with an endotracheal tube has a fever or leukocytosis, a new infiltrate on chest radiograph, and purulent tracheal secretions. However, these findings are not specific for pneumonia. Patients who undergo invasive (i.e., bronchoscopic) diagnosis of VAP have less antibiotic use and a lower 14-day mortality rate than patients in whom the diagnosis made by using a noninvasive, empiric approach. Protected brush specimens or BAL samples are sent for quantitative cultures; $>10^3$ and $>10^4$ colonies of bacteria, respectively, are generally considered diagnostic for VAP. A recent meta-analysis and large randomized trial suggested that nonquantitative endotracheal culture diagnosis of VAP may be equivalent to bronchoscopy, but lack of adherence to antibiotic protocols and extensive exclusion criteria in these other studies call this conclusion into question. Regardless of the method of obtaining the culture, narrowing empiric antibiotic coverage on the basis of culture results is key to responsible antibiotic use in the ICU.

14. **What are the alternatives to bronchoscopy for sample collection in the diagnosis of VAP?**

When bronchoscopy is unavailable, quantitative bacterial culture can be obtained by other methods. Blind protected brush sampling or nonbronchoscopic *(mini)* BALs may be viable and less-expensive alternatives. In both techniques, a catheter is inserted into the airways without bronchoscopic guidance until resistance is encountered. Then the protected brush is extended or saline solution is injected to obtain the sample, and the apparatus is withdrawn. The data to support these alternative methods of quantitative culture are not as well established, but some studies comparing the quality of samples obtained by these methods with standard bronchoscopic techniques have demonstrated similar sensitivity and specificity.

15. **Are transbronchial biopsies safe in patients receiving mechanical ventilation?**

Several studies have demonstrated higher complication rates in patients with mechanical ventilation. The largest case series showed a pneumothorax rate of 14%, compared with a previously reported 5% rate in spontaneously breathing patients. Other studies identified higher rates of bleeding and pneumothorax in patients with mechanical ventilation who undergo biopsies. However, no study has identified increased mortality, and valuable diagnostic information is obtained in the majority of patients. Mechanical ventilation is therefore not an absolute contraindication to transbronchial biopsy, which may provide a less morbid alternative to surgical lung biopsy in selected cases.

16. **Can BAL be safely performed in patients with the acute respiratory distress syndrome?**

Yes—if the partial arterial oxygen tension (PaO_2) is at least 80 mm Hg (with an FiO_2 as high as 1.0) and if the patient has no absolute contraindications for bronchoscopy. A study in 110 patients with acute respiratory distress syndrome who met these criteria found no significant morbidity or mortality associated with bronchoscopy and BAL. The protocol included sedation to improve patient cooperation and to minimize coughing during the procedure. The investigators found a nonsustained decrease in oxygen saturation (to $< 90\%$) in 4.5% of patients. Mild, self-limited bleeding followed the procedure in 34% of patients.

17. **How is bronchoscopy used in the evaluation and management of hemoptysis in the ICU?**

Flexible bronchoscopy can localize the site of bleeding and allows direct intervention to control bleeding by using local injection of cold saline solution, epinephrine, vasopressin, or fibrin. If these efforts are unsuccessful, bronchoscopy may be used to tamponade bleeding by using either the tip of the bronchoscope or a Fogarty balloon placed through the suction channel. Death by hemoptysis occurs via suffocation rather than exsanguination, and these efforts can prevent compromise of the unaffected lung until definitive action is taken to control bleeding with use of interventional radiology embolization or surgical resection. When bleeding is brisk, the small suction channel of the flexible bronchoscope may be overwhelmed; in such cases, rigid bronchoscopy may be preferable. Additional tools are available via rigid bronchoscopy, particularly laser and electrocautery.

18. **What is the role of bronchoscopy in potential lung donors?**

Bronchoscopy is routinely performed in potential lung donors before the decision is made to perform lung explantation. The purpose of this examination is threefold. First, the anatomy of the airways is assessed. Second, the operator searches for evidence of airway trauma, infection, or previous aspiration; it is likely that the lungs will be rejected if any of these is found. Third, samples are taken and sent for culture so that the microbiologic flora (if present) can be known before transplantation and covered in the recipient, who will soon have heavy immunosuppression.

19. **Is bronchoscopy indicated for management of patients with acute lobar atelectasis?**
Probably not. Bronchoscopy can be effective in improving atelectasis; however, studies have shown no added benefit of bronchoscopy over vigorous respiratory therapy alone, in patients either with intubation or spontaneously breathing. However, bronchoscopic intervention may be beneficial in some cases for the removal of retained, inspissated secretions or foreign bodies.

20. **How is bronchoscopy used in performing tracheostomy in the ICU?**
Bronchoscopy is often performed during percutaneous tracheostomy in the ICU to confirm tracheal puncture, to avoid injury to the posterior tracheal wall, and to ensure appropriate tracheostomy tube placement. Several studies suggest that bronchoscopic guidance reduces complications from percutaneous tracheostomy.

KEY POINTS: BRONCHOSCOPY

1. Complications of bronchoscopy may occur because of topical anesthesia, sedation, or the procedure itself and include hypoxia, pneumothorax, and hypotension.

2. Bronchoscopy samples can be obtained via BAL, protected brush specimen, cytology brush, or biopsy.

3. Flexible bronchoscopy is most commonly used in the ICU to diagnose and guide antibiotic choices for VAP.

4. Chest physiotherapy appears to be as effective as bronchoscopy in treating atelectasis, although bronchoscopy has a role in retained, inspissated secretions or foreign bodies.

5. Bronchoscopy can be safely performed in patients with mechanical ventilation, including those with acute respiratory distress syndrome.

BIBLIOGRAPHY

1. Annema JT, van Meerbeeck JP, Rintoul RC, et al: Mediastinoscopy vs endosonography for mediastinal nodal staging of lung cancer: a randomized trial. JAMA 304:2245-2252, 2010.
2. Fagon JY: Diagnosis and treatment of ventilator-associated pneumonia: fiberoptic bronchoscopy with bronchoalveolar lavage is essential. Semin Respir Crit Care Med 27:34-44, 2006.
3. Kreiker ME, Lipson DA: Bronchoscopy for atelectasis in the ICU. A case report and review of the literature. Chest 124:344-350, 2003.
4. Oberwalder M, Weis H, Nehoda H, et al: Videobronchoscopic guidance makes percutaneous dilational tracheostomy safer. Surg Endosc 18:839-842, 2004.
5. Shorr AF, Susla GM, O'Grady NP: Pulmonary infiltrates in the non-HIV-infected immunocompromised patient: etiologies, diagnostic strategies, and outcomes. Chest 125:260-271, 2004.
6. Steinberg KP, Mitchell DR, Maunder RJ, et al: Safety of bronchoalveolar lavage in patients with adult respiratory distress syndrome. Am Rev Respir Dis 148:556-561, 1993.
7. Wahidi MM, Rocha AT, Hollingsworth JW, et al: Contraindications and safety of transbronchial lung biopsy via flexible bronchoscopy. A survey of pulmonologists and review of the literature. Respiration 72:285-295, 2005.
8. Wang KP, Mehta AC (eds): Flexible Bronchoscopy, 2nd ed. Oxford, United Kingdom, Blackwell Science, 2004.

CHAPTER 18

PACEMAKERS AND DEFIBRILLATORS

Scott C. Streckenbach, MD, and Kenneth Shelton, MD

1. **What are the general principles of cardiovascular implantable electronic device (CIED) management according to the Heart Rhythm Society (HRS)–American Society of Anesthesiologists Consensus Statement published in 2011?**
    The primary recommendation is that the best prescription for the perioperative care of a patient with a CIED will be realized when that patient's CIED team (electrophysiologist or cardiologist) is asked for advice and that advice is effectively communicated to the procedural team. Thus the surgical or procedural team should communicate with the CIED team to identify the type of procedure and the likely risk of electromagnetic interference. The CIED team should then communicate with the procedure team to deliver information about the pacer or implantable cardiac defibrillator (ICD) and recommendations for the perioperative management of the patient and the device.

2. **How can one differentiate a pacemaker from an ICD?**
    Occasionally a patient is seen initially without information about his or her CIED. A critical step is to determine whether the device is a pacemaker or an ICD. The patient may be able to tell you why the device was inserted, and this might provide a clue. However, if the patient's history cannot help, the patient's chest radiograph can. The ICD leads, unlike pacer leads, have one or two radiodense shocking coils. Because of the shocking coils, the ICD leads (Fig. 18-1) are much larger than the pacer leads (Fig. 18-2), and this can be appreciated radiographically.

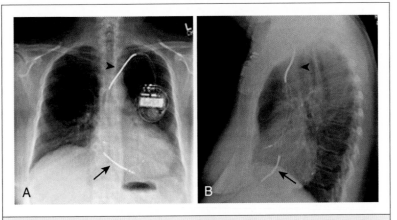

Figure 18-1. Chest radiographs (PA and lateral) of an ICD. *A,* The SVC shocking coil *(arrowhead)* and the RV shocking coil *(arrow)* are radiopaque and differentiate the ICD from a pacemaker radiographically. *B,* An atrial pace/sense lead is also noted in the lateral view.

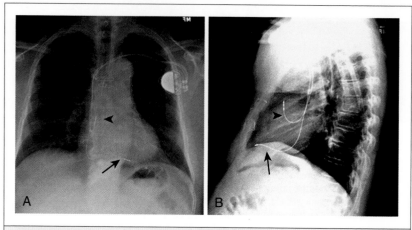

Figure 18-2. Chest radiographs (*A* and *B*, PA and lateral) of a pacemaker. The atrial pacing lead *(arrowhead)* and the ventricular pacing lead *(arrow)* are smaller in diameter and less radiopaque than the leads associated with an ICD.

3. **Describe the five-letter pacemaker code.**
   - First position of the code reflects the chamber(s) in which stimulation occurs.
   - Second position refers to the chamber(s) in which sensing occurs.
   - Third position refers to the mode of setting (or how the pacemaker responds to a sensed event).
   - Fourth position reflects rate modulation.
   - Fifth position of the code indicates whether multisite pacing is present.
     See Table 18-1.

TABLE 18-1. THE GENERIC PACEMAKER CODE				
POSITION 1: CHAMBER(S) PACED	**POSITION 2: CHAMBER(S) SENSED**	**POSITION 3: RESPONSE TO SENSING**	**POSITION 4: PROGRAMMABILITY**	**POSITION 5: MULTISITE PACING**
0 = none	**0** = none	**0** = none	**0** = none	**0** = none
A = atrium	**A** = atrium	**I** = inhibited	**R** = rate modulation	**A** = atrium
V = ventricle	**V** = ventricle	**T** = triggered		**V** = ventricle
D = dual (A + V)	**D** = dual (A + V)	**D** = dual (I + T)		**D** = dual (A + V)

4. **What is cardiac resynchronization therapy (CRT)?**
   CRT is the term applied to reestablishing synchronous contraction between the left ventricular (LV) free wall and the ventricular septum in an attempt to improve LV efficiency and subsequently to improve functional class. The LV pacing lead is usually placed in the posterior lateral LV wall via the coronary sinus circulation. CRT may be used with a pacemaker or with an ICD. Indications typically include a low ejection fraction ($<35\%$), a prolonged QRS (>120 ms), and class IV heart failure symptoms.

5. **Explain the following pacemaker codes: DOO, VVI, DDD, and DDDRV.**
   - DOO = asynchronous atrial-ventricular pacing with a constant A-V interval. Atrial and ventricular pacing pulses are emitted regardless of the underlying cardiac rhythm.
   - VVI = ventricular-only antibradycardia pacing. Failure of the ventricle to produce an intrinsic event within the appropriate time window results in ventricular pacing. With no atrial sensing, there can be no atrioventricular (AV) synchrony in a patient with any intrinsic atrial activity.
   - DDD = dual-chamber antibradycardia pacing. In the absence of intrinsic activity in the atrium, it will be paced. After any sensed or paced atrial event, an intrinsic ventricular event must occur before the expiration of the AV timer or the ventricle will be paced.
   - DDDRV = dual-chamber antibradycardia pacing with rate response mode circuitry (to increase the paced rate in setting of increased metabolic demand) and biventricular pacing capability.

6. **What is the effect of placing a magnet on a pacemaker?**
   Most pacemakers respond to a magnet by converting to an asynchronous pacing mode (e.g., DOO if pacer mode is DDD or VOO if VVI) at a rate dependent on the device manufacturer and the remaining battery life. For adequately charged pacemakers, the following is generally true:
   - Medtronic pacemakers pace at 85 beats/min
   - Biotronik, 90 beats/min
   - St. Jude, 98 beats/min
   - Boston Scientific, 100 beats/min
     See Table 18-2.

7. **What is a rate response mode?**
   The normal heart rate response to increased physiologic demand is linearly related to oxygen demand and consumption. Circumstances requiring heart rate variation include exercise, emotion, anxiety, baroreflexes, vagal maneuvers, hypovolemia, fever, and anemia. The two more common types of rate response sensors are based on patient movement (accelerometer) and patient ventilation (transthoracic impedance monitor). Both of these sensors will increase the patient's paced rate when increased patient activity is detected. The rate at which the heart rate changes is programmable. Typically the heart rate increase is slightly delayed and will return to baseline several minutes after the increased activity subsides. Because both of these sensors can be falsely activated in a hospital, knowledge of their presence is ideal for optimal patient care.

8. **How should one manage a patient with a minute ventilation rate response mode?**
   Minute ventilation sensors should be disabled while the patient is in the hospital. These monitors measure the rate and depth of change in thoracic impedance measured between one of the intracardiac pacing leads and the pulse generator. Increased frequency and depth of change in transthoracic impedance increase the paced rate to match the patient's increased minute ventilation. Electrocautery, ventilators, and patient monitors that measure respiratory rate can all cause significant changes in the paced rate if the minute ventilation rate response mode is not disabled. The rate response mode may be disabled with a device-specific programmer or a magnet.

9. **What is the mode switch function?**
   The automatic mode switching function describes the capability of a pacemaker both to detect the presence of atrial tachyarrhythmias and to switch automatically from a triggering mode (e.g., DDD) to a nontriggering one (e.g., DDI) for the duration of the tachyarrhythmia. In this manner, mode switching prevents the pacemaker-mediated conduction of an atrial tachyarrhythmia to the ventricle. During a mode switch the lower rate limit of the pacer usually increases (to compensate for the loss of the atrial kick). This may be interpreted as a pacer malfunction if the clinician is not aware of this programmed function.

TABLE 18-2. MAGNET EFFECT ON PACEMAKERS

MANUFACTURER TONE	BEGINNING OF LIFE	ERI	PROGRAMMABLE	AUDIBLE
Medtronic*	85 (DOO or VOO)	65 (VOO)	No	No
Biotronik†			Yes	No
Async	90 (DOO or VOO)	VOO 80		
Sync	No change	See user manual		
Auto	VOO for 10 beats	See user manual		
ELA/Sorin	96 (DOO or VOO)	80 (DOO or VOO)	No	No
St. Jude‡	98.6 (VOO or DOO) 100 (VOO or DOO)	86.3 <85	Yes§	No
Boston Scientific (Guidant)	100	85 (DOO or VOO)	Yes¶	No

Modified from Crossley GH, Poole JE, Rozner MA, et al: Heart Rhythm Society/American Society of Anesthesiologists expert consensus statement on the perioperative management of patients with implantable defibrillators, pacemakers and arrhythmia monitors: facilities and patient management. Heart Rhythm 8:1151-1152, 2011.

ERI, Elective replacement indicator.

*Medtronic Pacers: The first three beats with magnet application are at 100 beats/min with a change in pulse width on the third pulse to test threshold safety margin; then the rate is 85 beats/min.

†Biotronik pacers may be programmed in one of three ways as noted earlier.

‡St. Jude pacemakers: The majority of the devices will pace at 98.6 beats/min. Some models, including Microny, Microny II, Regency, Accent, Nuance, and Anthem, pace at 100 beats/min.

§Rarely, St. Jude pacers may be programmed to *off,* which will render the pacer unresponsive to a magnet.

¶Rarely, Boston Scientific pacers may be programmed to *electrogram,* and magnet application will not result in asynchronous pacing.

Table applies only to pacemakers not associated with an ICD. The pacemaker component of an ICD is unresponsive to a magnet.

10. **What is the rest or sleep mode?**

During sleep the native heart rate decreases to provide a *physiologic rest period* for the heart. Absence of this nightly rest period can decrease overall LV function. Therefore pacemaker manufacturers have created algorithms that allow the lower rate limit to drop at night. For example, the St. Jude rest mode activates whenever perceived patient activity decreases sufficiently for a specified duration of time. If the patient takes a nap at noon, approximately 15 minutes into the nap, the pacer's rate might drop from 60 to 50. The Medtronic sleep mode is time based, rather than activity based, and will activate at a preset time, e.g., from 9 PM to 5 AM. Both of these functions could confuse the clinician were he or she not aware of their presence.

11. **What is the "R on T" phenomenon, and how is it related to commotio cordis?**

"R on T" refers to a phenomenon in which the R wave of the QRS complex (ventricular depolarization) falls within the vulnerable part of ventricular repolarization (the 10- to 20-ms window immediately preceding the peak of the T wave) of the preceding electrical complex on the electrocardiogram (ECG). Clinically, this phenomenon may result in ventricular tachycardia or fibrillation, especially if the myocardium is ischemic or metabolically compromised. This was originally described in humans in 1949 by F. H. Smirk in an article reviewing 17 cases. Clinically, this explains the risk associated with using asynchronous pacing in a patient whose intrinsic heart rate exceeds the paced rate. If a ventricular pacing pulse were delivered in the high-risk window of the T wave, ventricular fibrillation (VF) can occur. A blow to the anterior chest in this similar vulnerable period can induce VF, an event known as commotio cordis.

12. **What are the options for establishing temporary cardiac pacing?**
The least invasive method is transcutaneous pacing with external defibrillation pads. This method typically provides ventricular pacing (either demand or asynchronous depending on the clinician's choice). It is uncomfortable for the awake patient because the energy required to pace is high. The next option is transesophageal pacing. This is typically limited to patients who have an endotracheal tube in place. Transesophageal pacing typically provides atrial pacing unless the pacing probe is inserted as far as possible. Transesophageal pacing uses long pulse wave duration to minimize the amount of pacing energy (and therefore prevent esophageal injury). This eventuates in significant ECG artifact. The last and most invasive method of pacing is transvenous pacing either directly through an introducer or through a pacing pulmonary artery (PA) catheter. This method is the most reliable and most flexible, that is, it allows the clinician to A-pace, V-pace, or AV-pace. This method should be used by only those with significant experience.

13. **How does an ICD work?**
An ICD detects the QRS signal of the patient. It measures the time between each QRS event. If the time interval is short (e.g., less than 300 ms, which corresponds to a heart rate of 200), the event counter starts. If there is a predetermined number of short intervals (e.g., eight out of the next 12), the device detects VF. Once detected, the ICD will charge its capacitors to 34 to 40 J. Most devices will reconfirm the presence of the dysrhythmia and then shock the patient. If the dysrhythmia has resolved during the reconfirmation period, the shock will be discharged slowly rather than shocking the patient, but battery life will be diminished.

14. **What is the meaning of primary and secondary prevention with respect to ICD therapy?**
Primary prevention refers to the use of an ICD to protect a patient from sudden cardiac death (SCD) who has already had a documented episode of VF, syncope. Secondary prevention refers to use of an ICD to prevent SCD in a patient at high risk for the same, for example, patients with hypertrophic obstructive cardiomyopathy and a family history of SCD, with an ejection fraction less than 35%, with arrhythmogenic right ventricular dysplasia, and with congenital long QT syndrome.

15. **How will a magnet affect an ICD?**
Magnets usually inhibit the antitachycardic functions (defibrillation, cardioversion, antitachy pacing) of an ICD. Because each manufacturer's device has some idiosyncrasies, the clinician must be sure to understand how the magnet will affect the ICD before magnet application. Removal of the magnet usually returns the ICD to the active mode. The rare exception may be the Boston Scientific Prizm series. Boston Scientific devices emit a tone for as long as the magnet is on the ICD. Medtronic devices emit a tone for approximately 30 seconds. The other devices do not emit a tone. A few devices in a specific scenario might not respond to a magnet. See Table 18-3.

TABLE 18-3.   MAGNET EFFECT ON ICDS

MANUFACTURER	MAGNET EFFECT ON TACHYCARDIA DETECTION OR THERAPY	IS MAGNET PROGRAMMABLE?	MAGNET EFFECT ON PACING	AUDIBLE TONE?
Biotronik	Suspends*	No	No	None
ELA/Sorin	Suspends	No	Rate changes to 96 beats/ min	None
Medtronic	Suspends	No	No	Yes[†]
St. Jude Medical	Suspends[‡]	Yes	No	None
Boston Scientific	Suspends[§]	Yes	No	Yes[§]

Modified from Crossley GH, Poole JE, Rozner MA, et al: Heart Rhythm Society/American Society of Anesthesiologists expert consensus statement on the perioperative management of patients with implantable defibrillators, pacemakers and arrhythmia monitors: facilities and patient management. Heart Rhythm 8:1153-1154, 2011.

*With the Biotronik Lumax series, a magnet placed continuously over the device will disable therapy for a maximum of 8 hours, at which point therapy will be reactivated. To inhibit ICD therapy for longer than 8 hours, the device will have to be reprogrammed.

[†]All devices have an audible tone for up to 30 seconds with magnet applied correctly over the device. A steady tone indicates normal magnet placement. Beeping or oscillating tones indicate an *alert* condition; notify ICD care provider.

[‡]There are two programmable options for St. Jude ICDs:
- Magnet response is nominally programmed to *normal* (ON).
- Response can be programmed to *ignore* (OFF).

[§]Boston Scientific (formally Guidant and CPI) devices are the most complex in this regard. For Vitality, Renewal, Confient and Livian, and Cognis and Teligen devices, there are two programmable modes:
- Enable magnet use ON/OFF
- Patient triggered EGM ON/OFF

If the device has *enable magnet use* programmed ON, then magnet application will inhibit the tachy detection–therapy function. This will be signaled by an audible R-wave synchronous tone. Removal of the magnet will reactivate the tachy detection–therapy. If the device has *enable magnet use* programmed OFF, then there will be no response of the ICD to the magnet; in other words, the tachy detection–therapy will remain ON. There will be no audible tone.

For Prizm/2/HE devices, there are three modes:
- Enable magnet use ON/OFF
- Change tachy mode with magnet ON/OFF
- Patient triggered EGM ON/OFF

The *enable magnet use* mode is the same as given earlier. If the device has the change tachy mode with magnet programmed ON, a very dangerous situation may occur. Magnet application for 30 seconds or more will permanently turn OFF tachy detection–therapy. The audible tone will convert from R-wave synchronous beeping to a continuous tone. The device will not reactivate when the magnet is removed.

16. **Why is it important to know when pacemaker or ICD leads were inserted when considering placement of a central line?**

Pacer or ICD leads take time to become secure after implantation. Active fixation leads, which are screwed into the endocardium, usually become secure sooner than passive fixation leads, which rely more on fibrosis for fixation. Coronary sinus leads used for cardiac resynchronization therapy are the least likely to become fixed. Insertion of a central line, and particularly a PA line, may dislodge the newly implanted lead. As a general rule of thumb, the risk for lead dislodgment is highest in the first 3 months after lead implantation. If a central line or PA catheter must be inserted in the first 3 months it should be done with fluoroscopic guidance, and backup pacing or defibrillation should be immediately available. All pacemakers and ICDs should be evaluated by a qualified specialist after the line has been inserted to ensure proper function.

17. **What are the considerations for placement of a PA line in a patient with an active ICD?**

Caution is required whenever a guidewire is inserted into a heart in the presence of an active ICD. Contact between the guidewire and a sensing electrode (atrial or ventricular) can trigger antitachycardia therapy. If the therapy is a defibrillation, the guidewire can short the proximal coil to the distal coil and cause serious myocardial injury. To prevent this, ensure that the guidewire does not enter the ventricle or temporarily inhibit the ICD.

18. **What are the considerations for cardioversion or defibrillation in a patient with a CIED?**

Theoretically, high-voltage cardioversion or defibrillation can damage the pulse generator or the lead-myocardial interface. It appears that application of the defibrillation pads in the anterior-posterior orientation with the anterior pad >8 cm away from the pulse generator minimizes this risk. The HRS recommends that if a patient with a CIED undergoes cardioversion or defibrillation, especially in an emergency setting, the patient's device should be interrogated before the patient's discharge from the intensive care unit.

19. **How can electrocautery affect a pacemaker?**

Electrocautery can affect a pacemaker in multiple ways. It can inhibit pacer output if the device is set in a demand mode. This is typically noticed if the electrocautery is sensed by the ventricular lead. The pulse generator presumes that the cautery signal represents native ventricular depolarization and inhibits the ventricular pacing output. Electrocautery may also be sensed by the atrial lead. This can cause rapid atrial tracking (rapid ventricular pacing in response to a sensed high intrinsic atrial rate) to rates up to the upper rate limit of the pacer if the pacemaker is in the DDD mode. Atrial oversensing can also trigger a mode switch if the atrial sensing rate exceeds the mode switch cutoff rate (usually 170-180 beats/min). Finally, prolonged electrocautery can temporarily convert the pacer to a noise reversion mode or cause permanent pacemaker reset.

20. **How can electrocautery affect an ICD?**

Electrocautery in close enough proximity to the ICD leads (usually anywhere above the umbilicus) can be detected by the ICD as VF. The device will charge and shock the patient shortly thereafter if the electrocautery persists during the reconfirmation period (at the end of the charging period). It takes only 3 to 4 seconds of electrocautery to fool the ICD into detecting VF. It takes another 4 to 10 seconds to charge before a shock can be delivered. If, during the reconfirmation period, electrocautery has stopped, the device will abort the charge. Although a shock is prevented, battery depletion is not. The electrocautery will also affect the ICD's pacer function as described previously.

KEY POINTS: PACEMAKERS AND DEFIBRILLATORS

How will a magnet affect a pacemaker?

1. Magnets convert most pacemakers to an asynchronous pacing mode.

2. The magnet-induced paced rate is manufacturer specific.

3. No audible sound is emitted from a pacemaker when a magnet is applied.

4. Magnets will inhibit any programmed rate response mode in a pacemaker.

5. Magnets do not affect the pacemaker component of an ICD.

WEBSITES

www.biotronik.com
www.bostonscientific.com
www.hrsonline.org (Heart Rhythm Society)
www.medtronic.com
www.PacerICD.com (go to Fundamentals of Pacing, Fundamentals of ICDs, or IBHRE Exam Study
  Materials for video lectures)
www.sjm.com

BIBLIOGRAPHY

1. American Society of Anesthesiologists: practice advisory for the perioperative management of patients with cardiac implantable electronic devices: pacemakers and implantable cardioverter-defibrillators. Anesthesiology 114:247-261, 2011.

2. Crossley GH, Poole JE, Rozner MA, et al: Heart Rhythm Society/American Society of Anesthesiologists expert consensus statement on the perioperative management of patients with implantable defibrillators, pacemakers and arrhythmia monitors: facilities and patient management. Heart Rhythm 8:1114-1152, 2011.

3. Lau W, Corcoran S, Mond H: Pacemaker tachycardia in a minute ventilation rate-adaptive pacemaker induced by electrocardiographic monitoring. Pacing Clin Electrophysiol 29:438-440, 2006.

4. Manegold JC, Israel CW, Erlich JR, et al: External cardioversion of atrial fibrillation in patients with implanted pacemaker or cardioverter-defibrillator systems: a randomized comparison of monophasic and biphasic shock energy application. Eur Heart J 28:1731-1738, 2007.

5. Maron BJ, Estes M: Medical progress: commotio cordis. N Engl J Med 362:917-927, 2010.

6. Smirk FH: R waves interrupting T waves. Br Heart J 11:23-36, 1949.

CHAPTER 19

CIRCULATORY ASSIST DEVICES

*Joseph L. Weidman, MD, Michael N. Andrawes, MD,
and Michael G. Fitzsimons, MD, FCCP*

1. **What is an intraaortic balloon pump (IABP)?**

   An IABP is a circulatory assist device that is intended to provide temporary support to a failing heart through synchronized actions focused on reducing afterload and augmenting diastolic pressure. The system consists of a 30- to 50-cc balloon attached to a catheter. The balloon rests within the lumen of the descending thoracic aorta, and the attached catheter snakes through the arterial vessels and out of the body. The catheter relays with an external console that monitors aortic pressure tracings and electrocardiogram (ECG) readings, inflating the internal balloon at the appropriate times. The balloon is inflated with either helium or CO_2. Although CO_2 has higher blood solubility and therefore a lower risk of embolization, helium is much more common because it is less dense and thus allows for faster filling and emptying times.

2. **How is an IABP placed?**

   The most common site for IABP placement is through the femoral artery via the percutaneous Seldinger technique. Alternative insertion sites include the iliac, axillary, and subclavian arteries. IABP placement may even be accomplished via the ascending aorta, as is occasionally done after cardiac surgery. The ideal location for the tip of the balloon is just distal to the aortic arch, 1 to 2 cm beyond the left subclavian artery. The other end of the balloon should sit proximal to the takeoff of the celiac axis. Correct positioning of the balloon may be confirmed at the time of placement with either transesophageal echocardiography or fluoroscopy. Alternatively, confirmation may be performed after placement by chest radiograph.

3. **What are the physiologic benefits of an IABP?**

   The IABP is designed to inflate during diastole and deflate during systole. It is beneficial in both phases of the cardiac cycle. During diastole, inflation of the balloon displaces blood proximally, increasing perfusion pressure to the coronary arteries and the critical vessels branching off the aortic arch. Perfusion and blood flow are equally improved in the aorta distal to the balloon through the vessels supplying blood to the mesentery and the lower extremities. In systole, deflation of the balloon creates a relative negative space within the aorta, which reduces afterload. As a consequence, not only is cardiac function improved because of lower systemic resistance, but the duration of isovolumic contraction, the most energy-demanding phase of the cardiac cycle, is also reduced.

4. **How is IABP inflation-deflation timing coordinated?**

   Three possible triggers are routinely used to coordinate IABP inflation-deflation:
   - An ECG tracing
   - An arterial pressure waveform or
   - A pacing device if one is being used

   The ideal time for balloon inflation is at the onset of diastole, just after the closure of the aortic valve. This moment corresponds with the middle of the T wave on the ECG and with the dicrotic notch on the arterial pressure waveform. Deflation ideally occurs at the beginning of systole, which coincides with the peak of the R wave on the ECG and with the point just before the systolic upstroke on the arterial waveform. Alternatively, an option exists to run the IABP in an asynchronous mode with a preset rate, but it is not routinely used. Some recent work has also been done on real-time dicrotic notch detection and prediction, which may improve IABP timing during both regular and irregular rhythms.

5. **What are the indications for IABP placement?**
Clinical conditions that may warrant initiation of IABP therapy can be broken down into two categories: those conditions that would benefit primarily from increased diastolic coronary perfusion and those that would benefit mainly from afterload reduction. Balloon pumps may also be placed prophylactically in high-risk patients undergoing cardiac surgery (Box 19-1). The most common condition for which IABP therapy is started is cardiogenic shock, accounting for approximately 20% of placements.

BOX 19-1. IABP COUNTERPULSATION INDICATIONS

Increase Diastolic Coronary Perfusion
Persistent angina refractory to medical management
Infarction or ischemia associated with PCI
Cardiogenic shock after MI

Afterload Reduction
Acute ventricular septal rupture
Acute mitral regurgitation (chordae tendineae or papillary muscle rupture)
Cardiogenic shock refractory to medical management
Bridge to transplantation
Postbypass low cardiac output syndrome

Prophylactic Indications
Significant left main coronary artery disease before surgery
High-risk PCI
High-risk electrophysical intervention (i.e., ablation of ventricular fibrillation)
High-risk patient undergoing noncardiac surgery

MI, Myocardial infarction; *PCI*, percutaneous coronary intervention.

6. **What are the contraindications for IABP placement?**
The contraindications for IABP placement include the following:
- Anything more than mild aortic insufficiency
- Aortic aneurysm
- Aortic dissection
- Severe aortoiliac atheromatous disease

7. **What are possible complications of IABP placement?**
Complications related to the use of IABP fall into three categories: vascular, positional, and balloon related.
- Vascular complications include hematoma, perforation, dissection, pseudoaneurysm, and aneurysm. These complications are more common in patients with diabetes or peripheral vascular disease, smaller patients, and females.
- Complications resulting from poor positioning of the balloon occur because of the unintended obstruction of arterial branches of the aorta. This results in compromised perfusion and/or ischemia to the upper extremities and brain (if the balloon is too proximal) or to the mesentery (if it is too distal). Poor positioning may also affect the ability of the IABP to maximally augment.
- Balloon-related complications include balloon rupture, gas embolization, and traumatic thrombocytopenia. Of note, the reduction in platelet count caused by the balloon pump is predictable and generally stabilizes after 4 days. Platelet counts return to baseline quickly after removal of IABP.

8. **Is anticoagulation necessary in a patient with an IABP?**
The standard of care is that unfractionated heparin be used for anticoagulation during the IABP use, with a partial thromboplastin time goal from 50 to 70 seconds. Data are inconclusive as to whether this actually decreases the incidence of limb ischemia; however, in animal studies an immobile, deflated balloon is subject to thrombus after 20 minutes. For this reason, a nonfunctional balloon should be removed promptly, as soon as anticoagulation has been reversed. For elective removals, it is recommended that heparin be discontinued for at least 2 hours before taking out the device.

9. **How is a patient weaned from an IABP?**
The amount of aid a balloon pump provides can be quantified as a ratio of native beats to assisted beats. Full support is at a ratio of 1:1; that is, every beat is augmented by the IABP. Weaning occurs by gradually reducing the augmentation ratios to 1:2, 1:4, and then 1:8. Time intervals between step-downs vary depending on the clinical situation but are usually on the order of 1 to 6 hours. During weaning, cardiac output, blood pressure, mental status, kidney function, and distal perfusion should be monitored. It may be necessary to commence inotropic support as the patient is weaned. As the augmentation ratio is reduced, the risk of thrombus formation on the balloon pump increases. Weaning may also be accomplished by gradually reducing the balloon volume.

10. **What are the clinical criteria for IABP removal?**
Actual criteria will vary from institution to institution. Some of the recommended clinical criteria for the removal of an IABP include the following:
- Cardiac index (CI) greater than 2 $L/min/m^2$
- Drop in CI less than 20% during IABP weaning
- Absence of angina
- Increase in left ventricular pressure no greater than 20%
- Minimal inotropic support
- Urine output greater than 30 mL/hr
- Heart rate less than 100 beats/min
- Fewer than six ectopic ventricular beats/min
- An absence of signs of systemic hypoperfusion
  Systemic anticoagulation should be corrected before removal of IABP. The balloon pump may be removed percutaneously, with direct pressure being applied to the insertion site for 20 to 30 minutes after removal to assure hemostasis.

11. **What does an arterial pressure tracing look like in a patient being assisted by an IABP?**
The function of an IABP during diastole results in an upswing in the arterial pressure waveform during diastole (Fig. 19-1). The peak created by the IABP is known as the peak augmented diastolic pressure. The upstroke created by the IABP, if timing is correct, correlates with the dicrotic notch. When maximal augmentation by the IABP is achieved, the peak augmented diastolic pressure will be greater than the unassisted systolic pressure. In addition, both the assisted aortic end-diastolic pressure and the assisted systolic pressure should be less than their unassisted counterparts, given appropriate IABP function.

12. **What are some common problems that may result in failure of the IABP to augment?**
Failure to augment may be associated with inadequate inflated balloon size, as a result of either a balloon that is too small or an appropriately sized balloon that is being underfilled. A balloon that is misplaced too proximal or too distal in the aorta might not augment appropriately, as will a balloon inadvertently placed in a false passage (possibly created with insertion of the device). Inappropriate timing of inflation or deflation of the balloon, which may be

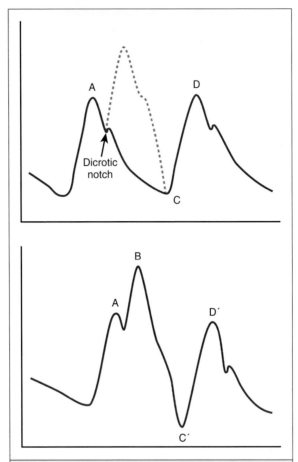

Figure 19-1. *A* and *D,* Unassisted systolic pressure. *B,* Diastolic pressure augmentation by IABP. *C,* Unassisted aortic end-diastolic pressure. *C',* Assisted (post-IABP) aortic end-diastolic pressure. *D',* Assisted (post-IABP) systolic pressure.

either too early or too late, can impair augmentation (Table 19-1). Improper timing can often be corrected manually on the IABP console. Both tachycardia and bradycardia can result in failure to augment, as can certain arrhythmias such as atrial fibrillation. These rhythm abnormalities should be treated to allow for maximal effectiveness of the IABP.

13. **What is a ventricular assist device (VAD)?**
    In general, VADs are mechanical devices inserted to assist cardiac function by offloading part or all of the pumping responsibilities from the ventricle. Placement of a VAD can be done on the left side of the heart to assist in left ventricular function (LVAD) or on the right to help with the right ventricle (RVAD). The presence of both an LVAD and an RVAD is referred to as biventricular support (BiVAD). A number of different VAD constructs exist, with major differentiators being pulsatile versus nonpulsatile (continuous), external versus internal, degree of assistance provided, ability to help the left or right sides, and the length of time it can be used (Table 19-2). Some VADs are intended to be used for only 7 to 10 days, whereas others have supported patients over a 7-year period.

TABLE 19-1. RESULTS OF INAPPROPRIATE IABP TIMING	
TIMING ISSUE	**RESULTING PROBLEMS**
Early IABP inflation	Early closure of aortic valve
	Reduction in cardiac output
	Increased oxygen consumption
Early IABP deflation	Reduction in duration of diastolic augmentation
Late IABP inflation	Reduction in duration of diastolic augmentation
Late IABP deflation	Increased left ventricular afterload
	Increased oxygen consumption

14. What are the end goals of VAD therapy?

When deciding the appropriateness of the placement of a VAD, multiple potential end points can be considered. A "bridge to recovery" implies temporary VAD support with the goal of removal once native heart function has returned to baseline. A "bridge to transplant" refers to the use of a VAD in a patient who ultimately will be best served by cardiac transplantation but needs temporary assistance until a heart becomes available. The term "destination therapy" means that the VAD itself is the end goal of therapy. These patients have irreversible heart conditions and, for whatever reason, are not eligible for transplantation.

15. What are common insertion sites for LVADs and RVADs?

The VAD inflow cannula permits blood flow to the pump. It may be placed in the right atrium for an RVAD or the left ventricular apex for an LVAD. After going through the VAD pumping system, blood exits the device by passing through an outflow conduit. For RVADs, these are attached and direct blood flow to the pulmonary artery. In LVADs, outflow conduits are usually connected to the ascending aorta. Newer LVADs exist that are entirely endovascular and sit across the aortic valve.

16. What are the differences between pulsatile and continuous systems?

VADs (and other bypass systems) can be divided into two classes based on how they eject blood from the pump: in a continuous or pulsatile manner. Continuous systems typically use either a roller pump or a rotary pump to propel blood. Roller pumps, while inexpensive, generally require continuous vigilance and tend to cause more trauma to blood components. As a result, they are rarely, if ever, used in VADs. The more practical rotary pumps can be further divided into subsets based on mechanism of propulsion. The two most popular subsets are axial (screwlike) and radial (better known as centrifugal) systems. Pulsatile VAD systems generally provide blood propulsion via pneumatically or electrically powered systems. They do not cause significant hemolysis and may have physiologic advantages over nonpulsatile systems. They do, however, tend to be larger than many of the continuous systems.

17. What is the difference between extracorporeal membrane oxygenators (ECMO) and a VAD?

ECMOs are very similar to VADs in terms of function and placement. The major difference is that a VAD requires that lung function be adequate, because it only helps with cardiac function, depending on the lungs to oxygenate the blood. ECMO incorporates an oxygenator that maintains gas exchange and is often used in clinical situations in which the lungs are no longer effective in maintaining oxygenation or ventilation. In addition, unlike ECMO, many VADs are created with portability in mind.

TABLE 19-2. SPECIFIC TYPES OF VADS

DEVICE	PROPULSION	LOCATION	DURATION	RV/LV/BIV	FLOWS (L/MIN)	ANTICOAGULATION
First generation						
Thoratec PVAD	Pneumatic pulsatile	Extracorporeal	Long	RV/LV/BiV	6.5	Yes
Thoratec IVAD	Electric pulsatile	Intracorporeal	Long	RV/LV/BiV	6.5	Yes
Thoratec HeartMate I	Electric pulsatile	Intracorporeal	Long	LV	10	Low dose
Abiomed BVS5000/AB5000	Pneumatic pulsatile	Extracorporeal	Short	RV/LV/BiV	5	Yes
Second generation						
Impella LP 2.5/5.0/LD	Microaxial continuous	Intravascular	Short	LV	2.5 or 5	Yes
Levitronix CentriMag	Centrifugal continuous	Extracorporeal	Short	RV/LV/BiV	9	Yes
TandemHeart Percutaneous VAD	Centrifugal continuous	Extracorporeal	Short	LV	5 to 8	Yes
Thoratec HeartMate II	Axial continuous	Intracorporeal	Long	LV	10	Yes
Jarvik 2000 Flowmaster	Axial continuous	Intracorporeal	Long	LV	7	Yes
MicroMed HeartAssist 5 (DeBakey)	Axial continuous	Intracorporeal	Long	LV	5	Yes

18. **What are the indications for VAD placement?**

No consensus criteria exist for placement of a VAD. As a result, indications may vary from institution to institution. However, guidelines do exist to assist in optimizing patient selection. Examples of parameters for consideration include the following:

- CI index <2.0 L/min/m^2
- Systemic hypotension with mean arterial pressure <60 mm Hg
- Cardiac filling pressures of either right or left atrium >20 mm Hg
- Persistent inotropic dependence
- VO$_2$ <12 mL/kg/min, all despite maximal medical therapy

Consideration may also be given to patients with cardiac function that is better than the parameters listed above but who have unpredictable, life-threatening ventricular arrhythmias.

19. **Are there any contraindications for VAD placement?**

Absolute contraindications include abdominal aortic aneurysm >5 cm, active systemic infection or high chronic risk of infection, severe pulmonary dysfunction (FEV$_1$ <1 L or fixed pulmonary hypertension), impending or actual renal or hepatic failure (including portal hypertension), inability to tolerate anticoagulation, or neurologic or psychosocial inability to manage the device. Clearly, a coexisting terminal condition contraindicates VAD placement in a patient. Relative contraindications include age >65 years (unless minimal other risk factors); chronic kidney disease; severe chronic malnutrition; morbid obesity; or uncorrected aortic regurgitation, mitral regurgitation, or mitral stenosis.

20. **What are the significant potential complications that arise in patients with VAD?**

Potential complications are not infrequent and can be quite serious. They include infection, neuroembolic events, and bleeding. As model design has improved, complication rates have decreased. Infection rates lessened with exploration of alternative implantation possibilities, which sometimes eliminated the need for external or peritoneal device components. Also, innovations such as sintered (ridged) titanium materials, which promote pseudointimal layer formation on device components, as well as investigation into axial flow mechanics, helped to decrease the incidence of thromboembolic complications. Secondary organ failure (respiratory, renal) does remain a concern.

21. **Why is it that some patients who have an LVAD placed subsequently require an RVAD?**

Placement of an LVAD offloads some or all of the work from the left ventricle (LV). It can increase cardiac output and, as a result, can increase the venous return to the right side of the heart. This increase in right ventricular preload, along with relative emptying of the LV, can result in right ventricle (RV) distention, worsening RV contractility, and increased tricuspid regurgitation, all of which decrease RV performance. In addition, significant cytokine release can take place during the perioperative period. These cytokines can mediate pulmonary vasoconstriction, placing further stress on the RV. It is important to monitor vigilantly for impending right-sided heart failure, because appropriate pharmacologic intervention may help avoid additional surgical intervention.

22. **List the major considerations for intensive care unit management of a patient directly after an LVAD placement.**

As mentioned above, optimization of right-sided heart function is critical in the immediate postoperative period after LVAD placement. Inotropic support should be provided as needed to assure optimal right-sided heart functionality. In addition, decreasing right-sided heart afterload through the pulmonary vasculature can assist in right side of the heart performance. Milrinone, epoprostenol, and nitric oxide all have their roles in decreasing pulmonary vascular resistance in the postoperative period. With continuous-flow LVADs, it is also important to be aware of and know how to manage suction events. These events can occur when the LVAD motor speeds are high and LV venous return is low and are a result of a collapse of the ventricle.

23. How is weaning attempted with a VAD?

When a VAD is used as a bridge to recovery, intermittent assessments of cardiac function are performed to determine the necessity of continued VAD use. Methods of assessment include echocardiography, radionucleotide studies, and exercise stress testing. As cardiac function returns, the amount of support, defined by the VAD flow rate, can gradually be reduced. As VAD flows are decreased, the RV is allowed to fill with blood. Indicators of successful weaning include ability to maintain cardiac output without increases in central venous or pulmonary artery pressures. Once VAD support is weaned to 1 to 1.5 L/min, patients can usually tolerate discontinuation of the device.

24. Do percutaneous options exist for ventricular assist systems?

Several devices can be inserted by cardiologists in the catheterization laboratory or percutaneously by cardiac surgeons in the operating room. One such device is the tubelike Impella, which is situated across the aortic valve and functions via a nonpulsatile axial flow mechanism. Another is the TandemHeart. This VAD's inflow cannula is placed through the femoral vein, and then, via transseptal puncture, the tip of the cannula is positioned in the left atrium. Blood taken from the left atrium is pumped by an external centrifugal pump back into circulation via a cannula placed in the femoral artery. Flow rates up to 5 L/min can be achieved, and this temporary device is typically used as a bridge to recovery or *bridge to bridge* therapy.

25. What is the REMATCH study?

The REMATCH (Randomized Evaluation of Mechanical Assistance for the Treatment of Congestive Heart Failure) study refers to a landmark *New England Journal of Medicine* article from Columbia University in 2001, entitled "Long-term Use of a Left-Ventricular Assist Device for End-stage Heart Failure." The article described a 3-year study in 129 patients with end-stage heart failure who were ineligible for cardiac transplantation and were randomly assigned to two groups: optimal medical management or LVAD therapy. Data showed significant increases in 1- and 2-year survival rates of the LVAD cohort over the medical therapy cohort (52% vs. 25% and 23% vs. 8%, respectively), as well as an improved quality of life.

KEY POINTS: CIRCULATORY ASSIST DEVICES

1. IABPs are effective circulatory assist devices because they both increase diastolic blood pressure and decrease systolic afterload.

2. Improper timing and/or positioning of an IABP can result in ineffective blood pressure augmentation, as well as ischemia to the end organs of blocked arteries.

3. VADs are placed for three reasons:

   a. As a bridge to recovery

   b. As a bridge to cardiac transplantation

   c. As a therapeutic means in and of itself (destination therapy)

4. A VAD can be used to augment the left ventricle (LVAD), the right ventricle (RVAD), or both ventricles (BiVAD) but does not help with blood oxygenation or ventilation.

5. With the incidence in the United States of new patients with cardiac failure each year being around 40,000 and the number of available donor hearts at only 2300, the role of VADs continues to increase, as does the pressure for technologic and industrial advances that will increase device effectiveness and improve the safety profile.

BIBLIOGRAPHY

1. Campbell LJ: Circulatory assist devices. In Parsons PE, Wiener-Kronish JP (eds): Critical Care Secrets, 4th ed. Philadelphia, Mosby, 2007.

2. Cohn L: Perioperative/intraoperative care. In Cardiac Surgery in the Adult, 3rd ed. New York, McGraw-Hill, 2008, pp 507-533.

3. Counterpulsation Applied: An Introduction to Intra-Aortic Balloon Pumping. Mount Holly, N.J., Arrow International, Inc, 2005, pp 1-158.

4. Donelli A, Jansen JR, Hoeksel B, et al: Performance of a real-time dicrotic notch detection and prediction algorithm in arrhythmic human aortic pressure signals. J Clin Monit Comput 17:181-185, 2002.

5. Fitzsimons MG, Ennis S, MacGillivray T: Devices for cardiac support. In Sandberg WS, Urman R, Ehrenfeld J (eds). The MGH Textbook of Anesthetic Equipment, 1st ed. Philadelphia, Saunders, 2010, pp 247-262.

6. Laish-Farkash A, Hod H, Matetzky S, et al: Safety of intra-aortic balloon pump using glycoprotein IIb/IIIa antagonists. Clin Cardiol 32:99-103, 2009.

7. Mitter N, Sheinberg R: Update on ventricular assist devices. Curr Opin Anaesthesiol 23:57-66, 2010.

8. Nicolosi AC, Pagel PS: Perioperative considerations in the patient with a left ventricular assist device. Anesthesiology 98:565-570, 2003.

9. Rose EA, Gelijns AC, Moskowitz AJ, et al: Long-term use of a left ventricular assist device for end-stage heart failure. N Engl J Med 345:1435-1443, 2001.

10. Roy SK, Howard EW, Panza JA, et al. Clinical implications of thrombocytopenia among patients undergoing intra-aortic balloon pump counterpulsation in the coronary care unit. Clin Cardiol 33:30-35, 2010.

11. Slaughter MS, Rogers JG, Milano CA, et al: Advanced heart failure treated with continuous-flow left ventricular assist device. N Engl J Med 361:2241-2251, 2009.

12. Song X, Throckmorton AL, Untaroiu A, et al: Axial flow blood pumps. ASAIO J 49:355-364, 2003.

13. Thunberg CA, Gaitan BD, Arabia FA, et al: Ventricular assist devices today and tomorrow. J Cardiothorac Vasc Anesth 24:656-680, 2010.

14. Trost JC, Hillis LD: Intra-aortic balloon counterpulsation. Am J Cardiol 97:1391-1398, 2006.

15. Wilson SR, Mudge GH Jr, Stewart GC, et al: Evaluation for ventricular assist device: selecting the appropriate candidate. Circulation 119:2225-2232, 2009.

ACUTE BACTERIAL PNEUMONIA

Kenneth Shelton, MD, Jeanine P. Wiener-Kronish, MD, and Aranya Bagchi, MBBS

CHAPTER 20

1. **Define severe community-acquired pneumonia (CAP).**
   Patients with severe CAP have a number of characteristics:
   - They generally require intensive care unit (ICU) management.
   - They have a higher mortality rate than do patients with nonsevere CAP.
   - Empiric antibiotic therapy in this group differs from that in patients with nonsevere CAP.

   Unfortunately, it is challenging to *prospectively* identify this cohort of patients. Of particular concern are patients who are initially triaged as having nonsevere CAP but subsequently need ICU admission (up to 50% of ICU admissions fall under this category in some studies). Such patients tend to have a higher mortality than equally sick patients who have been directly admitted to an ICU. A number of severity of illness scores have been developed to help define severe CAP, a popular one being derived from the joint Infectious Diseases Society of America–American Thoracic Society guidelines for the management of CAP in adults (Box 20-1), which incorporates elements of the **c**onfusion, **u**rea, **r**espiratory **r**ate, and **b**lood pressure (CURB) score. By this definition, patients with *one* major criterion *or* three minor criteria are designated as having severe CAP. Another widely used score is the Pneumonia Severity Index (PSI). However, none of these scores has been prospectively validated for individual patients. Clinical judgment remains critical; do not blindly follow scores! In recent years other approaches have been explored to identify patients with severe CAP; some of these are discussed below (see answer 9 on recent developments in CAP).

BOX 20-1. CRITERIA FOR SEVERE CAP

Minor Criteria
Respiratory rate >30 breaths/min
PaO_2/FiO_2 ratio <250
Multilobar infiltrates
Confusion or disorientation
Uremia (blood urea nitrogen level >20 mg/dL)
Leukopenia (WBC count <4000 cells per cubic millimeter as a result of infection alone)
Thrombocytopenia (platelet count $<100,000$ cells per cubic millimeter)
Hypothermia (core temperature $<36°$ C)
Hypotension requiring aggressive fluid resuscitation

Major Criteria
Invasive mechanical ventilation
Septic shock with the need for vasopressors

Modified from Mandell LA, Wunderink RG, Anzueto A, et al: Infectious Diseases Society of America/American Thoracic Society consensus guidelines on the management of community-acquired pneumonia in adults. Clin Infect Dis 44(2 Suppl):S27-S72, 2007.

2. **Which pathogens most commonly cause severe CAP?**
   The most common causes of severe CAP in ICU patients are (in order of decreasing incidence):
   - *Streptococcus pneumoniae*
   - *Legionella* sp
   - *Haemophilus influenzae*
   - Gram-negative rods (GNRs)
   - *Staphylococcus aureus*
   - *Pseudomonas aeruginosa*

   Pathogens are identified in fewer than 50% of cases. Specific therapy seems to have no particular advantage over empiric therapy *except* in ICU patients, where every effort should be made to reach an etiologic diagnosis and tailor therapy accordingly. A typical work-up for an ICU patient would include sputum Gram stain in addition to sputum and blood cultures. In addition urinary antigen tests for *Legionella* and pneumococcus should be considered. More invasive tests, such as bronchoscopic bronchoalveolar lavage, may be considered in individual patients.

3. **How is CAP diagnosed? Are the sputum Gram stain and culture diagnostically helpful for CAP?**
   CAP is diagnosed on the basis of the presence of a constellation of signs and symptoms (fever, cough, sputum production, and pleuritic chest pain) **with radiographic evidence of lung infiltrates**. Sputum Gram stain and culture can be obtained noninvasively and are inexpensive diagnostic tests. A sputum Gram stain specimen is considered satisfactory for interpretation when the neutrophil count is ≥25 and the epithelial cell count is ≤10 per low power field. Gram staining can have multiple benefits: the results can be used to broaden coverage to cover microorganisms that are typically not covered by empiric regimens, such as *S. aureus* and GNRs. Conversely, the absence of characteristic Gram stains and sputum culture is a strong argument for presumptively excluding *S. aureus* and GNRs as probable etiologies for the pneumonia. In addition, a positive Gram stain validates a subsequent sputum culture. Keep in mind the diagnostic limitations of sputum Gram stain and culture, including the inability to visualize atypical organisms, contamination by oral flora, and the difficulty encountered by some patients to provide adequate specimens.

4. **What determines the selection of empiric antimicrobial therapy for patients with severe CAP?**
   The initial empiric antibiotic regimen for patients in the ICU with severe CAP is outlined in Box 20-2. Broadly speaking, the general principles of antibiotic therapy are as follows:
   - Empiric treatment should cover the three most common pathogens causing severe CAP (see earlier), all atypical pathogens, and most relevant Enterobacteriaceae species. Broader coverage may be considered depending on epidemiologic considerations (see later).
   - Combination therapy is better than monotherapy.
   - Recent data strongly suggest that benefits of combination therapy are maximal when one of the agents is a macrolide. Therefore a macrolide should be included in all regimens unless a compelling reason exists not to do so.

5. **What risk factors would prompt broader coverage?**
   Risk factors that would prompt broader antimicrobial coverage can be conveniently considered by the type of organism to be covered:
   - ***Pseudomonas:*** Long-term oral steroids (>10 mg prednisone per day), underlying bronchopulmonary disease (bronchiectasis), severe chronic obstructive pulmonary disease, alcoholism, frequent antibiotic use. Note that the strongest justification for beginning antipseudomonal coverage is the presence of a consistent Gram stain of blood or sputum.

BOX 20-2. RECOMMENDED EMPIRIC ANTIBIOTICS FOR SEVERE CAP IN THE ICU

A β-lactam (cefotaxime, ceftriaxone, or ampicillin-sulbactam)
PLUS
Either azithromycin
OR
A respiratory fluoroquinolone (levofloxacin [750 mg], moxifloxacin, or gemifloxacin)
If *Pseudomonas* is a consideration:
An antipneumococcal, antipseudomonal β-lactam (piperacillin-tazobactam, cefepime, imipenem, or meropenem)
PLUS
Either ciprofloxacin or levofloxacin (750 mg)
OR
The previously mentioned β-lactam **plus** an aminoglycoside **and** azithromycin
OR
The previously mentioned β-lactam **plus** an aminoglycoside **and** an antipneumococcal fluoroquinolone (for penicillin-allergic patients, substitute aztreonam for previously mentioned β-lactam)
If CA-MRSA is a consideration: Add vancomycin or linezolid.
Penicillin allergy: Substitute **aztreonam** for the previously mentioned β-lactams.

Modified from Mandell LA, Wunderink RG, Anzueto A, et al: Infectious Diseases Society of America/American Thoracic Society consensus guidelines on the management of community-acquired pneumonia in adults. Clin Infect Dis 44(2 Suppl):S27-S72, 2007.

- **Community-acquired methicillin-resistant *S. aureus* (CA-MRSA):** Patients with cavitary lesions, patients who have had influenza, patients receiving long-term dialysis, intravenous (IV) drug abusers, and patients who have had recent antibiotic treatment (particularly with fluoroquinolones). Although a consistent sputum Gram stain is a strong reason to cover for *S. aureus*, a blood Gram stain may be falsely positive because of contamination.
- **Anaerobes:** Aspiration in the setting of alcohol or drug intoxication or in the presence of gingival disease or esophageal dysmotility.
- **Drug-resistant *S. pneumoniae* (DRSP):** Age >65 years, alcoholism, immunosuppression, exposure to antibiotics in the last 3 months (class-specific resistance), comorbidities, and exposure to children attending day care. In most cases, typical empiric therapy for CAP in the ICU (Box 20-2) should cover DRSP.

6. **When should antibiotics be initiated, and what is the optimal duration of treatment?**
Although earlier guidelines recommended initiation of antibiotics within 4 hours of diagnosis of CAP, more recent evidence has prompted a subtle shift in the current guidelines. They still recommend prompt initiation of antibiotics but do not specify a window of greatest benefit. The guidelines do recommend that patients admitted through the emergency department (ED) should receive their first dose of antibiotics while in the ED.
  Patients with CAP should be treated for a **minimum** of 5 days, should be afebrile for 48 to 72 hours, and should not have more than one CAP-associated sign of clinical instability (Box 20-3) before stopping treatment.

7. **When is it safe to switch a patient to oral therapy?**
Conversion to oral therapy may be considered in the hemodynamically stable patient who is improving clinically, can take oral medications, and has a normally functioning gastrointestinal tract.

> **BOX 20-3. CRITERIA FOR CLINICAL STABILITY IN RESOLVING CAP**
>
> Temperature $< 37.8°$ C
> Heart rate < 100 beats/min
> Respiratory rate < 24 breaths/min
> Systolic blood pressure > 90 mm Hg
> Arterial oxygen saturation $> 90\%$ or $PO_2 > 60$ mm Hg with room air

Modified from Mandell LA, Wunderink RG, Anzueto A, et al: Infectious Diseases Society of America/American Thoracic Society consensus guidelines on the management of community-acquired pneumonia in adults. Clin Infect Dis 44(2 Suppl):S27-S72, 2007.

8. **Discuss CA-MRSA infections.**
   An important trend in public health is the increasing prevalence of CA-MRSA infections. Here we will briefly discuss some of the salient features caused by CA-MRSA, particularly with reference to CAP.
   - CA-MRSA infections have reached epidemic proportions in the United States and are now the most common cause of infections in patients coming to EDs. The majority of infections are skin and soft tissue infections; approximately 2% of CA-MRSA infections present as CAP.
   - CAP caused by CA-MRSA tends to be severe, with a high incidence of necrotizing pneumonia, shock, respiratory failure, lung abscess, and empyema.
   - CA-MRSA–induced pneumonia has typically been more common in children but is being increasingly seen in adults. Risk factors that predispose to CA-MRSA were mentioned earlier.
   - CA-MRSA differs from the more typical health care–associated MRSA (HA-MRSA) at the genomic, phenotypic, and epidemiologic levels. However, CA-MRSA strains are beginning to be increasingly represented in nosocomial infections, and the distinctions between them may be blurring.
   - Two key features that distinguish CA-MRSA from HA-MRSA are the production of more virulence factors, including the Panton-Valentine leukocidin (PVL) toxin, and a greater susceptibility to non–β-lactam antibiotics in vitro. However, the role of PVL in human disease is unclear.
   - First-line treatment for CA-MRSA CAP remains vancomycin. Alternatives may include linezolid or clindamycin, which have the theoretic advantage of having some efficacy against CA-MRSA exotoxins.

9. **What are some recent developments in CAP?**
   Areas of active investigation in the field include biomarkers for the diagnosis and prognosis in CAP, using the genomic bacterial load as a marker of disease severity, and epidemiologic studies of long-term health effects of CAP. These will be briefly discussed.
   - **Biomarkers in CAP:** The potential applications of biomarkers in CAP include stratifying patients accurately into high- and low-risk groups and guiding antibiotic therapy (both initiation and duration). Examples of biomarkers that have been studied include procalcitonin and proadrenomedullin. Some studies have shown that combining these markers with existing severity of illness scores such as the PSI or CRB-65 (a modified form of the CURB score) has resulted in improved predictive capacity. However, the data are not convincing enough for these biomarkers to have entered routine clinical practice.
   - **Quantitative bacterial load:** Recently some investigators have been studying the use of quantitative bacterial load in blood as a marker of severity of illness, analogous to the use of viral load in the management of diseases such as hepatitis C and human immunodeficiency virus (HIV). Quantification of *S. pneumoniae* DNA in blood with use of real-time polymerase chain reaction was shown to be a strong predictor of the risk for shock and the risk for death in pneumococcal pneumonia. This test is more sensitive than blood cultures, with a specificity approaching 100%. It is rapid (turnover time < 3 hours), is inexpensive, and can

also determine susceptibility to penicillin. If validated by further studies, this test could have a major impact in the management of CAP.

- **Long-term consequences of CAP:** An important change in our understanding of the impact of CAP on patients has been the realization that the 2-year mortality of patients with an episode of CAP was significantly increased over that of controls, even in the *absence* of comorbid diseases. Although the cause of the increased mortality is not completely clear, some evidence suggests a predominantly cardiovascular cause. Epidemiologic data show a strong association between acute respiratory tract infections and subsequent acute myocardial infarctions. This gives rise to the possibility that the acute inflammatory and procoagulant state induced by CAP can destabilize atheromatous plaques and accelerate underlying cardiovascular disease. Further studies are needed to identify patients most at risk for delayed mortality, and potential treatments such as aspirin or 3-hydroxy-3-methyl-glutaryl (HMG) coenzyme A reductase inhibitors (such as statins) can perhaps be tried. It may therefore be helpful to view CAP as an acute illness with long-term health implications rather than a self-limiting process.

10. **What defines a treatment failure?**
The majority of patients receiving appropriate therapy show a favorable clinical response within 72 hours. Therefore initial antibiotic therapy should not be changed before 72 hours unless indicated by significant clinical worsening or microbiologic data. Remember that certain host factors, such as advanced age, alcoholism, and chronic obstructive pulmonary disease, have been associated with delayed resolution despite appropriate treatment. Radiographic resolution of pneumonia lags behind clinical improvement and in some cases may take up to 8 to 10 weeks to clear completely.

11. **Discuss the potential reasons why a patient may not respond favorably to empiric therapy.**
Clinical deterioration or a lack of response to empiric antimicrobial therapy within 3 days often indicates treatment failure, warranting thorough reassessment and additional investigation. The following should be considered:
1. Inappropriate antimicrobial therapy
   a. Is the dosing adequate?
   b. Are all potential bacterial pathogens covered by the empiric regimen?
   c. Are the organisms resistant or has a previously sensitive pathogen developed resistance?
   d. Is the pathogen bacterial? Consider other pathogens to include viruses, endemic fungi, and mycobacteria.
   e. Is the host immunocompromised and at risk for opportunistic infections such as *Pneumocystis jiroveci*?
   f. Is the disease infectious? Has the patient been misdiagnosed? (See question 13.)
2. Complications of lung infection or hospitalization
   a. Has a lung abscess or empyema developed?
   b. Does the patient have acute respiratory distress syndrome (ARDS)?
   c. Have the bacteria seeded extrapulmonary sites (e.g., endocarditis, septic arthritis, meningitis)?
   d. Has the patient acquired a new nosocomial infection (e.g., urinary tract infection, central line infection, sinusitis)?

12. **How should a patient with nonresolving pneumonia be evaluated?**
The clinician should review initial culture results and sensitivities and collect additional lower respiratory tract and blood cultures. Broadening empiric therapy may be indicated while awaiting results of additional testing. All patients should have a repeated chest radiograph at this time. Additional history may reveal HIV risk factors, tick exposure, travel history, or other diagnostic clues. Further testing, such as a chest computed tomographic or ultrasound scan, should be directed at the likely cause of treatment failure. If the procedure can be performed safely,

a thoracentesis of a pleural effusion can exclude a complicated effusion or empyema. Bronchoscopy has good diagnostic utility, and specimens should be sent for quantitative bacterial cultures and sensitivities, as well as for stains and cultures of unusual organisms (mycobacteria, viruses, endemic fungi, and *P. jiroveci*). If the diagnosis remains elusive, a trial of corticosteroids or a thoroscopic or open lung biopsy may be considered in the appropriate clinical setting.

13. **Which noninfectious processes can present with signs and symptoms of acute pneumonia?**

   Noninfectious conditions that can mimic acute pneumonia include ARDS, traumatic pulmonary contusion, pneumonitis resulting from connective tissue disease (e.g., systemic lupus erythematosus), acute hypersensitivity pneumonitis, drug-induced pneumonitis, diffuse alveolar hemorrhage (e.g., Goodpasture syndrome), Wegener granulomatosis, bronchiolitis obliterans organizing pneumonia, acute interstitial pneumonia (Hamman-Rich syndrome), acute eosinophilic pneumonia, pulmonary embolism with infarction, atelectasis, chemical pneumonitis (aspiration), and malignancy (e.g., bronchoalveolar carcinoma, lymphangitic carcinomatosis, Kaposi sarcoma).

14. **What are hospital-acquired pneumonia (HAP), health care–associated pneumonia (HCAP), and ventilator-associated pneumonia (VAP)?**

   - HAP is defined as pneumonia that occurs 48 hours or more after admission, which was not incubating at the time of admission.
   - HCAP refers to pneumonia that develops in a patient who lives in a nursing home or long-term care facility; undergoes hemodialysis; has received IV antimicrobial therapy, chemotherapy, or wound care within the preceding 30 days; or has been hospitalized for at least 2 days within the preceding 90 days. The causative pathogens in these patients are similar to those responsible for HAP and VAP and are often multidrug resistant (MDR).
   - VAP: Universally agreed-on diagnostic criteria for VAP do not exist; however, commonly used criteria include the presence of *all* of the following:
     1. Mechanical ventilation for >48 hours.
     2. A new and persistent infiltrate on chest radiograph or ARDS; in the setting of ARDS, it may be impossible to visualize a new infiltrate on chest radiograph.
     3. Two of the following three findings:
        a. Fever (temperature >38.3° C)
        b. Leukocytosis or leukopenia
        c. Purulent tracheal secretions
     4. Quantitative cultures of a lower respiratory tract specimen at or above the threshold defined as consistent with lung infection.

   The use of clinical criteria alone without microbiologic data tends to overdiagnose lung infection.

15. **How do you decide on the initial empiric antibiotic therapy for HAP, HCAP, or VAP?**

   If the patient has late-onset pneumonia development (≥5 days) or risk factors for MDR pathogens, then broad-spectrum antibiotic therapy is indicated. If neither of these criteria is met, limited-spectrum antibiotic therapy is appropriate. If HAP, VAP, or HCAP is suspected, disease severity is not considered in the initial empiric antibiotic decision.

16. **What are the risk factors for MDR pathogens causing HAP, HCAP, and VAP?**

   Risk factors for MDR causing HAP, HCAP, and VAP include antimicrobial therapy in the preceding 90 days, current hospitalization of 5 days or more, high frequency of antibiotic resistance in the community or in the specific hospital unit, immunosuppressive disease and/or therapy, or presence of risk factors for HCAP (hospitalization for 2 days or more in the preceding 9 days, residence in a nursing home or extended-care facility, home infusion therapy [including antibiotics], long-term dialysis within 30 days, home wound care, family member with MDR pathogen).

17. **What initial empiric antibiotic therapy is recommended for HAP, HCAP, or VAP in patients with no known risk factors for MDR, early onset pneumonia development, and any disease severity?**
Recommended antibiotics include ceftriaxone, levofloxacin (moxifloxacin or ciprofloxacin can replace levofloxacin), ampicillin-sulbactam, or ertapenem. Potential pathogens include *S. pneumoniae*, *H. influenzae*, methicillin-sensitive *S. aureus*, and antibiotic-sensitive enteric gram-negative bacilli (*Escherichia coli*, *Klebsiella pneumoniae*, *Enterobacter*, *Proteus*, *Serratia marcescens*.

18. **What initial empiric antibiotic therapy is recommended for HAP, HCAP, or VAP in patients with known risk factors for MDR, late-onset disease development, and any disease severity?**
Recommended combination antibiotic therapy includes an antipseudomonal cephalosporin (cefepime or ceftazidime), antipseudomonal carbapenems (imipenem or meropenem), or β-lactam–β-lactamase inhibitor (piperacillin-tazobactam) *plus* an antipseudomonal fluoroquinolone (ciprofloxacin or levofloxacin) or an aminoglycoside (amikacin, gentamicin, or tobramycin). Linezolid or vancomycin should be added if MRSA risk factors are present or there is a high incidence locally. Potential MDR pathogens include *P. aeruginosa*, *K. pneumoniae*, *Acinetobacter* species, and MRSA (Table 20-1).

19. **What are some specific treatment strategies for MDR *Pseudomonas*, *Acinetobacter*, and MRSA VAP?**
   - Combination therapy for *P. aeruginosa* pneumonia remains controversial. Resistance is mediated partly by multiple efflux pumps.
   - *Acinetobacter* species are most sensitive to the carbapenems, sulbactam, colistin, and polymyxin. More than 85% of isolates are susceptible to carbapenems, but resistance is increasing because of either integral membrane protein (IMP)-type metalloenzymes or carbapenemases of the oxacillinase (OXA) type.
   - MRSA produces a penicillin-binding protein with reduced affinity for β-lactam antibiotics. Linezolid is an alternative to vancomycin for the treatment of MRSA VAP.

20. **What measures can be taken to decrease the risk of VAP?**
   1. Avoid intubation when possible, and apply noninvasive positive-pressure ventilation when appropriate.
   2. Use orotracheal tubes preferentially over nasotracheal tubes.
   3. Minimize the duration of mechanical ventilation with the aid of weaning protocols.
   4. Apply continuous aspiration of subglottic secretions.
   5. Maintain an endotracheal tube cuff pressure >20 cm H_2O to prevent leakage of oropharyngeal secretions containing bacteria into the lungs.
   6. Avoid unnecessary manipulation of the ventilator circuit.
   7. Carefully discard contaminated condensate from the ventilator circuit.
   8. Keep the head of the bed elevated by 30 degrees.
   9. Avoid heavy sedation and paralytics because they impair the patient's ability to cough.
   10. It does not appear that sucralfate or therapies that decrease gastric acid increase the incidence of nosocomial pneumonia.

TABLE 20-1. INITIAL EMPIRIC THERAPY FOR HAP, VAP, AND HCAP: FOR PATIENTS WITH LATE-ONSET DISEASE OR RISK FACTORS FOR MDR PATHOGENS AND ALL DISEASE SEVERITY

POTENTIAL PATHOGENS	COMBINATION ANTIBIOTIC THERAPY
MDR pathogens	Antipseudomonal cephalosporin (cefepime, ceftazidime)
P. aeruginosa	*or*
*K. pneumoniae (ESBL⁺)**	Antipseudomonal carbapenem (imipenem or meropenem)
Acinetobacter species*	*or*
	β-Lactam/β-lactamase inhibitor (piperacillin–tazobactam)
	plus
	Antipseudomonal fluoroquinolone* (ciprofloxacin or levofloxacin)
	or
	Aminoglycoside (amikacin, gentamicin, or tobramycin)
	plus
MRSA	Linezolid or vancomycin[†]
*Legionella pneumophila**	

Modified from American Thoracic Society, Infectious Diseases Society of America: Guidelines for the management of adults with hospital-acquired, ventilator-associated, and healthcare-associated pneumonia. Am J Respir Crit Care Med 171:388-416, 2005.

ESBL, Extended-spectrum β-lactamase.

*If an ESBL⁺ strain, such as *K. pneumoniae,* or an *Acinetobacter* species is suspected, a carbapenem is a reliable choice. If *L. pneumophila* is suspected, the combination antibiotic regimen should include a macrolide (e.g., azithromycin), or a fluoroquinolone (e.g., ciprofloxacin or levofloxacin) should be used rather than an aminoglycoside.

[†]If MRSA risk factors are present or there is a high incidence locally.

21. **How do you decide when to continue, de-escalate, and discontinue the use of antibiotic treatment on the basis of clinical response and culture data?**
When HAP, VAP, or HCAP is suspected, consider obtaining lower respiratory tract samples for culture (quantitative or semiquantitative) and microscopy. Unless there is both a low clinical suspicion for pneumonia and negative microscopy of the lower respiratory tract sample, begin empiric antimicrobial therapy. At day 2 and 3, check cultures and assess clinical response (temperature, white blood cell [WBC] count, chest radiograph, oxygenation, purulent sputum, hemodynamic changes, and organ function). If no clinical improvement is seen after 2 to 3 days with negative cultures, search for other pathogens, complications, diagnoses, or sites of infection. If no improvement is seen but cultures are positive, adjust antibiotic therapy but also broaden infectious search as you would with negative cultures. If clinical improvement is noted after 2 to 3 days but cultures are negative, consider stopping antibiotics. If clinical improvement is noted and cultures are positive, de-escalate antibiotics, and consider treating selected patients for 7 to 8 days and reassess (Fig. 20-1).

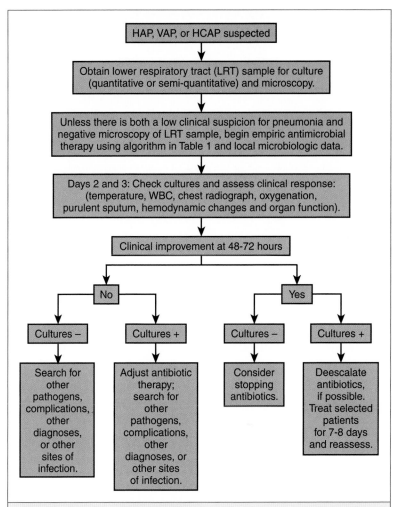

Figure 20-1. Algorithm for treatment of HAP, VAP, or HCAP. Data from American Thoracic Society, Infectious Diseases Society of America: Guidelines for the management of adults with hospital-acquired, ventilator-associated, and healthcare-associated pneumonia. Am J Respir Crit Care Med 171:388-416, 2005.

22. **How long should you continue antibiotic management for HAP, HCAP, or VAP?**
    In a prospective, randomized clinical trial, an 8-day treatment strategy for culture-proved VAP resulted in a significant decrease in multiresistant bacteria and more antibiotic-free days with no differences in mortality, ICU length of stay, or mechanical ventilator–free days when compared with a 15-day regimen. A higher rate of recurrence was documented with the 8-day regimen when the infection was due to *Acinetobacter* or *Pseudomonas*; therefore VAP due to these organisms should be treated for 15 days. Because the infecting pathogens are similar, HAP and HCAP can be treated similarly. Extended therapy (14-21 days) may be indicated in the setting of multilobar disease, cavitation, malnutrition, or necrotizing gram-negative infection.

KEY POINTS: INITIAL MANAGEMENT OF ACUTE BACTERIAL PNEUMONIA

1. Treat empirically if pneumonia is clinically suspected.

2. Select the initial empiric therapy on the basis of the current bacteriology and resistance patterns at each institution. Alternatively, published evidence-based practice guidelines may be used.

3. Obtain cultures of respiratory tract specimens to identify pathogen(s), preferably before initiation of antibiotics. However, the administration of antibiotic therapy should not be delayed for diagnostic testing.

4. Narrow the initial antibiotic regimen on the basis of quantitative culture results and clinical response (de-escalation).

5. Avoid excessive antibiotic use by de-escalating therapy when appropriate and prescribing the minimal duration of therapy required for efficacy.

BIBLIOGRAPHY

1. American Thoracic Society, Infectious Diseases Society of America : Guidelines for the management of adults with hospital-acquired, ventilator-associated, and healthcare-associated pneumonia. Am J Respir Crit Care Med 171:388-416, 2005.

2. Chastre J, Wolff M, Fagon J-Y, et al: Comparison of 8 vs 15 days of antibiotic therapy for ventilator-associated pneumonia in adults. JAMA 290:2588-2598, 2003.

3. Chow JW, Fine MJ, Shlaes DM, et al: *Enterobacter* bacteremia: clinical features and emergence of antibiotic resistance during therapy. Ann Intern Med 115:585-590, 1991.

4. Kobayashi SD, DeLeo FR: An update on community-associated MRSA virulence. Curr Opin Pharmacol 9:545-551, 2009.

5. Kruger S, Santiago E, Sven G, et al: Cardiovascular and inflammatory biomarkers to predict short- and long-term survival in community-acquired pneumonia. Am J Respir Crit Care Med 182:1426-1434, 2010.

6. Mandell LA, Wunderink RG, Anzueto A, et al: Infectious Diseases Society of America/American Thoracic Society consensus guidelines on the management of community-acquired pneumonia in adults. Clin Infect Dis 44(2 Suppl):S27-S72, 2007.

7. Messori A, Trippoli S, Vaiani M, et al: Bleeding and pneumonia in intensive care patients given ranitidine and sucralfate for prevention of stress ulcer: meta-analysis of randomized controlled trials. BMJ 321:1-7, 2000.

8. Nordmann P, Poirel L: Emerging carbapenemases in Gram-negative aerobes. Clin Microbiol Infect 8:321-331, 2002.

9. Rello J, Lisboa T, Lujan M, et al: Severity of pneumococcal pneumonia associated with genomic bacterial load. Chest 136:832-840, 2009.

10. Waterer GW, Rello J, Wunderink RG: Management of community-acquired pneumonia in adults. Am J Respir Crit Care Med 183:157-164, 2011.

11. Wunderink RG, Cammarata SK, Oliphant TH, et al: Continuation of a randomized, double-blind, multicenter study of linezolid versus vancomycin in the treatment of patients with nosocomial pneumonia. Clin Ther 25:980-992, 2003.

12. Wunderink RG, Rello J, Cammarata SK, et al: Linezolid vs vancomycin: analysis of two double-blind studies of patients with methicillin-resistant *Staphylococcus aureus* nosocomial pneumonia. Chest 124:1789-1797, 2003.

CHAPTER 21

ASTHMA

Ali Al-Alwan, MD, Gilman B. Allen, MD, and David A. Kaminsky, MD

1. **What are important factors to address when taking the history of patients with acute severe asthma?**

   Box 21-1 summarizes the important historical points in a patient with acute severe asthma. If the clinician is able to obtain a history from the patient, it is important to first exclude other possible causes of the patient's presentation. A history of heart failure may suggest wheezing and shortness of breath resulting from left ventricular failure and pulmonary edema. A history of allergies or prior anaphylactic reactions, along with a recent exposure to certain foods, new medications, or other known triggers, could be an important warning of potentially imminent upper airway inflammation and closure. A history of recent-onset cough, wheezing, and hemoptysis with unilateral inspiratory and expiratory wheezes could be clues to an intrabronchial tumor, such as a carcinoid or carcinoma. Pulmonary embolism can also mimic asthma and should especially be considered in the patient with dyspnea, anxiety, and hypoxemia but clear breath sounds. In a patient with dyspnea, anxiety, and inspiratory stridor, vocal cord dysfunction should be considered. Spirometry can be an especially useful tool in the emergency department (ED) when evaluating these patients, and flow-volume loops often show the characteristic truncated or flattened inspiratory loops.

   > **BOX 21-1. IMPORTANT HISTORICAL POINTS IN ACUTE ASTHMA**
   >
   > - History of asthma (i.e., when diagnosed, type of treatment, common triggers)
   > - Factors related to asthma control (e.g., frequency of use of medications, nocturnal symptoms, history of hospitalization, intubation, use of oral steroids)
   > - Timing of onset of symptoms (i.e., gradual versus sudden)
   > - Nature of symptoms (e.g., wheezing, chest pain, intermittent versus continuous, associated cough, sputum production, fever)
   > - Exclusion of other causes of shortness of breath (e.g., heart failure, pulmonary embolus)
   > - Exclusion of other causes of wheezing (e.g., bronchospasm from allergic reaction, endobronchial tumor)
   > - Consideration of paradoxical vocal cord closure on inspiration (i.e., vocal cord dysfunction)

2. **List some important indicators of a severe asthma attack.**
   - Use of accessory muscles
   - Inability to speak in full sentences
   - Heart rate > 130 beats/min
   - Pulsus paradoxus > 15 mm Hg
   - Respiratory rate > 30 breaths/min
   - Inability to lie down
   - A silent chest
   - Somnolence
   - Advancing fatigue
   - Normal or elevated $PaCO_2$
   - Inability to maintain oxygenation by mask (oxygen saturation $< 90\%$)
   - Cyanosis

3. **Which patients are at greatest risk for near-fatal or fatal asthma?**

A survey of North American adult patients with asthma seen in the ED identified a number of factors associated with a high number of ED visits, including nonwhite race, Medicaid, other public or no insurance, and markers of chronic asthma severity, such as history of prior hospitalization, intubation, or recent use of inhaled corticosteroids. Also at increased risk for near-fatal asthma are patients with a high degree of bronchial reactivity, those with a history of poor compliance with therapy and follow-up, and those judged to be poor at perceiving the severity of their own attack, as demonstrated by a poor correlation between reported symptoms and peak expiratory flow (PEF) values. These are patients for whom home monitoring of PEF is strongly indicated.

Patients in whom sudden, severe attacks develop or those who have severe, slowly progressive disease are both typically at risk. A history of marked diurnal variation in forced expiratory volume in 1 second (FEV_1) is also believed to be a risk factor, but this could simply be related to its being a marker for increased bronchial responsiveness. Historical data indicate that female sex, endotracheal intubation, and prolonged neuromuscular blockade are associated with more prolonged hospital stay, whereas elevated arterial CO_2 level and lower arterial pH within 24 hours of admission are associated with increased mortality.

Although not widely identified as a true marker of increased risk, the use of inhaled heroin is also frequently associated with near-fatal or fatal attacks of asthma. It is not known whether this is due to a direct effect of the inhaled drug (or its diluents), the degree of airflow limitation, or simply the impaired judgment of the user that delays arrival to the ED and initiation of appropriate care. However, opioids have long been known to cause bronchoconstriction via mast cell degranulation and histamine release. Although most reports of severe asthma attacks after inhalation of narcotics are in patients with known asthma, they have also been reported in patients without any history of asthma.

4. **How should one treat a severe asthma attack?**
   - **Oxygen therapy** to achieve an arterial oxygen saturation of 90% or greater.
   - **β-Agonists:** These are the first-line therapy in an acute asthma attack. It is now widely accepted that the inhaled forms of these drugs are superior to the subcutaneous or intravenous (IV) route, with fewer adverse affects, and their administration can be repeated up to three times within the first hour after presentation while monitoring for adverse effects such as tachyarrhythmia and lactic acidosis, the latter of which can be underrecognized. The subcutaneous route is still reserved for patients who have such severe dyspnea that they are unable to take deep-enough breaths, but these are usually the patients who later undergo intubation. It is also accepted that metered dose inhalers are as effective as aerosolized delivery, provided good technique is used with a spacer device. Nebulized or aerosolized delivery is still used frequently in the ED, in part from convention and in part because less instruction and observation are needed to ensure good delivery. The use of salmeterol as an outpatient monotherapy was recently shown to increase the risk of hospitalization. However, this increased risk was not seen among patients receiving combined therapy with inhaled corticosteroids and salmeterol (Table 21-1).
   - **Corticosteroids:** These drugs also play a key role in treatment, and typical dosage is 60 mg of IV or PO methylprednisolone every 12 to 24 hours for the first 24 hours. This must be delivered as soon as possible because peak onset of action can take several hours. Therapy is typically administered every 6 hours until the attack appears to be subsiding and then gradually tapered over days to weeks. Comparisons between oral prednisone and IV corticosteroids have not shown differences in the rate of improvement of lung function or in the length of the hospital stay. Thus the oral route is preferred for patients with normal mental status and without conditions expected to interfere with gastrointestinal absorption.
   - **Anticholinergics:** Many studies have shown a marginal benefit from adding inhaled ipratropium to β-agonist therapy (versus β-agonists alone) in the treatment of acute asthma.

TABLE 21-1. PRIMARY PHARMACOLOGIC TREATMENT OF ACUTE ASTHMA*

AGENT	DOSE	COMMENTS
β-Agonists	■ 4-8 puffs (90 mcg/puff) MDI + spacer, every 20 min up to 4 hr, then every 1-4 hr as needed or ■ 2.5-5 mg nebulized every 20 min for 3 doses, then every 1-4 hr as needed	■ Inhaled better than subcutaneous or IV ■ MDI + spacer works as well as nebulized ■ Levalbuterol similar to racemic albuterol, but with less tachycardia ■ Elevated lactate levels seen after high doses
Corticosteroids	■ 40-80 mg per day PO or IV in 1 or 2 divided doses until PEF = 70% of predicted or personal best ■ Continue for 3-10 days, tapering if dose continues for longer than 7 days	■ Single 160-mg intramuscular depot injection of methylprednisolone has been found to be as effective as an 8-day tapering course of the same dose of oral methylprednisolone once patients discharged
Anticholinergics	■ 8 puffs (18 mcg/puff) MDI + spacer, every 20 min as needed up to 3 hrs or ■ 0.5 mg (500 mcg) nebulized every 20 min for 3 doses, then as needed	■ Improves lung function and reduces rate of hospitalization when added to standard care ■ Combined use with inhaled β-agonists is beneficial
Oxygen	■ Titrate to $SaO_2 > 92\%$	■ Avoid excessive oxygenation, which can result in CO_2 retention ■ Use humidified oxygen

Other agents (magnesium sulfate, heliox, leukotriene antagonists, inhaled anesthetics) discussed in text.
MDI, Metered dose inhaler, *SaO₂*, oxygen saturation.
*Per EPR3 Guidelines for treatment of acute asthma in adult patients.

■ **Aminophylline:** Oral theophylline is a third-line agent in the outpatient management of asthma. This is in part due to the recognition of its intrinsic antiinflammatory properties, even at serum levels lower than those once thought necessary to achieve significant benefit. However, the use of IV aminophylline in the treatment of acute asthma remains controversial and is no longer recommended.

■ **Inhaled epinephrine:** A recent meta-analysis of using inhaled epinephrine in refractory asthma demonstrated a similar degree of bronchodilation and PEF improvement when compared with albuterol. The use of inhaled epinephrine is safer than IV epinephrine, which is associated with a higher risk of acute myocardial infarction and tachyarrhythmias.

■ **Inhaled anesthetic agents:** In patients receiving mechanical ventilation with ongoing severe bronchospasm despite aggressive conventional treatment, inhaled anesthetic agents can be used for their intrinsic properties of bronchodilation. Because their delivery requires a special apparatus and conventional therapy is usually more effective, their use is often considered as a rescue therapy only. Isoflurane or enflurane are the agents of choice.

- **Antibiotics:** There is no benefit to the routine use of antibiotics in the management of an acute asthma episode unless findings are suspicious for pneumonia or other bacterial infections.

5. **Does magnesium sulfate offer any benefit in the treatment of status asthmaticus?**

Although a small number of controlled trials have yielded mixed results, one controlled study suggests that patients with severe asthma (FEV_1 <25% predicted) treated with IV magnesium sulfate in the ED had significantly reduced admission rates compared with those treated with placebo. A more recent meta-analysis did not support these findings. Proposed mechanisms of possible benefit are as follows:

- Blockage of calcium channels and reduced calcium entry into smooth muscle cells, leading to bronchodilation
- Possible inhibition of mast cell degranulation
- Improving respiratory muscle function by correction of lower baseline serum levels

Because the only reported adverse side effects from a single dose of magnesium are flushing, mild fatigue, or burning at the IV site, its use in the treatment of persons with severe asthma may be warranted by its potential for lowering admission rates, but this remains a controversial topic. Magnesium sulfate is generally delivered as 2 gm in 50 mL of normal saline solution given IV over a 20-minute period. Interestingly, inhaled magnesium sulfate administered with inhaled β- agonist has also been shown to improve lung function and may reduce the rate of hospital admission.

6. **How can one best decide when to admit a patient and when to discharge a patient from the ED?**

Patients who have a poor response to treatment are defined by persistent wheezing, dyspnea, and accessory muscle use at rest despite 3 hours of treatment in the ED. Such patients should be admitted to the hospital. One study suggests that in persons with severe asthma (peak expiratory flow rate [PEFR] and FEV_1 <35% of predicted), improvement in PEFR measured 30 minutes after initiation of therapy may be an early predictor of response to treatment after 3 hours. Any patient with worsening PEFR, rising $PaCO_2$, or advancing fatigue should, at the very least, be monitored in the intensive care unit and possibly undergo intubation. A recent study developed a classification tree for use in risk stratification for hospital admission for acute asthma. This validated scheme involved three key variables, history of hospitalization, peak flow, and oxygenation, and was entitled the CHOP classification:

- **C**hange in PEF severity category
- History of prior **h**ospitalization for asthma
- **O**xygen saturation with room air
- Initial **p**eak expiratory flow

Signs of good response to therapy in the ED that would allow a patient to be discharged include a sustained response of at least 1 hour after the last treatment with FEV_1 or PEF ≥70% predicted, no distress, and improvement in physical examination results. The Expert Panel Report 3 (EPR3) guidelines emphasize that such patients be instructed to continue their therapy at home with inhaled short-acting β-agonists; be given a 3- to 10-day course of oral corticosteroids; consider initiation of inhaled corticosteroids; receive education on medications, inhaler technique, and use of a written action plan and possibly a PEF meter; and arrange for medical follow-up within the next 1 to 4 weeks.

7. **Which patients need to have an endotracheal tube (ETT) placed?**

Any patient with apnea, near apnea, or cardiopulmonary arrest should have an ETT placed. Any patient with progressive lethargy, somnolence, near exhaustion, or unresponsiveness should have an ETT placed. An elevated $PaCO_2$ level on admission, although shown to be associated with increased mortality, may not necessarily warrant immediate endotracheal intubation. Any patient with a progressive rise in $PaCO_2$ despite therapy and increasing fatigue most likely will require intubation. Other signs would include a silent chest, an inability to maintain oxygenation by mask (oxygen saturation <90%), and visible cyanosis. Other relative indications are coexistent medical conditions that can increase minute ventilation requirements or compromise oxygen delivery, such as sepsis, myocardial infarction, metabolic acidosis, or life-threatening arrhythmias.

8. **Is normocapnia or hypercapnia an absolute indication for intubation in a person with asthma?**
Most persons with severe asthma are initially seen with hypocapnia because of the hyperventilation associated with dyspnea and hypoxemia. A normal or elevated $PaCO_2$ is usually a sign of fatigue but can also be due to a high dead space–to–tidal volume ratio resulting from air trapping and ineffective ventilation of noncommunicating segments of lung. In either case, it should be taken seriously and can be a sign of impending respiratory failure. Studies indicate, however, that most patients with normal or elevated $PaCO_2$ on blood gas analysis at initial evaluation improve with time in response to conventional therapy and do not require intubation. Because mechanical ventilation in severe asthma can be complicated by increased air trapping and barotrauma, it is advisable not to perform intubation and mechanical ventilation in a patient with acute asthma merely on the basis of an elevated $PaCO_2$, unless concomitant somnolence, progressive fatigue, or worsening acidosis exists.

9. **Can noninvasive mechanical ventilation be used safely to avoid intubation in a person with asthma?**
Noninvasive positive-pressure ventilation (NIPPV) via face mask has been shown to be safe and effective when applied to a patient with severe asthma and hypercapnia whose condition fails to improve with conventional therapy. It can be effective in unloading respiratory muscles, improving dyspnea, lowering respiratory rate, and improving gas exchange. NIPPV has been shown to be an effective potential means of avoiding endotracheal intubation and may also help avoid the need for reintubation after extubation. However, it is also critical to determine early in a patient's course whether he or she is responding appropriately to NIPPV, because delays in endotracheal intubation may be associated with worse outcomes. NIPPV should not be used in persons with asthma who have life-threatening hypoxemia, somnolence, or hemodynamic instability, and it should be aborted in patients whose conditions fail to improve or who cannot tolerate the mask.

10. **Are helium admixtures of any proved benefit in treating severe asthma?**
When helium (He) is blended with oxygen (in a 20% O_2, 80% He or 30% O_2, 70% He mixture), the gas density becomes approximately one-third that of room air, but viscosity is increased, leading to increased laminar flow and a reduction in airway resistance in areas of greatest turbulent flow. This can result in a reduction in the work of breathing required to meet the same minute ventilation requirement when breathing room air. Because work of breathing is reduced, it would seem likely that respiratory fatigue might be delayed until conventional therapy has had time to take effect. Despite numerous trials and two recent meta-analyses, no evidence yet exists that helium-oxygen (heliox) admixtures can prevent the need for endotracheal intubation. However, heliox has been shown to improve PEFR and reduce the degree of pulsus paradoxus in acute asthma attacks. This is presumably due to the decrease in airway resistance and lower generated negative pleural pressures but also possibly caused by improved expiratory flow and less dynamic hyperinflation (DHI). The improved laminar flow afforded by heliox may also allow deeper lung deposition of inhaled aerosols. Because heliox mixtures typically include only 20% to 30% oxygen, hypoxemia is a barrier to use of heliox. However, when the patient does not have hypoxemia, it is safe and worthwhile to use, particularly in patients with fatigue and hypercapnia who are at risk for progressing to the point of requiring mechanical ventilation.

11. **Once a patient requires intubation, what is the best management strategy?**
   - **Intubation:** Blind nasoendotracheal intubation is often better tolerated by an awake patient, but oral endotracheal intubation is the preferred method of intubation because it permits the use of an ETT

with a larger internal diameter. This will lead to lower resistance within the respiratory circuit and allow easier deep suctioning of secretions and mucous plugs. It is important to remember that the resistance of a tube is indirectly proportional to its internal radius (to the fourth power), and the resistance of an 8-mm ETT is roughly one-half that of a 7-mm ETT. Oral intubation is indicated for patients with apnea and cyanosis. Because intubation in a person with asthma is often difficult and may induce laryngospasm or lead to increased bronchospasm, it should be performed by the most experienced person available, and rapid-sequence technique should be used. Because of its intrinsic sympathomimetic and bronchodilating properties, ketamine has been advocated by many as the induction agent of choice to avoid the possible loss of sympathetic tone and drug-induced vasodilation, thus helping to prevent cardiovascular collapse. The usual dose of ketamine for intubation is 1 to 2 mg/kg, given IV over a 2-minute period. Sedation is usually necessary, and, although sometimes warranted, paralysis should be avoided if possible. Barbiturates such as thiopental should not be used because of their association with histamine release and potential worsening of bronchoconstriction. Although the narcotic fentanyl is often useful because it inhibits airway reflexes and causes less histamine release than morphine, one should be aware of its potential to trigger bronchoconstriction and laryngospasm.

- **Avoiding potential complications:** Some authors advocate hand bag-ventilating patients with asthma immediately after intubation to assess the severity of bronchospasm and avoid dynamic hyperinflation by slowly delivering a rate of 4 to 5 breaths/min as a bridge to mechanical ventilation. Ensuring adequate humidification of inspired gas is particularly important to prevent thickening of secretions and drying of airway mucosa, which can promote mucous plugging and further bronchospasm.

- **DHI:** When airflow limitation is severe, the next ventilated breath can be initiated before the lungs can fully empty to a normal functional residual capacity, resulting in progressive air trapping. This leads to DHI and elevated end-expiratory alveolar pressures, referred to as *intrinsic positive end-expiratory pressure* ($PEEP_i$). Measuring $PEEP_i$ can be problematic, and it is often underestimated by the brief end-expiratory pause used to estimate it on the ventilator. This is due to the heterogeneous distribution of early airway closure that can prevent many hyperinflated segments from communicating their alveolar pressures to the transducer at the airway opening. Ideally, $PEEP_i$ should be kept below 15 cm H_2O. The key determinants of DHI are minute ventilation, tidal volume, exhalation time, and severity of airflow limitation. DHI can often be predicted by elevated plateau pressures and failure to achieve zero expiratory flow before the next delivered breath. DHI can lead to less effective respiratory muscle contraction and added work because of less optimal curvature of the diaphragm, which in turn can lead to less effective triggering of the ventilator. DHI can also lead to decreased venous return and right ventricular preload, increased right ventricular afterload (via extrinsic compression of the pulmonary vasculature), and decreased left ventricular compliance, which can all lead to diminished cardiac output and hypotension. When strongly suspected, the best immediate solution (and test) is to briefly disconnect the ETT from the ventilator circuit to allow for more complete exhalation. The other concern with DHI is that the high degree of associated $PEEP_i$ can ultimately lead to barotrauma.

- **Barotrauma:** High airway pressures can potentially lead to pulmonary interstitial emphysema, subcutaneous emphysema, pneumomediastinum, pneumothorax, and even pneumoperitoneum. Barotrauma correlates directly with the degree of DHI. Plateau pressures are traditionally thought to be a good indicator of the degree of DHI, and a level below 35 cm H_2O is still a widely recommended target for minimizing barotrauma. However, one study has shown that elevated end-inspiratory lung volume (the exhaled volume measured from end inspiration to the relaxation volume during a period of apnea) may be a more reliable predictor of barotrauma than are airway pressures. The most feared consequence of barotrauma is tension pneumothorax, typically characterized by a precipitous rise in airway pressures (peak and plateau), a drop in oxygen saturation, hypotension, tachycardia, unilaterally absent breath sounds and chest excursions, and possibly tracheal deviation. Tension pneumothorax is a clinical diagnosis and, if strongly suspected in a patient in unstable condition, should be treated immediately with needle thoracotomy followed by chest tube placement. Fatal air embolism may also occur because of barotrauma.

> ### BOX 21-2. PRINCIPLES OF MANAGEMENT OF MECHANICAL VENTILATION IN ACUTE ASTHMA
>
> The goal is to minimize DHI through the use of the following:
> - Minimal minute ventilation (low tidal volumes [e.g., 6-8 mL/kg]), low respiratory rate (8-10 beats/min)
> - Minimal (or zero) PEEP
> - Relatively high inspiratory flow rate (80-100 L/min), to reduce inspiratory time
> - Maintenance of plateau pressures $\leq$ 35 cm H_2O, and $PEEP_i$ $\leq$ 15 cm H_2O
> - Permissive hypercapnia up to 80 mm Hg (contraindicated in patients with intracranial bleeding, cerebral edema, or a space-occupying lesion), while trying to maintain pH $\geq$ 7.20

- **Ventilator settings in asthma** (Box 21-2): The best mode of ventilation is one that minimizes minute ventilation and allows for sufficient exhalation time to minimize DHI, while trying to maintain oxygen saturation > 92% (use 100% oxygen initially). This can generally be achieved with low tidal volumes of 6 to 8 mL/kg, a respiratory rate of 8 to 10 breaths/min, minimal added PEEP, and moderate inspiratory flow rates of 80 to 90 L/min. Decelerating flow waveforms may improve overall flow distribution and hence optimize gas exchange. Higher inspiratory flow rates with square waveforms allow for a shorter inspiratory time and hence, at the same respiratory rate, a longer expiratory time. It is the longer expiratory time, and not just the inspiratory-to-expiratory ratio, that is critical to limiting DHI. Lowering total minute ventilation is the most crucial goal, because a longer expiratory time and smaller burden of volume to be exhaled are what minimize DHI. Intentional hypoventilation with low minute volumes can significantly reduce the risk of DHI and barotrauma. Thus allowing for a maximum $PaCO_2$ of 80 mm Hg or a minimum pH of 7.20 is a safe and acceptable practice when performing ventilation in patients with severe airflow limitation. However, because an elevated $PaCO_2$ can increase cerebral perfusion, such use of "permissive hypercapnea" should be avoided in patients with intracranial bleeding, edema, or space-occupying brain lesions.
- **Sedation:** Agitation and inadequate sedation can lead to hyperventilation and asynchrony with the mechanical ventilator and hence DHI and unacceptably high airway pressures with increased risk of barotrauma. Deep anesthesia with benzodiazepines or propofol is often necessary to achieve optimal control to prevent dyssynchrony between patient and ventilator, especially when using intentional hypoventilation and permissive hypercapnia. Paralytics should and often can be avoided if sufficient levels of sedatives are used.

12. **Can added PEEP help reduce air trapping in patients with asthma who are receiving mechanical ventilation?**
    Some argue that added PEEP can help minimize air trapping by *stenting* open peripheral airways. Although this may be true to some extent in patients with emphysema and easily collapsible central airways, it is unlikely to be of much benefit in persons with severe asthma. In the classic model of airflow limitation, airway collapse occurs when the extraluminal pressure overcomes intraluminal pressures (and any architectural properties of the airway itself). In patients who already have significant $PEEP_i$, and in whom distal alveolar pressures already exceed extraluminal pressures at end-expiration, added PEEP will likely only increase distal alveolar pressures and worsen hyperinflation. It is important to remember that, because DHI can occur even in the absence of airflow limitation if the respiratory rate is high enough, the previously mentioned strategies are still best for minimizing DHI. However, once patients begin to recover and breathe spontaneously while using the ventilator, it is important to add sufficient PEEP to reduce the work of breathing necessary to trigger the next breath.

13. **What are some new pharmacologic strategies for treating acute asthma?**
    A recent Cochrane review found that the use of inhaled steroids in the ED reduces admission rates in patients with acute asthma, but this seems only to benefit those patients not already receiving

systemic corticosteroids. Inhaled budesonide has been shown to improve markers of airway inflammation and hyperresponsiveness as early as 6 hours after dosing. Another study demonstrated that inhaled fluticasone (3000 mcg/hr), administered as two puffs (500 mcg) every 10 minutes for 3 hours, can improve lung function and reduce hospitalization rate more than treating with 500 mg of IV hydrocortisone. The rapidity of the response suggests a noninflammatory mechanism of action that may involve topical vasoconstriction. Another potential therapy for acute asthma is leukotriene blockade. One study has found that IV delivery of montelukast improved FEV_1 more quickly than placebo when given with standard therapy, with an onset of action as early as 10 minutes, which was more rapid than the effect of oral montelukast. A trend was also seen toward a greater improvement in FEV_1 with IV versus oral montelukast. However, the use of leukotriene inhibitors in the setting of severe acute asthma still warrants further investigation.

KEY POINTS: ASSESSMENT AND TREATMENT OF ACUTE ASTHMA

1. Risk factors for acute asthma include poor perception of symptoms, poor compliance with therapy, lack of medical insurance, and previous hospitalization or intubation.

2. Examination findings suggesting impending respiratory failure in acute asthma include use of accessory muscles, inability to speak full sentences, inability to lie down, and a silent chest.

3. Patients with acute asthma should be admitted to the hospital when they have failed to respond to treatment in the ED within 3 hours or when they have a rising PCO_2.

4. Ventilator settings that minimize DHI and its complications include low minute ventilation (preferably via both reduced tidal volume and respiratory rate), high inspiratory flow rate to minimize inspiratory time, and no external PEEP.

BIBLIOGRAPHY

1. Camargo CA Jr, Gurner DM, Smithline HA, et al: A randomized placebo-controlled study of intravenous montelukast for the treatment of acute asthma. J Allergy Clin Immunol 125:374-380, 2010.

2. Edmonds ML, Camargo CA Jr, Pollack CV Jr, et al: Early use of inhaled corticosteroids in the emergency department treatment of acute asthma (Cochrane review). Cochrane Database Syst Rev 1; CD002308, 2001.

3. Gallegos-Solórzano MC, Perez-Padilla R, Hernandez-Zenteno RJ: Usefulness of inhaled magnesium sulfate in the coadjuvant management of severe asthma crisis in an emergency department. Pulm Pharmacol Ther 23:432-437, 2010.

4. Griswold SK, Nordstrom CR, Clark S, et al: Asthma exacerbations in North American adults: Who are the "frequent fliers" in the emergency department? Chest 127:1579-1586, 2005.

5. Hodder R, Lougheed MD, FitzGerald JM, et al: Management of acute asthma in adults in the emergency department: assisted ventilation. CMAJ 182:265-272, 2010.

6. Hodder R, Lougheed MD, Rowe BH, et al: Management of acute asthma in adults in the emergency department: nonventilatory management. CMAJ 182:E55-E67, 2010.

7. Holley AD, Boots RJ: Review article: management of acute severe and near-fatal asthma. Emerg Med Australas 21:259-268, 2009.

8. Lazarus SC: Emergency treatment of asthma. N Engl J Med 363:755-764, 2010.

9. Lugogo NL, MacIntyre NR: Life-threatening asthma: pathophysiology and management. Respir Care 53:726-735, 2008.

10. National Heart, Lung, and Blood Institute: Expert Panel Report 3 (EPR3): Guidelines for the Diagnosis and Management of Asthma. Section 5: Managing exacerbations of asthma. Bethesda, Maryland, National Heart, Lung, and Blood Institute, 2007.

11. Ram FS, Wellington S, Rowe BH, et al: Non-invasive positive pressure ventilation for treatment of respiratory failure due to severe acute exacerbations of asthma. Cochrane Database Syst Rev 3; CD004360, 2005.

12. Rodrigo GJ: Comparison of inhaled fluticasone with intravenous hydrocortisone in the treatment of adult acute asthma. Am J Respir Crit Care Med 171:1231-1236, 2005.

13. Rodrigo GJ, Nannini LJ: Comparison between nebulized adrenaline and beta2 agonists for the treatment of acute asthma. A meta-analysis of randomized trials. Am J Emerg Med 24:217-222, 2006.

14. Rodrigo G, Rodrigo C, Pollack CV, et al: Use of helium-oxygen mixtures in the treatment of acute asthma: a systematic review. Chest 123:891-896, 2003.

15. Tsai CL, Clark S, Camargo CA Jr: Risk stratification for hospitalization in acute asthma: the CHOP classification tree. Am J Emerg Med 28:803-808, 2010.

CHAPTER 22

CHRONIC OBSTRUCTIVE PULMONARY DISEASE

Anne E. Dixon, MA, BM, BCh

1. **What is chronic obstructive pulmonary disease (COPD)?**

   COPD is characterized by airflow limitation that is not fully reversible. Chronic airflow limitation results from a combination of small-airway disease and parenchymal destruction due to inflammatory processes. These inflammatory processes are often caused by exposure to noxious particles or gases.

2. **How many people are affected by COPD?**

   COPD is the fourth leading cause of mortality and morbidity in the United States. The number of people affected by COPD worldwide continues to increase because of exposure to tobacco smoke and aging of the population. Historically the prevalence of disease was higher in men, but, with changing patterns of exposure to tobacco, women are now affected as frequently as men. Worldwide, exposure to indoor pollution from heating and cooking fuels substantially contributes to COPD in women.

3. **What processes are involved in the pathogenesis of COPD?**

   COPD is characterized by chronic inflammation throughout the lung, with increased neutrophils, macrophages, and $CD8^+$ T lymphocytes. An imbalance between proteinase-antiproteinase activity and oxidative stress also contributes to the pathogenesis of this disease. Oxidative stress and proteinase-antiproteinase imbalance can be related to a combination of factors, including the inflammation itself, environmental exposures (e.g., oxidative substances in cigarette smoke), and genetics (e.g., α_1-antitrypsin deficiency).

4. **What are the major pathologic changes in COPD?**

   All structures of the lung are subjected to pathologic changes in COPD. In the central airways, inflammatory cells infiltrate the surface epithelium, edema is present, mucus-secreting glands are enlarged, and the number of goblet cells increases with mucus hypersecretion. In the peripheral airways (small bronchi and bronchioles with an internal diameter <2 mm), chronic inflammation leads to repeated injury and repair of the airway wall. In emphysema, destruction of alveolar septa leads to confluence of adjacent alveoli and enlarged terminal air spaces. Vascular changes include thickening of the vessel wall with increased smooth muscle, proteoglycans, and collagen deposition.

5. **How is severity graded in COPD?**

   The staging system should be regarded as an educational tool and a guide to management (Table 22-1).

6. **What are the benefits of smoking cessation for a patient with COPD?**

   Smoking cessation is the most important intervention. It is the most effective intervention to decelerate the decline in lung function characteristic of this disease. In addition to the modest improvement in forced expiratory volume in 1 second (FEV_1) seen with smoking cessation, the rate of decline in FEV_1 may be reduced, in some cases even to the rate found in healthy nonsmokers (± 30 mL/yr).

TABLE 22-1. CLASSIFICATION OF COPD BY SEVERITY	
STAGE	**SEVERITY**
0. At risk	Normal spirometry Chronic symptoms (e.g., cough, sputum production)
I. Mild COPD	$FEV_1/FVC < 70\%$ $FEV_1 \geq 80\%$ predicted
II. Moderate COPD	$FEV_1/FVC < 70\%$ $50\% \leq FEV_1 < 80\%$ predicted
III. Severe COPD	$FEV_1/FVC < 70\%$ $30\% \leq FEV_1 < 50\%$ predicted
IV. Very severe	$FEV_1/FVC < 70\%$

From the Global Initiative for Chronic Obstructive Lung Disease.
$FEV_1 < 30\%$ predicted or $FEV_1 < 50\%$ predicted plus chronic respiratory failure.
FEV_1, Forced expiratory volume in 1 second; *FVC*, forced vital capacity.

7. **Why are bronchodilators used in the treatment of COPD?**
   Bronchodilators treat airway obstruction in patients with COPD. By reducing bronchomotor tone, they decrease airway resistance, which can improve airflow. This will improve emptying of the lungs and tends to reduce dynamic hyperinflation during rest and exercise and thus improve exercise performance. Spirometric changes after bronchodilator therapy may be minimal, despite significant clinical benefit, as quantified by changes in quality-of-life measures and exercise tolerance (e.g., 6-minute walk).

8. **Which bronchodilators should be used in the treatment of COPD?**
   - **Anticholinergic agents:** These agents block cholinergic transmission. Ipratropium has a duration of action of 6 to 8 hours. Tiotropium bromide is more potent and has a longer duration of action, allowing once-daily administration. It is more convenient but more expensive.
   - **β_2-Adrenergic agents:** β_2-Adrenergic agents act on airway smooth muscle. Inhaled, short-acting β_2-adrenergic agents are readily absorbed systemically and can lead to numerous systemic adverse effects, such as tachycardia, tremor, and arrhythmias. Long-acting inhaled β_2-adrenergic agents are more effective and convenient but more expensive.
   - **Methylxanthines:** These are weak bronchodilators but have multiple other effects that might be important: an inotropic effect on diaphragmatic muscle, reduced muscle fatigue, increased mucociliary clearance and central respiratory drive, and some antiinflammatory effects. Because of the potential for toxicity with theophylline, other bronchodilators are preferred when available.

9. **Are inhaled corticosteroids beneficial in COPD?**
   Although regular use of inhaled corticosteroids does not prevent loss of lung function in patients with COPD, inhaled corticosteroids in combination with long-acting bronchodilators are recommended for patients with severe disease ($FEV_1 < 50\%$ predicted) and recurrent exacerbations. Data indicate that inhaled corticosteroids in combination with long-acting bronchodilators decrease the risk of exacerbations in patients with COPD. However, treatment with inhaled corticosteroids alone may increase the risk of pneumonia and does not reduce mortality.

10. **What other pharmacologic treatments may benefit patients with COPD?**
    - **α_1-Antitrypsin replacement:** This is recommended for patients with emphysema related to deficiency of α_1-antitrypsin.

- **Vaccines:** Patients with COPD are at risk for increased morbidity and mortality from respiratory tract infections. Pneumococcal and influenza vaccination, both alone and in combination, have been shown to reduce hospitalizations and mortality rates.
- **Phosphodiesterase-4 inhibitors:** Roflumilast has recently been approved for treatment of COPD in the United States. It reduces inflammation through inhibiting the breakdown of intracellular cyclic adenosine monophosphate and appears to reduce the risk of exacerbations. It cannot be used with methylxanthines.

11. **Who should get pulmonary rehabilitation?**
    Patients with all levels of COPD can benefit from exercise training programs. Pulmonary rehabilitation has been shown to improve functional status, decrease dyspnea, and reduce health care use. Pulmonary rehabilitation is currently recommended as part of the treatment plan for patients with moderate, severe, and very severe COPD.

12. **What are the indications for long-term oxygen therapy in patients with COPD?**
    For a patient at rest breathing room air in a stable condition:

    Arterial oxygen $(PaO_2) < 55$ mm Hg or arterial oxygen saturation $(SaO_2) \leq 88\%$

    or

    $$PaO_2 = 56 - 59 \text{ mm Hg}/SaO_2 = 89\%$$

    and one of the following:
    - Right-sided heart failure or polycythemia
    - Desaturation during sleep
    - Desaturation during exercise

13. **What level of oxygen should be prescribed for patients with the indications listed in question 12?**
    Oxygen should be prescribed in a dose sufficient to raise the PaO_2 to 65 to 80 mm Hg at rest during wakefulness. This PaO_2 usually is achieved with a 1- to 4-L/min oxygen flow through nasal prongs. The dose of O_2 should be increased by 1 L/min during sleep or exercise to prevent hypoxemic episodes. Oxygen should be given continuously at least 19 hours per day.

14. **Is lung volume reduction surgery effective in the treatment of COPD?**
    In lung volume reduction surgery, part of the lungs is resected to reduce hyperinflation. This has beneficial effects on the mechanical action of the respiratory muscles and improves elastic recoil, which facilitates emptying of the lungs. Lung volume reduction surgery does not improve long-term survival in COPD but does improve exercise capacity in a select group of patients. Patients who benefit from lung volume reduction surgery are those with predominantly upper lobe emphysema and a low exercise capacity.

15. **What factors predict death in patients with COPD?**
    Long-term prognosis is hard to predict in patients with COPD. Factors that have been shown to predict mortality include low body mass index, degree of airflow obstruction, dyspnea, and exercise capacity as measured by the 6-minute walk test.

16. **Are antibiotics useful in treating COPD exacerbations?**
    Giving antibiotics for COPD exacerbations is indicated when patients are seen with increased sputum purulence associated with increased sputum volume and/or dyspnea. For patients receiving mechanical ventilation for a COPD exacerbation, withholding antibiotics has been associated with increased mortality and hospital-acquired pneumonia.

17. **What organisms cause COPD exacerbations?**

Bacteria and viruses cause COPD exacerbations. In mild exacerbations *Streptococcus pneumoniae* is common. As severity of COPD increases, *Haemophilus influenzae* and *Moraxella catarrhalis* become more common, and, in severe COPD, *Pseudomonas aeruginosa* may occur.

18. **What is the role of steroids in the treatment of COPD exacerbations?**

Systemic glucocorticoids shorten the duration of the exacerbation and lead to faster improvements in lung function. A recent study suggested that nebulized budesonide may be an alternative to oral glucocorticoids in nonacidotic exacerbations but is likely to be more expensive.

19. **What are the causes of acute respiratory failure in patients with COPD?**

Causes include bronchial infection, pulmonary emboli, cardiac failure, pneumonia, pneumothorax, respiratory depression (usually by the injudicious use of sedatives or narcotic analgesic drugs), surgery (especially of chest and upper abdomen), stopping of medications, or occasionally malnutrition. In general, the criteria for the diagnosis of acute respiratory failure in patients with COPD include the following:

- Hypoxemia (PaO_2 <60 mm Hg)
- Hypercapnia ($PaCO_2$ >50-70 mm Hg)
- Respiratory acidosis (pH <7.35) associated with worsening of the patient's respiratory symptoms compared with baseline

20. **What is the initial treatment of a severe COPD exacerbation?**

Assess the patient's symptoms and signs, and obtain a chest radiograph and arterial blood gas analysis. Administer adequate oxygen: Death or irreversible brain damage results within minutes when severe hypoxemia is present, whereas hypercapnia may be well tolerated. The appropriate amount of oxygen is that which satisfies tissue oxygen needs: usually a PaO_2 >60 mm Hg, without worsening the respiratory acidosis and/or further depressing sensorium. Administer β_2-agonist and anticholinergic bronchodilators. Add glucocorticoids and antibiotics. Consider noninvasive ventilation.

21. **What is the role of noninvasive ventilation in the treatment of COPD exacerbations?**

Noninvasive ventilation has been used for patients with moderate to severe dyspnea and moderate to severe acidosis from a COPD exacerbation. A number of trials report improvements in acid-base balance, reduced $PaCO_2$, and decreased length of stay. Intubation rates are also reduced by noninvasive ventilation. Box 22-1 summarizes the indications and contraindications for noninvasive ventilation in COPD exacerbations; Box 22-2 summarizes indications for intubation and invasive mechanical ventilation in COPD exacerbation.

BOX 22-1. INDICATIONS AND CONTRAINDICATIONS FOR NONINVASIVE VENTILATION IN COPD EXACERBATION

Indications
- Moderate to severe dyspnea
- Moderate to severe acidosis and hypercapnia
- Respiratory rate >25 breaths/min

Contraindications
- Somnolence or altered mental status
- Severe hypoxemia
- Hemodynamic instability
- Craniofacial abnormalities
- High aspiration risk

> **BOX 22-2. INDICATIONS FOR INTUBATION AND INVASIVE MECHANICAL VENTILATION IN COPD EXACERBATION**
>
> - Severe dyspnea
> - Severe acidosis or hypercapnia
> - Respiratory rate >35 breaths/min
> - Severe hypoxemia
> - Failure of noninvasive ventilation
> - Hemodynamic instability

22. **What is the prognosis for a patient requiring mechanical ventilation?**
Many studies report reasonable short-term mortality rates (25%-30%) for patients with an endotracheal tube in place for a COPD exacerbation rate, and mortality is lower than among patients with an endotracheal tube for non-COPD causes. High mortality rates in the long term occur in patients with poor lung function (FEV_1 <30%) before intubation and those with significant other comorbidities.

23. **What is the role of positive end-expiratory pressure (PEEP) in mechanical ventilation during a COPD exacerbation?**
The presence of positive alveolar pressure at the end of exhalation (intrinsic PEEP) may prevent the patient from triggering the ventilator. The level of external PEEP should be set just below the level of intrinsic PEEP to allow the patient to trigger the ventilator with minimal effort.

24. **What is the preferred mode of mechanical ventilation in a COPD exacerbation?**
No mode of mechanical ventilation has been shown to be superior to another during a COPD exacerbation. In general, the principles of ventilation are to minimize hyperinflation by allowing adequate expiratory time and avoiding high tidal volumes. Oxygen should be titrated to maintain an arterial partial pressure of approximately 60 mm Hg. Overventilation should be avoided: These patients frequently have hypercapnia and a compensatory metabolic alkalosis at baseline.

KEY POINTS: CHRONIC OBSTRUCTIVE PULMONARY DISEASE

1. COPD is the fourth leading cause of morbidity and mortality in the United States.

2. Spirometry is required to grade the severity and make a diagnosis of COPD.

3. Systemic glucocorticoids are indicated only in acute exacerbations.

4. Noninvasive ventilation improves outcomes in patients with impending respiratory failure.

BIBLIOGRAPHY

1. Anthonisen NR, Manfreda J, Warren CP, et al: Antibiotic therapy in exacerbations of chronic obstructive pulmonary disease. Ann Intern Med 106:196-204, 1987.

2. Celli BR, Cote CG, Marin JM, et al: The body-mass index, airflow obstruction, dyspnea, and exercise capacity index in chronic obstructive pulmonary disease. N Engl J Med 350:1005-1012, 2004.

3. Eller J, Ede A, Schaberg T, et al: Infective exacerbations of chronic bronchitis: relation between bacteriologic etiology and lung function. Chest 113:1542-1548, 1998.

4. Esteban A, Anzueto A, Frutos F, et al: Characteristics and outcomes in adult patients receiving mechanical ventilation: a 28-day international study. JAMA 287:345-355, 2002.

5. Fabbri LM, Calverley PM, Izquierdo-Alonso JL, et al: Roflumilast in moderate-to-severe chronic obstructive pulmonary disease treated with long-acting bronchodilators: two randomized clinical trials. Lancet 374:695-703, 2009.

6. Fishman A, Martinez F, Naunheim K, et al: A randomized trial comparing lung-volume-reduction surgery with medical therapy for severe emphysema. N Engl J Med 348:2059-2073, 2003.

7. Gunen H, Hacievliyagil SS, Kosar F, et al: Factors affecting survival of hospitalised patients with COPD. Eur Respir J 26:234-241, 2005.

8. Niewoehner DE, Erbland ML, Deupree RH, et al: Effect of systemic glucocorticoids on exacerbations of chronic obstructive pulmonary disease. Department of Veterans Affairs Cooperative Study Group. N Engl J Med 340:1941-1947, 1999.

9. Nouira S, Marghli S, Belghith M, et al: Once daily oral ofloxacin in chronic obstructive pulmonary disease exacerbation requiring mechanical ventilation: a randomised placebo-controlled trial. Lancet 358:2020-2025, 2001.

10. Rabe KF, Hurd S, Anzueto A, et al: Global Initiative for Chronic Obstructive Lung Disease. Global strategy for the diagnosis, management, and prevention of chronic obstructive pulmonary disease: GOLD executive summary. Am J Respir Crit Care Med 176:532-555, 2007. Available at: http://www.goldcopd.org.

11. Sin DD, Wu L, Anderson JA, et al: Inhaled corticosteroids and mortality in chronic obstructive pulmonary disease. Thorax 60:992-997, 2005.

12. Singh S, Amin AV, Loke YK: Long term use of inhaled corticosteroids and the risk of pneumonia in chronic obstructive pulmonary disease: a meta-analysis. Arch Intern Med 169:219-229, 2009.

CHAPTER 23

COR PULMONALE

Luca M. Bigatello, MD, and Kay B. Leissner, MD, PhD

1. **What is cor pulmonale?**
    The term *cor pulmonale* was coined by Paul Dudley White in 1931 to indicate heart failure coexistent with a primary pathologic condition of the lung. Subsequent definitions have described pathologic aspects of the right ventricle, such as hypertrophy and dilatation. Recent literature has focused on pathophysiology, diagnosis, and therapy of the continuum of pulmonary hypertension and right ventricular failure. Currently, we can define cor pulmonale as acute or chronic pressure overload of the right ventricle in response to pulmonary artery (PA) hypertension of various causes.

2. **What are the subtypes of cor pulmonale?**
    Cor pulmonale can be acute or chronic.
    - In acute cor pulmonale the afterload to the right ventricle can rise in a matter of minutes (e.g., massive pulmonary embolism) giving very little room for compensation. The result will be acute right ventricular dilatation and failure, its severity depending primarily on the degree of acute PA hypertension.
    - In chronic cor pulmonale, an increase of right ventricular afterload in the face of slowly developing PA hypertension (e.g., hypoxemia in chronic obstructive pulmonary disease [COPD]) generates a compensatory response of the right ventricle (see later) that will preserve the stroke volume until either the afterload increases excessively or the myocardium fails because of ischemia or other pathologic condition.

3. **What is the pathophysiology of right ventricular failure?**
    Under normal conditions, the pulmonary circulation is a low-resistance circuit, and the right ventricle generates the same stroke volume as the left ventricle with end-systolic pressures that are just 20% to 25% of those in the left ventricle. The low pressure within the thin free wall of the right ventricle also allows myocardial perfusion to occur both in systole and in diastole. Because of its structure, similar to that of veins rather than arteries, the right ventricle accommodates well additional volume but not higher pressure. When pressure overload occurs acutely, the right ventricle can only dilate and, if the pressure is sufficiently elevated, fail. Chronically, in response to increased systolic workload the free wall of the right ventricle hypertrophies and becomes similar to the left ventricle. Laplace's law helps explaining the evolution from hypertrophy to dilatation and failure (Fig. 23-1): In a thin-wall chamber, an increase in intraluminal pressure increases wall stress unless thickness increases or the internal radius decreases. As the right ventricle hypertrophies, myocardial perfusion becomes limited to diastole, making its myocardium more susceptible to ischemia, and thus leading to dilatation and failure.

4. **What are the causes of cor pulmonale?**
    Any process that results in pulmonary hypertension can cause cor pulmonale. Pulmonary hypertension is defined as mean PA pressures >20 mm Hg at rest or >30 mm Hg with exercise. The most frequent cause of pulmonary hypertension and cor pulmonale is COPD, due to chronic hypoxia. In COPD the degree of hypertension is generally moderate, and oxygen supplementation may be effective in relieving some of the pressure load to the right ventricle and delaying failure. Additional causes of cor pulmonale include chronic pulmonary thromboembolic

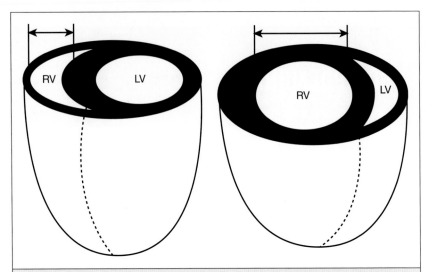

Figure 23-1. Diagrammatic cross-section of the right *(RV)* and left ventricular *(LV)* cavities. *Left,* Normal state. The right ventricle has a thin free wall and a characteristic crescentlike shape. *Right,* Right ventricular hypertrophy from pressure overload. The right ventricle assumes a spherical shape, thickened free wall, and an overall greater area than the left ventricle, which is normally the larger of the two ventricles. (From Voelkel NF, Quaife RA, Leinwand LA, et al. Right ventricular function and failure. Report of a National Heart, Lung, and Blood Institute working group on cellular and molecular mechanisms of right heart failure. Circulation 114:1883-1891, 2006. Copyright 2006 American Heart Association.)

disease, left-sided cardiac abnormalities, untreated obstructive sleep apnea (OSA), interstitial lung diseases, and primary pulmonary hypertension. A comprehensive classification of the diseases of the lung associated with PA hypertension and cor pulmonale is shown in Table 23-1.

5. **What is the pathophysiology of PA hypertension?**
   Hypoxemia and vascular occlusion are the major causes of pulmonary hypertension; both result in an increase in pulmonary vascular resistance and reduction of pulmonary blood flow. Hypoxemia causes local vasoconstriction (hypoxic pulmonary vasoconstriction), which in part corrects ventilation-perfusion match and improves gas exchange. However, chronic vasoconstriction also produces smooth muscle proliferation in the small arteries, leading to increased resistance and increased PA pressure. These architectural changes may promote platelet aggregation leading to thrombus formation that further increases pulmonary artery pressure and pulmonary vascular resistance.

6. **Discuss the epidemiology of cor pulmonale, with particular reference to COPD.**
   Cor pulmonale may account for approximately 10% of all admissions for congestive heart failure. COPD is the most frequent cause of cor pulmonale, but the actual incidence is unknown. Pulmonary hypertension in COPD has been reported to occur in 30% to 70% of the cases, a wide range that underlines the lack of large epidemiologic studies of patients with mild to moderate COPD. Severe pulmonary hypertension (mean pressure over 40 mm Hg) is uncommon and does not seem to be closely related to the degree of airflow limitation. Hence, when severe pulmonary hypertension is found in patients with COPD, further causes should be sought, such as chronic embolism, left-sided heart disease, and primary pulmonary hypertension. Regardless, the presence of pulmonary hypertension in COPD is associated with a reduced lifespan.

TABLE 23-1. CLASSIFICATION OF COR PULMONALE ACCORDING TO CAUSATIVE FACTOR

CATEGORY	EXAMPLE
Diseases affecting the air passages of the lung and alveoli	COPD
	Cystic fibrosis
	Infiltrative or granulomatous defects
	Idiopathic pulmonary fibrosis
	Sarcoidosis
	Pneumoconiosis
	Scleroderma
	Mixed connective tissue disease
	Systemic lupus erythematosus
	Rheumatoid arthritis
	Polymyositis
	Eosinophilic granulomatosis
	Radiation
	Malignant infiltration
Diseases affecting thoracic cage movement	Kyphoscoliosis
	Thoracoplasty
	Neuromuscular weakness
	Sleep apnea syndrome
	Idiopathic hypoventilation
Diseases affecting the pulmonary vasculature	Primary disease of the arterial wall
	Primary pulmonary hypertension
	Pulmonary arteritis
	Toxin-induced pulmonary hypertension
	Chronic liver disease
	Peripheral pulmonary stenosis
Thrombotic disorders	Sickle cell diseases
	Pulmonary microthrombi
Embolic disorders	Thromboembolism
	Tumor embolism
	Other embolic processes (amniotic fluid, air, fat)
	Schistosomiasis and other parasitic infections
Pressure on PAs	Mediastinal tumors
	Aneurysms
	Granulomata
	Fibrosis

Modified from Rubin LJ, ed: Pulmonary Heart Disease. Boston, 1984, Martinus Nijhoff, p 4.

7. **What are the signs and symptoms of cor pulmonale?**
   Signs and symptoms of cor pulmonale develop slowly over time, as the right ventricle compensates for the increased pressure load, and become more evident as failure sets in.
   Symptoms of cor pulmonale include the following:
   - Fatigability
   - Dyspnea
   - Light-headedness
   - Chest pain
   - Palpitations
   - Abdominal fullness, right upper quadrant pain
   Signs of cor pulmonale include the following:
   - Jugular veins distention
   - Prominent A and V waves in the jugular venous pulse trace
   - Accentuated pulmonic component of the second heart sound
   - Right-sided S_4
   - Murmurs of tricuspid and pulmonic insufficiency
   - Dependent peripheral edema and hepatomegaly

8. **What is the mortality associated with cor pulmonale?**
   Patients with COPD have a 62% 5-year survival rate, whereas patients with COPD and mean PA pressures in excess of 25 mm Hg have a 5-year survival of only 36% and of 30% if peripheral edema is present. It is unclear whether PA hypertension is the cause of death or whether it is a marker of increased mortality.

9. **What are the electrocardiographic (ECG) findings associated with right ventricular hypertrophy?**
   ECG criteria for right ventricular hypertrophy are neither highly specific nor highly sensitive, and in current practice the diagnosis is better made by echocardiography. However, recognizing ECG abnormalities that may be associated with right ventricular hypertrophy remains an important diagnostic tool in the preoperative anesthetic evaluation. ECG findings commonly associated with right ventricular hypertrophy include the following:
   - Right axis deviation: QRS negative in lead I, positive in aVR
   - Tall R waves in the right precordial leads, deep S waves in the left precordial leads
   - Right atrial enlargement: P pulmonale, large P wave, in II and V_1
   - ST-segment changes in the opposite direction of the QRS (i.e., wide QRS-ST angle)
   - Right bundle branch block: wide QRS (>1.12 seconds); RSR′ in V_1 and V_2

10. **How is the diagnosis of cor pulmonale made?**
    Once the suspicion of cor pulmonale is raised on clinical grounds (see earlier for signs and symptoms), a number of diagnostic tests are available.

11. **What tests can help determine the diagnosis of cor pulmonale?**
    Laboratory investigations to detect the underlying cause of cor pulmonale may include the following:
    - Arterial blood gas analysis with acid-base status.
    - Hematocrit to detect polycythemia.
    - Coagulation studies to diagnose hypercoagulability, including serum levels of proteins S and C, antithrombin III, factor V Leyden, homocysteine, anticardiolipin antibodies.
    - Antinuclear antibody level for connective tissue diseases, such as scleroderma.
    - Brain natriuretic peptide may be elevated to compensate right-sided heart failure by diuresis, natriuresis, and vasodilation.

Radiographic findings include the following:

- Chest radiograph
  - □ Enlargement of the central PAs (right PA >16 mm, left PA >18 mm) with oligemic peripheral lung fields (Westermark sign)
  - □ Enlargement of the right ventricle, presenting as an increased width of the cardiac silhouette in the posteroanterior view and increased retrosternal space in the lateral view
  - □ Distention of central veins including the azygous vein
  - □ General signs related to the primary lung condition
- Computed tomography and computed tomographic angiography
  - □ Dilation of the main PA diameter (≥29 mm has a reported sensitivity of 84% and a specificity of 75% for diagnosing pulmonary hypertension).
  - □ Cardiac dimensions may be evaluated.
  - □ Scans may help in diagnosing the underlying etiology of cor pulmonale, such as pulmonary embolism.
- Ultrafast, ECG-gated computed tomography (CT)
  - □ Ultrafast, ECG-gated CT has been evaluated to study right ventricular function: it may estimate ejection fraction and wall mass with high accuracy.
- Magnetic resonance imaging (MRI) and magnetic resonance angiography (MRA)
  - □ MRI can provide highly accurate information about right-sided heart mass, interventricular septal flattening, and biventricular function.
  - □ MRA has been used for the diagnosis of chronic thromboembolic pulmonary disease.
- Nuclear imaging
  - □ Radionuclide ventriculography and radionuclide angiography (gated blood pool scan) may determine ejection fraction of each ventricle noninvasively.

  Echocardiographic findings include the following:
- Transthoracic and transesophageal two-dimensional echocardiography (TTE and TEE, respectively) can be used to evaluate ventricular size and function, valvular dysfunction, and pulmonary hypertension.
  - □ Right ventricular myocardial thickness and dilation.
  - □ Paradoxical leftward motion and flattening of the interventricular septum during both systole and diastole.
  - □ In severe cases, the interventricular septum may bulge into the left ventricle during the entire cardiac cycle, resulting in reduced left ventricular filling and output.
- Doppler echocardiography is used to estimate PA pressure noninvasively.
  - □ The pressure difference between the right ventricle and right atrium can be calculated from the tricuspid valve regurgitant jet usually present in pulmonary hypertension.
  - □ The right atrial pressure needs to be estimated by the size and respiratory variation of flow in the inferior or superior vena cava. The PA pressure is then calculated by the modified Bernoulli equation:

  $$\text{PA systolic pressure} = 4 \times \text{Tricuspid jet velocity}^2 + \text{Right atrial pressure}$$

  - □ Other findings associated with cor pulmonale are midsystolic closure of the pulmonic valve and pulmonic insufficiency.

  Right-sided heart catheterization remains the gold standard for evaluation and diagnosis of pulmonary hypertension and cor pulmonale. Right-sided heart catheterization allows for precise measurement of pulmonary hemodynamics, including PA and right ventricle pressure, as well as the left ventricular end-diastolic pressure (PA "occlusion" pressure, or *wedge* pressure). It also allows for the initial assessment of response to treatments.

  MRI yields accurate dimensions of the right ventricle, although at this time it does not add a proved benefit to echocardiography.

12. **What are the indications for use of echocardiography in the evaluation of cor pulmonale?**
    Indications for TEE and diagnosis of pulmonary hypertension include the following:
    Class I: Conditions for which evidence and/or general agreement of an effective treatment exist
    1. Suspected pulmonary hypertension
    2. To distinguish cardiac versus noncardiac cause of dyspnea in patients in whom clinical and laboratory clues are ambiguous*
    3. To follow the response to treatment of pulmonary hypertension
    4. Lung disease with clinical suspicion of cardiac involvement (suspected cor pulmonale)

    Class II: Conditions for which conflicting evidence and/or a divergence of opinion exist about the usefulness or efficacy of a procedure or treatment
    Class IIa: Evidence or opinion is in favor of efficacy.
    Class IIb: Efficacy is less established.
    1. Pulmonary emboli and suspected clots in right atrium, ventricle, or large PA branches*
    2. Measurement of exercise PA pressure
    3. Evaluation of candidates for lung transplantation or other surgical procedure for advanced lung disease*

    Class III: Conditions for which evidence and/or general agreement exist that the treatment is not effective and in some cases may be harmful
    1. Lung disease without any clinical suspicion of cardiac involvement
    2. Reevaluation studies of right ventricular function in patients with chronic obstructive lung disease without a change in clinical status

13. **Discuss nonpharmacologic treatment options for patients with cor pulmonale.**
    - Lifestyle modifications. Although data are not available, it seems sensible that promoting a healthy lifestyle that includes moderate aerobic exercise and weight reduction should be beneficial. Strenuous activity should be avoided, and supplemental oxygen may be beneficial during even graded exercise, such as walking.
    - Oxygen therapy is considered a mainstay of treatment for patients with COPD. Large controlled trials demonstrate that long-term administration of oxygen improves survival in patients with hypoxemia and COPD. Oxygen therapy decreases pulmonary vascular resistance by diminishing pulmonary vasoconstriction and improves right ventricular stroke volume and cardiac output.
    - Phlebotomy may provide symptomatic relief of dyspnea to patients with pronounced polycythemia (hematocrit $> 60\%$). Although less frequently used than in the past, phlebotomy can be considered in patients with polycythemia with acute decompensation.
    - Noninvasive ventilation (NIV) is the first line of ventilatory support during exacerbation of COPD, and it is standard therapy for advanced OSA. It is reasonable to infer that by correcting hypoxemia and acidosis, NIV will also decrease PA pressure, ease the forward flow of the right ventricle, and improve stroke volume and cardiac output when right ventricle failure is present. However, no data exist on the outcome benefit of NIV in acute cor pulmonale.

14. **What are the pharmacologic therapies for patients with cor pulmonale?**
    - Diuretics are indicated to manage right ventricle failure and volume overload. No evidence exists of benefit of long-term diuretic therapy in compensated cor pulmonale.
    - Vasodilators are a mainstay of pharmacologic therapy of pulmonary hypertension. Vasodilators improve cardiac output by decreasing the afterload to the right ventricle, and their efficacy in cor pulmonale depends on their relative selectivity for the pulmonary circulation. Systemic hypotension, syncope, and myocardial infarction are all possible complications of vasodilator therapy. They are discussed in detail later.

---

*TEE is typically indicated when TTE studies are not diagnostic.

- Anticoagulation with warfarin (Coumadin) is indicated for those patients with cor pulmonale resulting from thromboocclusive pulmonary disease. In addition, and in the absence of the customary contraindications, it has been recommended for pulmonary hypertension associated with a variety of other diseases, such as collagen diseases, human immunodeficiency virus, and congenital left-to-right shunts.

  Additional therapies are specifically related to the primary lung disease, including surgical interventions, such as repair of intracardiac defects and lung transplantation.

15. **Discuss the different classes of vasodilators used in the treatment of cor pulmonale.**

    Long-term treatment of cor pulmonale includes the following:
    - Calcium channel blockers (nifedipine, diltiazem, amlodipine) have been used both in the short term as a test of pulmonary vascular responsiveness and in the long term as therapy.
    - Prostacyclins improve hemodynamics, symptoms, and outcome of patients with pulmonary hypertension of diverse etiology. Epoprostenol is administered as a continuous intravenous infusion through indwelling central venous access, and its use is limited to centers with the experience and structure to safely provide this treatment. Iloprost is a prostacyclin analogue that can be administered by inhalation. However, it requires a special nebulizer and six to nine administrations per day. Data on the long-term effect of iloprost therapy are still scarce.
    - Endothelin-receptor antagonists such as bosentan have shown significant improvements in symptoms and short-term composite outcomes. One advantage of bosentan is its oral administration. Disadvantages come from its common side effects, including headache, flushing, elevation of liver enzyme levels, dependent edema, and anemia, which may lead to discontinuation of treatment.
    - Phosphodiesterase inhibitors such as sildenafil improve exercise capacity but do not prevent clinical worsening over time. In many cases, the starting dose of sildenafil is 20 mg 3 times a day, but in many cases, a dose of 80 mg 3 times a day is needed, with significant systemic side effects.

    Vasodilators for acute cor pulmonale include the following:

    Inhaled nitric oxide (NO) is a selective pulmonary vasodilator available for a number of indications (often off-label) characterized by acute pulmonary hypertension and hypoxemia. Low doses of inhaled NO rapidly and reproducibly induce PA vasodilation and an increase in PaO_2 without systemic hypotension. However, its effect on pulmonary pressure and resistance in adults is modest and short-lived. Hence, the indications for inhaled NO are limited to the following:
    - Bridge treatment while other options are worked out and
    - Test of reactivity of the pulmonary circulation for chronic vasodilator therapy with other drugs.

    Inotropes with vasodilatory properties include the following:
    - Dobutamine is the prototype of these agents. Dobutamine is a catecholamine with β_1 and β_2 adrenergic vascular effects. Dobutamine enhances myocardial contractility and decreases vascular resistance, thus increasing stroke volume and decreasing pulmonary and systemic pressure. The balance of these actions determines the effectiveness of the drug in each individual patient. Ideally, it will decrease PA pressure and increase cardiac output enough to maintain an adequate systemic blood pressure. Its effect is limited by systemic hypotension and tachycardia. An advantage of this drug is that, like all catecholamines, it has a short half-life, and its effect regresses rapidly on discontinuation.
    - Milrinone is a phosphodiesterase inhibitor (different class from sildenafil) with hemodynamic actions similar to dobutamine, but longer-lived and possibly more effective (i.e., more inotropy and less arrhythmia). Given its different mechanism of action, milrinone can be added in the short term to catecholamines, such as dobutamine or norepinephrine, and further potentiate their inotropic effect.

16. **Is the function of the left ventricle affected in cor pulmonale?**

    Left ventricular dysfunction can occur as a mechanical consequence of the right ventricle pressure and volume overload. As the right ventricle adapts to a higher afterload, its end-diastolic volume increases, and the cross-sectional shape of the right ventricle changes from a crescent to a sphere, affecting the position and function of the interventricular septum. As the septum impinges onto the left ventricle, the diastolic volume of the left ventricle decreases, and the intracavitary pressure increases. Thus filling of the left ventricle is impaired, stroke volume decreases, and left-sided filling pressure increases, in a fashion similar to the mechanics that are seen in left ventricular hypertrophy of, for example, hypertensive cardiomyopathy or aortic stenosis.

17. **Discuss the considerations for ventilator management of patients with cor pulmonale.**
   Goals of mechanical ventilation in patients with pulmonary hypertension and cor pulmonale include the following:
   - Maintain adequate PaO_2 and $PaCO_2$ to optimize PA vasodilation.
   - Avoid excessive intrathoracic pressures, which may decrease venous return and increase afterload to the right ventricle, and consequent decreased filling and output of the left ventricle.
   - Limit intrathoracic pressure by controlling the level of mean airway pressure, which can be increased by increasing end-inspiratory pressure, end-expiratory pressure (PEEP, auto-PEEP), and inspiratory time. Careful administration of PEEP in patients with acute respiratory failure may be beneficial when it results in alveolar recruitment and consequent relief of hypoxemia.

KEY POINTS: COR PULMONALE

1. Any process that results in pulmonary hypertension can cause cor pulmonale.

2. COPD and untreated OSA are common causes of cor pulmonale.

3. The presence of cor pulmonale in advanced COPD has a poor 5-year survival rate.

BIBLIOGRAPHY

1. American College of Cardiology Foundation: 2003 Guideline Update for the Clinical Application of Echocardiography: a report of the American College of Cardiology/American Heart Association Task Force on Practice Guidelines. Washington, DC, 2003.

2. Bogaart HJ, Abe K, Noordergraf AV, et al: The right ventricle under pressure. Cellular and molecular mechanisms of right-heart failure in pulmonary hypertension. Chest 135:794-804, 2009.

3. Criner GJ: Effects of long-term oxygen therapy on mortality and morbidity. Respir Care 45:105-118, 2000.

4. Gordon C, Collard CD, Pan W: Intraoperative management of pulmonary hypertension and associated right heart failure. Curr Opin Anaesthesiol 23:49-56, 2010.

5. Haddad F, Couture P, Tousignant C, et al: The right ventricle in cardiac surgery, a perioperative perspective: I. Anatomy, physiology, and assessment. Anesth Analg 108:407-421, 2009.

6. Han MK, McLaughlin VV, Criner GJ, et al: Pulmonary diseases and the heart. Circulation 916:2992-3005, 2007.

7. Inglessis I, Shin JT, Lepore JJ, et al: Hemodynamic effects of inhaled nitric oxide in right ventricular myocardial infarction and septic shock. J Am Coll Cardiol 44:793-798, 2004.

8. McLaughlin VV, McGoon MD: Pulmonary arterial hypertension. Circulation 114:1417-1431, 2006.

9. Metha S, Hill NS: Noninvasive ventilation. Am J Respir Crit Care Med 163:540-577, 2001.

10. Minai OA, Chaouat A, Adnot S: Pulmonary hypertension in COPD: epidemiology, significance, and management: pulmonary vascular disease: the global perspective. Chest 137:39S-51S, 2010.

11. Oswald-Mammosser M, Weitzenblum E, Quoix E, et al: Prognostic factors in COPD patients receiving long-term oxygen therapy. Importance of pulmonary artery pressure. Chest 107:1193-1198, 1995.

12. Piazza G, Goldhaber SZ: Chronic thromboembolic pulmonary hypertension. N Engl J Med 364:351-360, 2011.

13. Scharf SM, Iqbal M, Keller C, et al: Hemodynamic characterization of patients with severe emphysema. Am J Respir Crit Care Med 166:314-322, 2002.

14. Simonneau G, Robbins IM, Beghetti M, et al: Updated classification of pulmonary hypertension. J Am Coll Cardiol 54:S43-S54, 2009.

15. Stobierska-Dzierzek B, Awad H, Michler RE: The evolving management of acute right-sided heart failure in cardiac transplant recipients. J Am Coll Cardiol 38:923-931, 2001.

16. Vizza CD, Lynch JP, Ochoa LL, et al: Right and left ventricular dysfunction in patients with severe pulmonary disease. Chest 113:576-583, 1998.

ACUTE RESPIRATORY FAILURE, ACUTE LUNG INJURY/ACUTE RESPIRATORY DISTRESS SYNDROME, AND ACUTE CHEST SYNDROME

Prema R. Menon, MD, and Gilman B. Allen, MD

1. **What is acute respiratory failure (ARF)?**

   ARF is a syndrome in which the respiratory system fails in gas exchange, in either oxygenation, carbon dioxide elimination, or both. ARF can occur within minutes or over hours.

2. **What are the types of ARF?**

   ARF can be either hypoxemic, hypercapnic, or a combination of both. Arterial blood gas analysis is the gold standard for diagnosis of respiratory failure. An arterial PO_2 of less than 50 mm Hg while breathing ambient air is considered hypoxemic, and hypercapnia is defined as a PCO_2 of greater than 50 mm Hg.

3. **What are the mechanisms and causes of hypoxemic respiratory failure?**

   Mechanisms of hypoxemia are as follows:
   - Low mixed venous oxygen (low cardiac output, anemia)
   - Ventilation-perfusion (V/Q) mismatch
   - Alveolar hypoventilation
   - Shunt: physiologic (alveolar level) and anatomic (proximal to lung)
   - Diffusion limitation
   - Low inspired oxygen fraction

   Common causes of hypoxemia and their respective primary mechanisms are as follows:
   - Chronic obstructive pulmonary disease: V/Q mismatch, diffusion limitation
   - Pneumonia, pulmonary edema, and acute respiratory distress syndrome: physiologic shunt
   - Pulmonary embolism: V/Q mismatch (physiologic dead space)
   - Pulmonary fibrosis: diffusion limitation
   - Obesity: alveolar hypoventilation

4. **What are the mechanisms and causes of hypercapnic respiratory failure?**

   Mechanisms (all related to alveolar hypoventilation) are as follows:
   - Decreased central respiratory drive
   - Abnormalities of the chest wall leading to excessive restriction
   - Airways abnormalities leading to excessive dead space or increased work of breathing and fatigue
   - Neuromuscular diseases (peripheral nervous system)

   Causes are as follows:
   - Severe asthma
   - Drug overdose
   - Myasthenia gravis
   - Cervical cord injuries
   - Brain stem injuries
   - Obesity-hypoventilation
   - Kyphoscoliosis

5. **What are the most important immediate goals of therapy for ARF?**
Hypoxia is the major immediate threat to organ function, and therefore initial goals should be directed toward oxygen supplementation and reversal or prevention of tissue hypoxia. Hypercapnia is generally better tolerated if not sudden or associated with severe acidosis. Supplemental oxygen should be delivered to achieve a $PaO_2 > 55$ mm Hg. This can be achieved with nasal prongs or face mask, but in many cases mechanical ventilation is required to reverse hypoxemia. Mechanical ventilation can maximize both inspired O_2 and alveolar ventilation (decrease $PaCO_2$).

6. **What are the main indications for endotracheal intubation and mechanical ventilation?**
Bradypnea, apnea, or respiratory arrest; acute respiratory distress syndrome; respiratory muscle fatigue; obtundation or coma; PaO_2 less than 55 mm Hg despite supplemental oxygen; PCO_2 greater than 50 mm Hg with arterial pH < 7.2.

7. **What are acute lung injury (ALI) and acute respiratory distress syndrome (ARDS)?**
The American-European Consensus Conference recommended the following criteria for definition of ARDS:
- Acute onset
- Bilateral infiltrates on chest radiograph
- Pulmonary artery wedge pressure ≤ 18 mm Hg or the absence of clinical evidence of left atrial hypertension
- PaO_2/FiO_2 ratio $\leq 200^*$ for ARDS
- Acute lung injury is defined by all of the above except a PaO_2/FiO_2 ratio $\leq 300^*$

8. **What is the pathogenesis of ARDS?**
The early phase of ALI or ARDS is characterized by injury and increased permeability of the endothelial and epithelial barriers of the lung leading to the accumulation of protein-rich edema fluid in the interstitium and alveolar airspace. This fluid contains plasma proteins, inflammatory cells (mostly neutrophils), and necrotic debris that can pack down into dense eosin-staining hyaline membranes, the latter of which are pathognomonic for the pathology of ARDS, termed *diffuse alveolar damage*. Leukocytes, fibroblasts, and epithelial cells release cytokines that enhance the inflammatory response. Because of up-regulation of procoagulant pathways diffuse intravascular thrombi formation and fibrin deposition occur. Patients usually begin to recover in the first 5 to 14 days of disease. During the later phase of injury, type II pneumocyte hyperplasia and collagen deposition occur and can serve to repopulate the epithelium during the healing process but can also progress to fibrosis. This latter *fibroproliferative phase* can lead to prolonged time using the ventilator and increased mortality but can also be self-limited and resolve entirely.

9. **What are risk factors for the development of ARDS?**
Several conditions can predispose one to the development of ARDS, such as aspiration of gastric contents, pneumonia, sepsis (most common cause), trauma, transfusion of blood products (particularly plasma-rich products), pancreatitis, fat emboli, and near-drowning. Comorbid conditions can be predictive of outcomes as well. Patients with a history of active malignancy, chronic alcoholism, liver disease, and right ventricular dysfunction have a higher likelihood of death from ALI and ARDS.

---

*Relevance of oxygenation index is questionable because it has not been shown to be prognostic and does not account for positive end-expiratory pressure, body position, inspiratory time, or other factors that might influence overall oxygenation.

10. **What is multiple-organ dysfunction syndrome (MODS)?**
    MODS is a process characterized by incremental degrees of physiologic derangement in individual organs, such as the liver, gut, kidney, brain, or cardiovascular and hematologic systems. Alterations in organ function can vary widely from a mild degree of organ dysfunction to irreversible organ failure. MODS is the single most important predictor of death in ALI and ARDS and a much more common cause of death in ALI or ARDS than is refractory hypoxemia.

11. **What is the mortality associated with ARDS?**
    When ARDS was first described in 1967, the mortality rate was approximately 58%. The overall mortality rate of patients with ARDS over the past several decades is approximately 43%. The mortality rate of ARDS has progressively declined over the last decade to approximately 30% but is still 41% to 45% in those between 65 and 84 years of age and approximately 60% in patients over the age of 85 years.

12. **How do patients with ARDS die?**
    Sepsis syndrome with multiorgan failure remains the leading cause of death in patients with ARDS. Unsupportable respiratory failure is a much less common cause of death.

13. **What medical therapy is available for the treatment of ARDS?**
    Despite many promising results from experimental animal studies, currently no specific therapies are proven to be effective in reducing ARDS mortality. Surfactant replacement therapy, *N*-acetylcysteine, ketoconazole, nitric oxide, steroids, lisofylline, activated protein C, β-agonists, and inhaled prostacyclins have all been studied in phase III randomized trials. Although some interventions such as recombinant surfactant protein C and prone positioning have been effective in improving oxygenation, but none of these therapies has demonstrated a reduction in mortality. The only interventions thus far shown to reduce ARDS mortality are the use of low tidal volumes and neuromuscular blockade (NMB). Although low tidal volumes have since been adopted as best practice, the data on NMB are limited, and controversy remains over whether paralysis should be uniformly applied to all patients with ARDS.

14. **How should the lungs of patients with ARDS be ventilated?**
    In the 1980s, animal studies revealed that ventilation with large tidal volumes and high inspiratory pressures led to the development of inflammatory infiltrates, alveolar flooding, and hyaline membranes. Since then several clinical studies have shown a benefit from using low tidal volumes in patients with ARDS. The most influential of these studies, conducted by the ARDS Network, showed a nearly 9% absolute reduction in the risk of death in patients with ARDS receiving ventilation with low tidal volumes (6 mL/kg predicted body weight) and targeted plateau pressures of ≤ 30 cm H_2O.

    Other modes of ventilation in ARDS have been and remain to be studied, such as higher positive end-expiratory pressure (PEEP), alveolar recruitment maneuvers, prone positioning, and high-frequency oscillatory ventilation (HFOV). None has demonstrated a reduction in mortality, but studies evaluating pressure-targeted PEEP and HFOV are ongoing.

15. **What is the role of alternate modes of ventilation?**
    Prone positioning has been shown to improve oxygenation but does not lead to a reduction in mortality. Although inverse ratio ventilation, airway pressure release ventilation, and HFOV may be considered as rescue modes in patients with life-threatening refractory hypoxemia receiving conventional low tidal volume ventilation, randomized controlled trials demonstrating their efficacy are lacking, and therefore these modes cannot be recommended for first-line management.

16. **What are the sequelae in survivors of ARDS?**

The spectrum of impairments in survivors of ARDS is broad. Surprisingly, limitations are minimal based on mean values of pulmonary function after 5 years. However, the range of values for forced vital capacity and diffusing capacity among survivors suggest a wide spectrum from moderate to no impairment at all. The majority of the physical impairment is related to decreased exercise capacity and musculoskeletal weakness. Quality of life among survivors is also negatively impacted by a large prevalence of cognitive deficits, depression, and anxiety as far as 2 years out from discharge, as well as musculoskeletal weakness, orthopedic injuries (heterotropic ossification, frozen shoulder), vocal cord dysfunction, and cosmesis (procedural scars from tracheostomy, chest tube insertions, and central and arterial lines).

17. **What is acute chest syndrome (ACS)?**

ACS is a frequent complication of sickle cell disease. It is defined as a combination of acute onset fever, chest pain, new pulmonary infiltrates, and signs and symptoms of pulmonary disease (i.e., tachypnea, dyspnea, and cough). ACS resembles bacterial pneumonia clinically but is entirely different in its pathology. It can be brought on by various physiologic insults or stressors, including infection, vasoocclusive crisis, embolization of marrow fat from infarcted bone, and lung infarction, but uniformly involves an acute occlusion of the pulmonary vascular bed by sickle erythrocytes.

18. **What are the treatment options for ACS?**

Blood transfusion, hydration, pain control, and antibiotics are the current mainstays of therapy. Red cell transfusion has no proven benefit over standard supportive care, but it can improve oxygenation and thus is still recommended. The role of corticosteroids is unclear. Studies examining the use of glucocorticoids have generated variable results. Some experts recommend the use of dexamethasone, primarily in patients with asthma and ACS. However, the risk for increased pain and subsequent readmission remains a limitation. A randomized controlled trial of dexamethasone in the treatment of ACS is currently underway.

19. **Is there a role for exchange transfusion in sickle cell disease?**

Simple or exchange transfusion successfully and rapidly increases oxygenation in patients with ACS. In patients requiring mechanical ventilation with multilobar processes who have already received simple transfusions, the current expert recommendation is to proceed with red cell exchange transfusions, but no randomized control studies have been done to date that demonstrate proven benefit from exchange transfusion in ACS.

20. **Is pulse oximetry reliable in patients with sickle cell disease?**

Pulse oximetry measurements may overestimate the oxygen saturation by including methemoglobin and carboxyhemoglobin, which are both slightly increased in hemoglobin (Hb) S disorders. Automated blood gas analyzers may also overestimate the saturation because they calculate O_2 saturation on the basis of standard HbA. Cooximetry is the most accurate method to analyze oxygen saturation in HbS disorders.

21. **What is the mortality for ACS?**

The overall mortality for ACS is 3%. However, adult patients have a higher overall mortality rate of 9%. The leading causes of death are respiratory failure and bronchopneumonia, but sepsis, pulmonary hemorrhage, hypovolemic shock, and intracranial hemorrhage are additional common causes of death in ACS.

KEY POINTS: ARF, ALI/ARDS, AND ACS

1. Definition of acute respiratory failure
   - Hypoxemic respiratory failure: PaO_2 <50 mm Hg
   - Hypercapnic respiratory failure: PCO_2 >50 mm Hg

2. Criteria for ALI or ARDS
   - Acute onset
   - Bilateral infiltrates on chest radiograph
   - Pulmonary capillary wedge pressure ≤ 18 mm Hg, no evidence of left atrial hypertension
   - PaO_2/FiO_2 ≤200 (ARDS)
   - PaO_2/FiO_2 ≤300 (ALI)

3. Treatment of ACS
   - Blood transfusion
   - Hydration
   - Pain control
   - Antibiotics
   - Exchange transfusion

BIBLIOGRAPHY

1. The Acute Respiratory Distress Syndrome Network: Ventilation with lower tidal volumes as compared with traditional tidal volumes for acute lung injury and the acute respiratory distress syndrome. N Engl J Med 342:1301-1308, 2000.

2. Bernard GR, Artigas A, Brigham KL, et al: The American-European Consensus Conference on ARDS. Definitions, mechanisms, relevant outcomes, and clinical trial coordination. Am J Respir Crit Care Med 149:818-824, 1994.

3. Esteban A, Fernandez-Segoviano P, Frutos-Vivar F, et al: Comparison of clinical criteria for the acute respiratory distress syndrome with autopsy findings. Ann Intern Med 141:440-445, 2004.

4. Graham LM Jr: The effect of sickle cell disease on the lung. Clin Pulm Med 11:369, 2004.

5. Herridge M, Tansey C, Cheung A, et al: Functional disability 5 years after acute respiratory distress syndrome. N Engl J Med 364:1293-1304, 2011.

6. Hudson LD, Milberg JA, Anardi D, et al: Clinical risks for development of the acute respiratory distress syndrome. Am J Respir Crit Care Med 151:293-301, 1995.

7. Papazian L, Forel JM, Gacouin A, et al: Neuromuscular blockers in early acute respiratory distress syndrome. N Engl J Med 363:1107-1116, 2010.

8. Rubenfeld GD, Caldwell E, Peabody E, et al: Incidence and outcomes of acute lung injury. N Engl J Med 353:1685-1693, 2005.

9. Slutsky AS: Mechanical ventilation. American College of Chest Physicians' Consensus Conference. Chest 104:1833-1859, 1993.

10. Stapleton RD, Wang BM, Hudson LD, et al: Causes and timing of death in patients with ARDS. Chest 128:525-532, 2005.

11. Suchyta MR, Orme JF, Morris AH: The changing face of organ failure in ARDS. Chest 124:1871-1879, 2003.

12. Tomashefski JF Jr: Pulmonary pathology of acute respiratory distress syndrome. Clin Chest Med 21:435-466, 2000.

13. Turner JM, Kaplan JB, Cohen HW, et al: Exchange versus simple transfusion for acute chest syndrome in sickle cell anemia adults. Transfusion 49:863-868, 2009.

14. Vichinsky EP, Neumayr LD, Earles AN, et al: Causes and outcomes of the acute chest syndrome in sickle cell disease. National Acute Chest Syndrome Study Group. N Engl J Med 342:1855-1865, 2000.

15. Ware LB, Matthay MA: The acute respiratory distress syndrome. N Engl J Med 342:1334-1349, 2000.

CHAPTER 25

HEMOPTYSIS

Michael E. Hanley, MD

1. **What is hemoptysis?**

   Hemoptysis is the expectoration of blood originating from the lower respiratory tract. It is classified on the basis of the volume of expectorated blood.
   - *Scant hemoptysis* refers to expectoration of sputa that are tinged or streaked with blood.
   - *Frank hemoptysis* is characterized by sputa that are grossly bloody but of a low volume (less than 100-200 mL in 24 hours).
   - *Massive hemoptysis* refers to bleeding that is potentially acutely life threatening. It is inconsistently defined but generally describes expectoration of at least 200 mL of blood within a 24-hour period. Most authors limit the definition of massive hemoptysis to expectoration of more than 600 mL of blood in 24 hours.

2. **How are hemoptysis and pseudohemoptysis different?**

   Pseudohemoptysis is expectoration of blood originating from a source other than the lower respiratory tract. It results from either aspiration of blood from the gastrointestinal tract or blood draining into the larynx and trachea from bleeding sites in the oral cavity, nasopharynx, or larynx.

3. **Describe the differential diagnosis of hemoptysis.**

   The differential diagnosis of hemoptysis is based on the site of bleeding. Hemoptysis in general results from either a focal or a diffuse tracheobronchial (airway) or pulmonary parenchymal process (Box 25-1). Occasionally nonpulmonary processes, in particular cardiac, vascular, or hematologic disorders, may result in bleeding in the lungs. The frequency with which hemoptysis is associated with these conditions is determined by the age of the patient, the population being studied (e.g., surgical vs. medical, veterans hospital vs. city or county indigent hospital), and the amount of expectorated blood. Approximately 30% of cases are cryptogenic, and no explanation for hemoptysis is determined despite extensive evaluation.

4. **What are the common causes of massive hemoptysis?**

   The most common causes of massive hemoptysis are bronchiectasis, active or inactive tuberculosis, necrotizing pneumonia (including lung abscess) and fungal infections. The latter include both mycetoma (aspergilloma) and, less commonly, chronic necrotizing pulmonary aspergillosis. The relative frequency of these causes has changed in the past few decades and depends on both the institution and country from which the data are reported. Pulmonary neoplasm, arteriovenous malformation, pulmonary vasculitis, valvular heart disease (especially mitral stenosis), and bleeding diathesis are also potential causes of massive hemoptysis but occur less frequently.

5. **Name the common iatrogenic causes of hemoptysis that occur in critically ill patients.**

   When hemoptysis begins after endotracheal intubation, upper airway trauma caused by the intubation procedure, endotracheal tube, or endotracheal suction catheters must be considered. If hemoptysis begins after a latent period of 1 or more weeks after intubation, a tracheoartery fistula may be the source of hemorrhage. This possibility is increased if a tracheostomy tube is present. Pulmonary artery rupture and pulmonary infarction should be considered when

BOX 25-1. CAUSES OF HEMOPTYSIS

Tracheobronchial Disorders
Acute tracheobronchitis
Amyloidosis
Gastric aspiration
Bronchial adenoma
Bronchial endometriosis
Bronchial telangiectasia
Bronchogenic carcinoma
Broncholithiasis
Chronic bronchitis
Cystic fibrosis
Endobronchial metastasis
Endobronchial tuberculosis
Foreign body aspiration
Bronchial mucoid impaction
Tracheobronchial trauma
Tracheoesophageal fistula

Localized Parenchymal Diseases
Nontuberculous pneumonia
Actinomycosis
Amebiasis
Ascariasis
Aspergilloma
Bronchopulmonary sequestration
Coccidioidomycosis
Congenital and acquired cyst
Cryptococcosis
Histoplasmosis
Hydatid mole
Lung abscess
Lipoid pneumonia
Lung contusion
Metastatic cancer
Mucormycosis
Nocardiosis
Paragonimiasis
Pulmonary endometriosis
Pulmonary tuberculosis
Sporotrichosis

Cardiovascular Disorders
Aortic aneurysm
Congenital heart disease
Congestive heart failure
Fat embolism
Mitral stenosis
Postmyocardial infarction syndrome
Pulmonary arteriovenous malformation
Pulmonary artery aneurysm
Pulmonary embolus
Pulmonary venous varix
Schistosomiasis
Superior vena cava syndrome
Tumor embolization

Hematologic Disorders
Anticoagulant therapy
Disseminated intravascular coagulation
Leukemia
Thrombocytopenia

Diffuse Parenchymal Diseases
Disseminated angiosarcoma
Farmer's lung
Goodpasture syndrome
Idiopathic pulmonary hemosiderosis
Mixed IgA nephropathy
Legionnaires disease
Mixed connective tissue disease
Mixed cryoglobulinemia
Polyarteritis nodosa
Scleroderma
Systemic lupus erythematosus
Wegener granulomatosis

Other
Idiopathic
Iatrogenic

Modified from Irwin RS, Hubmayr R: Hemoptysis. In Rippe JM, Irwin RS, Alpert JS, et al (eds): Intensive Care Medicine. Boston, 1985, Little, Brown. *IgA*, Immunoglobulin A.

hemoptysis occurs in a patient with a pulmonary artery catheter. Pulmonary infarction should be suspected if a wedge-shaped infiltrate is present distal to the catheter on the chest roentgenogram.

6. **Explain the significance of massive hemoptysis.**
   Massive hemoptysis is generally due to hemorrhaging from the bronchial artery (systemic pressure) circulation as opposed to the low-pressure pulmonary artery circuit and therefore is more capable of generating high-volume, life-threatening hemorrhage. Mortality from untreated massive hemoptysis in some studies is 75% to 100%.

7. **List the tests that should be included in a routine evaluation of patients with hemoptysis.**
   History, physical examination, complete blood cell counts including platelet count, coagulation studies, urinalysis, oxygenation by either pulse oximetry or arterial blood gas analysis, chest roentgenogram, and electrocardiogram.

8. **What is the initial approach to the evaluation of a patient with hemoptysis in the intensive care unit?**
   Evaluation should begin with the routine tests previously described. After the patient has been hemodynamically stabilized, the site, etiology, and extent of bleeding should be determined. Identifying the site of bleeding requires visualization of the airways of both the upper and lower respiratory tract and examination of the chest roentgenogram. Pernasal fiberoptic bronchoscopy allows examination of the nasopharynx, larynx, and major airways and may reveal whether hemorrhaging is focal or diffuse. The presence of an endotracheal tube may compromise this examination. In this instance, upper airway bleeding may be detected by aspirating the trachea free of blood with a bronchoscope while the endotracheal cuff is expanded and then observing fresh blood flow down from above the cuff when it is decompressed. Rigid bronchoscopy may be required if hemorrhaging is massive, such that blood cannot be adequately removed with a flexible bronchoscope.

9. **How does the chest roentgenogram assist in the evaluation of hemoptysis?**
   Examination of the chest roentgenogram often gives clues to both the site and etiology of hemoptysis. The presence of an infiltrate suggests the existence of a pulmonary parenchymal process. However, occasionally an infiltrate may occur after aspiration of blood coming from an airway source. Similarly, the presence of diffuse infiltrates suggests diffuse parenchymal disease, although this roentgenographic pattern may also occur with localized bleeding associated with severe coughing, which disperses blood throughout the lungs.

10. **Do all patients with hemoptysis require bronchoscopy?**
    No. Bronchoscopy may not be indicated if the initial evaluation strongly suggests that hemoptysis is due to a cardiovascular etiology, a lower respiratory tract infection, or a single episode of frank hemoptysis caused by acute or chronic bronchitis. However, bronchoscopy should be reconsidered in these clinical settings if the patient's hemoptysis does not improve or resolve after 24 hours of empiric therapy. Bronchoscopy is not indicated to make the specific diagnosis of a tracheoartery fistula.

11. **Describe the immediate management of massive hemoptysis.**
    The goals of immediate management of patients with massive hemoptysis are as follows:
    1. Maintain airway patency.
    2. Ensure adequate gas exchange.
    3. Establish hemodynamic stability.
    4. Stop ongoing hemorrhage.
    5. Prevent rebleeding.

Maintenance of airway patency is of paramount importance because death from massive hemoptysis more commonly results from asphyxiation due to major airway obstruction than from exsanguination. Several approaches have been advocated to maintain airway patency. If hemorrhage is occurring from a focal site and the site of hemorrhage is known, the patient should be positioned with the bleeding side dependent to prevent contamination of noninvolved airways. If the site of hemorrhage is unknown or diffuse, the patient should be placed in the Trendelenburg position. Other approaches to protect uninvolved airways include bronchoscopically guided selective intubation of the nonbleeding main stem bronchus or placement of a double-lumen endotracheal tube. The utility of double-lumen tubes is limited by the need for specialized training in their insertion and the tendency for double-lumen tubes to become dislodged.

12. **What specific therapies may be useful to stop ongoing hemorrhage?**
   If the etiology of hemorrhage is known, specific therapy directed at the cause (such as antibiotics for bronchiectasis or corticosteroids for pulmonary vasculitis) should be instituted to stop ongoing hemorrhage. Coagulopathies should be corrected with administration of appropriate blood products. If the patient is receiving anticoagulant therapy it should be discontinued.
   Life-threatening hemorrhage from a focal site requires more aggressive strategy. The most common of these is bronchial artery embolization (see question 14). Surgical resection may be considered in patients with adequate underlying lung function; however, because of the higher mortality associated with this approach when used emergently and the safety and efficacy of bronchial artery embolization it is usually reserved for those patients who have persistent bleeding despite other interventions. A number of bronchoscopic techniques are also available to control bleeding. These include the following:
   - Balloon tamponade with a Fogarty catheter placed under bronchoscopic guidance
   - Bronchoscopy-guided topical hemostatic tamponade therapy with use of either oxidized regenerated cellulose mesh or infusions of thrombin alone or fibrinogen with thrombin
   - Iced normal saline lavage of hemorrhaging lung segments
   - Regional instillation of vasoconstrictor agents such as epinephrine
   - If a focal airway lesion is the source of bleeding, electrocautery, laser photocoagulation, and cryotherapy

13. **Describe the management of a tracheoartery fistula.**
   The goals of immediate management are to control bleeding and to maintain a patent airway while preparing the patient for primary surgical correction. Bleeding from a tracheoartery fistula complicating a tracheostomy usually occurs at one of three sites: the tracheostomy tube stoma, the tracheostomy tube balloon, or the intratracheal cannula tip. Bleeding at the tracheostomy stoma can sometimes be tamponaded by applying forward and downward pressure on the top of the tracheostomy tube. Bleeding at the site of the balloon can be tamponaded by overinflating the balloon. These maneuvers should be performed immediately. However, they will not be helpful if bleeding is occurring at the cannula tip. If the bleeding stops or slows either spontaneously or subsequent to these efforts, an endotracheal tube should be placed distal to the bleeding site. However, the initial tracheostomy tube should not be removed without a surgeon present because a sudden increase in the rate of hemorrhage may necessitate blunt dissection down the anterior tracheal wall posterior to the sternum to attempt direct digital tamponade of the bleeding site.

14. **What is the role of bronchial artery embolization in the management of massive hemoptysis?**
   Bronchial artery embolization is important in the management of both surgical and nonsurgical causes of massive hemoptysis. It is a temporary measure for surgical lesions, facilitating the stabilization of patients while they undergo evaluation and preparation for surgery. It allows surgery to be performed in a more controlled setting. Bronchial artery embolization has become the primary mode of therapy for patients whose conditions are considered inoperable because of

either diffuse lung disease or poor pulmonary function. Such patients may undergo multiple episodes of embolization over many years if hemoptysis recurs.

15. **What is the success rate of bronchial artery embolization?**
Various studies have reported success rates in the initial 24-hour period after embolization from 73% to 98%. However, 16% to 30% of patients have rebleeding in the first year after embolization. Rebleeding tends to be bimodal in occurrence, with peaks in the first month (generally because of inadequate initial embolization) and at 1 to 2 years (because of progression of underlying disease).

16. **What complications are associated with bronchial artery embolization?**
Bronchial artery embolization is associated with low morbidity rates. The most common complications include pleuritic chest pain, fever, leukocytosis, and dysphagia. These symptoms may last for 5 to 7 days. Other complications are quite rare and are related to the vascular compromise of organs supplied from vessels that arise downstream from the site of catheter placement. Examples include spinal cord infarction, transverse myelitis, bronchial stenosis, bronchial-esophageal fistula, transient cortical blindness, and cerebrovascular accidents.

17. **When should surgery be considered in the management of massive hemoptysis?**
Bronchial artery embolization has largely replaced surgical resection as the initial therapy in massive hemoptysis. Embolization is associated with much lower morbidity and early mortality rates than emergent surgery. However, because of high rates of recurrence after embolization, surgery should be considered for patients who have hemoptysis due to focal lung lesions and good pulmonary reserve after their conditions have been stabilized with embolization. Surgery is contraindicated in patients with advanced lung disease that results in limited pulmonary reserve, significant comorbidity (especially advanced heart disease), or lung malignancies invading the trachea, mediastinum, heart, great vessels, and parietal pleura. In contrast, it remains the treatment of choice for patients with hemoptysis related to trauma, aortic aneurysm, and bronchial adenomas.

CONTROVERSY

18. **Should fiberoptic bronchoscopy be performed before bronchial artery embolization in patients with massive hemoptysis?**
For:
Fiberoptic bronchoscopy:
- Is important in guiding bronchial artery embolization by identifying the site of bleeding
- Is complementary to chest computed tomography in identifying the cause of hemoptysis, allowing the institution of specific therapy aimed at the underlying lung pathologic condition
- Facilitates the use of a number of techniques that can control bleeding

Against:
- A study of 29 patients who underwent bronchial artery embolization to control massive hemoptysis revealed that the site of bleeding could be identified in 80% of patients by chest radiograph alone. Bronchoscopy was essential to localizing the site of hemorrhage in only 10% of patients.
- The site of embolization is generally identified by angiography at the time of bronchial catheterization.
- Emergent bronchoscopy results in unnecessary delays before performance of bronchial artery embolization.
- Endobronchial tamponade is inferior to embolization as a temporary measure to control hemorrhage before the institution of more specific therapy and should be reserved for patients with contraindications to embolization.

KEY POINTS: MANAGEMENT GOALS IN MASSIVE HEMOPTYSIS

1. Maintain airway patency.

2. Ensure adequate gas exchange.

3. Establish hemodynamic stability.

4. Stop hemorrhage.

5. Prevent repeated hemorrhage.

BIBLIOGRAPHY

1. Bussières JS: Iatrogenic pulmonary artery rupture. Curr Opin Anaesthesiol 20:48-52, 2007.

2. Chun JY, Morgan R, Belli AM: Radiological management of hemoptysis: a comprehensive review of diagnostic imaging and bronchial arterial embolization. Cardiovasc Intervent Radiol 33:240-250, 2010.

3. Hsiao EI, Kirsch CM, Kagawaa FT, et al: Utility of fiberoptic bronchoscopy before bronchial artery embolization for massive hemoptysis. Am J Roentgenol 177:861-867, 2001.

4. Ibrahim WH: Massive haemoptysis: the definition should be revised. Eur Respir J 32:1131-1132, 2008.

5. Jean-Baptiste E: Clinical assessment and management of massive hemoptysis. Crit Care Med 28:1642-1647, 2000.

6. Johnson JL: Manifestations of hemoptysis: how to manage minor, moderate, and massive bleeding. Postgrad Med 112:101-113, 2002.

7. Jougon J, Ballester M, Delcambre F, et al: Massive hemoptysis: what place for medical and surgical treatment. Eur J Cardiothorac Surg 22:345-351, 2002.

8. Kalva SP: Bronchial artery embolization. Tech Vasc Interv Radiol 12:130-138, 2009.

9. Lordan JL, Gascoigne A, Corris PA: The pulmonary physician in critical care: illustrative case 7: assessment and management of massive haemoptysis. Thorax 58:814-819, 2003.

10. Menchini L, Remy-Jardin M, Faivre JB, et al: Cryptogenic haemoptysis in smokers: angiography and results of embolisation in 35 patients. Eur Respir J 34:1031-1039, 2009.

11. Praveen CV, Martin A: A rare case of fatal haemorrhage after tracheostomy. Ann R Coll Surg Engl 89(8):1-3, 2007.

12. Sakr L, Dutau H: Massive hemoptysis: an update on the role of bronchoscopy in diagnosis and management. Respiration 80:38-58, 2010.

13. Savale L, Parrot A, Khalil A, et al: Cryptogenic hemoptysis: from a benign to a life-threatening pathologic vascular condition. Am J Respir Crit Care Med 175:1181-1185, 2007.

14. Shigemura N, Wan IY, Yu SC, et al: Multidisciplinary management of life-threatening massive hemoptysis: a 10-year experience. Ann Thorac Surg 87:849-853, 2009.

15. Valipour A, Kreuzer A, Koller H, et al: Bronchoscopy-guided topical hemostatic tamponade therapy for the management of life-threatening hemoptysis. Chest 127:2113-2118, 2005.

16. Wang GR, Ensor JE, Gupta S, et al: Bronchial artery embolization for the management of hemoptysis in oncology patients: utility and prognostic factors. Vasc Interv Radiol 20:722-729, 2009.

17. Yoon W, Kim JK, Kim YH, et al: Bronchial and nonbronchial systemic artery embolization for lifethreatening hemoptysis: a comprehensive review. Radiographics 22:1395-1409, 2002.

CHAPTER 26

VENOUS THROMBOEMBOLISM AND FAT EMBOLISM

Madison Macht, MD, and Marc Moss, MD

1. **What are the sources of pulmonary embolism (PE)?**
   The majority of PEs arise from thromboses in the deep veins of the legs, particularly the iliac, femoral, and popliteal veins. Thromboses can also originate on central venous catheters and from the pelvic veins in women with a history of obstetric difficulties or recent gynecologic surgery. Nonhematologic sources of PE include fat particles, amniotic fluid, air introduced through central venous catheters, and foreign bodies such as talc and cotton fibers in intravenous drug users.

2. **What are some of the risk factors for PE and deep venous thrombosis (DVT)?**
   Three general conditions that increase the risk of venous thrombosis are called *Virchow's triad:* venous stasis, thrombophilia, and injury to the endothelium of vessel walls. Specific risk factors are listed in Box 26-1.

BOX 26-1. RISK FACTORS FOR VENOUS THROMBOEMBOLISM

Venous Stasis	Thrombophilia	Endothelial Injury
Prolonged bed rest	Malignancy	Major surgical procedures
Prolonged air travel	Factor V Leiden mutation	Trauma
(>8 hours)	Protein C or S deficiency	Prior venous thrombosis
Heart failure	Hyperhomocysteinemia	
	Antithrombin III deficiency	
	Antiphospholipid antibodies	
	High levels of factor VIII	
	Nephrotic syndrome	
	Inflammatory bowel disease	
	Pregnancy	
	Hormone replacement therapy	
	Oral contraceptives	
	Tamoxifen	

---

3. **How common is venous thromboembolism in critically ill patients?**
   DVT and PE are common and often underdiagnosed in critically ill patients. In prospective studies, 33% of medical patients in the intensive care unit (ICU) had DVTs on routine clinical screening, and 18% of trauma patients had proximal DVTs. In a retrospective series of respiratory ICU patients, 27% had PE on autopsy.

4. **How reliable is the physical examination for diagnosing DVT?**
   When patients complain of unilateral calf pain and swelling, a DVT is nearly always possible, and it is difficult to rule in or rule out its presence with physical examination alone. Furthermore,

asymptomatic DVT may occur 5% to 10% of the time. Specific physical examination maneuvers aimed at improving diagnostic accuracy include palpation for cords in the greater saphenous vein and its branches, detection of dilation of superficial tibial veins, checking for increased temperature in the lower extremity, squeezing specific parts of the leg to elicit tenderness, measuring the diameter of each leg, and checking for pain on passive ankle dorsiflexion (referred to as Homans sign). Unfortunately these maneuvers have limited sensitivity and specificity. Simplified clinical prediction models that combine many signs, symptoms, and historical features with serum D-dimer testing have been validated in outpatients. In these patients the combination of a low clinical probability of DVT and a low serum D-dimer level may effectively exclude DVT without ultrasonography. Importantly, these clinical prediction models have not been validated in critically ill patients.

5. **What are the signs and symptoms of an acute PE?**
The symptoms of an acute PE depend on the thromboembolic burden, the degree of underlying pulmonary parenchymal disease, and the ability of the right ventricle to accommodate acute pressure changes. Patients can present with syncope, shock, tachycardia, acute right ventricular failure, increased dead space, or refractory hypoxemia. However, patients may also be relatively asymptomatic. In patients with underlying cardiac or pulmonary disease, significant hemodynamic compromise may occur with less occlusion of the pulmonary vasculature. Common signs and symptoms of PE are listed in Box 26-2.

BOX 26-2. SIGNS AND SYMPTOMS OF ACUTE PE

Pleuritic chest pain
Tachypnea
Hemoptysis
Pleural friction rub
Acute onset of tachypnea
Tachycardia
Unexplained agitation
Hypotension
Unexplained hypoxia
Asymmetric leg swelling
Unilateral leg pain
Increased difference between pulmonary artery diastolic and wedge pressure

---

6. **What are some specific findings of PE visible on chest radiography?**
Chest radiography can neither be used to make nor to exclude the diagnosis of PE. However, the chest radiograph does assist in ruling out alternative diagnoses, determining the severity of the patient's illness, and identifying abnormalities that may require further evaluation. Contrary to common belief, the chest radiograph is frequently abnormal in patients with proven PE. Focal atelectasis, seen as linear streaks that run parallel above an elevated hemidiaphragm, may be seen (Fleischner lines). Small to moderate unilateral, exudative pleural effusions occur in approximately one third of patients. Although not specific for the diagnosis, patients with a pulmonary infarct may occasionally have a wedge-shaped opacity that abuts the pleura (Hampton hump). In addition, focal oligemia may be visible (Westermark sign) and when present should prompt further evaluation for PE.

7. **What are the electrocardiographic (ECG) findings associated with PE?**
ECG findings are also variable and relatively nonspecific. Sinus tachycardia and nonspecific ST-segment and T-wave changes occur frequently. The classic ECG findings of S_1, Q_3, T_3, or right bundle branch block occur in fewer than 15% of patients. The development of ECG findings of acute right ventricular strain (i.e., rightward shift of the QRS axis or peaked P waves in the inferior leads) in a critically ill patient should raise concern about potential PE.

8. **Are any laboratory test result abnormalities helpful in diagnosing PE?**
   No arterial blood gas values have adequate operating characteristics to exclude PE. Elevated serum D-dimer levels are highly sensitive but have low specificity. Although primarily validated in outpatients, when clinical suspicion for PE is low, the additional information of a serum D-dimer level below 500 ng/mL may be helpful to exclude the presence of PE without the need for further chest imaging.

9. **When should a ventilation-perfusion (V/Q) scan be ordered in the diagnostic work-up of PE?**
   V/Q scans can be particularly useful:
   - In patients for whom computed tomography angiography (CTA) is contraindicated (renal failure, radiocontrast allergy, concern for radiation exposure)
   - When a concern exists for chronic PE
   - At institutions with limited access or experience with CTA
     Eighty-seven percent of patients with a high-probability V/Q scan have a PE, whereas the diagnosis can essentially be excluded in patients with a normal V/Q scan. Unfortunately, more than 50% of V/Q scans are nondiagnostic (i.e., intermediate or low probability), and further testing is needed. Importantly, V/Q scans are more difficult to interpret in patients with preexisting lung disease.

10. **What about CTA for the diagnosis of PE?**
    The sensitivity and specificity of CTA exceed 90%. Higher imaging resolution and more experienced radiologists have contributed to this increase in CTA sensitivity and specificity. The sensitivity of CTA for small, subsegmental emboli is lower. However, several studies have demonstrated that subsequent DVT will develop in fewer than 1% of patients with a negative CTA for the diagnosis of PE over the next 3 months. Three additional advantages of CTA are the following:
    - Evaluation for alternative diagnoses in the chest
    - Direct visualization of emboli
    - Evaluation for inferior vena cava and lower extremity thromboses (when computed tomography venography is used in conjunction with CTA)
      A potential disadvantage of increased CTA sensitivity is the initiation of anticoagulation and an increased bleeding risk for patients with potentially insignificant emboli. Utility of CTA in the ICU is limited in patients with impaired renal function, the inability to lie flat, or illnesses that prohibit transportation.

11. **What is the role of echocardiography in the evaluation of PE?**
    Echocardiography is useful for risk stratification, and for those patients whose condition is too unstable for them to be transported for further imaging procedures. As many as 40% of patients with PE exhibit abnormalities of the right ventricle (RV). Findings of RV volume and pressure overload include abnormal motion of the intraventricular septum, RV dilation, and RV hypokinesis. Patients with signs of RV dysfunction by echocardiography may be at increased risk of death because of PE. Echocardiography also may diagnose conditions that simulate PE, such as aortic aneurysm, myocardial infarction, and pericardial tamponade.

12. **What is the recommended algorithm for the diagnosis of PE in the ICU for a patient who is hemodynamically stable?**
    In hemodynamically stable patients in whom PE is suspected the initial diagnostic test should be either a CTA or a V/Q scan. If these tests are nondiagnostic, a Doppler ultrasound scan of the legs should be performed. If the diagnosis is still not confirmed and the clinical suspicion for PE is high, pulmonary angiography should be performed.

13. **What is the recommended algorithm for the diagnosis of PE in the ICU for a patient who is hemodynamically unstable?**
    Anticoagulation should be started (if not contraindicated) as soon as PE is suspected. Because moving an unstable patient is difficult and potentially unsafe, the initial tests should be a Doppler ultrasound scan of the legs and cardiac echocardiography to look for signs of right ventricular dilatation, dysfunction, or thrombosis. A portable chest radiograph should be obtained to evaluate for alternative diagnoses.

14. **What are the goals of treatment for PE and DVT, and how are they achieved?**
    The major goals of PE and DVT therapy are to prevent further thrombotic and embolic complications and to promote resolution of the existing thrombosis. In the short term, unfractionated (UF) or low-molecular-weight (LMW) heparin should be administered. Oral anticoagulation therapy can be started when the patient's condition is stable and no invasive procedures are planned. If warfarin is used, in the absence of a mechanical heart valve or severe antiphospholipid antibody syndrome, the target international normalized ratio (INR) is 2.0 to 3.0. It is important to continue the heparin until the INR has been therapeutic for at least 2 days. The benefits of anticoagulation therapy need to be weighed against its risks. The most important complications include bleeding and thrombocytopenia. An often discussed but rare complication of warfarin therapy is skin necrosis caused by preexisting protein C or protein S deficiency.

15. **How long should a patient with PE or DVT be treated with anticoagulation?**
    - Patients with their first episode of PE or DVT due to a transient (reversible) risk factor (e.g., surgery, trauma, immobilization, pregnancy, venous catheter, hip fracture) should receive anticoagulation for 3 months.
    - Patients with their first episode of an unprovoked PE or DVT should be treated for *at least* 3 months, followed by an assessment and a discussion of the risks and benefits of long-term treatment.
    - Lifelong anticoagulation is recommended in those patients without contraindications who have the following:
        □ A second episode of PE or DVT
        □ An underlying hypercoagulable state
        □ An especially large thrombosis
        □ A thrombosis in an unusual site (i.e., cerebral vein)

16. **When should LMW heparin be used?**
    Patients with their first episode of an unprovoked PE or DVT should be treated for at least 3 months, followed by an assessment and a discussion of the risks and benefits of long-term treatment. Many patients and physicians opt for lifelong treatment in this situation.

17. **What is the role for newer oral anticoagulant agents in the treatment of DVT or PE?**
    In several clinical trials, patients taking warfarin have an INR within a therapeutic range only 60% of the time. In 2006, more than a half century after warfarin's initial approval, the Food and Drug Administration issued a black box warning for its bleeding risk. The bleeding risk, combined with warfarin's narrow therapeutic window, slow onset and offset, food and drug interactions, and monitoring requirements have prompted continued searches for an alternative oral anticoagulant. Although not approved for the treatment of venous thromboembolism, two new classes of oral anticoagulants, direct thrombin inhibitors and factor Xa inhibitors, are currently being studied in this disease. Early trials suggest that these agents may be effective and

safe in patients with near-normal renal function who are seen with acute DVT. A trial of these agents in acute symptomatic PE is ongoing.

18. **Which patients with PE should be treated with thrombolytic therapy?**
On the basis of limited clinical evidence, systemic thrombolytic therapy is recommended for patients with PE associated with significant hemodynamic compromise who lack contraindications related to bleeding risk (Box 26-3). Patients with significant hemodynamic compromise (systolic blood pressure < 90 mm Hg for at least 15 minutes or requiring inotropic support, not due to a cause other than PE) are often referred as having a *massive PE*. In contrast, *submassive PE* is often defined as PE with systolic blood pressure > 90 mm Hg but with either right ventricular dysfunction or evidence supporting cardiac ischemia. The use of systemic thrombolytic therapy in *submassive PE* is debated, and no strong guidelines exist.

BOX 26-3. CONTRAINDICATIONS TO THROMBOLYTIC THERAPY IN PE

Absolute	**Relative**
History of intracranial hemorrhage	Recent internal bleeding
Intracranial neoplasm, arteriovenous malformation, or aneurysm	Recent surgery or organ biopsy
Significant head trauma	Recent trauma, including cardiopulmonary resuscitation
Active internal bleeding (intracranial, retroperitoneal, gastrointestinal, genitourinary, respiratory)	Venipuncture at a noncompressible site
	Uncontrolled hypertension (systolic BP > 175 mm Hg and/or diastolic BP > 100 mm Hg)
Known bleeding diathesis	High risk of left-sided heart thrombosis
Intracranial or intraspinal surgery within 3 months	Acute pericarditis
Cerebrovascular accident within 2 months	Subacute bacterial endocarditis or septic thrombophlebitis
	Diabetic retinopathy
	Pregnancy
	Age > 75 years

BP, Blood pressure.

---

19. **When should the placement of an inferior vena cava (IVC) filter be considered?**
The most common and agreed-on indications for IVC filter placement are as follows:
1. An acute PE or proximal DVT with contraindication to anticoagulation
2. Recurrent acute PE despite therapeutic anticoagulation
    Patients with a large acute PE and poor cardiopulmonary reserve are often considered for IVC filter placement, although data to guide this decision are virtually absent, and decisions are often made on a case-by-case basis. Finally, in patients without an existing DVT or PE, but who have significant trauma (severe closed head injury, spinal cord injury, complex pelvic fracture, multiple long bone fractures) and high bleeding risk, some data suggest that prophylactic IVC filters may have a favorable risk/benefit ratio. Given the greatly increased risk for subsequent DVT (21%) and IVC thrombosis (2%-10%) in patients with IVC filters, resumption of anticoagulation is recommended when bleeding risk decreases, as long as the filter remains in place. The need for continued anticoagulation, combined with a finite window of time for safe

filter removal, necessitates a clinician's attention for the potential to remove the filter when appropriate. Other complications of IVC filter placement include device malposition (1.3%), pneumothorax (0.02%), hematoma (0.6%), IVC penetration (0.3%), filter migration or fracture (0.3%), and air embolism (0.2%).

20. **Are there important long-term sequelae of a PE?**
Symptomatic pulmonary hypertension occurs in approximately 4% of patients within 2 years after their first episode of PE.

21. **What is the recommended prophylactic therapy for patients at risk for the development of DVT or PE?**
Pharmacologic prophylaxis is recommended in all high-risk patients who lack contraindications and has been reported to decrease the incidence of DVT by 67%. Although mechanical methods of thromboprophylaxis (graduated compression stockings, intermittent pneumatic compression devices) are generally less efficacious, they are recommended in patients for whom anticoagulants are contraindicated. Importantly, the use of computerized electronic alert programs increased the use of prophylactic therapy and reduced the rate of DVT and PE in hospitalized patients.
The most common recommended medications for DVT or PE prophylaxis are as follows:
- UF heparin (5000 units subcutaneously every 8-12 hours).
- LMW heparin (dose depends on the specific drug and the patient's renal function).
- The once-daily, pentasaccharide factor Xa inhibitor fondaparinux is also approved for use in some high-risk patients.
A recent multicenter, randomized, double-blinded, placebo-controlled trial in 3746 ICU patients compared dalteparin (5000 units once daily) with UF heparin (5000 units twice daily). No difference was seen in the primary outcome of proximal leg DVT. Secondary outcomes included any DVT, PE, death, major bleeding, and HIT. No significant between-group difference was seen in the rates of major bleeding or death; however, significantly fewer PEs occurred in the dalteparin group. These results suggest that either UF or LMW heparin can be used, with similar risks for proximal DVT, major bleeding, and HIT.

22. **What is the fat embolism syndrome (FES)? Who is at risk for development of it?**
Embolism of fat occurs in nearly all patients with traumatic bone fractures and during orthopedic procedures. It can also occur in patients with pancreatitis or sickle cell crises and during liposuction. Most cases are asymptomatic. FES occurs in the minority of these patients who have signs and symptoms, usually affecting the respiratory, neurologic, and hematologic systems and the skin. Symptoms typically occur 12 to 72 hours after the initial injury. The presentation may be catastrophic with RV failure and cardiovascular collapse.

23. **How is FES diagnosed?**
Fat embolism is a clinical diagnosis. The use of bronchoscopy or pulmonary artery catheterization to detect fat particles in alveolar macrophages or blood from the pulmonary artery lacks both sensitivity and specificity for the diagnosis of FES. The Gurd criteria are the most widely used method of diagnosis (Box 26-4).

24. **What is the recommended treatment for FES?**
Treatment of FES is primarily supportive. Although it has been studied extensively, no compelling evidence exists that the use of corticosteroids is indicated for FES. Some studies have suggested that early stabilization of long bone fractures can minimize bone marrow embolization into the venous system.

BOX 26-4. GURD DIAGNOSTIC CRITERIA FOR FAT EMBOLISM SYNDROME

Major Criteria
(One Necessary for Diagnosis)
Petechial rash
Respiratory failure
Cerebral involvement

Minor Criteria
(Four Necessary for Diagnosis)
Tachycardia (heart rate > 120 beats/min)
Fever (temperature > 39° C)
Retinal involvement
Jaundice
Renal insufficiency

Additional Laboratory Criteria
(One Necessary for Diagnosis)
Thrombocytopenia
Anemia
Elevated erythrocyte sedimentation rate
Fat macroglobulinemia

KEY POINTS: VENOUS THROMBOEMBOLISM AND FAT EMBOLISM IN THE ICU

1. All high-risk patients in the ICU should receive prophylactic therapy for PE or deep venous thromboembolism.

2. Patients can have a PE without a significant increase in the A − a gradient.

3. No specific clinical, radiographic, or laboratory findings exist for PE. Therefore PE should be considered in any critically ill patient with deterioration of cardiopulmonary status.

4. Symptomatic pulmonary hypertension occurs in approximately 4% of patients within 2 years after the first episode of PE.

5. Thrombolytic therapy should be used in patients with massive PE associated with cardiogenic shock.

6. FES occurs in patients with traumatic bone fractures, pancreatitis, and sickle cell crises and during orthopedic procedures or liposuction.

BIBLIOGRAPHY

1. Anderson FA, Spencer FA: Risk factors for venous thromboembolism. Circulation 107:I9-I16, 2003.

2. Cook DJ, Donadini MP: Pulmonary embolism in medical-surgical critically ill patients. Hematol Oncol Clin North Am 24:677-682, 2010.

3. Dong BR, Hao Q, Yue J, et al: Thrombolytic therapy for pulmonary embolism. Cochrane Database Syst Rev 3; CD004437, 2009.

4. Fedullo PF, Tapson VF: The evaluation of suspected pulmonary embolism. N Engl J Med 349:1247-1256, 2003.

5. Goldhaber SZ: Echocardiography in the management of pulmonary embolism. Ann Intern Med 136:691-700, 2002.

6. Hirsh J, Guyatt G, Albers GW, et al: Antithrombotic and thrombolytic therapy: American College of Chest Physicians Evidence-based Clinical Practice Guidelines (8th edition). Chest 133:110S-112S, 2008.

7. Jaff MR, McMurtry MS, Archer SL, et al: Management of massive and submassive pulmonary embolism, iliofemoral deep vein thrombosis, and chronic thromboembolic pulmonary hypertension: a scientific statement from the American Heart Association. Circulation 123:1788-1830, 2011.

8. Kaufman JA, Kinney TB, Streiff MB, et al: Guidelines for the use of retrievable and convertible vena cava filters: report from the Society of Interventional Radiology multidisciplinary consensus conference. J Vasc Interv Radiol 17:449-459, 2006.

9. Kucher N, Rossi E, De Rosa M, et al: Prognostic role of echocardiography among patients with acute pulmonary embolism and a systolic arterial pressure of 90 mm Hg or higher. Arch Intern Med 165:1777-1781, 2005.

10. Merli G: Anticoagulants in the treatment of deep vein thrombosis. Am J Med 118(8A):13S-20S, 2005.

11. PROTECT Investigators for the Canadian Critical Care Trials Group and the Australian and New Zealand Intensive Care Society Clinical Trials Group : Dalteparin versus unfractionated heparin in critically ill patients. N Engl J Med 364:1305-1314, 2011.

12. Quiroz R, Kucher N, Zou KH, et al: Clinical validity of a negative computed tomography scan in patients with suspected pulmonary embolism: a systematic review. JAMA 293:2012-2017, 2005.

13. Rocha AT, Tapson VF: Venous thromboembolism in intensive care patients. Clin Chest Med 24:103-122, 2003.

14. Rodger MA, Carrier M, Jones GN, et al: Diagnostic value of arterial blood gas measurements in suspected pulmonary embolism. Am J Respir Crit Care Med 162:2105-2108, 2000.

15. Roy PM, Colombet I, Durieux P, et al: Systematic review and meta-analysis of strategies for the diagnosis of suspected pulmonary embolism. BMJ 331:1-9, 2005.

16. Smoot RL, Koch CA, Heller SF, et al: Inferior vena cava filters in trauma patients: efficacy, morbidity, and retrievability. J Trauma 68:899-903, 2010.

17. Stein PD, Yaekoub AY, Matta F, et al: Fat embolism syndrome. Am J Med Sci 336:472-477, 2008.

18. van Belle A, Büller HR, Huisman MV, et al: Christopher Study Investigators. Effectiveness of managing suspected pulmonary embolism using an algorithm combining clinical probability, D-dimer testing, and computed tomography. JAMA 295:172-179, 2006.

19. Wells PS, Owen C, Doucette S, et al: Does this patient have deep vein thrombosis? JAMA 295:199-207, 2006.

HEART FAILURE AND VALVULAR HEART DISEASE

Martin M. LeWinter, MD, and Neil Agrawal, MD

1. **What are the causes of cardiomyopathy resulting in the syndrome of heart failure (HF)?**
   - **Reduced ejection fraction** (HFREF, systolic HF, dilated cardiomyopathy): impaired contraction and/or loss of cardiomyocytes. Multiple causes but approximately 65% ischemic.
   - **Normal or preserved ejection fraction** (HFNEF, diastolic HF): abnormal relaxation and/or increased stiffness of the left ventricle (LV), most commonly associated with hypertension, type 2 diabetes mellitus, and aging. Comorbidities (e.g., chronic obstructive pulmonary disease, stroke, obstructive sleep apnea) are very common.
   - **Restrictive cardiomyopathy:** markedly decreased LV compliance leading to impaired diastolic filling. The usual cause is infiltrative disease.
   - **Hypertrophic cardiomyopathy:** LV hypertrophy usually with asymmetric septal thickening and often outflow tract systolic pressure gradient. The mechanisms of HF are complex, but the presumed cause is sarcomeric protein mutations.
   - **Right ventricular (RV) failure:** Most common causes are LV failure, obstructive sleep apnea, pulmonary hypertension, and RV myocardial infarction (MI).

2. **What are the causes of HFREF besides ischemic heart disease or MI?**
   See Table 27-1.

TABLE 27-1. CAUSES OF HFREF	
TYPE	**CAUSE**
Myocarditis	Infectious (viral) or inflammatory (e.g., systemic lupus erythematosus) giant cell (may require transplant)
Toxins	EtOH, cocaine, cancer chemotherapy, radiation
Stress-induced cardiomyopathy	Catecholamine surge from stress, apical ballooning (takotsubo syndrome)
Genetic	Idiopathic, familial (multiple mutations)
Valvular disease	Aortic, mitral (see valvular disease section)
Other	Peripartum, sustained tachycardia, HTN, DM, endocrine or nutritional, acidosis, sepsis

DM, Diabetes mellitus; *EtOH*, ethyl alcohol; *HTN*, hypertension.

3. **How do we classify HF by functional status or stage?**
See Table 27-2.

TABLE 27-2. CLASSIFYING HEART FAILURE BY FUNCTIONAL STATUS/STAGE

NYHA Functional Classification

Class I (mild)	No limitation of physical activity
Class II (mild)	Slight limitation of physical activity
Class III (moderate)	Marked limitation of physical activity
Class IV (severe)	Unable to carry out any physical activity without discomfort, symptoms at rest

ACC-AHA Staging System

Stage A	Patients at high risk for development of HF in the future but no functional or structural heart disease
Stage B	Structural heart disease but no symptoms
Stage C	Previous or current symptoms of HF in the context of underlying structural heart disease, adequately managed with medical treatment
Stage D	Advanced disease requiring hospital-based support, heart transplantation or mechanical support, or palliative care

ACC, American College of Cardiology; *AHA*, American Heart Association; *NYHA*, New York Heart Association.

4. **What is the role of brain natriuretic peptide in the diagnosis of HF?**
   - Not required to diagnose HF
   - Helpful when diagnostic uncertainty exists and for prognosis
   - Lower in HFNEF than in HFREF
   - Lower in obese patients

5. **How is acute decompensated HF treated?**
Treatment is based on systemic perfusion and evidence of vascular congestion.
See Table 27-3.
   Congestion: dyspnea, orthopnea, crackles, elevated venous pressure, ascites, peripheral edema
   Impaired perfusion: reduced pulse pressure, cold extremities, altered mentation

TABLE 27-3. SYSTEMIC PERFUSION AND CONGESTION

		CONGESTION (DRY-WET)	
		NO (DRY)	YES (WET)
Perfusion (warm-cold)	Yes (warm)	Dry and warm (1)	Wet and warm (3)
	No (cold)	Dry and cold (2)	Wet and cold (4)

The numbers in Table 27-3 can be defined as follows:

1. Normal and requires no intervention.
2. Pump failure without pulmonary edema. Usually represents end-stage HF. Patients require inotropic support: dobutamine (β_1-adrenergic agonist), milrinone (phosphodiesterase inhibitor), mechanical support (intraaortic balloon pump [IABP], LV assist device); consider cardiac transplantation.
3. Adequate perfusion with volume overload and increased filling pressures. The treatment focus is intravenous loop diuretics (most commonly furosemide) or bedside ultrafiltration. Reduction of preload with intravenous vasodilators (morphine sulfate, nitroglycerin or nitroprusside, angiotensin-converting enzyme inhibitors [ACEIs]) is another option.
4. Volume overload with pump failure. These patients require inotropes, vasodilators, diuretics, and consideration of mechanical support.

Notes:

- Ultrafiltration can remove large amounts of volume rapidly and is usually reserved for patients in whom an adequate response to IV diuretics is not achieved.
- Nesiritide is an alternative vasodilator therapy in patients whose blood pressure is normal and who continue to have dyspnea because of volume overload despite the use of intravenous loop diuretics.

6. **How is diastolic dysfunction diagnosed?**
   An elevated LV end-diastolic or pulmonary capillary wedge pressure in a patient with a normal LV EF and end-diastolic volume by echocardiography establishes the presence of diastolic dysfunction. Various two-dimensional echocardiographic-Doppler parameters are also used, including increased ratio of early transmitral flow velocity to early diastolic velocity of the mitral valve annulus (E/E'), left atrial enlargement, and concentric LV hypertrophy.

AORTIC STENOSIS

7. **What are the causes of aortic stenosis (AS)?**

   - Supravalvular (rarest)
   - Subvalvular (discrete, tunnel)
   - Valvular
   - Congenital
   - Age 1 to 30 years, unicuspid
   - Age 40 to 60 years, bicuspid
   - Rheumatic
   - Senile degenerative (>70 years) → most common in United States

8. **What is the pathophysiology of AS?**
   An increase in afterload caused by LV outflow obstruction causes concentric hypertrophy and increased wall thickness. By Laplace's law, the increased wall thickness normalizes systolic wall stress and maintains shortening (EF). These structural changes are associated with diastolic dysfunction (impaired relaxation, reduced chamber compliance), which increases LV filling pressures and, in turn, increases pressures in the pulmonary circulation. In a minority of patients, the ability to hypertrophy is exhausted, EF decreases, and the LV dilates.

9. **What is the classic triad of symptoms of AS, and what is its significance?**
   1. Increase in afterload
   2. Decrease in subendocardial blood flow
   3. Progressive hypertrophy with diastolic dysfunction
      This triad leads to the symptoms of dyspnea (HF), angina, and dizziness or syncope. The appearance of these symptoms directly correlates with mortality. Fifty percent of patients are dead 5 years after presentation with syncope, 3 years after presentation with angina, and 2 years after presentation with HF. The rate of progression of disease by valve gradient and area is another important predictor of mortality.

10. **How is the severity of AS graded with use of echocardiographic-Doppler methods?**
    See Table 27-4.

TABLE 27-4. GRADING AORTIC STENOSIS WITH USE OF ECHOCARDIOGRAPHIC-DOPPLER METHODS

SEVERITY	MEAN GRADIENT (mm Hg)	VALVE AREA (cm^2)
Mild	<25	>1.5
Moderate	25-40	1.0-1.5
Severe	>40	<1.0

11. **How is AS medically managed in the critically ill patient?**
    The only definitive treatment for AS is surgical valve replacement. Critically ill patients with adequate blood pressure can sometimes be managed with vasodilators, in particular nitroprusside. In carefully selected patients, nitroprusside increases cardiac index and stroke volume and reduces mean and diastolic arterial pressure and systemic vascular resistance. Vasodilator therapy should not be used without careful hemodynamic monitoring with a flow-directed pulmonary artery catheter. Excessive vasodilation causing systemic hypotension can cause severe deterioration by decreasing coronary perfusion. In some patients, dobutamine can be considered as an alternative.

12. **When should aortic valvuloplasty and percutaneous valve implantation be considered?**
    In carefully selected patients, balloon valvuloplasty can be used as a bridge to surgery for patients who are hemodynamically unstable. The procedure can also be used as palliation in patients with multiple comorbidities who are poor operative candidates. However, balloon valvuloplasty has a high rate of early restenosis and poor long-term survival, which prevent it from being a definitive treatment. Recently, interest has been great in transarterial aortic valve implantation, in which a replacement valve is inserted within the stenotic aortic valve with use of percutaneous techniques. This is currently not widely available but may well be a routine option in the future.

MITRAL STENOSIS

13. **What are the causes of mitral stenosis (MS)?**
    - Rheumatic disease (worldwide)
    - Congenital
    - Other: calcification related to aging and/or end-stage renal disease, obstructive left atrial myxoma, carcinoid heart disease

14. **How does MS affect cardiac function and hemodynamics?**
    As the mitral valve orifice narrows, the left atrial pressure rises and a diastolic pressure gradient develops between the left atrium (LA) and the LV. The latter is required to maintain forward flow. The increased LA pressure is transmitted backward, in turn increasing pressure in the pulmonary veins, capillaries, pulmonary artery, and RV. In the lungs, this results in congestion and symptoms of HF. Over time, the increased LA pressure and secondary increases in pulmonary artery pressure may result in RV overload with high filling pressures.

15. **How is mitral stenosis graded with use of echocardiographic-Doppler methods?**
See Table 27-5.

TABLE 27-5. GRADING MITRAL STENOSIS WITH USE OF ECHOCARDIOGRAPHIC DOPPLER METHODS

SEVERITY	MEAN GRADIENT (mm Hg)	MITRAL VALVE AREA (cm^2)
Mild	<5	>1.5
Moderate	5-10	1.0-1.5
Severe	>10	<1.0

16. **How are critically ill patients with MS managed?**
The most common cause of decompensation in patients with MS is a rapid heart rate associated with atrial fibrillation. If tachycardia is present, this should be the focus of treatment through the use of β-blockers or calcium channel antagonists such as diltiazem. Direct current cardioversion for atrial fibrillation often has a role but is usually contraindicated in the acute setting in patients who have not been receiving prior anticoagulant therapy. Diuretics should also be used if necessary to reduce circulatory congestion. Vasodilators and positive inotropic agents generally have no role. Patients with MS, even if critically ill, are candidates for percutaneous mitral balloon valvotomy.

17. **What are the indications for percutaneous mitral balloon valvotomy for MS?**
This is the preferred treatment for patients with moderate to severe MS who continue to have significant symptoms on medical management; who have pliable, noncalcified mitral valve leaflets; and who do not have moderate or worse mitral regurgitation. Contraindications to valvotomy include left atrial thrombus and more than moderate mitral regurgitation.

AORTIC REGURGITATION

18. **What are the causes of aortic regurgitation (AR)?**
See Table 27-6.

TABLE 27-6. CAUSES OF AORTIC REGURGITATION

VALVULAR DISEASE	AORTIC DISEASE
Rheumatic	—
Bicuspid	Type A aortic dissection
Endocarditis (bacterial or marantic)	Marfan
Degenerative or calcified	Degenerative
Vasculitis	Inflammatory (syphilis, Reiter syndrome)

19. **What is the pathophysiology of AR?**
AR represents combined volume and pressure overload. Regurgitant flow in diastole increases the end-diastolic pressure and volume. This initiates LV hypertrophy with both increased wall thickness and further increases in diastolic volume. This combination initially helps to maintain stroke volume. Approximately 50% of patients in whom severe AR is diagnosed progress to HF. Tachycardia reduces diastolic filling time and decreases the regurgitant fraction. In contrast, bradycardia does the opposite and is often poorly tolerated in patients with AR.

20. What is the management of acute, severe AR in the critical care setting?
Most acute, severe AR will require surgical intervention, depending on the cause
(e.g., endocarditis, valve vs. aortic disease). The first line of medical management in patients
with normal blood pressure is diuretics and nitroprusside to reduce LV filling pressure,
decrease the regurgitant fraction, and improve forward flow. Care must be taken not to
cause excessive hypotension. The LV is typically hyperdynamic and does not require
inotropic support. Pressors in general are contraindicated because they increase arterial
load and promote a higher regurgitant fraction. AR is also a contraindication for use of an
IABP. When AR is stabilized, treatment consists of vasodilators such as hydralazine, nifedipine,
and ACEIs.

21. What are the indications for surgery in AR?
Patients with prosthetic valve failure, aortic dissection, and most forms of acute, severe AR
should be considered for emergent surgical intervention. Patients with HF, symptoms provoked
by stress testing, EF <55%, or end-systolic dimension by echocardiography >55 mm should in
general have surgical intervention. With EF <50%, the 10-year survival after surgery is at best
56%. In the setting of endocarditis, surgical intervention should be balanced with antibiotic
sterilization. Active infection is not a contraindication for valve replacement in critically ill
patients.

MITRAL REGURGITATION

22. What are the causes of mitral regurgitation (MR)?
- Degenerative (mitral prolapse and/or chordal rupture): 65%
- Functional (dilated cardiomyopathy, LV and annular dilatation), ischemia of the posterior LV
  wall or the medial papillary muscle: 27%
- Rheumatic (in United States): 1%
- Other (endocarditis): 5%

23. What is the pathophysiology of MR?
The mitral apparatus (leaflets, chordae tendineae, papillary muscles, and underlying LV walls)
works in a coordinated fashion to maintain valve competence. In acute, severe MR, there are
increased LV filling and decreased afterload, which increase EF and total stroke volume (SV).
Forward SV is often reduced. The LV and LA chambers enlarge and become more compliant via
rearrangement of myocardial fibers (eccentric remodeling). This allows an increase in total and
forward SV. Eventually, the ventricle cannot meet the demands of worsening MR and volume
overload through hypertrophy. Further dilation occurs, which is associated with an increased
end-systolic volume and eventually a decrease in EF.

24. How is acute, severe MR managed?
In a patient with normal blood pressure, the goal of medical management is to pharmacologically
reduce MR. This can be done by reducing systemic vascular resistance with arterial dilators such
as nitroprusside and/or unloading the LV with diuretics. Acute MR often responds well to
vasodilators alone. In the patient whose condition is unstable or who has hypotension,
nitroprusside should be used in conjunction with an inotrope such as dobutamine or an IABP.
Almost all patients with severe MR will eventually require surgical treatment.

25. What are the indications for surgery in MR?
- Symptoms of HF, even if mild
- LV dysfunction (EF <50%, end-systolic dimension >40 mm)
- Severe, nonfunctional MR
  Note: EF <25% is usually prohibitive for surgery because of high operative mortality.

KEY POINTS: HEART FAILURE AND VALVULAR DISEASE ✓

1. The causes of cardiomyopathy
   - Systolic failure (reduced EF)
   - Diastolic failure (normal or preserved EF)
   - Restrictive cardiomyopathy
   - Hypertrophic cardiomyopathy
   - RV failure

2. Treatment of acute decompensated HF
   - Dry-cold → Inotropes
   - Wet-warm → Vasodilators or diuretics
   - Wet-cold → Inotropes, vasodilators, diuretics

3. AS and mortality
   - Syncope → 50% mortality after 5 years
   - Angina → 50% mortality after 3 years
   - Congestive HF → 50% mortality after 2 years

4. Treatment of AS in the critically ill
   - Valve replacement
   - Systolic blood pressure control

5. The pathophysiology of AR
   - Volume and pressure overload

BIBLIOGRAPHY

1. Bonow RO, Carabello BA, Chatterjee K, et al: 2008 Focused update incorporated into the ACC/AHA 2006 guidelines for the management of patients with valvular heart disease: a report of the American College of Cardiology/American Heart Association Task Force on Practice Guidelines (Writing Committee to Revise the 1998 Guidelines for the Management of Patients With Valvular Heart Disease): endorsed by the Society of Cardiovascular Anesthesiologists, Society for Cardiovascular Angiography and Interventions, and Society of Thoracic Surgeons. J Am Coll Cardiol 52:e1-e142, 2008.

2. Carabello BA: The current therapy for mitral regurgitation. J Am Coll Cardiol 52:319-326, 2008.

3. Carabello BA: Contemporary aortic valve therapy. Methodist DeBakey Cardiovasc J 6:33-39, 2010.

4. Felker GM, Thompson RE, Hare JM, et al: Underlying causes and long-term survival in patients with initially undiagnosed cardiomyopathy. N Engl J Med 342:1077, 2000.

5. Hunt SA, Abraham WT, Chin MH, et al: 2009 focused update incorporated into the ACC/AHA 2005 Guidelines for the Diagnosis and Management of Heart Failure in Adults: a report of the American College of Cardiology Foundation/American Heart Association Task Force on Practice Guidelines: developed in collaboration with the International Society for Heart and Lung Transplantation. Circulation 119:e391, 2009.

6. Nohria A, Mielniczuk LM, Stevenson LW: Evaluation and monitoring of patients with acute heart failure syndromes. Am J Cardiol 96:32G-40G, 2005.

CHAPTER 28

ACUTE MYOCARDIAL INFARCTION

Cameron Donaldson, MD, and Harold L. Dauerman, MD

1. **Who is at risk for acute myocardial infarction (AMI)?**
   - **Nonmodifiable:** older age, noncardiac atherosclerotic disease, first-degree relative with early atherosclerosis (male age <55 years, female age <65 years).
   - **Modifiable:** diabetes mellitus; hypertension; smoking; elevated low-density lipoprotein (LDL), high-density lipoprotein (HDL), and triglycerides; C-reactive protein; lipoprotein (a); low HDL; hypertriglyceridemia; metabolic syndrome; sedentary lifestyle; atherogenic diet.
   - **Unclear:** In more than 10% of patients, no obvious risk factor is seen for coronary artery disease (CAD).

2. **What causes an AMI?**
   Coronary arterial atherosclerotic plaque with a thin fibrous cap is the ideal substrate for myocardial infarction (MI). Shear stress created by turbulent flow through an irregular, diseased segment of coronary artery can result in sudden rupture of this thin-capped vulnerable plaque. Procoagulants from the plaque's lipid core are extruded into the bloodstream, forming an occlusive thrombus at the site of insult. Plaque rupture accounts for roughly three quarters of fatal AMIs. The remaining 25% are due to erosion of the endothelial monolayer, uncovering a nidus for clot formation and extension into the arterial lumen.

3. **How are patients typically seen initially with an AMI?**
   - Severe retrosternal pressure with radiation to arms, neck, or jaw. Usually ≥30 minutes in duration and associated with dyspnea, weakness, or diaphoresis. May be provoked by exertion, emotional stress, or extreme temperatures.
   - Rales, diaphoresis, hypotension, bradycardia or tachycardia, and transient murmur of mitral regurgitation are potential physical findings, though the examination results are most often unremarkable.
   - The key considerations in differential diagnosis are aortic dissection, pulmonary embolism, and pericarditis.

4. **Which biomarkers diagnose AMI?**
   The recently adopted universal definition of AMI includes elevation in cardiac biomarkers above the 99th percentile of the upper reference limit. See Table 28-1.

TABLE 28-1. BIOMARKERS TO DIAGNOSE AMI				
BIOMARKER	**ONSET/PEAK**	**DURATION**	**SENSITIVITY**	**SPECIFICITY**
Myoglobin	1-4 hr/6-12 hr	24-36 hr	Very high	Low
CK-MB	2-4 hr/5-9 hr	18-30 hr	High	High
Troponin T	4-6 hr/12-24 hr	7-10 days	Very high	Very high

CK-MB, Creatine kinase MB.

5. **How do you diagnose an ST-elevation MI (STEMI)?**
   - New left bundle branch block or $\geq$ 1-mm ST elevations in two or more contiguous leads. Absence of these electrocardiogram (ECG) changes leads to the alternative diagnosis: non–ST-elevation MI (NSTEMI). Both types of MI demonstrate positive cardiac biomarkers.
   - Formation of a fibrin-rich *red clot,* which adheres to activated platelets, causing total occlusion of the affected artery and probable transmural infarction.
   - This syndrome was formerly termed Q-wave MI, but this terminology has been abandoned in favor of the more specific STEMI term.

6. **In whom does cardiogenic shock develop?**
   - Shock complicating MI is most common among elderly patients.
   - Criteria for cardiogenic shock include persistent hypotension with a systolic blood pressure < 90 mm Hg, cardiac index < 1.8 $L/min^1/m^2$, left ventricular end-diastolic pressure > 18 mm Hg, or need for pressors or hemodynamic support.
   - Causes of cardiogenic shock include ventricular septal rupture, free wall or papillary muscle rupture, large MI, and nonischemic causes (myocarditis, takotsubo cardiomyopathy, valvular heart disease).

7. **What is the prognosis of a patient with AMI and out-of-hospital cardiac arrest?**
   - The cause of cardiac arrest is AMI in > 50% of patients. Other causes include nonischemic causes of arrhythmias (i.e., nonischemic cardiomyopathy).
   - Approximately 40% of patients with cardiac arrest may survive to hospital discharge. Predictors of discharge from hospital include witnessed arrest, initial ventricular tachycardia or ventricular fibrillation, bystander cardiopulmonary resuscitation, cooling or hypothermia, younger age, male sex, acute myocardial ischemia or heart failure, early invasive management of CAD, and absence of comorbidities.

8. **You diagnose a STEMI at a rural clinic without a catheterization laboratory; what do you do?**
   Reperfusion via percutaneous coronary intervention *(primary PCI)* is the preferred treatment for STEMI. A clear mortality benefit exists if this is done within 90 minutes of first contact with the medical system. In this case, door to balloon time is expected to exceed 120 minutes, and reperfusion should be achieved with fibrinolytics. In addition to fibrinolysis, adjunctive therapy with heparin, aspirin, and clopidogrel (600 mg) is warranted. Recent trials have demonstrated that a pharmacoinvasive approach leads to decreased risk of recurrent ischemia and infarction; thus all patients in the postlytic period should be transferred for cardiac catheterization and possible revascularization.

9. **Which antithrombotic therapy should be administered to the patient in question 8?**
   After receiving fibrinolytics, choices of anticoagulant include weight-based dosing of unfractionated heparin, enoxaparin, or fondaparinux. The most common regimen in patients being referred for early catheterization is unfractionated heparin, along with aspirin and clopidogrel. If the patient is being transferred for primary PCI, bivalirudin is an alternative to heparin-based therapy.

10. **Which antiplatelet therapies are indicated for the patient in question 8?**
    Aspirin (162-325 mg followed by 81 mg daily) and clopidogrel (600 mg loading dose followed by 75 mg daily) are the mainstays of antiplatelet therapy in STEMI and are indicated in our patient, who received full-dose fibrinolytic therapy. In the primary PCI population only, prasugrel (60 mg loading dose followed by 10 mg daily) reduces stent thrombosis compared with clopidogrel but is contraindicated in patients with prior stroke or transient ischemic attack. Addition of glycoprotein inhibition of platelets to unfractionated heparin or as bailout after bivalirudin (for slow flow in the culprit artery) is also possible.

11. **Which patients with unstable angina or NSTEMI have the highest mortality?**
Thrombolysis in Myocardial Infarction (TIMI), Global Registry of Acute Coronary Events (GRACE), and Platelet Glycoprotein IIb/IIIa in Unstable Angina: Receptor Suppression Using Integrilin (PURSUIT) are risk stratification schemes that aid in patient selection for early invasive versus conservative therapies. The TIMI risk score is composed of seven variables: age ≥ 65 years, three or more CAD risk factors, aspirin use within a week, two or more episodes of severe angina in the past day, elevated cardiac biomarkers, ST deviation ≥ 0.5 mm, and known $\geq 50\%$ coronary stenosis. The presence of three variables indicates intermediate risk (13% chance of death, MI, or need for urgent revascularization within 14 days), and five or more predicts a doubling of this risk.

12. **You are evaluating a patient with unstable angina. What patient characteristics would sway you to choose an early referral to the catheterization laboratory and possible invasive revascularization?**
See Table 28-2.

TABLE 28-2. RISK FACTORS ASSOCIATED WITH REFERRAL FOR INVASIVE MANAGEMENT STRATEGY

SYMPTOMS	TESTING	HISTORY	PHYSICAL EXAMINATION	OTHER
Refractory symptoms	New ST depressions	Prior PCI	Hemodynamic instability	Sustained ventricular tachycardia
—	Elevated biomarkers	Prior CABG	Heart failure	High risk score (i.e., TIMI)
—	EF $< 40\%$	—	New mitral regurgitation	High-risk noninvasive testing

Modified from O'Connor RE, Brady W, Brooks SC, et al: Part 10: acute coronary syndromes, 2010 American Heart Association Guidelines for Cardiopulmonary Resuscitation and Emergency Cardiovascular Care. Circulation 122(18 Suppl 3):S787-S817, 2010.
EF, Ejection fraction.

13. **What medications do you start in a patient initially seen with an NSTEMI?**
Aspirin (162-325 mg) should be administered to every patient. Intermediate- or high-risk patients should receive clopidogrel (300 or 600 mg) plus weight-adjusted unfractionated heparin, renal function–adjusted enoxaparin, or bivalirudin. In patients with renal insufficiency or elevated bleeding risk, bivalirudin may be recommended instead of heparin-glycoprotein inhibitors. For the early invasive strategy, pretreatment with a statin may decrease periprocedural infarction. Prasugrel (60 mg) should be loaded after coronary angiography and may be given in place of clopidogrel as long as the patient is not at high risk for bleeding (defined as age ≥ 75 years, previous stroke, or weight ≤ 60 kg). Relief of chest pain may be achieved with nitrates and morphine but should alert the care team to a high-risk situation.

Ongoing chest pain should warrant consideration for emergent catheterization because it may represent coronary occlusion and progression to STEMI.

14. **Your AMI patient is ready to go home. What prescriptions do you consider at discharge?**

Dual antiplatelet therapy should be continued in patients after MI, with clopidogrel (75 mg daily) 1 year after all acute coronary syndromes (STEMI, NSTEMI, or unstable angina) and aspirin (81 mg daily) indefinitely. More recently, 12 months of the new P2Y12 receptor antagonists (prasugrel) has been shown to decrease risk of recurrent ischemic events in patients with acute coronary syndrome, as compared with the older P2Y12 platelet receptor antagonist, clopidogrel, but with an increased risk of bleeding. β-Blockers, statins (goal LDL < 70 mg/dL), and angiotensin-converting enzyme (ACE) inhibitors (regardless of magnitude of blood pressure reduction) reduce cardiovascular morbidity and mortality and should be initiated in hospital. In addition, ACE inhibitors may reduce the risk of development of heart failure and mortality in select patients.

15. **Your AMI patient has cardiogenic shock. What is the only thing that can improve mortality?**

Early revascularization is recommended in all patients with AMI complicated by shock. The Should We Emergently Revascularize Occluded Arteries for Cardiogenic Shock (SHOCK) trial randomly assigned patients with cardiogenic shock due to acute MI and left ventricular failure to early revascularization with PCI and coronary artery bypass grafting (CABG) or initial medical stabilization and balloon pump placement. The 30-day mortality rate was lower in the early revascularization group (47% vs. 56%), with significantly better mortality and quality of life up to 6 years after MI. Of note, patients surviving their shock hospitalization were remarkably healthy at 1-year follow-up; 87% were class I or II New York Heart Association heart failure (none or minimal limitation of activity due to heart failure symptoms).

16. **Name the most appropriate first and second choice of vasopressor in cardiogenic shock.**

After PCI or early revascularization with CABG, pressors may be required for a period of time to allow hemodynamic stabilization. Dopamine and norepinephrine are the medications most often used for hypotension in cardiogenic shock. Both agents have α- and β-adrenergic properties, though to different degrees, resulting in disparate effects on renal and splanchnic perfusion. A recent multicenter randomized trial established norepinephrine as the first-line vasopressor in cardiogenic shock, with dopamine resulting in more arrhythmic events and a lower survival at 28 days. In patients with refractory hemodynamic instability, referral for left ventricular assist support devices and cardiac transplantation may be warranted.

17. **What are the indications for cooling or hypothermia after AMI and cardiac arrest?**

- Adult successfully resuscitated from a witnessed out-of-hospital or in-hospital cardiac arrest and now hemodynamically stable
- Patient with a presenting rhythm of ventricular fibrillation or nonperfusing ventricular tachycardia who remains comatose after restoration of spontaneous circulation

After cooling, patients should be monitored for electrolyte abnormalities, coagulation disturbances, pancreatitis, and leukopenia or thrombocytopenia. Contraindications to cooling include admission temperature < 30° C and patients who are pregnant, are terminally ill, have an inherited coagulopathy, or were comatose before arrest.

KEY POINTS: TREATMENT OF ACUTE MYOCARDIAL INFARCTION

1. Distinguish between unstable angina [UA]–NSTEMI and STEMI: STEMI is an occluded artery and requires immediate reperfusion with PCI or fibrinolysis; UA-NSTEMI requires medical therapy and invasive approach (within 4-48 hours of presentation) for all patients at increased risk.

2. Oral antiplatelet therapy should be initiated including aspirin and clopidogrel, prasugrel, or ticagrelor.

3. Antithrombotics (heparin, enoxaparin, fondaparinux, or bivalirudin) should be administered with weight- and glomerular filtration rate–adjusted dosing to avoid bleeding risks.

4. Statin, β-blocker, and ACE inhibitors should be considered in all patients with AMI regardless of baseline LDL level, blood pressure, and heart rate.

5. Revascularization (PCI, CABG) is warranted immediately (STEMI–primary PCI) or urgently (STEMI-postlytic, pharmacoinvasive approach) or within 4 to 48 hours of presentation (high-risk UA-NSTEMI).

BIBLIOGRAPHY

1. Antman EM, Cohen M, Bernink PJ, et al: The TIMI risk score for unstable angina/non-ST elevation MI: a method for prognostication and therapeutic decision making. JAMA 284:835-842, 2000.

2. Dauerman HL: Challenges in oral antiplatelet therapy: ST-segment elevation myocardial infarction. Am J Cardiol 104(5 Suppl):39C-43C, 2009.

3. Dauerman HL, Sobel BE: Synergistic treatment of ST-segment elevation myocardial infarction with pharmacoinvasive recanalization. J Am Coll Cardiol 42:646-651, 2003.

4. De Backer D, Biston P, Devriendt J, et al: Comparison of dopamine and norepinephrine in the treatment of shock. N Engl J Med 362:779-789, 2010.

5. Holzer M: Targeted temperature management for comatose survivors of cardiac arrest. N Engl J Med 363:1256-1264, 2010.

6. Redpath C, Sambell C, Stiell I, et al: In-hospital mortality in 13,263 survivors of out-of-hospital cardiac arrest in Canada. Am Heart J 159:577-583.e1, 2010.

7. Reynolds HR, Hochman JS: Cardiogenic shock: current concepts and improving outcomes. Circulation 117:686-697, 2008.

8. Sleeper LA, Ramanathan K, Picard MH, et al: Functional status and quality of life after emergency revascularization for cardiogenic shock complicating acute myocardial infarction. J Am Coll Cardiol 46:266-273, 2005.

9. Stone GW, Maehara A, Lansky AJ, et al: A prospective natural-history study of coronary atherosclerosis. N Engl J Med 364:226-235, 2011.

10. Thygesen K, Alpert JS, White HD, et al: Universal definition of myocardial infarction. J Am Coll Cardiol 50:2173-2195, 2007.

11. White HD, Chew DP: Acute myocardial infarction. Lancet 372:570-584, 2008.

12. Wiviott SD, Braunwald E, McCabe CH, et al: Prasugrel versus clopidogrel in patients with acute coronary syndromes. N Engl J Med 357:2001-2015, 2007.

CHAPTER 29

DYSRHYTHMIAS AND TACHYARRHYTHMIAS

Pierre Znojkiewicz, MD, and Peter S. Spector, MD

1. **How do you treat tachycardia in the intensive care unit (ICU)?**
   The first step in treating an arrhythmia in the ICU is determination of the urgency with which it must be resolved; hemodynamically unstable rhythms require immediate treatment at times not affording the clinician the luxury of full diagnostic assessment. Even in the patient whose condition is unstable a very quick look at a telemetry recording allows one to answer several key questions: Is this a wide (QRS > 120 ms) or narrow complex rhythm? Is the rhythm irregular or regular? **Unstable rhythms can be electrically cardioverted or defibrillated.** With better-tolerated rhythms it is important to gather some diagnostic information that may be required for both short- and long-term arrhythmia management.

2. **How do you determine the cause of wide complex tachycardias?**
   Whenever possible, a 12-lead electrocardiogram (ECG) should be obtained. The first distinction to make is between supraventricular and ventricular arrhythmias. A detailed description of how to make this distinction is beyond the scope of this chapter, but a few rules of thumb can be helpful. Narrow complexes indicate that the ventricles are being depolarized via the conduction system (His-Purkinje [HP]). A wide QRS complex indicates that ventricular activation is *not* entirely via the conduction system. This can occur with ventricular tachycardia (VT), ventricular pacing, bundle branch block (BBB), accessory pathway conduction, or rarely with ventricular conduction delay (e.g., hyperkalemia).

3. **How do you differentiate a VT from an aberrantly conducted supraventricular tachycardia (SVT)?**
   In wide complex tachycardia, one must distinguish SVT with aberrancy from VT. Step 1 is to identify P waves and assess the relationship between atrial and ventricular activation. A 1:1 relationship can occur with conduction between atria and ventricles (or vice versa and therefore does not distinguish SVT from VT). Atrioventricular (AV) dissociation, on the other hand, can identify VT (V faster than A) or SVT with aberrancy (A faster than V). Other indicators that suggest VT (though not definitively) are a very wide QRS (>160 ms), precordial concordance (leads V1-V6 all positive or all negative), and fusion beats (indicating intermittent conduction via the HP system during VT). Finally, inspection of an old ECG can help identify the prior presence of BBB or preexcitation. Irregularly irregular rhythms are likely to be atrial fibrillation.

4. **What rhythms produce a wide complex tachycardia that can be mistaken for VT?**
   SVTs that are conducted with BBB (preexisting or rate related) are referred to as SVT with aberrancy. In patients with an accessory pathway (AP) conduction from atria to ventricles over the AP will produce a wide complex. This will occur whether the AP is part of the arrhythmia circuit (antidromic AV reentrant tachycardia [AVRT]; conduction antegrade over the AP and retrograde over the AV node) or a *bystander* that simply conducts activation resulting from some other arrhythmia (e.g., atrial flutter).

5. **What should you think of when you see a very wide QRS (and no P waves)?**
   Hyperkalemia leads to baseline depolarization of cardiac cell membranes. This in turn results in an increased proportion of inactivated sodium channels. The global consequence of increased inactivation is decreased conduction velocity. In the atria this creates long low-amplitude P waves (which can be difficult to see), and in the ventricle it creates a very wide QRS. With sufficient hyperkalemia a sine wave–appearing rhythm can result. If the underlying rhythm is fast (e.g., sinus tachycardia) the wide QRS and apparent lack of P waves can be mistaken for VT. It is critical **not** to give sodium channel blocking antiarrhythmics (e.g., lidocaine) in this setting because they further increase sodium channel inactivation and can result in asystole and death. Treatment should be aimed at stabilizing the cell membrane (calcium) and reducing potassium (insulin, glucose, Kayexalate, and/or dialysis). See Figure 29-1.

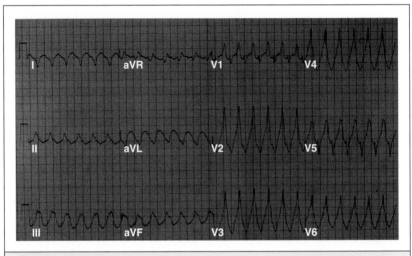

Figure 29-1. Example of a wide complex tachycardia in a patient with hyperkalemia. Note how this could easily be mistaken for VT.

6. **What is torsades de pointes, and what predisposes a patient to it?**
   Torsades de pointes, French for *twisting of the points*, is a specific polymorphic VT that is frequently self-limiting but can degenerate into ventricular fibrillation (VF). It must be distinguished from polymorphic VT due to ischemia. Torsades is defined by the following:
   - Constellation of one long QT interval (QTc >440 ms in men and >460 ms in women)
   - Initiation with a *long-short* interval (tachycardia begins after a pause [long cycle])
   - Premature ventricular contraction that begins during the T wave (short cycle)
     Long QT (and torsade) can result from a congenital ion channel abnormality or ion channel blocking medication (see Fig. 29-2) and can be exacerbated by hypomagnesemia, hypokalemia, and hypocalcemia.

7. **What drugs commonly used in the ICU can cause QT prolongation?**
   See Box 29-1. See also www.torsades.org.

8. **What is the Wolff-Parkinson-White (WPW) syndrome?**
   WPW syndrome occurs in patients who have an abnormal extra connection between the atria and the ventricles: an AP. This can result in evidence of preexcitation on surface ECG. The atrial wave

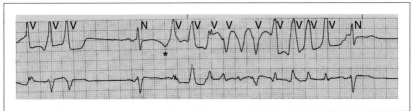

Figure 29-2. Example of torsades de pointes. Notice the long QT, long-short interval *(asterisk)*, and self-limited run of polymorphic VT with twisting of the points.

BOX 29-1. DRUGS COMMONLY USED IN THE ICU THAT CAN CAUSE QT PROLONGATION	
Amiodarone	Quinidine
Clarithromycin	Sotalol
Amitriptyline	Moxifloxacin
Haloperidol	Lithium
Methadone	Risperidone

front travels down the AP and begins depolarizing ventricular tissue before ventricular activation through the HP system, resulting in a short PR interval and initial slurring of the QRS (delta wave). This is followed by rapid activation of the remaining ventricular tissue through the HP system. A patient with preexcitation and documented AVRT is said to have WPW syndrome. Note that a subset of APs will only conduct retrograde and will not produce evident preexcitation; these are so-called concealed accessory pathways.

9. **What are the two forms of AV reentrant tachycardia (AVRT)?**
   In patients with an AP, a well-timed premature atrial contraction or premature ventricular contraction that conducts up or down through only one of the AV connections (either the AV node or the AP) but blocks in the other can then set up a reentrant arrhythmia called AVRT (not to be confused with AV nodal reentrant tachycardia [AVNRT]). The two forms of AVRT are described by the conduction through the AV node as either *orthodromic*, meaning that the tachycardia propagates down the AV node and back up to the atria via the AP, or *antidromic* when conducting down to the ventricles via the AP and retrograde over the AV node.
   Note: Orthodromic AVRT will produce a narrow complex tachycardia with loss of preexcitation; antidromic AVRT will produce a wide complex tachycardia.

10. **Why are patients with WPW syndrome at increased risk for sudden cardiac death?**
    Patients who have an accessory pathway lack the protection offered by AV node refractoriness. If their accessory pathway can conduct antegrade (from the atria to the ventricles) at high frequency they are at risk for very rapid ventricular rates should AF develop. Such rapid rates can lead to VT or VF. Any patient who is initially seen with an irregularly irregular wide complex tachycardia should raise the suspicion of preexcited AF. AV nodal blocking agents should be avoided in such patients because they can increase conduction down the AP leading to increased risk for VF or VT. Drugs that slow conduction of the pathway such as procainamide or amiodarone should be considered.

11. **What is the main effect of adenosine on cardiac conduction?**
    Adenosine's main clinically relevant effect on cardiac conduction is transient AV nodal block. As such it can be used in the diagnosis of various narrow complex tachycardias where the P waves are difficult to discern on the surface ECG. A bolus of adenosine produces rapid-onset, short-duration AV block. This can result in *unmasking* of P waves previously obscured by the QRST complex. In AV node–dependent rhythms (such as AVRT and AVNRT [described later]) adenosine will cause termination of tachycardia. Thus adenosine injection can be a diagnostic and therapeutic maneuver. Termination of a narrow complex tachycardia by adenosine strongly suggests an AV node–dependent rhythm but rarely can indicate adenosine-sensitive focal atrial tachycardias. It is important always to have a 12-lead ECG running when giving adenosine. See Figure 29-3.

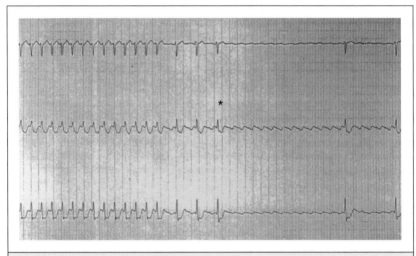

Figure 29-3. Example of narrow-complex tachycardia with unmasking of flutter waves once the transient AV block is achieved with adenosine *(asterisk)*.

12. **What are common causes of atrial fibrillation in a critical care patient?**
    Although the exact causes of atrial fibrillation are unknown, a number of factors are commonly associated with atrial fibrillation: pulmonary disease, pulmonary emboli, systemic inflammatory response, hyperthyroidism, alcohol *(holiday heart)*, valvular heart disease, and atrial enlargement.

13. **How do you treat hemodynamically stable tachycardias?**
    There are two issues to consider when identifying arrhythmias:
    1. Is the rhythm symptomatic (and hence treatment is aimed at relief from symptoms)? and/or
    2. Does the rhythm identify an underlying risk (e.g., an increased risk for sudden cardiac death or stroke)?

    Atrial fibrillation and rapid atrial tachycardias (e.g., atrial flutter) are associated with increased risk for stroke, and measures must be taken to reduce this risk *independent of* whether the rhythm is controlled. In some patients (e.g., those with decreased ventricular function), VT can indicate an increased risk for sudden cardiac death. Finally, preexcitation (antegrade conduction via an accessory pathway) *may* indicate an increased risk for sudden death depending on the refractory properties of the accessory pathway. Such patients may require an electrophysiologic study to assess the pathway's refractory period.

14. **What drugs can be used to control ventricular response rate in a patient with hypotension and atrial fibrillation?**

An unfortunate side effect of most rate-controlling medications such as β-blockers and calcium channel blockers is that they are vasodilators and negative inotropes and hence can lead to lowered systemic blood pressure. For this reason physicians are often hesitant to give these medications to a patient with AF and rapid ventricular response rate who have low pressure. In the vast majority of cases repeated small doses of intravenous (IV) medication (e.g., 5 mg of diltiazem) will reduce heart rate without decreasing blood pressure (the increased diastolic filling time offsets the vasodilatory and negative inotropic effects). Direct current cardioversion (DCCV) is the treatment of choice for hemodynamically unstable rapid AF.

15. **How should you treat AF in a hemodynamically stable patient?**

A patient with highly symptomatic atrial fibrillation should have attempts made at restoring and maintaining sinus rhythm. Cardioversion (chemical or electrical) is the usual first step in a patient who has new-onset atrial fibrillation of less than 48 hours. After 48 hours of AF without adequate anticoagulation, the risk for thromboembolic events increases. Under these circumstances the patient should have rate control and adequate anticoagulation for at least 4 weeks and then cardioversion. If the patient cannot tolerate AF for that period of time and if transesophageal echocardiography reveals no thrombus, cardioversion can be performed and anticoagulation started. Antiarrhythmic agents can be used for patients with symptoms either in whom DCCV has failed or who are going in and out of AF (in which case DCCV is not appropriate). Long-term management for patients with symptoms in whom antiarrhythmic therapy fails should involve consideration of AF ablation. In patients without symptoms it is reasonable to allow AF to continue and control ventricular response rates. Management of anticoagulation *is independent of rhythm control*.

16. **Who needs anticoagulation?**

In patients with new-onset AF of less than 48 hours duration the need for anticoagulation before and after cardioversion may be based on the patient's long-term risk for thromboembolism (see Table 29-1). For patients with AF of more than 48 hours duration anticoagulation should be initiated before cardioversion (for at least 3 weeks if possible or IV heparin if requiring immediate cardioversion for hemodynamic instability) and continued for 4 weeks. The decision for long-term anticoagulation is based on the CHA_2DS_2-VASc score. Patients with a score of 1 can receive either aspirin or full anticoagulation; patients with a score of 2 or more should receive long-term anticoagulation.

17. **Are there nonpharmacologic approaches to acute rate control with atrial tachycardias?**

In patients with atrial tachycardia who have atrial pacing leads in place a nonpharmacologic alternative to AV node–blocking drugs exists for controlling ventricular response rate. In an atrial tachycardia that cannot be otherwise rate controlled, efforts can be made to pace the atria *faster* than the rate of the atrial tachycardia; this can lead to a higher degree of block in the AV node (i.e., 3:1 vs. 2:1) and therefore paradoxically lower the ventricular rate.

18. **How do you treat rapid regular narrow-complex tachycardias?**

Adenosine can be a helpful diagnostic maneuver (see earlier). Typical atrial flutter can be recognized by its characteristic appearance: "sawtooth" P waves in the inferior leads and a narrow upright P wave in V_1. This ECG pattern reliably indicates counterclockwise reentry around the tricuspid annulus, a rhythm with a very high rate of cure with catheter ablation. Other atrial tachycardias can be treated with antiarrhythmic medication or ablation. Ablation of SVT has a high success rate and low complication rate. AV nodal–blocking agents can also be used for long-term suppression of SVT.

TABLE 29-1. CHA$_2$DS$_2$-VASc SCORE	
RISK FACTOR	**SCORE**
Congestive heart failure/LV dysfunction	1
Hypertension	1
Age >75 y	2
Diabetes mellitus	1
Stroke/TIA/TE	2
Vascular disease (prior myocardial infarction, peripheral artery disease, aortic plaque)	1
Age 65-74 y	1
Sex category (i.e., female gender)	1

From Lip GY, Nieuwlaat R, Pisters R, et al: Refining clinical risk stratification for predicting stroke and thromboembolism in atrial fibrillation using a novel risk factor-based approach—The Euro Heart Survey on Atrial Fibrillation. Chest 137:263-272, 2010.
LV, Left ventricular; *TE*, thromboembolism; *TIA*, transient ischemic attack.

19. **How do you decide which antiarrhythmic medication to use?**
   The choice of antiarrhythmic medication can be complex, but one should know major contraindications to the various antiarrhythmic agents. Amiodarone is contraindicated in patients with chronic lung disease and baseline thyroid dysfunction; patients taking amiodarone should have annual chest radiographs and biannual liver and thyroid function tests. Dronedarone is contraindicated in patients with congestive heart failure. Flecainide is contraindicated in patients with coronary artery or structural heart disease. Dofetilide and sotalol should be avoided in patients with renal insufficiency; with preserved renal function, therapy should be started in the hospital where the QTc can be monitored until steady states have been achieved.

20. **How are bradycardias described?**
   Bradycardia can result from abnormalities of impulse formation (e.g., sinus bradycardia, sinus arrest) or from failure of impulse conduction (i.e., AV node or HP system disease).

21. **How do you describe the different degrees of AV block?**
   - **First-degree** heart block: conduction delay with PR interval >200 ms. First-degree AV *block* is therefore a misnomer, and electrophysiology purists will use the term first-degree AV *delay*.
   - **Second-degree** heart block: periodic interruptions of AV conduction, leading to nonconducted beats. Second-degree heart block is divided into Mobitz type I (Wenckebach: progressive PR prolongation followed by a nonconducted beat) and Mobitz type II (intermittent nonconducted beats with a fixed PR interval that is typically not prolonged).
   - **Third-degree** heart block: complete interruption of AV conduction, with AV dissociation (if there are ventricular escape beats) or ventricular asystole.

22. **Which type of second-degree heart block is worrisome and why?**
   Second-degree AV block is rarely symptomatic and by itself is not dangerous. The question is whether second-degree block indicates increased risk for complete AV block, and if so whether asystole is likely to occur. AV node block rarely progresses to third-degree block and often has a reliable escape rhythm if it does. HP block is more likely to progress to complete block and is more likely to result in asystole. AV node suppression typically results in Mobitz I block, whereas HP

block leads to Mobitz II block. Therefore Mobitz II block is an indication for permanent pacemaker placement. In the presence of 2:1 AV block Mobitz I and II cannot be distinguished; widened QRS and normal PR interval suggest that block is at the HP level. Atropine improves AV node conduction. It has no direct effect on HP conduction but by causing increased sinus rate can *paradoxically* increase HP block and therefore should be avoided in this setting.

23. **How would you know whether transcutaneous pacing pads are capturing?**
Transcutaneous pacing is a temporary solution for hemodynamically unstable bradycardia. Electric current is delivered between the pacing/defibrillation pads on the patient's chest. It can be difficult to assess whether myocardial capture has been achieved; the surface electrogram and telemetry are frequently obscured by a large-amplitude pacing artifact, and palpation of the pulse can be misleading because of contraction of the skeletal muscles mimicking cardiac pulsation. One can look for T waves on the cardiogram, monitor arterial blood pressure, or palpate the femoral pulse. **Note:** the default setting on most external pacing machines is to start pacing at the machine's **minimum** output current.

KEY POINTS: DYSRHYTHMIAS AND TACHYARRHYTHMIAS

1. Characteristics that point toward a wide complex tachycardia being VT
   - AV dissociation
   - Very wide QRS complex
   - Precordial lead concordance
   - Fusion beats

2. Characteristics of torsades de pointes
   - Long QT
   - Long-short coupling initiation
   - Twisting of the points during VT

Torsades should be distinguished from ischemic polymorphic VT because treatment is very different.

3. Second-degree Mobitz II heart block indicates conduction system disease distal to the AV node and is an indication for evaluation for permanent pacemaker.

WEBSITES

http://ms.fletcherallen.org/ep_education/
http://www.torsades.org

BIBLIOGRAPHY

1. Jalife J, Delmar M, Davidenko J, et al: Basic Cardiac Electrophysiology for the Clinician. New York, Futura/Wiley-Blackwell, 1999.
2. Zipes DP, Jalife J: Cardiac Electrophysiology: From Cell to Bedside. Philadelphia, Saunders, 2009.

CHAPTER 30

AORTIC DISSECTION

Asheesh Kumar, MD, and Rae M. Allain, MD

1. **Define aortic dissection.**

   An aortic dissection is a tearing of the layers within the aortic wall, classically associated with sudden-onset chest or back pain, a pulse deficit, and mediastinal widening on a chest radiograph. Depending on size and degree of aortic involvement, it may result in marked hemodynamic instability and, often, a rapid death. Prompt diagnosis and appropriate treatment are critical to maximize the possibility of survival. Significant dissections are often fatal and rarely survive to clinical attention; the majority of dissections seen in the critical care environment are either subacute, contained, or sparing the major aortic vessels.

2. **What is the anatomy of injury in aortic dissection?**

   The tear usually originates in the *intima*. It then propagates into the media creating a false channel for blood to flow and hematoma to form. The dissection process may alternatively originate with hemorrhage in the media that secondarily causes disruption of the intima. In approximately 70% of patients, the intimal tear, which is the beginning of the dissection, occurs in the *ascending aorta*. In 20% of patients it occurs in the descending thoracic aorta, and in 10% of patients it occurs in the aortic arch. Only rarely is an intimal tear identified in the abdominal aorta.

3. **Describe the DeBakey and Stanford classifications of aortic dissection.**

   The two classification systems most commonly used both have anatomic as well as management implications.

   The **DeBakey** classification describes **three** types of dissection (Fig. 30-1):
   - *Type I*: extends from aortic root to beyond the ascending aorta
   - *Type II*: involves only the ascending aorta
   - *Type III*: begins distal to the takeoff of the left subclavian artery and has two subtypes
     - Type IIIA: limited to the thoracic aorta
     - Type IIIB: extends below the diaphragm

   The **Stanford** classification has **two** types of dissection (Fig. 30-2):
   - *Type A*: involves the ascending aorta
   - *Type B*: involves the descending aorta, distal to the left subclavian artery

4. **What is the epidemiology of dissection, including mortality?**

   Aortic dissection is a relatively rare but a highly lethal disease. The estimated incidence is 5 to 30 cases per million people per year. Population-based studies suggest that the incidence of acute dissection ranges from 2 to 3.5 cases per 100,000 person-years, which correlates with 6000 to 10,000 cases annually in the United States. It may be that two to three times as many patients die of dissections as of ruptured aortic aneurysms; approximately 75% of patients with ruptured aortic aneurysm will reach an emergency department alive, whereas for aortic dissection 40% die immediately. Furthermore, only 50% to 70% will be alive 5 years after surgery depending on age and underlying cause.

   For untreated acute dissection of the ascending aorta the mortality rate is 1% to 2% per hour after onset. For type A dissections treated medically it is approximately 20% within the first 24 hours and 50% by 1 month after presentation. Even with surgical intervention, the mortality rate for type A dissection may be as high as 10% after 24 hours and nearly 20% 1 month after repair.

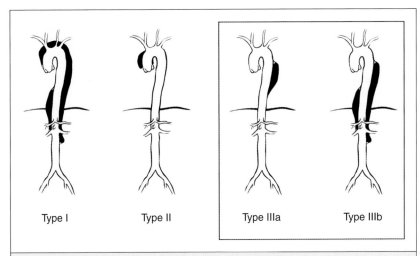

Figure 30-1. DeBakey classification. Illustration by Samuel Rodriguez, MD.

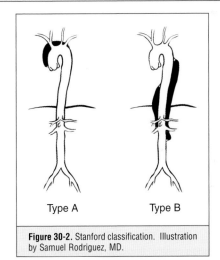

Figure 30-2. Stanford classification. Illustration by Samuel Rodriguez, MD.

Although type B dissection is less dangerous than type A, it is still associated with an extremely high mortality. The 30-day mortality rate for an uncomplicated type B dissection approaches 10%. However, patients with type B dissection who have complications such as limb ischemia, renal failure, or visceral ischemia have a 2-day mortality upwards of 20% and may prompt the need for surgical intervention.

5. **What are the risk factors and associated conditions for dissection?**
   The prevalence of aortic dissection appears to be increasing, independent of the aging population, as noted by Olsson and colleagues, who found that the incidence of dissection among Swedish men has increased to 16 per 100,000 yearly. Risk factors include the following:
   - **Hypertension:** Present in **70% to 90%** of patients with acute dissection.
   - **Advanced age:** Mean of 63 years in the International Registry of Acute Aortic Dissection (IRAD).

- **Male sex:** Represented by **65%** of patients in the IRAD.
- **Family history:** Recently recognized is a genetic, nonsyndromic familial form of thoracic aortic dissection. Studies of patients referred for repair of thoracic aortic dissections and aneurysms who did not have a known genetic mutation have indicated that between 11% and 19% of these patients have a first-degree relative with thoracic aortic disease.
- **Trauma (deceleration/torsional injury)**
- **Congenital and inflammatory disorders:** present as Marfan syndrome in almost **5%** of total patients in the IRAD and half of those patients under age 40 years. Other associated congenital disorders include Ehlers-Danlos syndrome, Loeys-Dietz syndrome, bicuspid aortic valve, aortic coarctation, Turner syndrome, Takayasu and giant-cell aortitis, relapsing polychondritis (Behçet disease, spondyloarthropathies), or confirmed genetic mutations known to predispose to dissections (*TGFBR1, TGFBR2, FBN1, ACTA2,* or *MYH11*).
- **Pregnancy:** Associated with 50% of dissections in women under age 40 and most frequently occurring in the **third trimester**. This might be attributable to elevations in cardiac output during pregnancy that cause increased wall stress.
- **Circadian and seasonal variations:** Producing a higher frequency of dissection in the morning hours and in the winter months.
- **Iatrogenic:** Occurring as a consequence of invasive procedures or surgery, especially when the aorta has been entered or its main branches have been cannulated, such as for cardiopulmonary bypass.

6. **Describe the common clinical signs and symptoms of aortic dissection.**
   - **Pain:** The most common presenting symptom is chest pain, occurring in up to 90% of patients with acute dissection. Classically, for type A dissections, sudden onset of *severe anterior chest pain with extension to the back* occurs that is described as *ripping* or *tearing* in nature. However, in the IRAD, pain was more often described as *sharp* rather than ripping or tearing. The pain is usually of maximal intensity from its inception and is frequently unremitting. It may migrate along the path of the dissection. The pain of aortic dissection may mimic that of myocardial ischemia. Patients with type B dissections are more likely to be seen with back pain (64%) alone.
   - **Syncope:** Syncope is a well-recognized clinical feature of dissection, occurring in up to 13% of cases. Impairments of cerebral blood flow can be due to acute hypovolemia, low cardiac output, or dissection-involvement of the cerebral vessels. Patients with a presenting syncope were significantly more likely to die than were those without syncope (34% vs. 23%), likely because of the frequent correlation with associated cardiac tamponade, stroke, decreased consciousness, and spinal cord ischemia.

7. **Describe the common clinical findings associated with aortic dissection.**
   A systems-based approach can be used to describe the wide range of clinical findings that can be associated with aortic dissection.
   - **Neurologic symptoms.** The reported frequency of neurologic symptoms in pooled data of type A and B dissections approaches 17%; in type A alone, 29% of patients were seen initially with neurologic symptoms, 53% of which represented ischemic stroke. Neurologic complications may result from hypotension, malperfusion, distal thromboembolism, or nerve compression. Acute paraplegia as a result of spinal cord malperfusion has been described as a primary manifestation in 1% to 3% of patients. Up to 50% of neurologic symptoms may be transient.
   - **Cardiovascular manifestations.** The heart is the most frequently involved end-organ in acute proximal aortic dissections.
     - □ **Acute aortic regurgitation** may be present in 41% to 76% of patients with proximal dissection and may be caused by widening of the aortic annulus resulting in incomplete valve closure or actual disruption of the aortic valve leaflets from the dissection flap. Clinical

manifestations of dissection-related aortic regurgitation span from mere diastolic murmurs without clinical significance to overt congestive heart failure and cardiogenic shock.

☐ **Myocardial ischemia or infarction** may result from compromised coronary artery flow by an expanding false lumen that compresses the proximal coronary or by extension of the dissection flap into the coronary artery ostium. This occurs in 7% to 19% of patients with proximal aortic dissections. Clinically, these present as electrocardiographic changes consistent with primary myocardial ischemia and/or infarction. Appropriate treatment of myocardial ischemia ought to be initiated without delay and concomitantly with aortic imaging to evaluate for dissection when both diagnoses are suspected.

☐ **Cardiac tamponade** is diagnosed in 8% to 10% of patients seen with acute type A dissections. It is associated with a high mortality and should prompt consideration for emergent drainage and aortic repair.

☐ **Hypertension** occurs in greater than 50% of patients with dissection, more commonly with distal disease. Ongoing renal ischemia can produce severe hypertension.

☐ **Hypotension/shock** may present in up to 20% of patients with dissection. This may be a result of cardiac tamponade from aortic rupture into the pericardium, dissection, or compression of the coronary arteries, acute aortic regurgitation, acute blood loss, true lumen compression by distended false lumen, or an intraabdominal catastrophe. Cardiogenic shock is a relatively uncommon complication, found to occur in approximately 6% of cases. This can be due to acute aortic regurgitation or ongoing myocardial ischemia.

■ **Peripheral vascular complications** can manifest as pulse and/or blood pressure differentials or deficits and occur in approximately one third to one half of patients with proximal dissection. Etiology is partial compression, obstruction, thrombosis, or embolism of the aortic branch vessels, resulting in cerebral, renal, visceral, or limb ischemia. Peripheral pulse deficits should alert the clinician to possible ongoing renal or visceral ischemia unable to be detected from physical examination or laboratory values alone.

■ **Pulmonary complications** may manifest as pleural effusions, which occur most frequently on the left. Causes include rupture of the dissection into the pleural space or weeping of fluid from the aorta as an inflammatory response to the dissection.

8. **What common laboratory abnormalities are associated with aortic dissection?**
Laboratory data are usually unrevealing, but *anemia* from blood loss into the false lumen can occur. A moderate *leukocytosis* (10,000-14,000 white cells per milliliter) is sometimes seen. Lactic acid dehydrogenase and bilirubin levels may be elevated because of hemolysis within the false lumen. Disseminated intravascular coagulation has been reported. Currently, randomized controlled data do not support the use of D-dimers or experimental serum markers (plasma smooth muscle myosin heavy chain protein, high-sensitivity C-reactive protein).

9. **Describe imaging modalities used to diagnose aortic dissection.**
In 2010, the American Heart Association and American College of Cardiology released guidelines for the diagnosis and management of patients with thoracic aortic disease, which identified high-risk clinical features to assist in the early detection of acute aortic dissection. On the basis of clinical risk factors and conditions, presentation, and associated examination findings, patients are stratified into low-, intermediate-, or high-risk categories. Further work-up is dictated by this pretest probability index. Some patients with acute dissection initially have no high-risk features, creating a diagnostic dilemma. According to most recent guidelines, if a clear alternative diagnosis is not established after the initial evaluation, then obtaining a diagnostic aortic imaging study should be considered.

Although lacking specificity, a chest radiograph should be obtained as part of the initial diagnostic evaluation. A radiograph abnormality is seen in up to 90% of patients with aortic dissection; most frequent is widening of the aorta and mediastinum. Other findings may include a localized hump on the aortic arch, displacement of calcification in the aortic knob, and pleural effusions. However, approximately 40% of radiographs in acute dissection lack a widened mediastinum, and as many as 16% are normal. Thus a negative radiograph must not delay definitive aortic imaging in patients deemed at high risk for aortic dissection by initial screening.

Computed tomography (CT) scanning, magnetic resonance imaging (MRI), and transesophageal echocardiography (TEE) are all highly accurate imaging modalities that may be used to make the diagnosis; all can provide acceptable diagnostic accuracy. Transthoracic echocardiography has limited diagnostic accuracy. Aortography, which was once the test of choice, is no longer used routinely because it is invasive and time-consuming and involves exposure to intravenous contrast dye. The most recent comparative study with nonhelical CT, MRI, and TEE showed 100% sensitivity for all modalities, with better specificity of CT (100%) as compared with TEE or MRI. A recent meta-analysis found that all three imaging techniques provided equally reliable results. Although each imaging modality offers advantages and disadvantages, the choice among CT, MRI, and TEE is probably best based on which is most readily available. It should be noted, however, that the diagnosis of acute aortic dissection can be difficult and occasionally cannot be absolutely excluded by a single imaging study. If a high clinical suspicion exists despite initially negative imaging, then consideration should be given to a second imaging modality. Regardless, prompt surgical consultation should be initiated in any patient with a suspected dissection.

10. **What diagnoses can be confused with aortic dissection?**

- Acute myocardial infarction
- Cerebrovascular accidents
- Thoracic nondissecting aneurysm
- Pericarditis
- Pleuritis
- Atherosclerotic emboli
- Pulmonary embolism
- Acute aortic regurgitation
- Mediastinal cysts or tumors
- Cholecystitis
- Musculoskeletal pain

11. **Differentiate between the management of Stanford type A and type B dissections.**
An acute type A dissection is a **surgical emergency**. However, medical management is critical to halt the progression of the dissection while the diagnostic work-up takes place and while preparations are made to bring the patient to the operating room for definitive treatment. While the diagnosis work-up proceeds and a cardiothoracic surgeon is consulted, the patient's condition should be carefully monitored and stabilized in an intensive care unit. Pain management and gradual down-titration of blood pressure are critical to prevent extension of the dissection. Sufficient blood products and intravascular access should be available in the event of aortic rupture.

Patients with uncomplicated type B dissection are preferably managed medically with β-blockers and other antihypertensive agents. Surgical intervention has no demonstrable superiority except in cases of failed medical management manifesting as malperfusion, aortic expansion with potential for imminent rupture, or intractable pain. Ongoing advances with less-invasive interventions (endovascular stent grafts and endovascular fenestration procedures) suggest an expanded role for interventional management in the treatment of acute type B dissection, especially in experienced centers.

12. **What are the strategies for medical management of dissection and commonly used medications?**
The goals of medical therapy are to treat pain, to aggressively control blood pressure, and to determine need for surgical or endovascular intervention. Patients who are seen with hypotension should receive the following:

- Prompt but judicious volume resuscitation and hemodynamic support with intravenous vasopressors to maintain a goal mean arterial pressure of 70 mm Hg
- Rapid search for underlying etiology (tamponade, myocardial dysfunction, acute hemorrhage)
- Emergent surgical consultation for operative management

In those who are seen initially with hypertension, the blood pressure should generally be lowered to a systolic of 100 to 120 mm Hg, to a mean of 60 to 65 mm Hg, or to the lowest level that is compatible with perfusion of the vital organs. The aortic wall stress is affected by the heart rate, blood pressure, and velocity of ventricular contraction (dP/dt).

The ideal antihypertensive regimen must decrease blood pressure without increasing cardiac output through peripheral vasodilatation. This is because an increased cardiac output can increase flow rates producing higher aortic wall stress and thus propagating the dissection. Intravenous β-blockers (commonly esmolol, labetalol, propranolol, or metoprolol) are considered the first-line medical stabilization regimen because they affect all three parameters without increases in cardiac output and aortic wall stress. In patients who are unable to tolerate β- blockade, nondihydropyridine calcium channel antagonists (verapamil, diltiazem) offer an acceptable alternative.

Often, single-drug therapy alone is inadequate to optimize blood pressure management. Adequate pain control is essential not only for patient comfort but also to decrease sympathetic-mediated increases in heart rate and blood pressure. This may be accomplished with intravenous opioid analgesics. If β-blockade and adequate pain control are ineffective to control blood pressure, the addition of a rapidly acting, easily titratable intravenous vasodilator, such as *nitroprusside*, should be considered. Other agents, such as nicardipine, nitroglycerin, and fenoldopam, are also acceptable. Vasodilator therapy without prior β-blockade may cause reflex tachycardia and increased force of ventricular contraction leading to greater wall stress and potentially causing false lumen propagation; therefore adequate β-blockade must be established first, ***before*** the vasodilator is initiated.

13. **Describe the surgical approach for repair of Stanford type A dissection.**
The purpose of surgery is to resect the aortic segment containing the proximal intimal tear, to obliterate the false channel, and to restore aortic continuity with a graft or by reapproximating the transected ends of the aorta. For patients with aortic insufficiency, it may be possible to resuspend the aortic valve, but in some cases replacement of the aortic valve is necessary. In some cases of proximal dissection, reimplantation of the coronary arteries is required. If a DeBakey type II dissection is present, the entire dissected aorta should be replaced. Surgery to repair an aortic dissection generally requires cardiopulmonary bypass and, often, deep hypothermic circulatory arrest.

14. **What is a more recent alternative to surgical repair of aortic dissection?**
An *endovascular* technique of stent-grafting and/or balloon fenestration may be used for initial surgical treatment of some dissections. Indications for open or endograft treatment are based on the anatomic features of the lesion, clinical presentation and course, patient comorbidities, and anatomic constraints related to endograft technology. Dissections pose a complex situation because the branches of the aorta may be perfused from either the true or false lumen. Often, both the true and false lumens are patent and some of the visceral, renal, or lower extremity vessels are fed by one channel and the remainder by the other. Consideration must be given to how blood flow reaches vital organs before considering treatment of a dissection with an endovascular stent-graft. For type B dissection, an increasing number of reports show better results with endovascular repair versus open surgical repair. The role of endovascular stent-graft versus optimal medical therapy was recently examined in the literature, but no difference was noted in survival or number of adverse events. However, longer-term (5 year) data are needed to fully assess the potential impact of stent-grafting for acute dissection, including effects on survival, clinical outcomes, and long-term aortic remodeling.

15. **What is the future direction for repair of aortic dissections?**
The use of *fenestrated endografts* will likely herald a new era in the treatment of aortic dissections. Unsuitable anatomy is a significant barrier to the use of endovascular stent-grafts for most forms of aortic disease, where the ostia of major vessels would otherwise be partially

or completed covered with the deployment of a stent-graft. Using preoperative three-dimensional CT aortic reconstruction, customized stents can be constructed, featuring holes (fenestrations) or side-branches matched to patient-specific anatomy to ensure perfusion to major aortic branch vessels. Current trials are underway in Europe and the United States for their use for complex aneurysmal disease, and expectations are high for similar application to aortic dissection.

Acknowledgment

Drs. Kumar and Allain wish to acknowledge Peter M. Schulman, MD, and Rondall Lane, MD, the authors of this chapter from the previous edition.

KEY POINTS: DIAGNOSIS AND TREATMENT OF ACUTE AORTIC DISSECTION

1. Aortic dissection is classically associated with sudden chest or back pain, a pulse deficit, and mediastinal widening on chest radiograph.

2. The imaging modality (CT, MRI, or TEE) that is most readily available should be the one selected to confirm the diagnosis of acute aortic dissection.

3. An acute type A aortic dissection is a surgical emergency. Although type B dissections are usually managed medically, one third of these patients eventually require surgery because of worsening of the dissection, rupture, malperfusion, or intractable pain. In either case, prompt surgical consultation is recommended.

4. When managing acute aortic dissection, adequate β-blockade must be established *before* the initiation of nitroprusside to prevent propagation of the dissection from a reflex increase in cardiac output.

5. The use of endovascular stent-grafts will likely play a large role in the management of dissections.

BIBLIOGRAPHY

1. Akin I, Kische S, Rehders TC, et al. Thoracic endovascular stent-graft therapy in aortic dissection. Curr Opin Cardiol 25:552-559, 2010.

2. Clouse WD, Hallett JW Jr., Schaff HV, et al: Acute aortic dissection: population-based incidence compared with degenerative aortic aneurysm rupture. Mayo Clin Proc 79:176-180, 2004.

3. Eggebrecht H, Nienaber C, Neuhauser M, et al. Endovascular stent-graft placement in aortic dissection: a meta-analysis. Eur Heart J 27:489-498, 2006.

4. Ehrlich MP, Dumfarth J, Schoder R, et al. Midterm results after endovascular treatment of acute, complicated type B aortic dissection. Ann Thorac Surg 90:1444-1448, 2010.

5. Estrera AL, Miller CC III, Safi HJ, et al: Outcomes of medical management of acute type B aortic dissection. Circulation 114(Suppl 1):I384-I389, 2006.

6. Hagan PG, Nienaber CA, Isselbacher EM, et al. The International Registry of Acute Aortic Dissection (IRAD): new insights into an old disease. JAMA 283:897-903, 2000.

7. Hiratzka LF, Bakris GL, Beckman JA, et al. 2010 CCF/AHA/AATS/ACR/ASA/SCA/SCAI/SIR/STS/SVM guidelines for the diagnosis and management of patients with thoracic aortic disease. Circulation 121:e266-e369, 2010.

8. Khoynezhad A, Plestis KA: Managing emergency hypertension in aortic dissection and aortic aneurysm surgery. J Card Surg 21(Suppl 1):S3-S7, 2006.

9. Leurs LJ, Bell R, Degrieck Y, et al. Endovascular treatment of thoracic aortic diseases: combined experience from the EUROSTAR and United Kingdom Thoracic Endograft registries. J Vasc Surg 40:670-680, 2004.

10. Nienaber C, Rousseau H, Eggebrecht H: Randomized comparison of strategies for type-B aortic dissection. The Investigation of Stent Grafts in Aortic Dissection (INSTEAD) trial. Circulation 120:2519-2528, 2009.

11. Olsson C, Thelin S, Stahle E, et al. Thoracic aortic aneurysm and dissection: increasing prevalence and improved outcomes reported in a nationwide population-based study of more than 14,000 cases from 1987 to 2002. Circulation 114:2611-2618, 2006.

12. Parsa CJ, Schroder JN, Daneshmand MA, et al. Midterm results for endovascular repair of complicated acute and chronic type B aortic dissection. Ann Thorac Surg 89:97-102, 2010.

13. Trimarchi S, Nienaber CA, Rampoldi V, et al. Role and results of surgery in acute type B aortic dissection: insights from the International Registry of Acute Aortic Dissection (IRAD). Circulation 14(Suppl 1):I357-I364, 2006.

14. Yagdi T, Atay Y, Engin C, et al. Impact of organ malperfusion on mortality and morbidity in acute type A aortic dissections. J Card Surg 21:363-369, 2006.

15. Zoli S, Etz CD, Roder F, et al. Long-term survival after open repair of chronic distal aortic dissection. Ann Thorac Surg 89:1458-1466, 2010.

PERICARDIAL DISEASE (PERICARDITIS AND PERICARDIAL TAMPONADE)

Stuart F. Sidlow, MD, and C. William Hanson, III, MD

1. **What is the structure of the pericardium?**
   The pericardium is a two-layered structure surrounding the heart and consisting of the fibrous and serous layers. The fibrous layer is a stiff, inelastic structure, which has little ability to accommodate fluid accumulation over a short time course. The serous layer consists of two layers, the parietal and visceral pericardium. The parietal layer is adherent to the fibrous pericardium, and the visceral layer is part of the epicardium or external layer of the heart wall. When pericardial effusion occurs, it normally is between the parietal and visceral layers of the serous pericardium. The pericardial space normally holds 15 to 50 mL of an ultrafiltrate of plasma.

2. **Why do hemodynamic changes occur with the buildup of fluid between the layers of the serous pericardium?**
   When fluid accumulates in the pericardial space, the fibrous pericardium has little ability to stretch. As the volume increases in this space, further inflow into the right side of the heart is impaired, which results in decrease in filling of the left side of the heart, and thus preload is decreased.

3. **What general types of pericardial disease exist?**
   - Acute fibrinous pericarditis (acute pericarditis)
   - Pericardial effusion without hemodynamic compromise
   - Cardiac tamponade
   - Constrictive pericarditis

4. **What are the major causes of acute pericarditis (greatest to least common)?**
   - Neoplastic or radiation
   - Viral-adenovirus, enterovirus, cytomegalovirus, influenza, hepatitis B virus, herpes simplex virus
   - Autoimmune or collagen vascular disease
   - Bacterial
   - Uremia
   - Tuberculosis (TB) (most common worldwide)
   - Idiopathic
   - Drugs or toxins

5. **Describe the clinical manifestation of acute pericarditis (history and physical examination).**
   Patient may complain of pleuritic chest pain worse on inspiration. Pain is exacerbated by supine position and relieved by sitting up. Dyspnea may be present. A pericardial friction rub is highly specific to acute pericarditis. Many are seen initially with high fever (temperature >38° C) and new cardiomegaly on chest radiograph. Pleural effusions are frequently observed.

6. **What is on the differential diagnosis of acute pericarditis?**
Differential diagnosis of acute pericarditis consists of acute myocardial infarction, pulmonary embolus, gastroesophageal reflux, and musculoskeletal pain.

7. **How is acute pericarditis manifested on electrocardiography (ECG)?**
There is a progression of four stages on ECG, but for diagnosis one should evaluate for concave-up ST segments throughout most leads (exceptions include aV_R and V_1).

8. **What other diagnostic tests are useful in diagnosis of acute pericarditis?**
Serum cardiac troponin I and creatine kinase, myocardial bound (CKMB) levels should be evaluated. Usually mild troponin increases occur in the absence of increased CKMB levels. The increase is due to inflammation of myocardium. Other tests may include (on the basis of suspicion and other findings) antinuclear antibodies, tuberculin skin test, human immunodeficiency virus serology, and blood cultures.

9. **How is pericardiocentesis used in diagnosing or treating acute pericarditis?**
Pericardiocentesis or surgical drainage should be performed for one of three reasons:
   - If moderate to severe tamponade is present, resulting in hemodynamic compromise (class I recommendation)
   - If purulent, TB or neoplastic effusion is suspected (class IIa recommendation)
   - If a persistently symptomatic effusion is present

10. **Does echocardiography play a role in the diagnosis of acute pericarditis?**
Echocardiography should be performed in all patients suspected of having acute pericarditis. The echo is often normal, but when an effusion is seen it supports the diagnosis of acute pericarditis. The absence of effusion does not rule it out. The use of echocardiography was given a class I recommendation by the American Heart Association, American College of Cardiology, and American Society of Echocardiography.

11. **How is therapy decided for treatment of acute pericarditis?**
Treatment is based on the cause of acute pericarditis as follows:
   - **Neoplastic:** Drainage if hemodynamic compromise, and appropriate chemotherapy.
   - **Viral:** Symptomatic and supportive care.
   - **Autoimmune:** Nonsteroidal antiinflammatory drugs (NSAIDs) are the mainstay of treatment (class I); corticosteroids may be used if refractory to NSAID therapy.
   - **Bacterial or TB:** Antibiotics as appropriate by blood or pericardial fluid culture.
   - **Uremia:** Reversal of uremic state.

12. **What is constrictive pericarditis?**
Constrictive pericarditis is a chronic condition by which the parietal and visceral layers of the pericardium fuse and are often calcified. Causes are similar to those with acute pericarditis. It is usually well tolerated until advanced stages, at which point diastolic filling becomes impaired. Patients have dyspnea and Kussmaul sign (described in question 15), peripheral edema is usually present, and a pericardial knock may be heard.

13. **What is pericardial tamponade?**
Pericardial tamponade is a process in which fluid (blood or serous fluid) accumulates in the pericardial space, either acutely or over time.

14. **What is Beck triad?**
Beck triad consists of falling arterial blood pressure, elevated systemic central venous pressure (CVP), and a small, quiet heart.

15. **What is Kussmaul sign?**

Kussmaul sign is a paradoxical increase in CVP with inspiration. It is observed in any condition that restricts venous return to the heart.

16. **List common settings for acute pericardial tamponade.**

After cardiac operations, blunt or penetrating mediastinal trauma (especially stab wounds), acute myocardial infarction with free wall rupture, endovascular catheterization (including aortograms and carotid arteriograms) with perforation, and, uncommonly, central venous catheter placement (due to erosion of the catheter through a vessel wall)

17. **Describe the changes in hemodynamic monitoring seen in a patient with pericardial tamponade.**

Generally referred to as pulsus paradoxus, on arterial line tracing one may see first subtle, then dramatic respiratory variation in the systolic pressure (>10 mm Hg difference between expiration and inspiration). In a patient who does not have an endotracheal tube in place, as venous return increases to the right side of the heart with negative intrathoracic pressure during inspiration, the free wall of the right ventricle (RV) cannot expand outward into the pericardial space because of the fluid accumulation. The intraventricular septum is displaced into the left ventricle (LV) as the RV distends. As a result, filling of the LV is impaired, causing a decrease in LV preload. During pulmonary artery (PA) catheter monitoring, one sees equalization of diastolic pressures. The pressures of Right atrium = RV = PA diastolic = Wedge pressure (difference <5 mm Hg).

18. **What is the differential diagnosis in a patient with pulsus paradoxus by arterial line tracing?**

- Obesity
- Asthma
- Pulmonary embolism
- Constrictive pericarditis
- Pericardial tamponade
- Cardiogenic shock

Sensitivity and specificity are 79% and 40% for tamponade. Always use clinical suspicion when diagnosing this or other life-threatening conditions. See Figure 31-1.

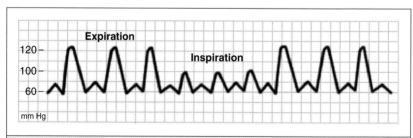

Figure 31-1. Pulsus paradoxus on arterial line tracing.

19. **How is pericardial tamponade diagnosed?**

Tamponade is a clinical diagnosis based on history and physical examination results. It usually represents an emergency and can lead to pulseless electric activity (PEA) cardiac arrest if left undiagnosed and untreated. Some common features include jugular venous distention with increased CVP (Kussmaul sign), faint heart sounds, sinus tachycardia, and pulsus paradoxus. If one is unsure of the diagnosis, some studies are helpful in diagnosis. The ECG may demonstrate electrical alternans or sinus tachycardia with low-voltage QRS complexes. Chest radiograph may show an enlarged cardiac silhouette. Echocardiography is extremely useful in diagnosis of this condition and has been given a class I recommendation. On echo, right atrial collapse is more sensitive but less specific than RV collapse. If tamponade is highly suspected, one should not wait for an echo before instituting therapy. See Figure 31-2.

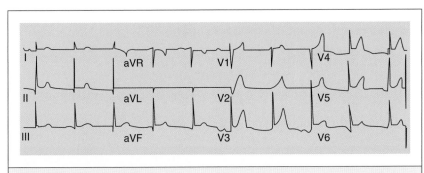

Figure 31-2. Electrical alternans.

20. **Briefly describe the hemodynamic strategy in a patient with suspected pericardial tamponade.**
    The hemodynamic strategy consists of "fast, full, and tight."
    - *Fast* means allow the patient to have tachycardia (no β-blockers, please).
    - *Full* means to increase preload (fluids wide open).
    - *Tight* indicates treatment that allows the patient's blood pressure to rise either by volume resuscitation or with vasopressors (norepinephrine, epinephrine, or phenylephrine) as indicated. This strategy should be used until definitive management of the tamponade can be performed. Intubation should be avoided until the last possible moment to avoid cardiovascular collapse during anesthetic induction.

21. **Why should intubation be avoided during initial treatment of tamponade?**
    Intubation should be deferred until the last possible moment because increasing intrathoracic pressure with positive pressure ventilation, and myocardial depression or vasodilation resulting from anesthetic agents, can decrease cardiac output by up to 25%, which may eliminate cardiac output in some patients.

22. **What therapeutic maneuvers should be performed in a patient with pericardial tamponade?**
    After determination of the cause and rapidity with which the fluid accumulated, either pericardiocentesis, pericardial window (pericardotomy), or sternotomy (as in patients after cardiac surgery) should be performed.

23. **List the contraindications for bedside pericardiocentesis.**
    - Severe coagulopathy or low platelet count
    - Stable effusion (i.e., blind, bedside pericardiocentesis should be performed only with impending cardiovascular collapse or during cardiopulmonary resuscitation)

24. **What other conditions are included in the differential diagnosis of pericardial tamponade?**
    Other conditions to be considered when tamponade is suspected include massive pulmonary embolus, tension pneumothorax, massive myocardial contusion or myocardial ischemia resulting in cardiogenic shock, exacerbation of severe chronic obstructive pulmonary disease with air trapping, and constrictive pericarditis.

KEY POINTS: CHARACTERISTICS OF PERICARDIAL TAMPONADE

1. It is usually a true medical emergency.

2. If left unnoticed or untreated, it results in PEA cardiac arrest.

3. It is a clinical diagnosis.

4. Most useful diagnostic tool is echocardiography, if time permits.

5. Life-saving measure consists of needle pericardiocentesis in emergent situation.

WEBSITES

UpToDate online version 13.3 (www.uptodate.com):
Schiller N, Foster E: Echocardiographic evaluation of the pericardium
Shabetai R, Hoit B: Cardiac tamponade
Shabetai R, Imazio M: Evaluation and management of acute pericarditis
Shabetai R, Soler-Soler J, Corey GR: Etiology of pericardial disease

BIBLIOGRAPHY

1. Benumof J: Anesthesia and Uncommon Diseases, 4th ed. Philadelphia, Saunders, 1998.

2. Moore K: Clinically Oriented Anatomy, 3rd ed. Philadelphia, Williams & Wilkins, 1992.

3. Murray M, Coursin D, Pearl R, et al: Critical Care Medicine—Perioperative Management, 2nd ed. Philadelphia, Lippincott Williams & Wilkins, 2002.

SEPSIS, SEVERE SEPSIS, AND SEPTIC SHOCK

David Shimabukuro, MDCM, Richard H. Savel, MD, FCCM, and Michael A. Gropper, MD, PhD

CHAPTER 32

1. What is sepsis?

Sepsis is an overwhelming inflammatory and coagulopathic response to a source of infection, usually from the lung or abdomen. If not recognized early, or not treated properly and aggressively, it is often a lethal syndrome. Please note that it is different from *bacteremia*, which only refers to the presence of bacteria in the bloodstream.

2. Explain the nomenclature for disorders related to sepsis.

In 1991, the American College of Chest Physicians and the Society of Critical Care Medicine determined the nomenclature for disorders related to sepsis. The following terms describe the progression of signs and symptoms regarding this somewhat confusing terminology:

- **Systemic inflammatory response syndrome (SIRS):** characterized by
  □ Temperature $>38°$ C or $<36°$ C
  □ Heart rate >90 beats/min
  □ Respiratory rate >20 breaths/min or the need for mechanical ventilation
  □ White blood cell count $>12,000$ cells/mm^3 or <4000 cells/mm^3
- **Sepsis:** a suspected or documented source of infection plus two or more SIRS criteria.
- **Severe sepsis:** sepsis with acute sepsis-induced organ dysfunction of one or more organ systems.
- **Septic shock:** a subset of severe sepsis syndrome in which the organ dysfunction is cardiovascular, that is, a subset of severe sepsis in which there is cardiovascular dysfunction. Specifically, sepsis-induced hypotension (mean arterial pressure [MAP] <65 mm Hg) that persists despite adequate and aggressive volume resuscitation. Patients will often require vasopressors to keep MAP ≥ 65 mm Hg.
- **Multiple organ dysfunction syndrome (MODS):** Failure in more than one organ system that requires acute intervention. Once the patient reaches this degree of illness, the chances of making a meaningful recovery can often be quite low.

In 2001, the International Sepsis Definitions Conference convened to once again address the difficulties in defining sepsis. During this meeting, conference members expressed the need for a better, more sophisticated way to stage the severity of sepsis. At this time **PIRO** was introduced. Over the past several years, several studies have been published correlating a total PIRO score with mortality. However, the studies are not identical, and they still need to be corroborated by other investigators. In brief, PIRO represents the following:

Predisposition: age, medical history, genotype (in the future)
Infection/insult: location of infection, organism, and/or cause of infection
Response: SIRS criteria
Organ dysfunction: location and number of organ dysfunction

3. What is the incidence of sepsis?

Septic shock and MODS are relatively common and associated with substantial mortality and consumption of health care resources. In 2007, an estimated 700,000 cases of severe sepsis or MODS occurred in the United States alone. This was a substantial increase over 2003. The numbers continue to rise every year. The incidence of sepsis is substantially higher in elderly than in younger people. The projected growth of the elderly population in the United States will contribute to an increase in incidence of 1.5% per year, yielding an estimated 934,000 and 1,110,000 cases by the years 2010 and 2020, respectively. The present annual cost of severe sepsis and septic shock in the United States is estimated at $25 billion.

4. **How does the nomenclature relate to outcome?**
Previous studies have shown that as the disorder progresses from SIRS to septic shock, the mortality rate increases. Of interest, some data support the concept that, although the degree of illness at presentation may have some correlation with outcomes, it is the change in clinical status from baseline that may have the closest correlation with outcomes. Regardless, sepsis progresses to MODS with tragic consequences. The mortality rate for patients with acute renal failure in the setting of sepsis ranges from 50% to 80%. For most patients with sepsis syndrome, the failure of three or more organ systems results in a mortality rate >90%. The organ systems most often affected early in the process are pulmonary, hematologic, renal, and cardiovascular. Despite the growing number of patients with septic shock and increase in likelihood of death with multiple organ failure, overall mortality appears to be declining in recent years. This could be related to an improvement in therapy and improvement in supportive measures but is more likely related to medical coding issues and the heterogeneity of the disease and the available data.

5. **Discuss current understanding of the pathogenesis of sepsis and septic shock.**
Sepsis syndrome begins with the invasion and growth of microorganisms (gram positive, gram negative, fungal, or viral) in a normally sterile tissue space. The endothelium is damaged by infection, trauma, or other insult, and activation of the host immune response begins. Tumor necrosis factor α, interleukin (IL)-6, and IL-8 are associated with the activation of an inflammatory cascade and chemotaxis of leukocytes, monocytes, and macrophages. Antiinflammatory substances such as IL-4, IL-10, prostaglandins, and other components of the immune system work to maintain homeostasis in the face of an infectious insult. Sepsis syndrome develops when the balance between the proinflammatory and antiinflammatory substances is lost.

The coagulation pathway plays a critical role in sepsis. The complement system, vasoregulatory system (nitric oxide, bradykinin, prostaglandins), the coagulation cascade (tissue factor, protein C, thrombin, antithrombin III), and fibrinolysis (fibrin, plasmin, and plasminogen-activating factor) play roles as well. The result is the development of a vicious circle that promotes, both locally and systemically, further inflammation, release of oxygen free radicals, and deposition of microvascular thrombi, resulting in a cycle of ischemia, reperfusion injury, and tissue hypoxia. Global tissue hypoxia independently contributes to endothelial activation and further disruption of the homeostatic balance among coagulation, vascular permeability, and vascular tone. These are key mechanisms leading to microcirculatory failure, refractory tissue hypoxia, and organ dysfunction.

It is becoming clear that the processes of coagulation and inflammation are tightly linked. Recent studies have shown that patients with severe sepsis have depleted levels of protein C, protein S, and antithrombin III.

6. **Which microorganisms are most commonly associated with sepsis?**
A recent study of nosocomial bloodstream infections found the following infecting organisms in the intensive care unit (ICU):
- **Gram positive (65%):** coagulase-negative staphylococci (36% of isolates), *Staphylococcus aureus* (17%), enterococci (10%).
- **Gram negative (25%):** *Escherichia coli* (4%), *Klebsiella* sp. (4%), *Pseudomonas aeruginosa* (5%), *Enterobacter* sp. (5%), *Serratia* sp. (2%), *Acinetobacter* sp. (2%). Clinically, however, the problem of resistant gram-negative organisms in the ICU is rapidly becoming a serious one nationwide.
- **Fungi (9%):** primarily *Candida* species (*albicans* 54%, *glabrata* 19%, *parapsilosis* 11%, *tropicalis* 11%).

Coagulase-negative staphylococci, *Pseudomonas* species, *Enterobacter* species, *Serratia* species, and *Acinetobacter* species were more likely to cause infections in patients in ICUs. The proportion of *S. aureus* isolates with methicillin resistance increased from 22% in 1995 to 57% in 2001.

7. **What are the most common primary sources of infection?**
    In decreasing order of incidence, there are lung, blood, abdomen, urinary tract, skin, and other sites.

8. **What clinical signs and symptoms should raise suspicion of SIRS, sepsis, and underlying organ dysfunction?**
    - **Respiratory:** cyanosis, tachypnea, orthopnea, increased sputum (yellow or green, frothy), hypoxemia (PaO_2/FiO_2 <300), oxygen saturation <90%.
    - **Cardiovascular:** need for vasopressors, chest pain, pulmonary edema, arrhythmias, cardiac index <2.5, heart rate >100 beats/min, decreased systemic vascular resistance, increased cardiac output.
    - **Renal:** urine output <0.5 mL/kg/hr, increased blood urea nitrogen level, increased creatinine level, acute renal failure, acidosis, worsening base deficit.
    - **Hepatic:** elevated aspartate aminotransferase, alanine aminotransferase, or γ-glutamyl transferase levels; prolonged bleeding time; asterixis; encephalopathy; elevated bilirubin level. This is often referred to as ischemic hepatopathy or *shock liver*.
    - **Immunologic:** fever with temperature >38° C or hypothermia, chills, leukocytosis with or without left shift, neutropenia.
    - **Hematologic:** weakness, pallor, poor capillary refill, easy bruising, spontaneous bleeding, anemia, increased prothrombin or partial thromboplastin time, decreased fibrinogen, disseminated intravascular coagulation (elevated D-dimer levels).
    - **Gastrointestinal:** anorexia, ileus, inability to tolerate tube feedings, nausea, vomiting, hypoalbuminemia.
    - **Endocrine:** hyperglycemia, hypoglycemia, adrenal insufficiency, weight loss.
    - **Neurologic:** weakness, confusion, delirium, psychoses, seizures.
    - **Metabolic:** elevated serum lactate level.

9. **What are the Surviving Sepsis Campaign Guidelines? What are some of the high points?**
    This document was originally published in 2004 and was codified by 11 international critical care organizations. It was updated in 2008. It provides a state-of-the-art evidence-based approach to the management of severe sepsis and septic shock. Some of the highlights of this important document are in Box 32-1.

10. **What is an evidence-based approach to the use of the pulmonary artery catheter (PAC)?**
    Since its initial description in the *New England Journal of Medicine* in 1970, the PAC has been an important tool for the critical care clinician. Its major roles have been to
    1. Distinguish cardiogenic from noncardiogenic pulmonary edema
    2. Determine which particular shock state (cardiogenic, distributive, hypovolemic) a patient may be in
    3. Serve as a guide for therapeutic interventions for patients in shock
        Recent data from large randomized trials have been unable to document a particular subgroup of patients in which the use of the PAC has been associated with improved outcomes. Multiple complex reasons are behind these results, which are still being debated in the literature. Nevertheless, it can be stated with some certainty that the placement of a PAC is no longer a requirement for the successful diagnosis and management of a patient with sepsis.

BOX 32-1. HIGHLIGHTS OF THE SURVIVING SEPSIS CAMPAIGN GUIDELINES

Initial Resuscitation

The initial resuscitation phase of a patient with severe sepsis or in septic shock should be completed within 6 hours of identification, usually signified by an elevated serum lactate level. Current recommendations are to rapidly place a catheter with central venous access, although this is not essential before fluid administration. Regardless of type of venous access, aggressive fluid therapy with a challenge of 1 L (10-20 mL/kg) of crystalloid over a 30-minute period should be performed. The target central venous pressure (CVP) is between 8 and 12 mm Hg in a patient breathing spontaneously; for a patient receiving mechanical ventilation a higher CVP goal is likely needed. The goal blood pressure is a MAP $\geq$ 65 mm Hg. If after adequate volume resuscitation has occurred (typically after 3-5 L of crystalloid) and the patient continues to have hypotension, vasopressors should be started to keep the MAP at goal. Vasopressors may also be needed during the fluid resuscitation. It is currently recommended that norepinephrine or dopamine be used as first-line agents when vasopressors are required to maintain an adequate MAP. Vasopressin and/or epinephrine infusions can be added if the norepinephrine or dopamine is ineffective. Inotropic agents should be used only if clear evidence of myocardial dysfunction exists (elevated filling pressures and low cardiac output). These agents should be delivered through a central venous catheter as soon as possible. Immediately after the start of the fluid challenge, samples for blood cultures should be drawn, if not already done. Appropriate intravenous broad-spectrum antibiotic therapy should be administered within the first hour of the initial resuscitation phase. If possible, a source should be identified and measures taken to control the infection (i.e., drainage of an abscess). Clearance of lactate (and resolution of metabolic acidosis) from the blood during resuscitation suggests that the resuscitation has been effective.

Adjunctive Therapy Within the First 24 Hours
Bicarbonate Therapy

It has been common practice to give bicarbonate therapy for vasopressor-dependent patients to improve hemodynamics. However, it is important to state that—to the extent that it has been studied—no data support this intervention. Current recommendations are not to give bicarbonate for hypoperfusion-induced lactic acidosis unless the serum pH is < 7.15.

Blood Product Administration

Red blood cell transfusions should only occur when the hemoglobin level has fallen to < 7.0 g/dL, with a target hemoglobin level of 7.0 to 9.0 g/dL. However, it may need to be higher in special circumstances (i.e., myocardial ischemia, acute hemorrhage, acute stroke). Fresh frozen plasma should not be administered to correct coagulation abnormalities unless the patient is bleeding.

Glucose

Recent data in critically ill patients—primarily patients who have had cardiac surgery—revealed multiple improved outcomes with the use of "tight glucose control." Current recommendations for critically ill patients, including those with severe sepsis, include some form of a glucose control protocol using low-dose insulin infusion. Though the precise glucose target for the critically ill patient remains controversial, $\leq$ 150 mg/dL is the current recommendation in the Surviving Sepsis Guidelines.

Mechanical Ventilation of Sepsis-Induced Acute Lung Injury or Acute Respiratory Distress Syndrome

The lungs are the most common organ system to fail in patients with sepsis, many of whom eventually require mechanical ventilation. The lungs are the most likely source of initial infection as well, and patients are at great risk for nosocomial and ventilator-associated pneumonias.

BOX 32-1   HIGHLIGHTS OF THE SURVIVING SEPSIS CAMPAIGN GUIDELINES—*cont'd*

The recent definitions and guidelines for management of acute lung injury (ALI) and acute respiratory distress syndrome (ARDS) have made a significant impact on identification of patients with these disorders. Diagnosis of ALI and ARDS is based on the following criteria: bilateral infiltrates, PaO_2/FiO_2 <300 (ALI) or <200 (ARDS), and no evidence of a cardiac source (e.g., left atrial hypertension) for respiratory distress. The ARDS Network (a multicenter organization aimed at treating ARDS) has identified a protective ventilation strategy, based on lower tidal volumes and use of positive end-expiratory pressure, which significantly decreases the mortality rate of patients with ARDS. It is currently recommended that patients with ALI or ARDS receive mechanical ventilation with a goal tidal volume of 6 mL/kg of predicted body weight and/or with plateau pressures $\leq$30 cm H_2O. The head of the bed should also be kept elevated between 30 and 40 degrees.

Steroids
The use of intravenous steroids in patients with persistent vasopressor-dependent septic shock is controversial but may be considered for refractory shock. At this time, laboratory testing of serum cortisol levels is not recommended.

Consideration for Limitation of Support
Severe sepsis and septic shock are serious diseases with significant mortality. It is important for the multidisciplinary critical care team to be in frequent communication with the family with appropriate updates regarding the status and prognosis of their loved one so that the family can set realistic expectations. It is paramount that the team be aware of any previous wishes the patient may have had regarding resuscitation, heroic measures, and artificial life support.

KEY POINTS: SEPSIS, SEVERE SEPSIS, AND SEPTIC SHOCK

1. Sepsis = Infection + Two or more SIRS criteria.

2. Severe sepsis = Sepsis plus acute organ dysfunction.

3. Heterogenous disease leads to difficulties with intervention trials.

4. Complex pathophysiology involves the immune system and coagulation homeostasis.

5. The Surviving Sepsis Campaign Guidelines provide a reasonable evidence-based approach to the current management of severe sepsis and septic shock.

WEBSITES

Society of Critical Care Medicine: www.sccm.org
Surviving Sepsis Campaign: www.survivingsepsis.org

BIBLIOGRAPHY

1. Dellinger RP, Carlet JM, Masur H, et al: Surviving Sepsis Campaign: International guidelines for management of severe sepsis and septic shock: 2008. Crit Care Med 36:296-327, 2008.

2. Lagu T, Rothberg MB, Shieh MS, et al: Hospitalizations, costs, and outcomes of severe sepsis in the United States 2003 to 2007. Crit Care Med 40:754-761, 2012.

3. Levy MM, Macias WL, Vincent JL, et al: Early changes in organ function predict eventual survival in severe sepsis. Crit Care Med 33:2194-2201, 2005.

4. Richard C, Warszawski J, Anguel N, et al: Early use of the pulmonary artery catheter and outcomes in patients with shock and acute respiratory distress syndrome: a randomized controlled trial. JAMA 290:2713-2720, 2003.

5. Sandham JD, Hull RD, Brant RF, et al: A randomized, controlled trial of the use of pulmonary-artery catheters in high-risk surgical patients. N Engl J Med 348:5-14, 2003.

6. Wisplinghoff H, Bischoff T, Tallent SM, et al: Nosocomial bloodstream infections in US hospitals: analysis of 24,179 cases from a prospective nationwide surveillance study. Clin Infect Dis 39:309-317, 2004.

CHAPTER 33

ENDOCARDITIS

Louis B. Polish, MD

1. **What are the important clinical manifestations of endocarditis?**

   Several processes contribute to the clinical signs and symptoms of infective endocarditis, including valvular involvement with intracardiac complications, high-grade and persistent bacteremia (which may lead to metastatic foci), bland or septic embolization to any organ, and immune complex formation. Fever occurs in 80% of patients, and nonspecific symptoms, including anorexia, weight loss, malaise, fatigue, chills, weakness, nausea, vomiting, and night sweats, are very common. Although heart murmurs are common, the so-called changing murmur is relatively uncommon.

   The incidence of peripheral manifestations has decreased. Osler nodes, although not specific for endocarditis, may occur in 10% to 25% of all cases and are generally seen in subacute cases. Janeway lesions (i.e., macular, painless plaques on the palms and soles) are seen in fewer than 10% of cases. Clubbing may be seen if the disease is long-standing and may occur 10% to 20% of the time. Splenomegaly occurs in 25% to 60% of cases, generally those with subacute disease. Joint complaints may occur in approximately 40% of patients and may be relatively innocuous with low back pain or myalgias and arthralgias. Musculoskeletal symptoms may also be quite severe, including frank septic arthritis and severe low back pain. Other less common musculoskeletal manifestations include septic bursitis, sacroiliitis, septic diskitis, and polymyalgia rheumatica. Long-standing subacute endocarditis may present as chronic wasting syndrome mimicking cancer or human immunodeficiency virus infection. Signs and symptoms of embolic episodes are determined by the location of the embolism. Patients with splenic emboli may have left upper quadrant pain, left-sided pleural effusions, or a rub. Renal infarction from a septic embolus may present as flank pain and hematuria. Immune complex formation may lead to renal insufficiency. Cough and shortness of breath with chest pain often accompany pulmonary emboli. Coronary emboli occur rarely and may present with myocarditis, arrhythmias, myocardial infarction, or a combination thereof. Extension into the myocardial space may lead to purulent pericarditis with severe chest pain and hemodynamic compromise. Unexplained heart failure in a young patient without prior cardiac disease should prompt an investigation for infectious endocarditis.

2. **Are there differences in the manifestations of endocarditis in elderly patients?**

   There does appear to be an increased incidence of endocarditis in elderly patients that may be related to an increased life span in patients with rheumatic and other cardiovascular diseases, with a commensurate increase among patients with calcific and degenerative heart disease. In addition, the increase in prolonged catheter use, implantable devices, and dialysis catheters increases the incidence of nosocomial endocarditis. Endocarditis in elderly persons is more likely to occur in men, with a ratio of approximately 2 to 8:1 in patients older than 60 years of age. Staphylococci and streptococci account for approximately 80% of the cases in elderly persons, and *Streptococcus bovis* may be noted more frequently in elderly patients associated with underlying colonic malignancy. The clinical presentation of endocarditis may be nonspecific, including lethargy, fatigue, malaise, anorexia, failure to thrive, and weight loss (which may be attributed to aging or other medical illnesses common in the elderly). In addition, fever, which occurs in roughly 80% of patients with endocarditis, is more likely to be absent in elderly patients. Worsening heart failure and murmurs may be attributed to underlying disease and therefore erroneously neglected. Consequently, a high index of suspicion is necessary.

3. **What are the Duke criteria for the diagnosis of endocarditis? How have they been modified?**

    The original Duke criteria for the diagnosis of infective endocarditis stratified patients into three categories:

    - **Definite:** identified by using clinical or pathologic criteria (Box 33-1)
    - **Possible:** findings consistent with infective endocarditis that fall short of definite, but the diagnosis cannot be rejected
    - **Rejected:** firm alternative diagnosis for manifestations of endocarditis *or* resolution of manifestations of endocarditis, with antibiotic therapy for 4 days or less, *or* no pathologic evidence of infective endocarditis at surgery or autopsy, after antibiotic therapy for 4 days or less

---

BOX 33-1. ORIGINAL DUKE PATHOLOGIC AND CLINICAL CRITERIA FOR DIAGNOSIS OF ENDOCARDITIS

Pathologic Criteria

Pathologic criteria include microorganisms demonstrated by culture *or* histology in a vegetation *or* in a vegetation that has embolized *or* in an intracardiac abscess *or* pathologic lesions, including vegetation or intracardiac abscess, confirmed by histologic analysis showing active endocarditis.

Clinical Criteria

Clinical criteria include either two major criteria *or* one major and three minor criteria *or* five minor criteria from the following list:

Major criteria are the following:

- Positive blood culture results with a typical microorganism for infective endocarditis from two separate blood cultures (viridans streptococci, including nutritionally variant strains; *S. bovis,* HACEK group, or community-acquired *S. aureus* or enterococci in absence of a primary focus)
- Persistently positive blood culture result, defined as recovery of a microorganism consistent with infective endocarditis from blood cultures drawn more than 12 hours apart *or* all of three or a majority of four or more separated blood cultures with first and last drawn at least 1 hour apart
- Echocardiogram result positive for infective endocarditis, including one of the following:
  - □ Oscillating intracardiac mass on valve or supporting structures, in the path of regurgitant jets, or on implanted material in the absence of an alternative anatomic explanation
  - □ Abscess
  - □ New partial dehiscence of prosthetic valve
  - □ New valvular regurgitation (increase or change in preexisting murmur not sufficient)

Minor criteria are the following:

- **Predisposition:** predisposing heart condition or IV drug use
- **Fever:** body temperature $>38°$ C (100.4° F)
- **Vascular phenomena:** major arterial emboli, septic pulmonary infarcts, mycotic aneurysm, intracranial hemorrhage, conjunctival hemorrhages, Janeway lesions
- **Immunologic phenomena:** glomerulonephritis, Osler nodes, Roth spots, rheumatoid factor
- **Microbiologic evidence:** positive blood culture result but not meeting major criterion as noted previously *or* serologic evidence of active infection with organism consistent with infective endocarditis
- **Echocardiogram:** consistent with infective endocarditis but not meeting major criterion as noted previously

Since the original Duke criteria were published in 1994, several refinements have been made based on studies evaluating the sensitivity and specificity of the criteria:

- Bacteremia with *Staphylococcus aureus* was included as a major criterion only if it was community acquired. Subsequent research has shown that a significant proportion of patients with nosocomially acquired staphylococcal bacteremia will have documented infective endocarditis. Consequently, *S. aureus* bacteremia is now included as a major criterion regardless of whether the infection is nosocomial or community acquired.
- An additional major criterion was added as follows: single blood culture result positive for *Coxiella burnetii* or anti–phase 1 immunoglobulin G antibody titer >1:800.
- An additional statement was added to the major criteria regarding endocardial involvement and an echocardiogram positive for infective endocarditis. The statement now includes the following: Transesophageal echocardiography (TEE) is recommended for patients with prosthetic valves, diagnoses rated at least "possible infective endocarditis" by clinical criteria, or complicated infective endocarditis (paravalvular abscess); transthoracic echocardiography (TTE) should be the first test in other patients.
- The echocardiogram minor criterion was eliminated.
- The category of "possible endocarditis" was adjusted to include the following criteria: one major and one minor criterion or three minor criteria. This so-called floor was designated to reduce the proportion of patients assigned to the "possible" category.

4. What are the organisms that most often cause endocarditis?

The etiologic agents of infective endocarditis include the following:

- Streptococci: 60%-80%
- Viridans streptococci: 30%-40%
- Enterococci: 5%-18%
- Other streptococci: 15%-25%
- Staphylococci: 20%-35%
- Coagulase-positive organisms: 10%-27%
- Coagulase-negative organisms: 1%-3%
- Gram-negative aerobic bacilli: 1%-13%
- Fungi: 2%-4%

S. aureus tends to be the most common etiologic agent of infective endocarditis in intravenous (IV) drug users. *Pseudomonas aeruginosa* is also more commonly seen in patients using IV drugs. In patients with prosthetic valves, the microbiology is somewhat dependent on whether they have early (<2 months after valve replacement) versus late (>12 months) endocarditis. Staphylococci account for 40% to 60% of the cases of early onset prosthetic valve endocarditis. Coagulase-negative staphylococci account for approximately 30% to 35% of cases, and *S. aureus* accounts for approximately 20% to 25%. Patients who have late-onset prosthetic valve endocarditis are more likely to have the organisms most commonly seen in patients with native valve endocarditis, with one exception: coagulase-negative staphylococci are seen more frequently (approximately 10%-12%) in patients with prosthetic valves. Patients who have fungal endocarditis are often IV drug users, have recently undergone cardiovascular surgery, or have received prolonged IV antibiotic therapy.

5. What are the HACEK organisms? How often do they cause endocarditis?

HACEK is an acronym for a group of fastidious, slow-growing, gram-negative bacteria:

- **H:** *Haemophilus parainfluenzae, Haemophilus aphrophilus, Haemophilus paraphrophilus, Haemophilus influenzae*
- **A:** *Actinobacillus actinomycetemcomitans*
- **C:** *Cardiobacterium hominis*
- **E:** *Eikenella corrodens*
- **K:** *Kingella kingae, Kingella denitrificans*

These organisms account for approximately 5% to 10% of cases of community-acquired endocarditis. Because an increasing number of these organisms produce β-lactamase, they should be considered resistant to ampicillin. The treatment of choice is ceftriaxone or other third- or fourth-generation cephalosporins.

6. **What is the prevalence of health care–associated endocarditis?**

   Recent data from the International Collaboration on Endocarditis–Prospective Cohort Study (ICE-PCS) suggested that health care–associated native valve endocarditis was present in 34% of non–IV drug–using patients (557 of 1622 patients). Of these 557 patients, 54% had nosocomial and 46% had nonnosocomial infections (infections developing outside the hospital but with extensive health care contact [i.e., dialysis centers, outpatient antibiotic programs, nursing homes]). Patients with health care–associated native valve endocarditis and without a history of injection drug use were more likely to have *S. aureus* (including methicillin-resistant *S. aureus* [MRSA]) and had a higher mortality rate than those with community-acquired infections.

7. **What is the appropriate role of echocardiography in the diagnosis and management of endocarditis?**

   Echocardiography is an essential tool in the diagnostic work-up of a patient with suspected endocarditis. The primary objective is to identify, localize, and characterize valvular vegetations. However, echocardiography is also potentially important in the management of endocarditis. Identification of an abscess may indicate the need for surgical intervention. Patients may also benefit from repeating the echocardiography once a definitive diagnosis has been established to assess complications, including congestive heart failure and atrioventricular block, which suggest worsening valvular and myocardial function. It is important to emphasize that echocardiographic findings should always be interpreted in coordination with clinical information.

   The TEE is more sensitive than a TTE for the diagnosis of endocarditis. Sensitivities of the different modalities have ranged from 48% to 100% for TEE and from 18% to 63% for TTE. This is in part related to the fact that the transesophageal approach allows closer proximity to the heart and therefore can be performed at higher frequencies, providing greater spatial resolution. It can identify structures as small as 1 mm. TEE is the preferred modality in patients with prosthetic valves. The spatial resolution of the TTE may be limited by overlying fat in obese patients or hyperinflated lungs from chronic obstructive pulmonary disease or mechanical ventilation. The TTE may only be able to identify structures as small as 5 mm. Both modalities however are highly specific in the range of 95%.

   A cost-effectiveness analysis study conducted by Heidenreich and colleagues suggested that the prior probability of endocarditis was the most important factor in choosing the appropriate modality. TEE is the preferred modality in patients with a higher pretest probability of disease or in patients in whom the TTE would be less sensitive, that is, with obesity, lung hyperinflation, or prosthetic valves. Recently, Kaasch suggested that echocardiography is highly recommended in patients with at least one of the following clinical prediction criteria: prolonged bacteremia (>4 days elapsed between the first blood culture to yield *S. aureus* and first negative follow-up blood culture, or if the blood cultures were not performed), presence of a permanent intracardiac device, hemodialysis dependency, spinal infection, and nonvertebral osteomyelitis. However, in the subset of patients without any of the above criteria, TEE evaluation may not be necessary although physician discretion is paramount, and these data will need to be validated in a prospectively controlled study.

   Although echocardiography has become an essential diagnostic tool in patients with suspected endocarditis, no definitive echocardiographic features can reliably distinguish infection from those lesions that are noninfective. Cardiac computed tomography (CT) and magnetic resonance imaging have been used in diagnosing complications of infective endocarditis, and in at least one study cardiac multislice CT was shown to be as effective as TEE. However, at this time they are not part of the current standard of care in diagnosing infective endocarditis.

8. **Is there a way to clinically predict the presence of a perivalvular abscess in patients with endocarditis?**

   The presence of a perivalvular abscess should be considered in patients with pericarditis, congestive heart failure (CHF), IV drug use, *S. aureus* infection, prosthetic valve endocarditis, aortic valve disease, or persistent fever or bacteremia while taking appropriate antibiotics. Formal evaluation has suggested that previously undetected atrioventricular or bundle branch block may be a significant correlate of a perivalvular abscess. Aortic valve involvement and IV drug use have also been found to be significant factors in predicting the presence of a perivalvular abscess.

9. **What is the optimal timing, volume, and number of blood cultures for a patient in whom infective endocarditis is suspected?**

Multiple blood cultures are necessary. Two blood cultures performed with adequate volumes of blood will identify approximately 99% of patients with culture-positive bacteremia. However, this does not apply to patients who have received empirical antibiotics, patients with fungal endocarditis, or organisms that are difficult to culture. Multiple blood cultures increase the yield, help distinguish between contamination and true bacteremia, and prove continuous bacteremia characteristic of infective endocarditis. If the first set of blood culture results is negative, it is important to realize that repeating blood cultures may be important if the pretest probability of endocarditis remains high. If the clinical situation evolves and endocarditis appears less likely, repeating blood cultures may be counterproductive. Although it makes sense that the optimal time to obtain blood culture specimens is during the hour before the onset of chills or fever spikes, in reality this is not practical. Because of the continuous bacteremia associated with endocarditis, timing is less important, and waiting to initiate therapy in a patient with acute disease with a particularly virulent organism such as *S. aureus* is not warranted. Two to three blood cultures should be obtained within 5 minutes of each other before initiation of antimicrobial therapy. However, if the patient has a clinical course suggestive of subacute endocarditis, obtaining blood cultures over several hours to document continuous bacteremia would be prudent. In general, 20 mL of blood should be obtained for each two-bottle blood culture set. It should also be stressed that each blood culture set requires a separate venipuncture site.

10. **How do you distinguish a case of *S. aureus* endocarditis from uncomplicated *S. aureus* bacteremia?**

In a classic 1976 study, Nolan and Beaty suggested that, among 105 patients with *S. aureus* bacteremia retrospectively identified, most of the 26 patients with endocarditis could be identified on the basis of three characteristics: community-acquired infection, absence of a primary focus of infection, and presence of metastatic foci of infection. However, in prospectively identified patients with *S. aureus* bacteremia who undergo early echocardiography, approximately 25% will have evidence of endocarditis by TEE. Clinical findings and predisposing heart disease did not distinguish those with or without endocarditis. In addition, a substantial portion of these patients had hospital-acquired *S. aureus* bacteremia.

11. **What is nonbacterial thrombotic endocarditis (NBTE)?**

NBTE refers to small, sterile vegetations on cardiac valves from platelet-fibrin deposits. The cardiac lesions most commonly resulting in NBTE include mitral regurgitation, aortic stenosis, aortic regurgitation, ventricular septal defect, and complex congenital heart disease. NBTE may also result from a hypercoagulable state, and sterile vegetations can be seen in systemic lupus erythematosus (i.e., Libman-Sacks endocarditis), antiphospholipid antibody syndrome, and collagen vascular diseases. Noninfectious vegetations can also be seen in patients with malignancy (e.g., renal cell carcinoma or melanoma), burns, or even acute septicemia. Other lesions that may be somewhat misleading include myxomatous valves, benign cardiac tumors, and degenerative thickening of the valves. Lambl excrescences, which are multiple small tags on heart valves seen in a large number of adults at autopsy, can also be confused with infectious vegetations; however, these tend to be much more filamentous in appearance.

12. **What are the causes of culture-negative endocarditis?**

Approximately 2% to 30% of patients with infective endocarditis will have sterile blood culture specimens; however, it is more likely to be 5% with use of strict diagnosis criteria. Potential causes of culture-negative endocarditis include the following:
- Prior antibiotic usage
- NBTE or an incorrect diagnosis
- Slow growth of fastidious organisms, including anaerobes, HACEK organisms, nutritionally variant streptococci, or *Brucella* species

- Obligate intracellular organisms, including rickettsia, chlamydiae, *Tropheryma whippelii*, or viruses
- Other organisms, including *C. burnetii* (the etiologic agent of Q fever) and *Legionella, Bartonella,* or *Mycoplasma* species
- Subacute right-sided endocarditis
- Fungal endocarditis
- Mural endocarditis, as in patients with ventricular septal defects, post–myocardial infarction thrombi, or infection related to pacemaker wires
- Culture specimens taken at the end of a long course, usually >3 months

13. **What conduction abnormalities can be associated with endocarditis?**

Right and left bundle branch blocks, second-degree atrioventricular block, and complete heart block. Heart block generally is the result of extension of infection to the atrioventricular node or the bundle of His. Most patients with heart block have involvement of the aortic valve. In one series, conduction abnormalities occurred in approximately 10% of patients with native valve endocarditis. Mitral valve endocarditis may cause first- or second-degree heart block, but third-degree heart block would be unusual. Aortic valve endocarditis can cause first- or second-degree heart block as well as bundle branch blocks, hemiblocks, and complete heart blocks. It should be remembered that the electrocardiogram (ECG) is specific but not sensitive for involvement of the conduction system. Consequently, one could have a valve ring abscess but not have conduction abnormalities on the ECG. Complete heart block may be preceded by prolongation of the PR interval or a left bundle branch block. Conduction abnormalities in the setting of endocarditis may occur for other reasons as well, including myocardial infarction (rarely), myocarditis, or pericarditis. ECG findings may also have prognostic implications because patients with persistent conduction abnormalities have an increased 1-year mortality compared with patients who have normal ECG findings.

14. **What valves are most commonly affected in patients with endocarditis?**

This depends on the etiology of the endocarditis. In patients with native valve endocarditis, the mitral valve alone is involved in 28% to 45% of cases, 5% to 36% for the aortic valve alone, and 0% to 35% for both valves combined. The tricuspid valve is involved alone 0% to 6% of the time, and the pulmonic valve is involved in <1% of the cases of endocarditis. Endocarditis occurs in approximately 5% to 15% of injection drug users admitted to the hospital for acute infection. In these patients, the frequency of valvular involvement is as follows: tricuspid valve alone or in combination, 50%; aortic valve alone, 19%; mitral valve alone, 11%; and aortic plus mitral, 12%. In patients with prosthetic valve endocarditis, a difference does not seem to exist in the incidence of endocarditis at the aortic compared with the mitral location. The overall risk of endocarditis is similar with a mechanical valve compared with a bioprosthetic valve; however, slight differences exist in the risk on the basis of the length of time after surgery. Within the first 6 postoperative months, mechanical valves have a slightly increased risk of infection; however, no significant increased risk was seen within the first 5 years after surgery with mechanical valves compared with bioprosthetic valves. After 5 years, the risk for endocarditis for bioprosthetic valves is slightly greater than that for mechanical valves. In patients with fungal endocarditis, the aortic valve was involved 44% of the time either alone or in combination with other valves; the mitral valve, 26% alone or in combination; and the tricuspid valve, 7%; other locations were documented in 18% of patients.

15. **What are the clinical differences between right-sided and left-sided endocarditis?**

In patients with right-sided endocarditis (either the tricuspid or pulmonic valve), particularly injection drug users with tricuspid valve endocarditis, only 35% will have an audible murmur. In general, symptoms and complications arise from involvement of the pulmonary vasculature and are characterized by multiple pulmonary septic emboli that may cause pulmonary infarction, abscesses, pneumothoraces, pleural effusions, or empyema. In addition, multiple pulmonary emboli may result in right-sided heart failure with chamber dilatation and worsening tricuspid regurgitation. Clinical symptoms associated with these complications may include chest pain, dyspnea, cough, and hemoptysis. Peripheral embolic phenomena and neurologic involvement are generally absent in patients with right-sided endocarditis, and, when they do occur in the setting of right-sided endocarditis, involvement of the left side or paradoxical embolization should be considered. Patients with left-sided endocarditis (aortic or mitral) generally have greater hemodynamic consequences and are more likely to have congestive heart failure. Systemic embolization (brain, kidney, spleen) is more common with left-sided lesions.

16. **What is the appropriate empirical therapy (cultures pending) for patients with presumptive infective endocarditis?**
Several regimens considered by authorities to be appropriate would include the following:
- **Acute:** nafcillin or oxacillin, 2 g IV every 4 hours, plus gentamicin or tobramycin, 1 mg/kg IV every 8 hours, *or* vancomycin, 15 mg/kg every 12 hours IV (dosing interval based on creatinine clearance) plus gentamicin, 1 mg/kg every 8 hours. Some experts would add ampicillin, 2 g IV every 4 hours, to the previously described nafcillin regimen to cover the possibility of enterococci.
- **Subacute:** ampicillin and sulbactam, 3 g IV every 4 to 6 hours, plus gentamicin or tobramycin, 1 mg/kg every 8 hours IV, *or* vancomycin, 15 mg/kg every 12 hours IV (dosing interval based on creatinine clearance), plus ceftriaxone, 2 g every 12 hours IV.
- **Prosthetic valve:** vancomycin, 15 mg/kg every 12 hours (dosing interval based on creatinine clearance), plus gentamicin, 1 mg/kg every 8 hours IV, plus rifampin, 600 mg/day orally.

17. **What are the indications for surgical therapy?**
Clinical situations that warrant surgical intervention include moderate and severe (i.e., New York Heart Association class III or IV) or progressive and refractory CHF, valve dehiscence, rupture, or fistula. Although CHF has a worse prognosis with medical therapy alone, an increased surgical risk also exists. Delay in surgery may also lead to worsening cardiac decompensation or perivalvular extension, which will increase operative mortality as well as secondary complications. Several studies have shown benefits in mortality statistics with surgical intervention. Progressive heart failure in the presence of aortic or mitral valve regurgitation requires surgery. Right-sided endocarditis with tricuspid regurgitation is reasonably well tolerated if the pulmonary vascular resistance is not increased, and surgery is often not required. Other indications for surgery include perivalvular extension of infection, persistent bacteremia without evidence of an extracardiac source of bacteremia, mechanical valve obstruction, fungal endocarditis, prosthetic endocarditis, and difficult-to-treat organisms, including *Pseudomonas* species, *C. burnetii, Brucella* species, and *Staphylococcus lugdunensis.* Surgery may also be indicated to avoid embolizations. Conventional wisdom has been that indications for surgery to avoid embolization have been two or more major embolic events during therapy. However, determining the number and timing of embolic events may be difficult, given that the detection of damage may occur well after the actual embolism. The risk of embolization also decreases significantly during the first 1 to 2 weeks of antibiotic therapy.

18. **Is there a relationship between duration of antibiotic therapy before surgery and operative mortality?**
Although it is important to have adequate antibiotic coverage during surgery, the duration of antibiotic therapy does not generally influence operative mortality. The incidence of reinfection of newly implanted valves is approximately 3% and may be as high as 10%.

19. **What are the neurologic manifestations of endocarditis?**
Overall, the incidence of central nervous system involvement during the course of infective endocarditis ranges between 20% and 40%. Neurologic symptoms are the presenting manifestations in endocarditis approximately 16% to 23% of the time; however, there are generally other clues to the diagnosis. Neurologic complications usually occur within the first 2 weeks after starting antibiotics, but later complications—months to as long as 2 years after successful therapy—have been documented. The most common neurologic manifestation is stroke, and this accounts for approximately 50% to 60% of all neurologic complications. Stroke generally occurs from cerebral emboli with infarction, but hemorrhage or abscess may occur as

well. Other neurologic manifestations with their associated main clinical presentations include encephalopathy (decreased level of consciousness), seizures, severe or localized headache, psychiatric syndromes from minor personality changes to more severe psychiatric syndromes (generally in elderly patients), various dyskinesias, visual disturbances, spinal cord involvement (paraplegia or tetraplegia), peripheral nerve involvement (mononeuropathy), and meningitis, which is more common with *S. aureus* and *Streptococcus pneumoniae* (with or without focal signs). Ocular complications include acute embolic occlusion of the central retinal artery, which may result in sudden vision loss. Other complications that have been well documented include involvement of cranial nerves III, IV, and VI, which can lead to diplopia, deviation of the eyes, nystagmus or unequal pupils, retinal hemorrhages, and endophthalmitis.

20. **How often do intracranial mycotic aneurysms (ICMAs) occur?**
    ICMAs are uncommon, and although they constitute only 2% to 6% of all intracranial aneurysms, 80% of these are identified in the setting of infective endocarditis. Among patients with endocarditis, only 1% to 5% will have a recognized ICMA. The mortality rate is approximately 60%, and many patients are seen initially with a sudden subarachnoid or intracerebral hemorrhage. Rupture of an ICMA may occur while the patient is being treated for endocarditis or after completion of therapy.

21. **What are the warning signs of ICMA? How is it diagnosed?**
    Serious warning signs that should prompt further investigation for the possibility of an ICMA include severe localized headache and other focal neurologic signs, such as seizures, ischemic deficits, and cranial nerve abnormalities. Although sudden rupture is not an uncommon presentation of an ICMA, some aneurysms may leak slowly before rupture and produce meningeal irritation manifested by cerebrospinal fluid that is sterile but shows a moderate number of red cells and a neutrophilic reaction. When hemorrhage is suspected, either a CT angiogram or magnetic resonance angiography (MRA) should be obtained. Recent studies have shown that CT angiography and MRA have similar results in the detection of noninfectious intracranial aneurysms, and it is likely that the same would be true for infectious intracranial aneurysms. If hemorrhage has been confirmed and surgery is considered, conventional angiography is still the most appropriate diagnostic procedure to pinpoint location and anatomic relationships.

KEY POINTS: ENDOCARDITIS

1. The Duke criteria for the diagnosis of endocarditis include either two major criteria (i.e., positive blood culture results plus positive echocardiographic evidence of endocarditis), one major and three minor criteria (i.e., predisposition, fever, vascular or immunologic phenomena, and microbiologic evidence), or five minor criteria.

2. The HACEK organisms are fastidious, slow-growing, gram-negative bacteria and include *Haemophilus, Actinobacillus, Cardiobacterium, Eikenella,* and *Kingella* species.

3. *S. aureus* endocarditis cannot be distinguished from bacteremia on the basis of community-acquired infection, lack of a primary focus, and presence of metastatic foci of infection.

4. Symptoms and complications of right-sided endocarditis generally result from involvement of the pulmonary vasculature, whereas complications of left-sided endocarditis are generally characterized by greater hemodynamic consequences, congestive heart failure, and systemic embolization.

5. Nervous system involvement occurs in 20% to 40% of patients and may be the presenting symptom in approximately 20% of the cases of infective endocarditis.

BIBLIOGRAPHY

1. Baddour LM, Wilson WR, Bayer AS, et al: Infective endocarditis: diagnosis, antimicrobial therapy and management of complications. A statement for healthcare professionals from the Committee on Rheumatic Fever, Endocarditis and Kawasaki Disease, Council on Cardiovascular Disease in the Young, and the Councils on Clinical Cardiology, Stroke and Cardiovascular Surgery and Anesthesia, American Heart Association. Circulation 111:e394-e433, 2005.

2. Blumberg EA, Karalis DA, Chandrasekaran K, et al: Endocarditis-associated paravalvular abscesses: Do clinical parameters predict the presence of abscess? Chest 107:898-903, 1995.

3. Cavassini M, Meuli R, Francioli P: Complications of infective endocarditis. In Scheld WM, Whitley RJ, Marra CM (eds): Infections of the Central Nervous System, 3rd ed. Philadelphia, Lippincott Williams & Wilkins, 2004, pp 537-568.

4. Chun JY, Smith W, Halbach VV, et al: Current multimodality management of infectious intracranial aneurysms. Neurosurgery 48:1203-1213, 2001.

5. Dhawan VK: Infective endocarditis in the elderly. Clin Infect Dis 34:806-812, 2002.

6. DiSalvo G, Habib G, Pergola V, et al: Echocardiography predicts embolic events in infective endocarditis. J Am Coll Cardiol 37:1069-1076, 2001.

7. Ellis ME, Al-Abdely H, Sandridge A, et al: Fungal endocarditis: evidence in the world literature, 1965-1995. Clin Infect Dis 32:50-62, 2001.

8. Fowler V, Scheld WM, Bayer A: Endocarditis and intravascular infections. In Mandell GL, Bennett JE, Dolin R (eds): Principles and Practice of Infectious Diseases, 7th ed. New York, Churchill Livingstone, 2004, pp 1067-1112.

9. Gonazales-Juanatey C, Gonzalez-Gay M, Llorca J, et al: Rheumatic manifestations of infective endocarditis in non-addicts: a 12 year study. Medicine 80:9-19, 2001.

10. Heidenreich PA, Massoudi FA, Maini B, et al: Echocardiography in patients with suspected endocarditis: a cost-effectiveness analysis. Am J Med 107:198-208, 1999.

11. Kaasch A, Fowler VG, Rieg S, et al: Use of a simple criteria set for guiding echocardiography in nosocomial *Staphylococcus aureus* bacteremia. Clin Infect Dis 53:1-9, 2011.

12. Mehta NJ, Nehra A: A 66 year old man with fever, hypotension and complete heart block. Chest 120:2053-2056, 2001.

13. Natividad B, Miro JM, de Lazzari E, et al: Health care–associated native valve endocarditis: importance of non-nosocomial acquisition. Ann Intern Med 150:586-594, 2009.

14. Nolan CM, Beaty HN: *Staphylococcus* bacteremia—current clinical patterns. Am J Med 60:495-500, 1976.

15. Olaison L, Pettersson G: Current best practices and guidelines: indications for surgical intervention in infective endocarditis. Infect Dis Clin North Am 16:453-475, 2002.

16. Petti CA, Fowler VG Jr: *Staphylococcus aureus* bacteremia and endocarditis. Infect Dis Clin North Am 16:413-435, 2002.

17. Rosen AB, Fowler AG, Corey GR, et al: Cost-effectiveness of transesophageal echocardiography to determine the duration of therapy for intravascular catheter–associated *Staphylococcus aureus* bacteremia. Ann Intern Med 130:810-820, 1999.

18. Sachdev M, Peterson GE, Jollis JG: Imaging techniques for diagnosis of infective endocarditis. Infect Dis Clin North Am 16:319-337, 2002.

19. Townes ML, Reller LB: Diagnostic methods: current best practices and guidelines for isolation of bacteria and fungi in infective endocarditis. Infect Dis Clin North Am 16:363, 2002.

CHAPTER 34

MENINGITIS AND ENCEPHALITIS IN THE INTENSIVE CARE UNIT

Cindy Noyes, MD, and Christopher D. Huston, MD

MENINGITIS

1. **Describe the most common signs and symptoms of acute meningitis syndrome.**
   Fever, neck stiffness, and altered mental status are the classic triad, but they occur together only approximately 45% of the time. In a systematic review, 95% of patients had two of the three classic signs. The onset is hours to days, although historical detail may be limited if the patient's sensorium is altered.

2. **What is the pathophysiology of meningitis?**
   The pathogen gains entry via attachment on epithelial mucosal cells, endocytosis by dendritic cells, or direct vascular access. In the setting of bacterial meningitis, infection causes cytokine production and influx of inflammatory cells. The blood-brain barrier may have changes in permeability, allowing for protein entry in addition to inflammatory cells and fluid. Vasculature initially vasodilates but then becomes stenotic with infiltration of inflammatory cells. This vasculitis can result in ischemia and/or infarction. Glucose metabolism is increased and transport across the blood-brain barrier possibly decreased.

3. **What is the distinction between acute versus chronic meningitis?**
   Acute meningitis syndrome consists of fever, neck stiffness, and altered mental status with an onset of hours to days. Patients with acute bacterial meningitis may have rapid progression of signs and symptoms. This is in contrast to chronic meningitis, which is defined by presence of symptoms and abnormal cerebrospinal fluid (CSF) that persists for 4 weeks or more. The two syndromes have very distinct causes.

4. **What host factors are important to consider regarding risk and cause for acute bacterial meningitis?**
   Factors such as age, immune deficiency or suppression, recent central nervous system (CNS) instrumentation, and possible exposures should be considered and will influence empirical therapy. See Table 34-1.

5. **What are the most common causes of community-acquired acute bacterial meningitis in adults?**
   Table 34-2 includes the most common organisms in descending order based on case series with preferred antimicrobial therapy and suggested duration of treatment.

6. **What is adequate empirical therapy while awaiting culture results?**
   Empirical therapy should reflect suspected pathogens on the basis of host factors as well as local antibiotic susceptibility patterns. For example, *Streptococcus pneumoniae* is commonly known to have resistance to penicillin. Some strains are also resistant to third-generation cephalosporins. As a result, empirical therapy for *S. pneumoniae* should include high-dose third-generation cephalosporin as well as vancomycin. Empirical therapy with third-generation cephalosporin is also suggested for *Neisseria meningitidis*. For *Listeria monocytogenes*, preferred treatment is ampicillin, although trimethoprim-sulfamethoxazole is another option

TABLE 34-1. IMPORTANT CONSIDERATIONS REGARDING RISK AND CAUSE FOR ACUTE BACTERIAL MENINGITIS

HOST FACTORS	COMMON PATHOGENS				EMPIRICAL THERAPY
Age					
<1 mo	Streptococcus agalactiae	Escherichia coli	L. monocytogenes	Klebsiella species	Ampicillin + third-generation cephalosporin
1-23 mo	S. agalactiae	E. coli	Haemophilus influenzae	N. meningitidis	Vancomycin + third-generation cephalosporin
2-50 yr	S. pneumoniae	N. meningitidis			Vancomycin + third-generation cephalosporin
>50 yr	S. pneumoniae	N. meningitidis	L. monocytogenes	Aerobic gram-negative bacilli	Vancomycin + third-generation cephalosporin + ampicillin
Immune Suppression	S. pneumoniae	N. meningitidis	L. monocytogenes	Aerobic gram-negative bacilli, including nosocomial organisms	Vancomycin + carbapenem or fourth-generation cephalosporin + ampicillin
Post Neurosurgery	S. aureus (including methicillin resistant)	Coagulase-negative staphylococci	Aerobic gram-negative bacilli		Vancomycin + carbapenem or fourth-generation cephalosporin or ceftazidime

TABLE 34-2. MOST COMMON CAUSES OF COMMUNITY-ACQUIRED BACTERIAL MENINGITIS IN ADULTS

PATHOGENS	PREFERRED ANTIMICROBIAL	SUGGESTED DURATION OF THERAPY
S. pneumoniae		
PCN MIC < 0.1 mcg/mL	PCN or ampicillin	10-14 days
PCN MIC 0.1-1 mcg/mL	Third-generation cephalosporin	
PCN MIC ≥ 2 mcg/mL	Vancomycin + third-generation cephalosporin	
N. meningitidis		
PCN MIC < 0.1 mcg/mL	PCN or ampicillin	7 days
PCN MIC > 0.1 mcg/mL	Third-generation cephalosporin	
L. monocytogenes	Ampicillin or PCN	≥ 21 days
Streptococcus agalactiae, pyogenes	Ampicillin or PCN	21 days
S. aureus	MSSA → nafcillin, oxacillin	14 days
	MRSA → vancomycin	
H. influenzae		
β-Lactamase negative	Ampicillin	7 days
β-Lactamase positive	Third-generation cephalosporin	

MIC, Minimum inhibitory concentration; *MSSA*, methicillin-sensitive *S. aureus*; *PCN*, penicillin.

if the patient is penicillin allergic. Thus in an adult older than 50 years, an initial empirical regimen including vancomycin, high-dose ceftriaxone, and ampicillin would be suggested to treat the most likely community-acquired pathogens.

In the event that a patient has undergone recent neurosurgical instrumentation and has risk for nosocomial pathogens, one would also want to include therapy directed at methicillin-resistant *Staphylococcus aureus* (MRSA) and resistant nosocomial gram-negative bacilli, such as *Pseudomonas aeruginosa*.

Risk factors that may additionally influence empiricism must be identified with each patient. Prompt and detailed history should be explored. Factors including exposures, such as contaminated food consumption, travel, and sick contacts should be identified. Presence of immune suppression should also be elicited. The type and degree of immune suppression, including medications, absence of spleen, advanced HIV, and administration of chemotherapy should be sought. Risk factors for nosocomial pathogens, including recent neurosurgical procedures, presence of a foreign body within the CNS (such as a ventricular drain), and trauma are also important to determine, as noted earlier.

7. **When and to whom should steroids be administered?**
Adults suspected of having bacterial meningitis should receive steroids before or with the administration of antibiotics. On the basis of a prospective, randomized, placebo-controlled trial, dexamethasone was shown to reduce morbidity and mortality in adults who received corticosteroid therapy before or at the same time as administration of antibiotics. This had the

greatest benefit in patients with pneumococcal meningitis. The dose used in the study was 10 mg of dexamethasone every 6 hours for 4 days. Shorter durations and alternative dosing regimens have not been evaluated in adults.

8. **What are the contraindications to lumbar puncture (LP)?**
   LP is critical to diagnostic evaluation. If clinical suspicion for meningitis exists, one should perform an LP. Conditions such as elevated intracranial pressure, mass lesion, uncorrected coagulopathy, and skin infection overlying intended puncture site are to be considered before LP.

9. **When would one consider imaging before LP?**
   Most patients do not require imaging before LP. Computed tomography (CT) of the head should occur before LP if the patient has any signs or symptoms that suggest elevated intracranial pressure. These include new-onset neurologic deficits, new-onset seizure, and papilledema. Consideration should also be given to imaging in patients with moderate to severe cognitive impairment and immune compromise.

10. **Is there harm in awaiting CT and LP results before initiating therapy?**
    Yes. Delay in initiating antimicrobial therapy has been associated with increase in mortality. If imaging is needed before LP:
    - Obtain blood cultures.
    - Initiate antibiotic therapy and steroids.
    - Obtain CT of head, and perform LP if safe. CSF cultures may be affected by pretreatment with antibiotics before lumbar puncture, but CSF findings including cell counts, chemical analyses, and Gram stain should remain helpful. Van de Beek, in his review, noted that yield of Gram stain was similar in patients who had been treated with antibiotics before LP as compared with those who had not.

11. **What CSF studies are important?**
    A number of guides help determine likelihood for bacterial meningitis based on various CSF markers, although it is important to know that none are absolute. See Table 34-3 for specific indicators.

    A positive Gram stain confirms bacterial meningitis. However, culture data remain important for speciation (especially if morphology is not characteristic) and antimicrobial sensitivities. Low glucose level can be very helpful in indicating acute bacterial meningitis, but it is important to remember that other factors can contribute to a low glucose finding. For example, *Mycobacterium tuberculosis* meningitis, which is typically chronic, is commonly associated with low CSF glucose level. Malignancies are also associated with low CSF glucose level.

TABLE 34-3.   TYPICAL CSF FINDINGS IN BACTERIAL AND ASEPTIC MENINGITIS

	BACTERIAL DISEASE LIKELY	EARLY BACTERIAL/ VIRAL/SYPHILIS	MENINGITIS UNLIKELY
White blood cell count	>1000 cells/mcL	100-1000 cells/mcL	<5 cells/mcL
White blood cell differential	Neutrophil predominance (although 10% have 50% lymphocytes)	Lymphocyte predominance	
Glucose	<34 mg/dL	>45 mg/dL	Normal
Protein	>250 mg/dL	50-250 mg/dL	Normal

In addition, other tests have been studied to improve performance when trying to distinguish bacterial versus nonbacterial causes of meningitis. One such marker, CSF lactate, was shown to add predictive value when trying to distinguish between bacterial meningitis and nonbacterial meningitis shortly after neurosurgery. In a study of patients after neurosurgery by Lieb and colleagues, a cutoff of 4 mmol/L CSF lactate was 88% sensitive and 98% specific for diagnosis of bacterial meningitis. Of interest, CSF lactate levels did not vary with the presence or absence of red blood cells (RBCs), nor was there a correlation with days after surgery.

12. **How does one correct for a suspected traumatic LP?**
In the event of traumatic LP, one general guideline is subtraction of one white blood cell (WBC) for every 500 to 1500 RBCs. More precise calculation would be to tabulate the predicted CSF WBC count per microliter. The formula:

$$\text{Predicted CSF WBC count/mcL}^* =$$
$$\text{CSF RBC} \times (\text{Peripheral WBC count}/\text{Peripheral RBC count})$$

13. **In the setting of documented bacterial meningitis, who gets postexposure prophylaxis?**
The goal of postexposure prophylaxis is to eradicate nasopharyngeal carriage. There are two pathogens for which one would consider postexposure prophylaxis with specific indications listed as follows.
1. *N. meningitidis*
   1. Extended period of contact (>8 hours) in close proximity (within 3 feet)
   2. Contact with oral secretions, with such as activities as kissing, mouth-to-mouth resuscitation, intubation
   3. Household contacts, including communal living (military recruits, college dormitory residents)

   Exposure 1 week before symptom onset until after 24 hours of effective antibiotic therapy is considered significant. Postexposure prophylaxis should occur despite history of vaccination, because not all people respond to vaccination and there is one serotype not included in the vaccine.
   Suggested regimens:
   - Ciprofloxacin 500 mg orally (PO) × 1
   - Rifampin 10 mg/kg PO every 12 hours for 2 days (or 600 mg every 12 hours in adults)
   - Ceftriaxone 250 mg intramuscularly (IM) × 1 in adults; 125 mg IM × 1 in children
2. *H. influenzae*: If there is a partially vaccinated child or child younger than 4 years of age, prophylaxis is suggested for all household contacts, including adults. Prophylaxis of day-care contacts can be considered if applicable. The highest risk is in children under the age of 2 years.
   Suggested regimen: Rifampin 20 mg/kg per day for 4 days

14. **What is aseptic meningitis?**
Aseptic meningitis is defined by a syndrome of meningeal symptoms accompanied by abnormal CSF, usually with lymphocytic pleocytosis, in the setting of negative routine stains and cultures. Symptoms can be severe. Differential diagnosis includes infectious as well as noninfectious causes. This syndrome is usually associated with viral pathogens but can be caused by bacteria such as *M. tuberculosis, Treponema pallidum*, and *Borrelia burgdorferi*. This constellation of findings could also reflect a partially treated bacterial meningitis or a parameningeal focus.

---

*Ten times this predicted count has been shown to be a sensitive and specific indicator of meningitis in the setting of traumatic LP.

Medications, connective tissue disorders, and malignancy can also cause aseptic meningitis. It is imperative that the common bacterial causes be excluded.

15. **What are important historical data to obtain to help determine possible etiologic viral pathogens?**
The list of possible causes is extensive. Various factors can help narrow the possibilities. See Box 34-1.

BOX 34-1. DETERMINING POSSIBLE ETIOLOGIC VIRAL PATHOGENS FOR ASEPTIC MENINGITIS

Time of year or season
Exposures
    Animal
    Insect (tick, mosquito)
    Travel
    Water
    Sick contacts
    Environmental (day care, college dormitory, military recruit)
    Sexual history
Skin rash
Genital lesions
HIV status
    As primary cause
    As a risk for secondary cause

---

16. **What are the most common viral causes of meningitis?**
The most common viruses associated with meningitis are nonpolio enteroviruses. These include various coxsackievirus, echovirus, and enterovirus strains. Diagnosis was historically made by viral culture, although polymerase chain reaction (PCR) evaluation of CSF is now readily available in many laboratories. Treatment is supportive in nature, and the illness is usually self-limited with complete recovery. Exceptions to this are neonates less than 2 weeks of age and persons with immune deficiencies, such as agammaglobulinemia, in whom severe disease can develop. Other common viruses include flaviviruses, such as St. Louis encephalitis (SLE) and West Nile virus (WNV), and herpes family viruses, such as herpes simplex virus 2 (HSV-2) and varicella-zoster virus (VZV). These too can be confirmed by PCR. It is important to note that other viral illnesses can cause meningitis. These include acute HIV infection and various respiratory viruses such as influenza and parainfluenza. It is important to remember that, to diagnose acute HIV, viral load RNA quantification is necessary because antibody testing is usually negative during acute seroconversion.

ENCEPHALITIS

17. **What symptoms and signs are commonly associated with encephalitis?**
Encephalitis is defined by inflammation of brain parenchyma. Most causal pathogens are viral and gain access to the CNS via the bloodstream, although some viruses such as herpes simplex virus 1 (HSV-1) and rabies directly invade via neuronal transport. Acute encephalitis usually occurs over a brief period of time (days) as compared with chronic encephalitis, which can progress over weeks to months. Many patients will be seen with a prodromal illness with symptoms of fever, myalgias, and anorexia, which corresponds to viremia. Neurologic

manifestations can range from headache, focal neurologic defect, and behavioral changes to seizure and coma. Meningeal inflammation can also occur resulting in symptoms suggestive of meningitis. Various viruses may have slightly different neural tropism, which can suggest cause based on presentation. For example, HSV-1 has a predilection for the temporal lobe. Encephalitis is associated with high morbidity and mortality.

18. **What are the most common causes of acute encephalitis?**
    Despite often aggressive diagnostics, the cause of encephalitis in the majority of patients remains unknown. Any epidemiologic clues should be identified to guide diagnostic work-up as well as to initiate prompt empirical therapy. In the United States, when a cause is identified, the most common pathogens are HSV-1, WNV, and enteroviruses.
    Possible infectious causes include but are not limited to the following:
    - Viral: HSV-1, enterovirus, WNV, VZV, SLE, influenza, HIV, Epstein-Barr virus, measles, rabies, cytomegalovirus (CMV)
    - Bacterial: *Bartonella henselae*, *L. monocytogenes*
    - Rickettsial: *Ehrlichia*, *Rickettsia rickettsii*, *Anaplasma*
    - Parasitic: *Toxoplasma gondii*, *Naegleria fowleri*
    - Fungal: *Histoplasma capsulatum*, *Cryptococcus neoformans*, *Coccidioides immitis*

    Up to 5% to 10% of sporadic cases of encephalitis, when diagnosis is available, are attributable to HSV-1. Postinfectious, postimmunization, and noninfectious causes, such as connective tissue disease and paraneoplastic phenomena, must also be explored if diagnosis is elusive. Acute disseminated encephalomyelitis may follow a viral illness or vaccine and is important to differentiate from an infectious cause.

19. **What should the initial diagnostic work-up include?**
    After careful history and physical examination, neuroimaging is recommended. This can suggest possible causes, dependent on regions of involvement, and may also exclude other possible causes, such as brain abscess. The most sensitive neurologic imaging is magnetic resonance imaging (MRI). If MRI cannot be performed, CT with contrast is the next preferred method. CSF evaluation is also suggested, unless contraindicated. CSF studies should include the usual cell count with differential, protein, and glucose markers. CSF should be sent for PCR evaluation for HSV and enteroviruses. A positive test is helpful, but a negative first test does not exclude infection if the clinical suspicion is high. Repeated testing within 3 to 7 days is suggested. Of note, the presence of hemoglobin can interfere with HSV PCR and cause a false negative result. PCR can also be performed to evaluate for VZV and CMV. If acute HIV is considered, one would need to obtain serum quantification of HIV RNA levels, because initial antibody testing may be negative. CSF cultures have not been helpful in elucidating viral causes but should be obtained if concern exists for nonviral causes, including bacteria and fungal organisms. Brain biopsy is usually reserved for those cases in which initial evaluation has been unrevealing and the patient continues to have clinical decline.
    Additional studies should be obtained in the context of a patient's epidemiologic risks. For example, travel to endemic areas could heighten concern for rickettsial disease or flaviviruses. An animal bite, particularly in a developing nation, could increase suspicion for rabies.

20. **What empirical therapy is suggested?**
    In any person with suspected encephalitis, acyclovir should be initiated at 10 mg/kg every 8 hours. If a patient has had travel to regions where rickettsial disease is endemic, doxycycline should also be administered. Given the overlap of encephalitis and meningitis syndromes, in the appropriate clinical context, empirical therapy for bacterial meningitis can be considered. However, the combination of tetracyclines and β-lactam antibiotics should be used cautiously because historical data suggest this combination to have static-cidal inhibition and an increase in mortality when used in patients with pneumococcal meningitis.

KEY POINTS: DELAYED LUMBAR PUNCTURE

When LP is delayed during evaluation for acute bacterial meningitis, the following diagnostic and management actions are suggested:

1. Obtain blood cultures.

2. Initiate antibiotic and steroid therapy.

3. Obtain head CT.

4. Perform LP if safe.

BIBLIOGRAPHY

1. Attia J, Hatala R, Cook D, et al. Does this adult patient have acute meningitis? JAMA 281:175-181, 1999.

2. Durand M, Calderwood S, Weber D, et al. Acute bacterial meningitis in adults: a review of 493 episodes. N Engl J Med 328:21-28, 1993.

3. Gans JD, Van de Beek D: Dexamethasone in adults with bacterial meningitis. N Engl J Med 347:1549-1556, 2002.

4. Hasbun R, Abrahams J, Jekel J, et al. Computed tomography of the head before lumbar puncture in adults with suspected meningitis. N Engl J Med 345:1727-1733, 2001.

5. Leib S, Boscacci R, Gratzl O, et al. Predictive value of cerebrospinal fluid (CSF) lactate levels versus CSF/blood glucose ratio for the diagnosis of bacterial meningitis following neurosurgery. Clin Infect Dis 29:69-74, 1999.

6. Lepper MH, Dowling HF: Treatment of pneumococcic meningitis with penicillin compared with penicillin plus aureomycin; studies including observations on an apparent antagonism between penicillin and aureomycin. AMA Arch Intern Med 88:489-494, 1951.

7. Mayefsky JF, Roghmann KJ: Determination of leukocytosis in traumatic spinal tap specimens. Am J Med 82:1175-1181, 1987.

8. Sawyer MH, Rotbart HA: Viral meningitis and aseptic meningitis syndrome. In Scheld WM, Whitley RJ, Marra CM (eds): Infections of the Central Nervous System, 3rd ed. Philadelphia, Lippincott Williams & Wilkins, 2004, pp 75-93.

9. Tunkel AR, Glaser CA, Bloch CB, et al. The management of encephalitis: clinical practice guidelines by the Infectious Disease Society of America. Clin Infect Dis 47:303-327, 2008.

10. Tunkel AR, Hartman BJ, Kaplan SL, et al. Practice guidelines for the management of bacterial meningitis. Clin Infect Dis 39:1267-1284, 2004.

11. Tunkel AR, Van de Beek D, Scheld WM: Acute meningitis. In Mandell G, Bennett J, Dolin R (eds): Mandell, Douglas, and Bennett's Principles and Practice of Infectious Diseases, 7th ed. Philadelphia, Churchill Livingstone, 2010, pp 1189-1229.

CHAPTER 35

DISSEMINATED FUNGAL INFECTIONS

Themistoklis Kourkoumpetis, MD, and Eleftherios E. Mylonakis, MD, PhD, FIDSA

1. **What is the definition of disseminated fungal infection?**
   We define *disseminated fungal infection* as the presence of a fungal pathogen in the blood (fungemia) and/or any other sterile deep-seated structure because of hematogenous seeding. This distinguishes disseminated infection from superficial infection, which mostly involves the mucocutaneous structures, that is, dermatitis, onychitis, stomatitis, esophagitis, and keratitis, as well as from simple colonization, which is the isolation of a fungal pathogen from a nonsterile site without any sign of infection attributable to the specific pathogen. Invasive fungal infection is a more general term and refers to fungemia and other fungal infections such as disseminated candidiasis, endocarditis, meningitis, and hepatosplenic infection.

2. **What are the most clinically important fungal pathogens?**
   Candida spp., *Aspergillus* spp., and *Cryptococcus* spp. are by far the most common fungal pathogens encountered in the hospital setting, with *Candida* being the leading fungal pathogen. Of note is that *Aspergillus* spp. have been steadily increasing in the intensive care unit (ICU) setting.

3. **What is the epidemiology of fungal infections in hospitalized patients?**
   In the last 25 years the total number of fungal infections in hospitalized patients has increased from 6% in 1980 to 10.4% in 1990 and currently may be as high as 25%. *Candida* species are the fourth most commonly recovered blood culture isolates in the United States.

4. **Why has the incidence of fungal infection increased so dramatically?**
   Fungi generally do not cause invasive infection in healthy individuals. Robust cellular and antibody-mediated immunity and intact mucosal barriers play a major role in shielding the human body from opportunists such as *Candida* spp., which seek a way of passing through tissues and entering the bloodstream and other deep-seated organs. With the numbers of immunosuppressed patients increasing through cancer and chemotherapy, transplantation, and HIV infection, as well as with the increased use of vascular and urinary catheters and broad-spectrum antibacterial agents, an alarming increase of deep-seated fungal infections has been seen in clinical practice.

5. **What fungi are responsible for invasive infection in humans?**
   C. albicans accounts for the majority (mostly >50%-60%) of all *Candida* infections, but this percentage is declining to 45%. *C. tropicalis, C. glabrata,* and *C. krusei* account for most of the remainder. This is particularly important because certain *Candida* spp. such as *C. krusei* can be resistant to fluconazole. On the other hand, *Aspergillus* spp. account for at least 15% to 20% of all fungal infections; however, the rate can be higher in patients after lung transplantation. Other less-common but increasing mycoses include blastomycoses, coccidioidomycoses, cryptococcosis, histoplasmosis, and sporotrichosis.

6. **What are the most important risk factors for disseminated *Candida* infection?**
   - ICU stay
   - Immunosuppression (hematologic malignancy, hematopoietic stem cell transplantation, immunosuppressive therapy such as steroids and chemotherapeutic regimens, neutropenia, and HIV infection)
   - Total parenteral nutrition
   - Comorbidities and a high APACHE (Acute Physiology, Age, and Chronic Health Evaluation) score
   - Broad-spectrum antimicrobial agents
   - *Candida* colonization in multiple sites
   - Acute renal failure especially requiring hemodialysis
   - Foreign bodies (central venous, arterial, or urinary catheters)
   - General and especially abdominal surgery

7. **List the diagnostic criteria for disseminated fungal infection.**
   Definitive:
   - Single positive blood culture (never mistake a positive fungal blood culture as a contaminant)
   - Fungus cultured from biopsy specimen
   - Burn wound invasion
   - Endophthalmitis
   - Fungus cultured from peritoneal or cerebrospinal fluid

   Suggestive: three confirmed colonized sites (should be regarded as a risk factor rather than a definite sign of infection)

8. **How reliable are these diagnostic criteria?**
   The preceding criteria are positive in only 30% to 50% of patients with disseminated fungal infection. Therefore a high index of suspicion must be maintained.

9. **Should asymptomatic candiduria be treated?**
   Among low-risk individuals no treatment is recommended. Amphotericin bladder irrigation is no longer recommended. Usually a change of urinary catheter should suffice. Among high-risk patients (patients with neutropenia or with urologic manipulations, low-birth-weight infants) treatment is similar to the one used for invasive candidiasis.

10. **Should a central venous catheter be removed once candidemia is confirmed?**
    Practice guidelines indicate that all central venous catheters should be removed once candidemia is confirmed (Table 35-1). Of note is that a recent randomized controlled trial and other studies question the benefit of early removal of central venous catheters in the onset of candidemia for some selected patients. We recommend following the standard practice guidelines.

11. **When should you suspect disseminated candidiasis?**
    Unfortunately, disseminated candidiasis has a wide spectrum of manifestations from a mild fever to a sepsis syndrome with multiorgan failure. On certain occasions the hematogenous spread of *Candida* produces visible changes throughout the body including muscle, skin, and eyes, making a bloodstream process clinically apparent. However, this is not always the case, and that is why there must be a low threshold for the disease especially in patients with multiple risk factors for candidiasis.

12. **If disseminated candidiasis is suspected, where should you look for it?**
    The first consideration is to perform blood cultures. Then examine the retina for endophthalmitis. However, recent reports show that rate of hematogenous endophthalmitis is considerably lower (2%-3%) compared with older studies that reported a 30% rate of such complication. Keep in mind that patients with neutropenia may have no symptoms until they regain their normal counts.

TABLE 35-1. RECOMMENDATION ON CVC REMOVAL IN PATIENTS WITH CANDIDEMIA

VENOUS ACCESS	RECOMMENDATION
Normal venous access	*Remove* CVC, and send tip for culture.
Limited venous access (impossible to remove catheter)	*Exchange* CVC over a guidewire, and perform catheter tip cultures. If catheter is colonized with the same *Candida* sp. that is found in the blood, then it is prudent to remove catheter.

Modified from www.guidelines.gov and Mermel LA, Allon M, Bouza E, et al: Clinical practice guidelines for the diagnosis and management of intravascular catheter-related infection: 2009 update by the Infectious Diseases Society of America [published errata appear in: Clin Infect Dis 50:457, 2010, and Clin Infect Dis 50:1079, 2010]. Clin Infect Dis 49:1-45, 2009.
CVC, Central venous catheter.

You can also search for *Candida* in the heart valves for endocarditis; the bone for osteomyelitis; and the liver, spleen, and kidneys for renal abscesses and candiduria. Also make sure to perform a biopsy of skin lesions to add extra yield to the diagnosis along with blood cultures. This is important because blood cultures are only 50% to 60% sensitive.

13. **What is the overall mortality associated with candidemia?**
The overall mortality associated with candidemia is 40% to 68%, with an attributable mortality of 25% to 40%. However, the earlier the initiation of antifungal agents, the better the prognosis. Early targeted antifungal therapy is difficult to accomplish because cultures take 24 to 48 hours to yield the species and antifungal resistance profiles. That is why empirical therapy should take into account risk factors for antifungal resistance, that is, prolonged exposure to antifungal agents or long length of hospital stays, and also risk factors for non-*albicans* species intrinsically resistant to fluconazole.

14. **Should antifungal therapy be delayed until blood cultures are positive for fungus?**
Absolutely not! Early therapy means lower mortality. Blood cultures have been found to be only 40% to 70% sensitive. Systemic antifungal therapy should be strongly considered, especially in a patient who is at high risk for disseminated fungal infection, if:
- Fever persists despite antibacterial agents and negative blood cultures
- High-grade funguria occurs in the absence of a bladder catheter
- Funguria persists after removal of a bladder catheter
- Fungus is cultured from at least two body sites
- Visceral fungal lesions are confirmed

15. **What are the major classes of antifungal drugs in use today?**
Antifungal drugs in clinical use today fall into three broad categories: polyene antifungals (amphotericin B), antifungal azoles, and the echinocandins.

16. **So, how do we treat?**
According to recent guidelines, physicians should choose among an echinocandin, fluconazole, an amphotericin B preparation, or combination of amphotericin B with flucytosine. The therapeutic strategy should take into account any previous use of antifungal agents (because it

can select resistant species), the epidemiology of fluconazole-resistant or non-*albicans* strains in the community, and any comorbid conditions (which could influence drug pharmacokinetics or worsen coexisting conditions such as renal failure). An echinocandin or amphotericin B should be preferred over fluconazole among patients with neutropenia and critically ill patients, as well as those known to be exposed to fluconazole-resistant strains. Of course the physician can always switch to fluconazole whenever an antifungal resistance profile becomes available.

17. How do amphotericin B and flucytosine work?
Amphotericin B, a polyene, is fungicidal. It binds irreversibly to ergosterol (but not to cholesterol, the major sterol in mammalian cell membranes), creating a membrane channel that allows leakage of cytosol leading to cell death. Flucytosine is sometimes used in conjunction with amphotericin B and is synergistic *Cryptococcus*. Flucytosine acts directly on fungal organisms by competitive inhibition of purine and pyrimidine uptake.

18. What antifungal azoles are available, and how do they work?
Fluconazole, itraconazole, voriconazole, and posaconazole, which are triazoles, are fungistatic against *Candida* spp. They inhibit C-14 α-demethylase, a cytochrome P-450–dependent fungal enzyme required for synthesis of ergosterol, the major sterol in the fungal cell membrane. This alters cell membrane fluidity, decreasing nutrient transport, increasing membrane permeability, and inhibiting cell growth and proliferation.

19. How do echinocandins work, and are they being used?
The target for echinocandins is the complex of proteins responsible for synthesis of cell wall polysaccharides. Caspofungin, anidulafungin, and micafungin are used in the treatment of candidemia and other forms of disseminated *Candida* infections.

20. What advantages does fluconazole offer over amphotericin B in the treatment or prevention of disseminated fungal infections?
- Fluconazole is available in both intravenous (IV) and oral (PO) forms; patients have been successfully treated with 7 days of IV fluconazole followed by PO if the patient is able. Administration by mouth is both easier and less costly than IV administration.
- Fluconazole is not nephrotoxic and has fewer overall adverse effects than amphotericin B, which can cause hypokalemia, fever, and chills.

21. Are there any limitations to the use of fluconazole?
Yes. Fluconazole is not active against *Aspergillus* spp. or *C. krusei* and other resistant *Candida* spp. Also, remember that fluconazole may inhibit the P-450 detoxification system and cause hepatotoxicity, increasing phenytoin and cyclosporin levels and potentiating warfarin's anticoagulant effects. Fluconazole has fewer overall adverse effects than amphotericin B.

22. What should be done when a *Candida* infection fails to respond to fluconazole?
An echinocandin agent or an amphotericin B preparation should be considered. Make sure that the diagnosis is confirmed, the dosage is appropriate, and drug-drug interactions are ruled out (for example, rifampin decreases fluconazole levels). Keep in mind that resistance can happen to all antifungal agents. For example, *C. krusei* and *C. glabrata* can be resistant to azoles, *C. lusitaniae* can be resistant to amphotericin B, and *C. parapsilosis* can have higher minimum inhibitory concentration to echinocandins.

23. Are there less toxic forms of amphotericin B available?
Yes. To reduce the toxicity associated with amphotericin B, lipid formulations have been produced. The earliest and most widely studied of these is AmBisome, which in randomized trials has been shown to be safer than amphotericin B with many fewer side effects. Other

lipid-associated, nonliposomal products are amphotericin B lipid complex (Abelcet) and amphotericin B colloidal dispersion (Amphocil). The disadvantage of these alternative forms of amphotericin B is their currently high cost.

24. **Can health care providers help prevent the spread of fungal colonization in the ICU?**
Easily. Wash hands and wear gloves when working directly with patients. *Candida* species were found on the hands of 33% to 75% of ICU staff in one study.

CONTROVERSY

25. **Does the strategy of *presumptive* or *preemptive* treatment of high-risk patients prevent severe candidiasis in critically ill surgical patients?**
The effectiveness of fluconazole in treating overt candidiasis has unfortunately provoked its widespread, unjustified use in patients without neutropenia in the ICU setting. This practice has likely led to an increase in non-*albicans* species, which are resistant to fluconazole. Several studies have shown decreased incidence of colonization and the risk of candidiasis with such empirical treatment but have failed to show decreased mortality in any group other than high-risk patients who have received a transplant. Recent reviews have suggested that targeted preemptive strategy may be of benefit in preventing candidiasis in the ICU. This concept requires further study before continued practice. Of note is that fluconazole should be given as secondary prophylaxis in patients with HIV with CD4 <200 cells/mm^3 who survived cryptococcosis.

Acknowledgment

Dr. Mylonakis has received research support from Astellas Pharma US and T2 Biosystems.

KEY POINTS: DISSEMINATED FUNGAL INFECTIONS

1. Fungal infections are an increasing source of morbidity and mortality in ICUs.

2. Simple colonization does not require treatment.

3. *Candida* species and *Aspergillus* account for more than 90% of disseminated fungal infections.

4. Fluconazole is comparable to amphotericin B for most forms of disseminated candidiasis without the toxicity caused by amphotericin.

5. Do not wait for confirmation by culture to treat, because up to 50% of lethal infections may be culture negative before death.

6. Presumptive or preemptive therapy may be useful in selected high-risk groups.

7. The earlier the administration of antifungal treatment the lower the mortality.

BIBLIOGRAPHY

1. Horn DL, Neofytos D, Anaissie EJ, et al: Epidemiology and outcomes of candidemia in 2019 patients: data from the prospective antifungal therapy alliance registry. Clin Infect Dis 48:1695-1703, 2009.

2. Kourkoumpetis TK, Velmahos GC, Ziakas PD, et al: The effect of cumulative length of hospital stay on the antifungal resistance of Candida strains isolated from critically ill surgical patients. Mycopathologia 171:85-91, 2011.

3. Nucci M, Anaissie E, Betts RF, et al: Early removal of central venous catheter in patients with candidemia does not improve outcome: analysis of 842 patients from 2 randomized clinical trials. Clin Infect Dis 51:295-303, 2010.

4. Piarroux R, Grenouillet F, Balvay P, et al: Assessment of preemptive treatment to prevent severe candidiasis in critically ill surgical patients. Crit Care Med 32:2443-2449, 2004.

5. Rex JH, Bennett JE, Sugar AM, et al: A randomized trial comparing fluconazole with amphotericin B for the treatment of candidemia in patients without neutropenia. N Engl J Med 331:1325-1330, 1994.

6. Richardson MD: Changing patterns and trends in systemic fungal infections. J Antimicrob Chemother 56(Suppl 1):i5-i11, 2005.

7. Spanakis EK, Aperis G, Mylonakis E: New agents for the treatment of fungal infections: clinical efficacy and gaps in coverage. Clin Infect Dis 43:1060-1068, 2006.

CHAPTER 36

MULTIDRUG-RESISTANT BACTERIA

Christopher Grace, MD, FACP

1. **What is multidrug resistance?**

   Antibiotic classes include the β-lactams, aminoglycosides, quinolones, tetracyclines, sulfonamides, polymyxins, glycopeptides, and the newer agents with gram-positive bacterial activity such as the lipopeptides, oxazolidinones, streptogramins, and lipoglycopeptides. The definition of multidrug-resistant (MDR) bacteria has not been universally agreed on but generally denotes bacteria that are resistant to at least three of these classes.

2. **Why are MDR bacteria such a concern?**

   With increasing bacterial resistance our therapeutic options lessen. Patients with antimicrobial resistance have been shown to have higher rates of hospital-acquired infections, higher APACHE (Acute Physiology, Age, and Chronic Health Evaluation) III scores, longer hospital stays, increased intensive care unit (ICU) admissions, increased mortality, and higher hospital costs. Increasing antibiotic resistance has become a serious public health issue. In contrast to a large number of newer gram-positive coccal (GPC) agents that have been developed over the past 15 years, very few new agents are in the pharmaceutical pipeline with activity against MDR gram-negative rods (GNR). The development of new GNR agents may take 8 to 10 years and cost billions of dollars.

3. **What are the risk factors for MDR infections?**

   Major risk factors for colonization or infection with MDR organisms are as follows:
   - Long-term antibiotic exposure
   - Prolonged ICU stay
   - Nursing home residency
   - Severe illness
   - Residence in an institution with high rates of ceftazidime and other third-generation cephalosporin use
   - Instrumentation or catheterization

4. **How do mutations in cell wall synthesis contribute to MDR?**

   Almost all bacteria have cell walls that are located outside of the inner membrane and are composed of repeating carbohydrate units of *N*-acetylmuramic acid and *N*-acetylglucosamine. See Figure 36-1. The key structural stabilizing step is the cross-linking between the carbohydrate layers. Penicillin-binding proteins (PBP) are the bacterial enzymes that accomplish this cross-linkage. β-Lactam antibiotics (penicillins, cephalosporins, carbapenems, and monobactams) bind to PBP, inactivating them, thus interfering with the cross-linkage. Gram-positive bacteria can become MDR by mutations in the PBP such that the β-lactam cannot bind to them. Methicillin-resistant *Staphylococcus aureus* (MRSA), penicillin-resistant *Streptococcus pneumoniae,* and vancomycin-resistant enterococcus (VRE) all have evolved mutated PBP.

5. **Why are β-lactamases so important in causing MDR infections?**

   β-Lactamases are bacterial enzymes that inactivate β-lactam antibiotics by opening the amide bond of the β-lactam ring. See Figure 36-1. These enzymes are the most common cause of MDR in GNR. The β-lactamases causing the most common MDR in the ICU include the following:
   - **Extended-spectrum β-lactamases (ESBL)** cause resistance to most β-lactam antibiotics with the exceptions of the cephamycins (cefoxitin, cefotetan) and carbapenems. The most common

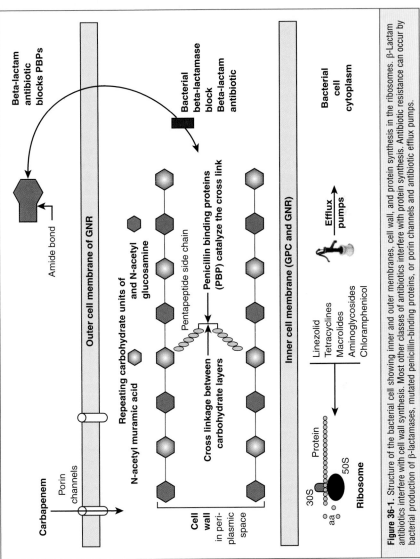

Figure 36-1. Structure of the bacterial cell showing inner and outer membranes, cell wall, and protein synthesis in the ribosomes. β-Lactam antibiotics interfere with cell wall synthesis. Most other classes of antibiotics interfere with protein synthesis. Antibiotic resistance can occur by bacterial production of β-lactamases, mutated penicillin-binding proteins, or porin channels and antibiotic efflux pumps.

bacteria carrying ESBL are *Klebsiella* spp. and *Escherichia coli.* Less commonly *Enterobacter, Serratia, Morganella, Proteus,* and *Pseudomonas aeruginosa* spp. may harbor these genes. The genes for these enzymes are carried on chromosomes or plasmids and are thus transferrable between bacteria. ESBL-producing bacteria are also often resistant to aminoglycosides and quinolones. These enzymes are usually inhibited by β-lactamase inhibitors such as clavulanic acid, sulbactam, and tazobactam.

- **AmpC cephalosporinases** are β-lactamases that confer resistance to cephalosporin antibiotics (including cephamycins) by *Enterobacter, Nitrobacteria, Morganella, Serratia,* and *P. aeruginosa.* In contrast to ESBL enzymes, they are most often chromosomally encoded and not transferable. Paradoxically they are inducible by third-generation cephalosporins. More recently these genes have been found on transferable plasmids but are not inducible. These enzymes are often resistant to β-lactamase inhibitors.

- **Carbapenemases** are enzymes that can inactivate the carbapenems (meropenem, imipenem-cilastatin, ertapenem, and doripenem). These enzymes may also be able to inactivate all classes of β-lactam antibiotics and are resistant to β-lactamase inhibitors. Organisms found to carry these MDR genes include *P. aeruginosa, Acinetobacter, Stenotrophomonas, Klebsiella, Serratia, Enterobacter, E. coli,* and *Citrobacter.* In 2009, a new carbapenemase was isolated in pathogens from New Delhi, India, called the New Delhi metallo-β-lactamase-1 (NDM-1). Bacteria harboring the NDM-1 include *Klebsiella, E. coli, Enterobacter, Nitrobacteria, Morganella, Providencia, Acinetobacter,* and *P. aeruginosa.* The resistance gene is carried by a plasmid and is thus transferable between bacteria. Isolates have now been found in Europe and the United States. Transmission of aminoglycoside and quinolone resistance may be carried by other genes on the plasmid.

6. **What other resistance mechanisms cause MDR in the ICU?**
   Bacterial enzymes can modify aminoglycosides, chloramphenicol, macrolides, or tetracyclines before the antibiotic reaches its ribosomal target. Decreased permeability of carbapenems through the porin channel of the GNR outer membrane can occur. Removal of the antibiotic by bacterial efflux pumps can cause resistance to tetracyclines, macrolides, β-lactams, quinolones, and linezolid. Alteration of the bacterial ribosomes leads to resistance to tetracyclines, macrolides, aminoglycosides, and linezolid. Mutations of the bacterial DNA topoisomerase cause resistance to all quinolones. Sulfonamides lose activity when mutations of the bacterial dihydropteroate synthetase occur.

7. **How do bacteria become multiresistant?**
   Bacteria become resistant to antibiotics by DNA mutation at select points or by insertions or deletions that alter microbial enzymes or the antibiotic targets. Genetic material can be transferred between bacteria by plasmids (extrachromosomal double-stranded circular DNA) via direct cell-to-cell contact. Bacteria may also acquire new resistance genes by infection with bacteriophage viruses that carry resistance genes with them when they infect bacteria. Once bacteria develop or acquire new resistance genes they have a selective advantage when antibiotics are used. As more mutations or transferred genetic material accumulates, the more classes of antibiotics the bacteria become resistant to, inducing MDR.

8. **What MDR gram-positive bacteria pose the greatest risk in the ICU?**
   - **MRSA** is resistant to all penicillins and cephalosporins and often resistant to clindamycin and quinolones. Long known as a nosocomial pathogen, MRSA is now appearing as community-acquired infections. MRSA can cause pneumonias, severe abscesses with cellulitis, and bloodstream and central line infections. It is not a classic urinary pathogen, and its presence in the urine should raise the suspicion of bacteremia. Vancomycin remains the "go to" drug although resistance is emerging more commonly. For those isolates with a minimum inhibitory

concentration of >1 mcg/mL, vancomycin may not be effective, especially for endocarditis, bloodstream infections, and pneumonia.
- **VRE** have become increasingly common. They can be part of bowel flora and colonize the urinary tract. They can be nosocomial pathogens causing blood, urinary tract, and central catheter infections and endocarditis.

9. **What are the treatment options for these MDR gram positives?**
- **Vancomycin** interferes with bacterial cell wall synthesis by blocking penicillin-binding proteins. It is active against MRSA and vancomycin-sensitive enterococci. Vancomycin-intermediate *S. aureus* (VISA) isolates have been found clinically, and fear remains concerning vancomycin-resistant *S. aureus* (VRSA) isolates.
- **Daptomycin** is the first of a new class of antibiotics called lipopeptides that interfere with gram-positive bacterial cell membrane function. It has activity against MRSA, some VISA, and VRE. Daptomycin may cause myositis, and creatine phosphokinase levels need to be monitored. Daptomycin is inactivated by pulmonary surfactant and should not be used to treat pneumonia.
- **Linezolid** is the first oxazolidinone antibiotic. It interferes with bacterial protein synthesis by binding to the 50 S ribosome. It is bacteriostatic with activity against MRSA and VRE. It can be used orally or intravenously. Linezolid can cause thrombocytopenia.
- **Quinupristin-dalfopristin** (Synercid) is a combination streptogramin antibiotic that interferes with the bacterial 50 S ribosome. It has activity against MRSA. Although it does not have activity against *Enterococcus faecalis*, it does work against *Enterococcus faecium* including VRE.
- **Ceftaroline fosamil** is a new cephalosporin with activity against MRSA and penicillin-resistant *S. pneumoniae*. As with all cephalosporins, there is no enterococcal activity including VRE.
- **Televancin** is a new lipoglycopeptide antibiotic that inhibits cell wall synthesis and disrupts bacterial cell membrane function. It has activity against MRSA and enterococci but not VRE.
- Older agents, such as **doxycycline,** may have activity against both MRSA and VRE. **Trimethoprim-sulfamethoxazole** (TMP-SMX) may have activity against MRSA. **Clindamycin** may have MRSA activity, but it is important to check for erythromycin resistance because that may predict inducible clindamycin resistance.

10. **What MDR gram-negative bacteria pose the greatest risk in the ICU?**
- **Enterobacteriaceae** that have increasing MDR include *E. coli, Klebsiella,* and *Enterobacter.* Resistance is most often conferred by ESBL, AmpC cephalosporinases, and carbapenemases. These organisms may be urinary, wound, or respiratory colonizers but also cause a wide array of nosocomial infections including pneumonia, bacteremia, and urinary tract infections. Agents with possible activity include carbapenems, aminoglycosides, tigecycline, and colistin.
- ***P. aeruginosa*** has the greatest ability to develop resistance. It has minimal nutritional requirements, which accounts for its successful growth in many environments and its ability to colonize endotracheal tubes and urinary catheters in the ICU. *P. aeruginosa* may cause pulmonary, bloodstream, central line, and urinary tract infections. In the host with neutropenia, necrotic skin lesions, ecthyma gangrenosum, can occur. Resistance is mediated by ESBL, AmpC cephalosporinases, carbapenemases, efflux pumps, and outer membrane porin mutations. See Figure 36-1. No evidence exists that using two antibiotics for synergy improves outcomes or reduces emerging resistance. Antibiotics that may retain activity against MDR *P. aeruginosa* include colistin and, in some situations, doripenem.

- ***Acinetobacter*** *calcoaceticus* (80% of clinical isolates) and *Acinetobacter baumannii* have limited nutritional requirements, are resistant to many disinfectants, and can easily contaminate environmental surfaces. Approximately 25% of the healthy population are colonized. All of these factors contribute to colonization and infection in the ICU. Infections may occur in the lung, bloodstream, urinary tract, and traumatic wounds. *Acinetobacter* have multiple β-lactamases, loss of outer-membrane porin channels, and efflux pumps causing MDR to most β-lactams, quinolones, and aminoglycosides. Isolates may be sensitive to carbapenems, tigecycline, ampicillin-sulbactam, TMP-SMX, rifampicin, and colistin.
- ***Stenotrophomonas maltophilia*** is most often encountered in the nosocomial setting in patients with prior broad-spectrum antibiotic exposure. It is often isolated in patients with cystic fibrosis. The most common infections include bacteremias related to central venous catheters and pneumonia. Resistance is mediated through β-lactamases, efflux pumps, and outer-membrane porin channel mutations. Although TMP-SMX and ticarcillin-clavulanic acid are often effective, reports are increasing of TMP-SMX resistance. Other agents that may have activity include ceftazidime, aztreonam, minocycline, tigecycline, and ciprofloxacin.

11. **What are the treatment options for these MDR gram negatives?**
    - **Carbapenems** should remain active against ESBL and AmpC-producing bacteria. Rates of *P. aeruginosa*, *Acinetobacter*, and *S. maltophilia* resistance are increasing.
    - **Colistin** is polymyxin E, a cationic polypeptide antibiotic that binds to the lipopolysaccharides of the GNR outer membrane to disrupt it and cause cell death. It has been used successfully intravenously and as an aerosol to treat MDR *Acinetobacter*. It may be used for MDR *P. aeruginosa* and carbapenemase-producing Enterobacteriaceae. *Serratia*, *Proteus*, and *S. maltophilia* are resistant. Nephrotoxicity and neurotoxicity are the major toxicities.
    - **Tigecycline** is a parenteral derivative of minocycline. It may have activity against ESBL and carbapenemase-producing Enterobacteriaceae, *S. maltophilia*, and *Acinetobacter*. *P. aeruginosa* and *Proteus* are resistant. Because of low urinary concentrations, it should not be used to treat urinary tract infections.

12. **Control of MDR bacteria**
    Because the emergence of MDR bacteria is related to selective antibiotic pressure, the best means of reducing or controlling MDR bacteria is by limiting antimicrobial exposure. Although challenging in the ICU setting because of the critical nature of illness, antibiotic usage can be curtailed by careful differentiation of colonization from true infection and narrowing of *broad-spectrum* empiricism once cultures are available. Minimizing the duration of antimicrobial use will also decrease exposure. Guidance developed by the Infectious Diseases Society of America and the American Thoracic Society suggests that 5 days of an active antibiotic for community-acquired pneumonia and 7 days for uncomplicated hospital- or ventilator-acquired pneumonia are adequate. Limitation of excess culturing can also avoid repeated sampling of universally positive cultures from endotracheal tubes and urinary catheters. Strict use of infection control measures can also limit health care worker transfer of resistant bacteria from one patient to another. This is especially true for hand washing before and after each patient contact. Patients with MDR bacteria (GPC and GNR) should be placed in a private room and contact precautions (gown and gloves) be practiced by all those entering the room. On a more societal level, removing antibiotics from animal feed products will also lessen antibiotic pressure and selection of resistant strains.

    MDR bacteria are becoming an increasing threat to ICU patients. Although a large array of agents with activity against the resistant *Staphylococcus* and *Enterococcus* now exists, there are very few options for patients infected with MDR GNR. It is feared these options will only become more limited as times goes on. Newer agents to fill the breach are not on the horizon. For the foreseeable future our best defense against this growing menace will be the judicious use of our current limited resources.

KEY POINTS: MULTIDRUG-RESISTANT BACTERIA

1. GNR and GPC MDR bacteria are becoming an increasingly greater problem.

2. Increasing bacterial resistance is caused by excessive antibiotic usage both by physicians and in animal feeds.

3. Before initiating antibiotic therapy it is vital to differentiate between colonization and infection.

4. Many new agents exist with activity against MDR staphylococcus and enterococcus.

5. Because of the lack of new agents with activity against MDR GNR, older drugs such as colistin will be required more often.

BIBLIOGRAPHY

1. Garnacho-Montero J, Amaya-Villar R: Multiresistant *Acinetobacter baumannii* infections: epidemiology and management. Curr Opin Infect Dis 23:332-339, 2010.

2. Hoa J, Tambyaha PA, Paterson DL: Multi-resistant gram-negative infections: a global perspective. Curr Opin Infect Dis 23:546-553, 2010.

3. Kumarasamy KK, Toleman MA, Walsh TR, et al: Emergence of a new antibiotic resistance mechanism in India, Pakistan, and the UK: a molecular, biological, and epidemiological study. Lancet Infect Dis 10:597-602, 2010.

4. Niederman MS, Craven D, Bonten MJ, et al: Guidelines for the management of adults with hospital-acquired, ventilator-associated, and healthcare-associated pneumonia. Am J Respir Crit Care Med 171:388-416, 2005.

5. Nikaido H: Multidrug resistance in bacteria. Annu Rev Biochem 78:119-146, 2009.

6. Overdevest I, Willemsen I, Rijnsburger M, et al: Extended-spectrum β-lactamase genes of Escherichia coli in chicken meat and humans, the Netherlands. Emerg Infect Dis 17:1216-1222, 2011.

7. Roberts RR, Hota B, Ahmad I, et al: Hospital and societal costs of antimicrobial-resistant infections in a Chicago teaching hospital: implications for antibiotic stewardship. Clin Infect Dis 49:1175-1184, 2009.

8. Toleman MA, Bennett PM, Bennett DMC, et al: Global emergence of trimethoprim/sulfamethoxazole resistance in *Stenotrophomonas maltophilia* mediated by acquisition of *sul g*enes. Emerg Infect Dis 13:556-565, 2007.

CHAPTER 37

BIOTERRORISM

Sarah Mooney, MBBCh, MRCP, and Christopher Grace, MD, FACP

1. **What is the definition of bioterrorism?**
   A bioterrorism attack has been defined by the Centers for Disease Control and Prevention (CDC) as "the deliberate release of viruses, bacteria or other agents used to cause illness or death in people, animals or plants." An attack would most likely be occult and have occurred days to weeks before the first patients presenting to the intensive care unit (ICU). Many of the agents are contagious via person-person spread, which may lead to secondary and tertiary waves of ill patients over weeks to months. The intent of an attack is not only to cause significant morbidity and mortality but also to spread terror and panic throughout the population.

2. **What are some possible agents that might be used in an attack?**
   The CDC classifies six pathogens as class A bioterrorism agents: smallpox, plague, botulism, tularemia, viral hemorrhagic fever (VHF), and anthrax. These agents are considered to have the greatest potential for mass casualties, large-scale dissemination, and public panic and social disruption. All of them except VHF have been developed as biological weapons. They are stable in aerosol form and would be most likely delivered in this manner. Most of the civilian population remains susceptible to them, and most cause illnesses not typically seen by providers, causing delayed or missed diagnoses. The major clinical syndromes are summarized in Table 37-1.

3. **What are clues to a biological attack?**
   Recognition of a biological attack may be delayed until patients begin accessing medical care, which may be days to weeks after the event depending on the incubation period of the pathogen (Table 37-1). Features that might suggest a biological attack include the following:
   - Any unusual increase or clustering of patients being seen with clinical symptoms that suggest an infectious disease outbreak
   - A suspected or confirmed communicable disease in a nonendemic area, for example, plague in New England
   - An unusual age distribution of a common disease
   - An unusual temporal and/or geographic clustering of illness, for example, persons who attended the same ball game or parade
   - Simultaneous outbreaks in humans and animals (all class A agents with the exception of smallpox infect animals)
   - An unusual seasonal distribution of illness, for example, influenza-like symptoms in summer

4. **What pathogens would present with respiratory failure?**
   - *Anthrax:* Pneumonic anthrax is caused by the inhalation of the spore form of *Bacillus anthracis*. It begins as a nonspecific influenza-like illness with fever, cough, malaise, headache, and vomiting. Rapid progression occurs to hemorrhagic mediastinitis, hilar lymph node enlargement, respiratory failure, hemodynamic collapse, and death. Although chest radiographs classically show only a widened mediastinum without pulmonary infiltrates, several of the victims from the anthrax letter attacks in the fall of 2001 did have pulmonary infiltrates and pleural effusions. Bacteremia and meningitis can occur.

TABLE 37-1. CATEGORY A BIOTERRORISM AGENTS

BIOLOGICAL AGENT	INCUBATION PERIOD (DAYS)	CLINICAL PRESENTATION	LABORATORY DIAGNOSIS
Anthrax			
Cutaneous	2-5	Necrotic painless edematous ulcer	Blood, sputum, cutaneous lesion Gram stain and culture
Inhalational	1-6	Widened mediastinum and hilar lymphadenopathy	
		Pleural effusions	
		Rapid progression to respiratory failure	
Gastrointestinal	2-5	Abdominal pain	
		Bloody diarrhea	
Smallpox	7-17	Fever before rash	Skin scraping for viral culture, EM, and pathology
		Centrifugal rash progressing synchronously from macules to papules to deep-seeded pustules	
Plague			
Bubonic	2-8	Enlarged , tender, necrotic regional lymph nodes that may drain	Serology
			Blood, sputum, lymph nodes Gram stain and culture
			IF for Fraction 1 (F1) capsular antigen
Pneumonic	1-3	Pneumonia, hemoptysis with rapid progression to respiratory failure	
Septicemic	Bacteremia from bubonic or pneumonia	Fever, shock, petechiae, purpura, and ecchymosis	
Botulism	0.5-3	Symmetric descending paralysis	Toxin identification in stool or serum by mouse neutralization bioassay
		Cranial palsies	
		Dilated pupils, dry mouth	
		Abnormal results of nerve stimulation studies	

(Continued)

TABLE 37-1.   CATEGORY A BIOTERRORISM AGENTS—*cont'd*

BIOLOGICAL AGENT	INCUBATION PERIOD (DAYS)	CLINICAL PRESENTATION	LABORATORY DIAGNOSIS
Tularemia			
Ulceroglandular	3-5	Cutaneous ulceration and regional lymphadenopathy	Sputum and pharyngeal washings for Gram stain and culture
Pneumonia		Initial flulike illness with pharyngitis, bronchitis, conjunctivitis Pneumonia may progress to respiratory failure	Direct FA, PCR, ELISA on sputum Serum antibody for epidemiologic investigation
VHFs	2-21, depending on the virus	Initial flulike illness, conjunctivitis Maculopapular rash Mucocutaneous bleeding Shock	IgM antibody or fourfold rise in IgG Viral isolation

ELISA, Enzyme-linked immunosorbent assay; *EM*, electron microscopy; *FA*, fluorescent antibody; *IF*, immunofluorescent antibody; *IgG*, immunoglobulin G; *IgM*, immunoglobulin M; *PCR*, polymerase chain reaction.

- *Plague:* Pneumonic plague, caused by *Yersinia pestis*, can develop secondarily from bubonic plague via hematogenous dissemination from involved lymph nodes or primarily from inhalation of the plague bacillus. Patients are seen with the sudden onset of headache, fever, shortness of breath, cough, and hemoptysis. Chest radiographs most often reveal bilateral bronchopneumonia. There may be leukocytosis, disseminated intravascular coagulation (DIC), and elevated liver function test results. Rapid progression to respiratory failure and shock ensues.
- *Tularemia:* If *Francisella tularensis* is inhaled, a syndrome similar to community-acquired pneumonia develops with fever, myalgias, headache, pleuritic chest pain, and a dry cough. Concomitant pharyngitis may be present. Some patients demonstrate a pulse-temperature deficit, where an increase in temperature is not accompanied by a relative increase in heart rate. Chest radiographs may have a variety of findings including unilateral or bilateral pneumonia, hilar lymphadenopathy, pleural effusions, and, less often, parenchymal cavitation.

5. **What pathogens would present with shock?**
   - Anthrax and plague may present with shock coupled with pneumonia and respiratory failure.
   - VHF can be caused by a diverse group of RNA viruses including Ebola, Marburg, Lassa fever, and Rift Valley fever from sub-Sahara Africa, in addition to Junin virus, Machupo virus,

Guanarito virus, and Sabia virus from South America. These are all capable of causing a wide spectrum of illness ranging from asymptomatic to life threatening. As the name implies, these viruses cause fever and a bleeding diathesis. Patients typically are seen with an acute febrile illness associated with headache, fatigue, myalgias, abdominal pain, diarrhea, rash, pharyngitis, and hypotension. Bleeding can range from mild conjunctival hemorrhage to severe mucocutaneous bleeding. Progression to shock occurs in severe cases, and patients typically die of septic shock rather than blood loss.

6. **What pathogens would present with paralysis?**
Botulism is caused by a toxin released by *Clostridium botulinum*. The toxin may be ingested from infected food or released from bacteria infecting a wound. Botulism presents as a progressive paralysis, which begins with the bulbar musculature and descends to the extremities and trunk. Typical initial symptoms include diplopia, ptosis, dilated pupils, facial weakness, dysarthria, and dysphagia. Over hours to days, the paralysis descends to the arms, the diaphragm resulting in respiratory failure, and finally the legs. Features that are not consistent with botulism are extremity weakness without bulbar weakness, impaired consciousness, fever except when an aspiration pneumonia has developed, or sensory abnormalities.

7. **What pathogens may present with predominantly cutaneous manifestations?**
   - Smallpox, caused by the DNA virus variola major, is acquired via inhalation of infectious droplets aerosolized by affected patients. Typically a prodrome of fever, chills, myalgias, and headache occurs over 2 to 4 days, followed by the eruption of intraoral macules. A maculopapular rash develops on the face, which then progresses in a centrifugal manner to involve the extremities and finally the trunk. The rash progresses to deep-seated vesicles and pustules over 8 to 10 days. Complications include bacterial superinfections, fluid and electrolyte abnormalities, desquamation, panophthalmitis, residual scarring, and death. Secondary bacterial infections involving the skin or lungs may occur and are often complicated by bacteremia and sepsis.
   - Bubonic plague presents as an acute bacterial lymphadenitis with fever and chills. Enlarged lymph nodes, called buboes, can enlarge to up to 10 cm and may suppurate and drain. A secondary bacteremic phase may follow with sepsis, DIC, purpura, and gangrene of the distal extremities.
   - VHF may present with a diffuse maculopapular rash.

8. **What initial steps should be taken if a patient is suspected to be a victim of a bioterrorist attack?**
If the biological agent is known, appropriate isolation and infection control measures should be implemented as outlined in Table 37-2.
  If the agent of a presumed biological attack is unknown, maximum precautions should be taken including negative pressure room isolation and the use of contact and airborne precautions including N95 respirators or powered air purifying respirators (PAPR). The hospital laboratory should be notified to assist with microbiology work-up and the regional or state health department notified. The names, addresses, and phone numbers of all persons who have been in contact with the patient should be collected.

9. **What infection control measures need to be taken in the ICU?**
The biological agents that pose a transmission threat to health care workers in the ICU include smallpox, plague, and VHFs. Anthrax, botulism, and tularemia are not transmissible to health care workers in the ICU setting. See Table 37-2. Infection control precautions include the following:
   - *Standard:* Gown and/or gloves if contact with body secretions is expected and mask or face shield if facial splash may occur. Hand hygiene before and after patient contact is required.

TABLE 37–2. INFECTION CONTROL FOR CATEGORY A BIOLOGICAL WEAPONS

DISEASE	MODE OF TRANSMISSION	PRECAUTIONS
Anthrax		
Pulmonary	Inhalation of spores	**No person-to-person transmission** Standard precautions Initial decontamination of patient is appropriate
Cutaneous	Direct cutaneous contact with spores into broken skin	**No person-to-person transmission** Standard precautions
Gastrointestinal	Ingestion of contaminated food	**No person-to-person transmission** Standard precautions
Botulism	Ingestion or inhalation of toxin if aerosolized	**No person-to-person transmission** Standard precautions
Plague		
Pneumonic	Inhalation of organism if aerosolized; droplet transmission from an infected person; bite of an infected flea	**Person-to-person transmission** Droplet precautions until patient has received 72 hours of antibiotic therapy
Bubonic		**No person-to-person transmission** Standard precautions
Smallpox	Inhalation of organism if aerosolized; airborne transmission from an infected person (contagious from onset of rash until scabs separate); contact transmission from lesions and clothing or linen	**Person-to-person transmission** Airborne and contact precautions Use negative-pressure rooms Wear N95 respirator or PAPR Exposed individuals should be quarantined during the incubation period Clothing and linen must be isolated

TABLE 37-2.	INFECTION CONTROL FOR CATEGORY A BIOLOGICAL WEAPONS— cont'd	
DISEASE	**MODE OF TRANSMISSION**	**PRECAUTIONS**
Tularemia	Inhalation of organism if aerosolized; contact with infected animals	**No person-to-person transmission** Standard precautions
VHFs	Contact with infected blood or secretions; possibly airborne during end-stage disease	**Person-to-person transmission** Contact and airborne precautions Use negative-pressure isolation rooms Wear N95 respirator or PAPR

- *Contact:* Standard precautions *plus* the wearing of gowns and gloves when entering the room and mask or face shield if facial splash expected.
- *Droplet:* Standard precautions *plus* wearing a surgical mask if within 3 to 6 feet of the patient in a private room.
- *Airborne:* Place patient in negative pressure room, and use fit-tested N95 respirator or PAPR.

10. **How should the patient be treated (Table 37-3)?**
    - *Anthrax:* Cutaneous anthrax can usually be treated with prolonged oral antibiotics for 60 days. Pneumonic anthrax and severe cutaneous disease should initially be treated with intravenous ciprofloxacin or doxycycline coupled with one or two additional agents such as vancomycin, rifampin, or imipenem-cilastatin. Transition to oral ciprofloxacin or doxycycline can be made when the patient is clinically stable. Total treatment should last for 60 days.
    - *Smallpox:* Supportive care is the mainstay. Both cidofovir and imatinib mesylate (Gleevec) may have activity.
    - *Plague:* Intravenous antibiotics should be administered for 7 days.
    - *Tularemia:* Intravenous antibiotics should be given for 10 to 14 days.
    - *Botulism:* Although passive immunization with equine antitoxin is helpful in naturally occurring botulism, it may be of limited usefulness in a terrorist attack because it may not be effective if used more than a few hours after exposure.
    - *VHF:* Therapy is limited. Ribavirin intravenously may have some efficacy against Lassa fever, New World arenaviruses, and Rift Valley fever.

11. **What postexposure prophylaxis (PEP) should be used?**
    PEP against the category A agents is summarized in Table 37-3.

TABLE 37-3. TREATMENT AND POSTEXPOSURE PROPHYLAXIS

PATHOGEN	TREATMENT	POSTEXPOSURE PROPHYLAXIS (ALL ADMINISTERED ORALLY)
Anthrax		
Cutaneous	Ciprofloxacin PO 500 mg bid	Ciprofloxacin 500 mg bid × 60 days
	or	*or*
	Doxycycline PO 100 mg bid	Doxycycline 100 mg bid × 60 days
	or	*or*
	Amoxicillin PO 500 mg tid	Amoxicillin 500 mg tid × 60 days
Pneumonic	Ciprofloxacin IV 400 mg/ 12 hr	
	or	
	Doxycycline IV 100 mg/12 hr	
	and	
	IV vancomycin, rifampin, or imipenem-cilastatin	
Smallpox	Supportive	Vaccination
	Cidofovir	
	or	
	Imatinib mesylate (Gleevec)	
Plague	Ciprofloxacin IV 400 mg/12 hr	Ciprofloxacin 500 mg bid × 7 days
	or	*or*
	Doxycycline IV 100 mg/12 hr	Doxycycline 100 mg bid × 7 days
	or	
	Gentamicin IV 7 mg/kg/day	
Tularemia	Gentamicin 7 mg/kg IV daily	Ciprofloxacin 500 mg bid × 14 days
	or	*or*
	Ciprofloxacin IV 400 mg/12 hr	Doxycycline 100 mg bid × 14 days
	or	
	Doxycycline IV 100 mg/12 hr	
Botulism	Supportive	None
	and	
	Passive immunization with equine antitoxin	
VHFs	Supportive	None
	and	
	Ribavirin	

bid, Twice daily; *IV*, intravenously; *PO*, orally; *tid*, three times daily.

12. What web-based resources can I access?
Resources are listed in Table 37-4.

TABLE 37-4. WEB-BASED RESOURCES		
SOURCE	WEBSITE	COMMENT
U.S. Army Medical Research Institute of Infectious Diseases, Fort Detrick, Md.	www.usamriid.army.mil	Reference materials: Medical Management of Biological Casualties Handbook, "Blue Book"
CDC Public Health Emergency Preparedness and Response	www.bt.cdc.gov	Biological agents Latest BT news Fact sheets Frequently asked questions Links to *MMWR* Preparation and planning Emergency response Laboratory information
CDC National Center for Infectious Diseases	http://emergency.cdc.gov/bioterrorism	Information about specific pathogens
Center for Biosecurity of UPMC	www.upmc-biosecurity.org	BT agents medical summary Fact sheets Review of Dark Winter (smallpox) Links to BT-related journal articles
Infectious Diseases Society of America	www.idsociety.org	BT agents Treatment algorithms Slide sets
Journal of the American Medical Association	jama.ama-assn.org	Key review articles: Smallpox. 281:1735-1745, 1999 Anthrax. 287:2236-2252, 2002 Plague. 283:2281-2290, 2000 Botulism. 285:1059-1070, 2001 Tularemia. 285:2763-2773, 2001 VHF. 287:2391-2405, 2002

(Continued)

TABLE 37-4. WEB-BASED RESOURCES—*cont'd*

SOURCE	WEBSITE	COMMENT
American College of Physicians (ACP)	www.acponline.org/clinical_information/resources/bioterrorism	Overview of BT agents Links to news services ACP testimony Links to federal BT-related websites
Association for Professionals in Infection Control and Epidemiology	www.apic.org	BT agents, diagnosis, and therapy Isolation precautions Patient fact sheets Hospital readiness plans
World Health Organization	www.who.int	Health topics: smallpox Health aspects of biological and chemical weapons
Food and Drug Administration	www.fda.gov	Links to many good BT-related sites
National Institute for Allergy and Infectious Diseases Biodefense Research	www.niaid.nih.gov/dmid/bioterrorism	Research efforts for BT-related immunology, vaccines, and antibiotics
Federal Bureau of Investigation	www.fbi.gov	Summary statements of anthrax investigation

BT, Bioterrorism.

KEY POINTS: CLUES TO RECOGNITION OF A BIOLOGICAL ATTACK

1. Unusual increase or cluster in clinical syndromes

2. Unusual age distribution of disease

3. Unusual temporal and/or geographic clustering of disease

4. Unusual seasonal distribution of disease

5. Suspected or confirmed communicable disease in a nonendemic area

6. Simultaneous outbreaks in humans and animals

BIBLIOGRAPHY

1. Arnon SS, Schechter R, Ingelsby TV, et al: Botulinum toxin as a biological weapon. JAMA 285:1059-1070, 2001.

2. Dennis DT, et al: Tularemia as a biological weapon. In Henderson DA, Inglesby TV, O'Toole T (eds): Bioterrorism: Guidelines for Medical and Public Health Management. Chicago, American Medical Association Press, 2002, pp 611-626.

3. Franz DR, Jahrling PB, Friedlander AM, et al: Clinical recognition and management of patients exposed to biological warfare agents. JAMA 278:399-411, 1997.

4. Henderson DA, Inglesby TV, Bartlett JG, et al: Smallpox as a biological weapon: medical and public health management. JAMA 281:2127-2137, 1999.

5. Inglesby TV, Dennis DT, Henderson DA, et al: Plague as a biological weapon: medical and public health management. JAMA 283:2281-2290, 2000.

6. Inglesby TV, O'Toole T, Henderson DA, et al: Anthrax as a biological weapon, 2002: updated recommendations for management. JAMA 287:2236-2252, 2002.

7. Jernigan DB, Ragunathan PL, Bell BP, et al: Investigation of bioterrorism-related anthrax, United States, 2001: epidemiologic findings. Emerg Infect Dis 8:1019-1028, 2002.

8. Management of patients with suspected viral hemorrhagic fever—United States. MMWR Morb Mortal Wkly Rep 44:475-479, 1995.

9. Miller JM: Agents of bioterrorism. Preparing for bioterrorism at the community level. Infect Dis Clin North Am 15:1127-1156, 2001.

10. Waterer GW, Robertson H: Bioterrorism for the respiratory physician. Respirology 14:5-11, 2009.

CHAPTER 38

SKIN AND SOFT TISSUE INFECTIONS

Erica S. Shenoy, MD, PhD, and David C. Hooper, MD

GENERAL PRINCIPLES

1. **If patients with skin or soft tissue infection are seen with signs of systemic toxicity, what laboratory studies should be undertaken?**

   Blood cultures, cultures of drainage from skin infection site, complete blood cell count with differential, and serum creatinine, bicarbonate, creatine phosphokinase, glucose, albumin, and calcium levels should be obtained. (See Table 38-1.)

2. **What are clinical signs of potential severe deep tissue infection?**
   - Pain disproportionate to physical findings
   - Skin findings: violaceous bullae, ecchymoses, cutaneous hemorrhage, sloughing, anesthesia
   - Rapid progression
   - Gas in tissue
   - Edema beyond the margin of erythema
   - Signs and symptoms of systemic involvement

3. **Which common causative organisms have shown emerging antibiotic resistance?**
   - *Staphylococcus aureus* (methicillin resistance with resistance to all β-lactams except ceftaroline): Assume resistance because of high prevalence of methicillin-resistant *S. aureus* (MRSA), both community and hospital acquired.
   - *Streptococcus pyogenes* (erythromycin resistance): Resistance is increasing to macrolides (approximately 7% in the United States, 2% to 32% reported in Europe), although the majority remain susceptible to clindamycin, and all are susceptible to penicillin.

CELLULITIS

4. **What are the common presentation patterns of cellulitis caused by *S. aureus* or *S. pyogenes*?**
   - *S. aureus*: cellulitis with associated furuncles, carbuncles, or subcutaneous abscesses
   - *S. pyogenes*: cellulitis that is more diffuse and can spread rapidly

5. **What distinguishes impetigo from cellulitis?**

   Impetigo is characterized by discrete purulent lesions, usually on the face, arms, and legs. Bullous and nonbullous forms exist. Whereas impetigo is superficial, cellulitis involves the deep dermis and subcutaneous fat.

6. **Lack of response to initial therapy could signify what?**
   - If a patient does not respond to initial therapy, consider the possibility of resistant strains, atypical organisms, deeper processes such as necrotizing fasciitis or abscess (which may

TABLE 38-1. EVALUATION OF CELLULITIS AND SOFT TISSUE INFECTIONS

	STUDY	FINDING	COMMENTS
Microbiology	Culture and sensitivity	Identification of causative organism and antimicrobial susceptibility data to guide therapeutic choices	When possible, obtain before administration of antibiotics
Laboratory	CBC with differential	Leukocytosis with left shift suggests deep-seated or systemic infection	*Clostridium sordellii*: associated with leukemoid reaction and hemoconcentration
		Thrombocytopenia suggests bacteremia, TSS, or gas gangrene	*C. perfringens*: associated with low hematocrit, elevated LDH, and intravascular hemolysis
	Serum creatinine	Elevation	Seen in group A streptococcal or clostridial myonecrosis, TSS
	Serum CPK	Elevation	Seen in rhabdomyolysis, clostridial or streptococcal myonecrosis, or necrotizing fasciitis
	Serum calcium	Decreased	Seen in staphylococcal or streptococcal TSS or necrotizing fasciitis
Radiology	CT or MRI	Localization of infections and extent of involvement	Useful in early diagnosis of necrotizing infections
	Ultrasound	Necrotizing fasciitis caused by group A streptococcus may reveal thickening of the fascia	CT preferred to ultrasound in adults to define extent of disease

Modified from Stephens DL, Eron LL: In the clinic: cellulitis and soft-tissue infections. Ann Intern Med 150:ITC1-16, 2009.
CBC, Complete blood cell count; *CPK*, creatinine phosphokinase; *CT*, computed tomography; *LDH*, lactate dehydrogenase; *MRI*, magnetic resonance imaging.

require surgical intervention), as well as underlying conditions such as diabetes, chronic venous insufficiency, or lymphedema (which may slow the clinical response to antimicrobial therapy).
- Timely administration of appropriate antibiotic therapy is essential. One study found that each hour of delay between documented hypotension and administration of antibiotics was associated with an average decrease in survival of 7.6% across all sources of infection; subgroup analysis for patients with skin and soft tissue infections demonstrated a significant increase in the adjusted odds ratio of death. This same study found that time to initiation of effective antimicrobial therapy was the strongest predictor of hospital survival. Despite the impact of delayed therapy, the study found that the median time to effective therapy was 6 hours.

7. **What risk factors predispose individuals to development of cellulitis?**
- Obesity
- Previous episodes of cellulitis in the same location (may result in damage to lymphatics)
- Toe-web abnormalities (i.e., maceration, tinea pedis)
- Breach in skin barrier, such as ulcers, trauma, fungal infection, eczema
- Surgical procedures that affect lymphatic drainage such as radical mastectomy with lymph node dissection or coronary artery bypass graft for which the saphenous vein has been harvested
- Chronic medical conditions such as diabetes, arterial insufficiency, chronic venous insufficiency, chronic renal disease, neutropenia, cirrhosis, hypogammaglobulinemia

8. **What organisms are associated with cellulitis in:**
- Cat or dog bites? *Pasteurella multocida, Capnocytophaga canimorsus*
- Fresh water exposure? *Aeromonas hydrophila*
- Saltwater exposure? *Vibrio vulnificus* and other vibrios
- Exposure to fish farming and aquaculture? *Streptococcus iniae*
- Exposure to meatpacking or shellfish? *Erysipelothrix rhusiopathiae*
- Preorbital cellulitis in children? *Haemophilus influenzae*
- Hosts with deficiencies in cell-mediated immunity? *Cryptococcus neoformans*
- Combat trauma patient? *Acinetobacter baumannii*
  See Table 38-2.

TABLE 38-2.	ANTIMICROBIAL THERAPY FOR MSSA AND MRSA SKIN AND SOFT TISSUE INFECTIONS		
ORGANISM	**ANTIBIOTIC**	**ADULT DOSING**	**PEDIATRIC DOSING**
MSSA	Nafcillin or oxacillin	1-2 g IV every 4 hr	100-150 mg/kg/day IV in four divided doses
	Cefazolin	1 g IV every 8 hr	50 mg/kg/day in three divided doses
	Clindamycin	600 mg IV every 8 hr or 300-450 mg PO every 8 hr	25-40 mg/kg/day IV in three divided doses or 10-20 mg/kg/day PO in three divided doses

TABLE 38-2. ANTIMICROBIAL THERAPY FOR MSSA AND MRSA SKIN AND SOFT TISSUE INFECTIONS—cont'd

ORGANISM	ANTIBIOTIC	ADULT DOSING	PEDIATRIC DOSING
	Dicloxacillin	500 mg PO every 6 hr	25 mg/kg/day PO in four divided doses
	Cephalexin	500 mg PO every 6 hr	25 mg/kg/day PO in four divided doses
	Doxycycline, minocycline	100 mg PO every 12 hr	Not recommended in children <8 years old
	TMP-SMZ	1 or 2 DS tabs PO every 12 hr	8-12 mg/kg (based on TMP component) IV in four divided doses or PO in two divided doses
MRSA	Vancomycin	30 mg/kg IV in two divided doses	40 mg/kg/day IV in four divided doses
	Linezolid	600 mg IV or PO every 12 hr	10 mg/kg IV or PO every 12 hr
	Clindamycin	600 mg IV every 8 hr or 300-450 mg PO every 8 hr	25-40 mg/kg/day IV in three divided doses or 10-20 mg/kg/day PO in three divided doses
	Daptomycin	4-6 mg/kg IV every 24 hr	N/A
	Doxycycline, minocycline	100 mg PO every 12 hr	Not recommended in children <8 years old
	TMP-SMZ	1 or 2 DS tabs PO every 12 hr	8-12 mg/kg (based on TMP component) IV in four divided doses or PO in two divided doses

Modified from Stevens DL, Bisno AL, Chambers HF, et al: Practice guidelines for the diagnosis and management of skin and soft-tissue infections. Clin Infect Dis 41:1373-1406, 2005.
DS, Double strength; *MRSA,* methicillin-resistant *S. aureus; MSSA,* methicillin-sensitive *S. aureus; N/A,* not applicable; *PO,* oral; *TMP-SMZ,* trimethoprim/sulfamethoxazole. Note that doses are not adjusted for renal function.

CUTANEOUS ABSCESSES

9. **How are abscesses managed?**
   - Large abscesses should be incised and drained, with careful attention to the potential for loculated cavities (and the disruption of these cavities through probing of the pus pocket).
   - Once drained, the lesion can be left packed or unpacked depending on its extent.
   - In the absence of multiple lesions, gangrene, impaired host defenses, fever, or systemic signs and symptoms of infection, once a cutaneous abscess is drained, systemic antimicrobial therapy may not be needed.

10. **What are the common organisms implicated in cutaneous abscesses?**
    - Monomicrobial infection with *S. aureus* occurs in approximately 25% of cases.
    - Consider polymicrobial infection given predisposing conditions (i.e., diabetes mellitus, trauma resulting in a *dirty wound*) or the location of the abscess (i.e., perianal).

NECROTIZING SKIN AND SOFT TISSUE INFECTIONS

11. **Is necrotizing fasciitis usually monomicrobial or polymicrobial?**
    - Both. Organisms seen in monomicrobial infection include *S. pyogenes*, *V. vulnificus*, *A. hydrophila*, *S. aureus,* and anaerobic streptococci. An average of five different organisms is cultured in the case of polymicrobial infections. Surgical procedures involving the bowels, penetrating abdominal trauma, decubitus ulcer, perianal abscesses, infection at the site of injection drug use, and spread for a Bartholin abscess are associated with polymicrobial necrotizing fasciitis.
    - Necrotizing fasciitis is categorized as type I (usually mixed aerobic and anaerobic) and type II (caused usually by group A *Streptococcus* but also *S. aureus*).
    - *Vibrio* infections have been associated with saltwater exposures. Individuals with hepatic dysfunction are at greater risk for *Vibrio* infection.

12. **Which organisms cause gas gangrene?**
    - Clostridial gas gangrene, or myonecrosis, is caused by *Clostridium perfringens, Clostridium septicum, Clostridium histolyticum,* and *Clostridium novyi*.
    - Predisposing factors include penetrating trauma, crush injuries, and intravenous (IV) drug abuse.
    - *C. perfringens* is the most common cause of trauma-related gas gangrene—symptoms develop within 24 hours of infection. *C. septicum* is the most common cause of spontaneous gangrene and is associated with neutropenia and gastrointestinal malignancies.
    - Antimicrobial therapy includes clindamycin and penicillin because 5% of strains of *C. perfringens* are clindamycin-resistant.
    - Rapid surgical debridement is the most important determinant of outcome.

13. **What is appropriate antimicrobial therapy for necrotizing skin and soft tissue infections?**
    - For mixed infection, ampicillin-sulbactam plus clindamycin plus ciprofloxacin or a third-generation cephalosporin. For patients with severe allergies to penicillin, clindamycin or metronidazole plus an aminoglycoside or fluoroquinolone can be substituted.
    - For streptococcal infections, including streptococcal toxic shock syndrome (TSS), treat with penicillin plus clindamycin. In patients with severe allergies to penicillin, vancomycin, linezolid, quinupristin-dalfopristin, or daptomycin can be substituted for penicillin.
    - The value of IV immunoglobulin (IVIG) in these circumstances has yet to be fully defined. One study showed no improved survival in patients with TSS randomly assigned to receive IVIG, whereas a retrospective cohort analysis did demonstrate improved outcomes. A more recent study in the pediatric population found no difference in outcomes for patients treated for TSS with and without IVIG.

- For *S. aureus* infections, nafcillin, oxacillin, or cefazolin are drugs of choice for susceptible strains. If concern exists for methicillin resistance, vancomycin or clindamycin are options.

INFECTIONS AFTER ANIMAL BITES

14. **Which organisms are commonly isolated after cat bites?**
   Pasteurella spp., most commonly, but these infections are usually polymicrobial. Common organisms found in the oral cavity of cats include *Bartonella henselae*, *Moraxella* spp., staphylococci, streptococci, and anaerobes. Cats with outdoor exposure can additionally carry *Leptospira*, *Listeria*, and *Nocardia* spp. as well as *Francisella tularensis*, *Streptobacillus moniliformis*, *Erysipelothrix rhusiopathiae*, and *Coxiella burnetii*, but these organisms are uncommon causes of cat-bite infections. (See Table 38-3.)

15. **Which organisms are commonly isolated after dog bites?**
   As in cat bites, *Pasteurella* spp. are most common, followed by staphylococci, streptococci, *Moraxella*, corynebacteria, *Neisseria,* and *Capnocytophaga canimorsus.*

16. **Which antibiotics should be administered after a cat or dog bite?**
   Oral amoxicillin-clavulanate, with activity against both *Pasturella* and anaerobes, is a first choice; IV ampicillin-sulbactam or ertapenem can be chosen if IV therapy is required. In cases of invasive disease in patients with severe penicillin allergies, aztreonam has been reported to be successful.

17. **What are the infectious complications of animal bite wounds?**
   - Septic arthritis
   - Osteomyelitis
   - Abscess
   - Tendinitis
   - Bacteremia

18. **What are other considerations after animal bite wounds?**
   - Rabies prophylaxis—in the case of unvaccinated domestic, feral, or wild animal bites
   - Tetanus prophylaxis—in cases in which the last tetanus booster was >5 years previously or unknown

TABLE 38-3. MAJOR PATHOGENS ISOLATED FROM CAT AND DOG BITES		
	AEROBES	**ANAEROBES**
Cat bites	*Pasteurella* spp., *Streptococcus* spp., *Staphylococcus* spp., *Moraxella* spp.	*Fusobacterium* spp., *Bacteroides* spp., *Porphyromonas* spp.
Dog bites	*Pasteurella* spp., *Streptococcus* spp., *Staphylococcus* spp., *Neisseria* spp.	*Fusobacterium* spp., *Bacteroides* spp., *Porphyromonas* spp., *Prevotella* spp., *Capnocytophaga* spp.

Data from Oehler RL, Velez AP, Mizrachi M, et al: Bite-related and septic syndromes caused by cats and dogs. Lancet Infect Dis 9:439-447, 2009.
Note: Most infections include a mix of aerobes and anaerobes.

INFECTIONS AFTER HUMAN BITES

19. **What are the common bacteria responsible for infections after human bites?**
    Streptococci are found in 80% of human bite wounds. Other common organisms include
    staphylococci, *Haemophilus* spp., *Eikenella corrodens*, *Fusobacterium* spp., peptostreptococci,
    Prevotella spp., and *Porphyromonas* spp.

20. **What viruses can be transmitted by human bites?**
    Herpesviruses, hepatitis B and C viruses, and HIV.

21. **Should antibiotics be administered after a human bite?**
    Yes. Prophylactic antibiotics should be given to all patients as early as possible after a human
    bite. Attention should be paid to wound cleaning and the need for debridement as well.

22. **What are the potential complications of human bite infections?**
    - Deep infection of the synovium, joint capsule, and bone in the case of closed-fist
      injuries—early evaluation by a hand surgeon is recommended. Hospitalization for empiric IV
      antibiotics may be needed and should be directed at *S. aureus*, *Haemophilus* spp.,
      E. corrodens, and β-lactamase–producing anaerobes.
    - Radiographs can be useful in identifying foreign bodies (i.e., retained teeth).

SURGICAL SITE INFECTIONS

23. **How common are surgical site infections (SSIs), and what factors are related to
    their incidence?**
    - The development of a SSI depends on a variety of factors, including location and type of
      surgery; duration of the surgery; whether or not the wound was classified as "clean," "clean-
      contaminated," "contaminated," or "dirty," and a series of patient-related risk factors,
      including diabetes, obesity, smoking, colonization or nasal carriage with *S. aureus*, and
      systemic steroids, among other factors.
    - The most commonly isolated organism is *S. aureus*.

24. **What techniques have been shown to reduce the risk of SSI?**
    - Proper skin preparation: avoidance of preoperative use of a razor for removing hair at the
      incision site (clippers should be used if hair removal is needed), use of chlorhexidine-alcohol or
      iodophor-alcohol skin antiseptics
    - Surgical techniques: gentle traction during surgery, effective hemostasis,
      removal of devitalized tissues, obliteration of dead space, irrigation of tissues, use of
      nonabsorbable monofilament suture material, closed-suction drains, and wound closure
      without tension
    - Antimicrobial prophylaxis: preoperative administration of antibiotics within 1 hour before the
      incision is recommended. Cefazolin is a common choice, with clindamycin or vancomycin
      in patients allergic to penicillin. Vancomycin should also be considered in the case of
      institutions where the rate of MRSA is high and in patients with known history of or current
      infection with MRSA (See Table 38-4).

TABLE 38-4. EMPIRIC ANTIBIOTIC THERAPY FOR INTESTINAL/GENITAL TRACT AND NONINTESTINAL SSIs

SURGICAL SITE	SINGLE-AGENT THERAPY	COMBINATION THERAPY	
		FACULTATIVE AND AEROBIC ACTIVITY	ANAEROBIC ACTIVITY
Intestinal or genital tract	• Cefoxitin, or • Ceftizoxime, or • Ampicillin/sulbactam, or • Ticarcillin/clavulanate, or • Piperacillin/tazobactam, or • Imipenem/cilastatin, or • Meropenem, or • Ertapenem	• Fluoroquinolone, or • Third-generation cephalosporin, or • Aztreonam, or • Aminoglycoside	• Clindamycin, or • Metronidazole, or • Chloramphenicol, or • Penicillin agent plus β-lactamase inhibitor
Nonintestinal: trunk and extremities	• Oxacillin, or • First-generation cephalosporin		
Nonintestinal: axillae or perineum	• Cefoxitin, or • Ceftizoxime, or • Ampicillin/sulbactam, or • Ticarcillin/clavulanate, or • Piperacillin/tazobactam, or • Imipenem/cilastatin, or • Meropenem, or • Ertapenum		

Modified from Stevens DL, Bisno AL, Chambers HF, et al: Practice guidelines for the diagnosis and management of skin and soft-tissue infections. Clin Infect Dis 41:1373-1406, 2005.
PCN, Penicillin.

KEY POINTS: SKIN AND SOFT TISSUE INFECTIONS

1. Selection of empiric antimicrobial therapy. In a patient with skin and soft tissue infection, consider host factors including comorbidities, prior microbiologic history, and epidemiologic background.

2. Risk factors that predispose to cellulitis. Obesity, prior cellulitis in the same location, toe-web abnormalities, breach in skin barrier, surgical procedures that affect lymphatic drainage, diabetes, arterial insufficiency, chronic venous insufficiency, chronic renal disease, neutropenia, cirrhosis, and hypogammaglobulinemia are predisposing factors.

(Continued)

3. Appropriate antimicrobial therapy for streptococcal TSS. Penicillin and clindamycin are first-line therapy for patients with severe allergies to penicillin, vancomycin, linezolid, quinupristin-dalfopristin, or daptomycin can be substituted. For *S. aureus* TSS, use vancomycin if concern exists for MRSA.

4. Human bites. Always treat with prophylactic antibiotics; involve surgical service early if complications including deep infection are suspected.

5. SSI rates. SSI rates depend on many factors, including location and type of surgery; duration of the surgery; surgical classification of the wound, and a series of patient-related risk factors.

BIBLIOGRAPHY

1. Anaya DA, Dellinger EP: Necrotizing soft-tissue infection: diagnosis and management. Clin Infect Dis 44:705-710, 2007.

2. Chen I, Kaufisi P, Erdem G: Emergence of erythromycin- and clindamycin-resistant *Streptococcus pyogenes* emm 90 strains in Hawaii. J Clin Microbiol 49:439-441, 2011.

3. Henry FP, Purcell EM, Eadie PA: The human bite injury: a clinical audit and discussion regarding management of this alcohol-fueled phenomenon. Emerg Med J 24:455-458, 2007.

4. Kumar A, Roberts D, Wood KE, et al: Duration of hypotension before initiation of effective antimicrobial therapy is the critical determinant of survival in human septic shock. Crit Care Med 34:1589-1596, 2006.

5. Liu C, Bayer A, Cosgrove SE, et al: Clinical practice guidelines by the Infectious Diseases Society of America for the treatment of methicillin-resistant *Staphylococcus aureus* infections in adults and children. Clin Infect Dis 52:1-38, 2011.

6. Mangram AJ, Horan TC, Pearson ML, et al: Guideline for prevention of surgical site infection, 1999. Infect Control Hosp Epidemiol 20:247-278, 1999.

7. Oehler RL, Velez AP, Mizrachi M, et al: Bite-related and septic syndromes caused by cats and dogs. Lancet Infect Dis 9:439-447, 2009.

8. Seaton RA: Daptomycin: rationale and role in the management of skin and soft tissue infections. J Antimicrob Chemother 62(suppl 3):iii15-iii23, 2008.

9. Sebeny PJ, Riddle MS, Peterson K: *Acinetobacter baumannii* skin and soft-tissue infection associated with war trauma. Clin Infect Dis 47:444-449, 2008.

10. Shah SS, Hall M, Srivastava R, et al: Intravenous immunoglobulin in children with streptococcal toxic shock syndrome. Clin Infect Dis 49:1369-1376, 2009.

11. Stevens DL, Bisno AL, Chambers HF, et al: Practice guidelines for the diagnosis and management of skin and soft-tissue infections. Clin Infect Dis 41:1373-1406, 2005.

12. Stevens DL, Eron LL: In the clinic: cellulitis and soft-tissue infections. Ann Intern Med 150:ITC1-16, 2009.

13. Talan DA, Citron DM, Abrahamian FM, et al: Bacteriologic analysis of infected dog and cat bites. N Engl J Med 340:85-92, 1999.

14. Tsai YH, Wen-Wei Hsu R, Huang KC, et al: Comparison of necrotizing fasciitis and sepsis caused by *Vibrio vulnificus* and *Staphylococcus aureus*. J Bone Joint Surg Am 93:274-284, 2011.

15. Winner JS, Gentry CA, Machado LJ, et al: Aztreonam treatment of *Pasteurella multocida* cellulitis and bacteremia. Ann Pharmacother 37:392-394, 2003.

CHAPTER 39

INFLUENZA

Christopher Grace, MD, FACP

1. What is influenza?

Influenza is a respiratory illness caused by an RNA virus that comes in two forms: influenza A and influenza B. Although generally self-limited, influenza can cause significant morbidity and mortality especially in those at risk (see answer 4 below). Influenza is most common during the fall and winter months because of increased indoor crowding and low humidity, though illness can continue through April and May in the Northern hemisphere.

2. How are influenza A strains designated?

Influenza A is described by the surface glycoproteins: hemagglutinin (H) and neuraminidase (N). The hemagglutinin, of which there are 16 structurally different types, allows attachment to host respiratory epithelium. The neuraminidase, of which there are nine different types, acts as an enzyme that facilitates release of newly replicated viruses from the infected cell. Humans are most often infected with influenza viruses having H1, H2, or H3 and N1 or N2.

The H and N terminology is also used to name the influenza strains spreading yearly. Generally each year one or two influenza A strains and an influenza B strain circulate. During the 2010-2011 season, the circulating strains included A H1N1, A H3N2, and influenza B.

3. What are the symptoms of influenza?

Influenza is characterized by the abrupt onset of fever, nonproductive cough, sore throat, rhinitis, headache, myalgia, and fatigue. Children may also have otitis media. Symptoms generally resolve within 5 to 7 days though the cough may persist for several weeks. During the flu season, an otherwise healthy adult with fever and cough has an 80% to 90% chance of having influenza. Such a simple case definition though may not accurately diagnose influenza in young children, the elderly, or those with comorbid cardiopulmonary illness.

4. Who is at risk for more severe or complicated influenza?

The Centers for Disease Control and Prevention (CDC) has warned that influenza can be especially serious and life threatening for patients with the risk factors as follows:

- Aged 6 months to 4 years
- Aged 50 years and older
- Chronic pulmonary (including asthma), cardiovascular (except hypertension), renal, hepatic, neurologic, hematologic, or metabolic disorders (including diabetes mellitus)
- Immunosuppression caused by medications, organ transplantation, malignancy, or HIV
- Pregnancy during the influenza season
- Aged 6 months to 18 years and receiving long-term aspirin therapy (Reye syndrome)
- Residents of nursing homes and other long-term–care facilities
- American Indians and Alaska Natives
- Morbidly obese (body mass index is 40 or greater)

5. What complications can occur from influenza?

According to the CDC on average in excess of 36,000 deaths and 226,000 hospitalizations are attributable to influenza during each yearly flu season. Influenza can cause a primary viral hemorrhagic pneumonia characterized by progressive dyspnea and leukocytosis, potentially progressing to respiratory failure and acute respiratory disease syndrome. A secondary bacterial pneumonia may develop in older patients and those with chronic cardiopulmonary illness. After a period of improvement the patient appears to worsen with signs and symptoms of bacterial pneumonia, most often caused by *Streptococcus pneumoniae, Haemophilus influenzae,* or *Staphylococcus aureus.*

In addition, patients may have exacerbations of chronic cardiopulmonary illnesses. Less-common complications include myositis, myocarditis, pericarditis, encephalitis, a toxic shock–like illness, Guillain-Barré syndrome, and Reye syndrome.

6. **What other infections can mimic influenza?**
   The symptoms of influenza are very nonspecific and can be caused by a large array of viruses and bacteria. Because these pathogens can cause an illness similar to influenza, any febrile respiratory illness may be referred to as influenza-like illness (ILI). Causes of ILI, in addition to influenza, include respiratory syncytial virus, parainfluenza, rhinovirus, and coronavirus (agents of the common cold); adenovirus; metapneumovirus; group A streptococcus; mycoplasma; chlamydia; and *Bordetella pertussis.*

7. **How do you diagnose influenza?**
   Influenza is often a clinical diagnosis. For those without risks for complications or requiring hospitalization, no further diagnostics are required. The most accurate way to confirm that a patient does or does not have influenza is to obtain a nasopharyngeal swab. The swab is the same one used to collect and transport bacterial culture samples. The swab needs to be inserted through the nose to the pharynx. Testing by polymerase chain reaction (PCR) is most accurate. Testing by rapid influenza diagnostic tests (RIDT) is not very sensitive (50%-70%) but is reasonably specific (90%-95%). A negative RIDT is not helpful. A positive RIDT can be helpful, and most people with a positive RIDT have influenza A.

8. **What is the approach to the patient with an ILI?**
   The approach to the patient with ILI can progress in a stepwise manner. The patient should be assessed for degree of illness and presence of risk factors for complications.

   Those with mild symptoms (no shortness of breath and able to maintain hydration) and no risks for complications do not need further testing and can be treated symptomatically. Those with moderate symptoms (some shortness of breath, difficulty maintaining hydration, signs and symptoms of pneumonia) should be tested and treated with antiviral medications. Those with severe symptoms (respiratory distress, altered mental status) need immediate assessment in the emergency department. Pregnant women with influenza, especially those in the third trimester, have a high rate of complications and should be urgently assessed in the emergency department also. See Figure 39-1.

9. **How do you treat influenza?**
   M2 channel blockers, such as amantadine and rimantadine, are not often used because of emergence of resistance and central nervous system toxicity. Neuraminidase inhibitors such as oseltamivir and zanamivir act by blocking the surface neuraminidase. Both are active against influenza A and B. Oseltamivir is oral and dosed at 75 mg twice daily for 5 days for treatment. Zanamivir is a nasal spray and has been approved for persons aged ≥ 7 years. These agents have been shown to shorten the duration of influenza symptoms but only modestly; if started within 48 hours of symptoms, the duration of the illness may be decreased by approximately 1 day. Several intravenous (IV) formulations are in research such as IV zanamivir and peramivir that may be used in critically ill persons who are unable to use or absorb the conventional agents.

10. **How do you manage a patient admitted to the hospital with ILI?**
    All patients with ILI during the fall-winter flu season admitted to the hospital should be presumed to have influenza until ruled out by nasopharyngeal PCR. Until that test result is back, they should:
    - Be isolated in a private room.
    - Have standard and droplet precautions used.

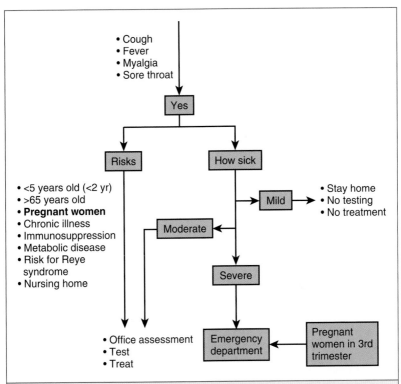

Figure 39-1. Approach to the patient with an ILI. When testing and treatment are being decided on, the patient's risk for complications and severity of illness need to be taken into account.

- Be treated with neuraminidase inhibitors. Consideration should be given to treating with antibiotics such as ceftriaxone and vancomycin to cover potential streptococcal, staphylococcal, and *Haemophilus* superinfection.
  If the nasopharyngeal PCR returns negative, influenza treatment and isolation can be stopped. Keep in mind that a negative RIDT does not rule out influenza.

11. **What are epidemics and pandemics?**
    The hemagglutinin (H) and neuraminidase (N) undergo small changes in structure called antigenic drift on a yearly basis, which allows the virus to partially evade humans' past immune response and cause yearly epidemics. Larger changes in the H and N, called antigenic shift, occur infrequently. When antigenic shift occurs, much of the population has essentially no or limited immunity to the new strain, and a pandemic may occur as was seen in 1918, 1956, 1967, and 2009. Pandemic refers to a new viral type and worldwide spread but not severity. The 1918 pandemic was very severe, causing an estimated 50 to 100 million deaths worldwide, whereas the 2009 pandemic was no more severe than a usual epidemic year, though it disproportionately affected younger adults and children.

12. **What have we learned from past pandemics?**
    The influenza virus can mutate and reassort frequently and randomly making occurrence of pandemics unpredictable. Over the past 300 years there has been no regular periodicity with

times between pandemics varying from 8 to 42 years. Pandemics often unfold in waves of severity over several years as occurred in 1918. Pandemics disproportionately affect the young as occurred in both 1918 and 2009. Pandemics may not follow seasonal (fall-winter) patterns as evidenced by the 2009 pandemic's springtime arrival.

13. What is "bird flu"?

Viral strains that affect predominately birds including aquatic fowl and domestic poultry are referred to as bird flu and generally do not infect humans. In 1997, a bird flu, H5N1, infected 18 people in Hong Kong, resulting in six deaths. It reappeared in 2003 infecting persons in Vietnam, Cambodia, Laos, Thailand, Indonesia, China, Egypt, and central Asia. As of March 16, 2011, there have been 534 confirmed human infections with H5N1 with 316 deaths, a startling 59% mortality. The great majority of these patients had extensive direct contact with infected poultry. Several limited episodes of human-to-human transmission have occurred but no sustained transmission. Although the H5N1 virus is still circulating and continues to cause illness and death in these countries, it has not attained the ability, yet, to be easily transmitted to or between people.

14. What was the pandemic of 2009?

During the 2009-2010 influenza season, a large change in the H and N structure occurred, leaving much of the population, especially those younger than 65 years old, with inadequate immunity. This new structure was the result of a reassortment of bird, swine, and human influenza strains resulting in an antigenically new H1N1 strain. It appeared to start simultaneously in Southern California and Mexico in the spring of 2009 and spread rapidly worldwide with the World Health Organization declaring a pandemic on June 11, 2009. Young adults and children were particularly affected. In Argentina, for example, pediatric hospitalization rates doubled. Of hospitalized children, 19% were admitted to the intensive care unit (ICU), 17% required mechanical ventilation, and 5% died. In the United States, 45% of patients admitted to the hospital were under the age of 18 years. Seventy-three percent of patients had at least one underlying condition including asthma, diabetes, heart, lung and neurologic diseases, and pregnancy.

15. How severe was the pandemic of 2009?

Fortunately the 2009 pandemic was a *mild* pandemic as compared with that in 1918. The severity has been estimated to be similar to that of the 1957 and 1968 pandemics. Many countries including Australia, Spain, and the United States reported more ICU admissions, patients requiring mechanical ventilation, and deaths. Those admitted to ICUs often had extensive multifocal pneumonias on chest radiograph. In one study of those admitted to the ICU, 36% had pulmonary emboli on chest computed tomography. Early in the pandemic, Spain noted that 91% of the patients admitted to the ICU had primary viral pneumonia, 75% had multiorgan failure, 75% required mechanical ventilation, and 22% needed renal replacement therapy. In the Australia and New Zealand experience, one third of patients receiving mechanical ventilation were treated with extracorporeal membrane oxygenation (ECMO), and 21% died. In Canadian experience, 81% of critically ill patients received mechanical ventilation for a median of 12 days. The 28-day mortality of these patients was 14.3%. Lung rescue therapies included neuromuscular blockade (28%), inhaled nitrous oxide (13.7%), high-frequency oscillatory ventilation (11.9%), ECMO (4.2%), and prone-positioning ventilation (3.0%). The 90-day mortality was 17.3%.

16. How should the patient admitted to the ICU be managed?

Any patient admitted to the ICU with a respiratory illness during the influenza season should be presumed to have influenza until proved otherwise by nasopharyngeal swab PCR. Patients may be seen with exacerbations of underlying cardiopulmonary diseases, primary viral pneumonia, or secondary bacterial pneumonias. All patients should be given treatment with a neuraminidase inhibitor and antibiotics. Antibacterial therapy should be directed primarily against *S. pneumoniae*, *S. aureus*, and *H. influenzae*. Possible initial regimens may include ceftriaxone and vancomycin. Once respiratory and blood culture results are known, the empiric antibiotics should be narrowed or stopped.

17. **What infection control measures are needed?**
    Influenza is most often spread by large-particle respiratory droplets created by patient coughing or sneezing. This mode of transmission generally requires close contact (3-6 feet) because these larger and heavier respiratory particles quickly fall out of the air. Hand contact with environmental surfaces contaminated with the virus can also transmit influenza when those hands come in contact with mucosal surfaces such as touching the eye, nose, or mouth. Concern has been expressed that influenza may be airborne transmitted by small-particle aerosols, though it is not clear how much this mode of transmission contributes to community spread. For the office and hospital, the CDC recommends standard and droplet precautions as follows:
    - Placing the patient in a private room.
    - Wearing a surgical mask when entering the patient room.
    - Wearing gloves and gowns if you should expect contact with patient's blood, body fluids, or secretions (including respiratory).
    - If participating in an aerosol-generating procedure such as intubation, extubation, bronchoscopy, or autopsy, a fit-tested N95 respirator or a powered air-purifying respirator (PAPR) should be worn.

      All health care workers need to practice good hand hygiene before and after patient contact.

18. **Who should get the influenza vaccine?**
    The CDC now recommends that all persons older than 6 months get yearly vaccination. This is especially true for those at high risk for complications of influenza as outlined earlier. The subcutaneous injectable form uses inactivated hemagglutinin antigen from three circulating vaccine strains. For those between 2 and 49 years of age who are in good health and not pregnant, a nasal aerosol of live attenuated viruses is available. Both forms are safe and effective. In children and adults younger than 65 years, approximately 90% developed protective levels of antibodies, though that may be less effective in the elderly and immune compromised. All health care workers need to be vaccinated yearly so as to remain healthy and not risk spreading influenza to the more vulnerable patients.

KEY POINTS: INFLUENZA

1. Influenza can cause severe respiratory illness requiring ICU care.

2. Influenza may exacerbate underlying cardiopulmonary conditions.

3. All patients admitted to the hospital for presumed influenza should be treated with antiviral medications.

4. Secondary bacterial pneumonias may develop and should be looked for and treated.

5. All persons aged older than 6 months should be vaccinated yearly.

BIBLIOGRAPHY

1. Fiore AE, Fry A, Shay D, et al: Antiviral agents for the treatment and chemoprophylaxis of influenza. Recommendations of the Advisory Committee on Immunization Practices (ACIP). MMWR Recomm Rep 60:1-24, 2011.

2. Girard MP, Tam JS, Assossou OM, et al: The 2009 A (H1N1) influenza virus pandemic: a review. Vaccine 28:4895-4902, 2010.

3. Homsi S, Milojkovic N, Homsi Y: Clinical pathological characteristics and management of acute respiratory distress syndrome resulting from influenza A (H1N1) virus. South Med J 103:786-790, 2010.

4. Kumar A, Zarychanski R, Pinto R, et al: Critically ill patients with 2009 influenza A (H1N1) infection in Canada. JAMA 302:1872-1879, 2009.

5. Tang JW, Shetty N, Tsan-Yuk Lam T: Features of the new pandemic influenza A/H1N1/2009 virus: virology, epidemiology, clinical and public health aspects. Curr Opin Pulm Med 16:235-241, 2010.

CHAPTER 40

IMMUNOCOMPROMISED HOST

Kristen K. Pierce, MD

1. **What is the initial approach to the immunocompromised host in the intensive care unit (ICU)?**
   The approach in the ICU setting relies on several factors:
   - High index of clinical suspicion: Immune-compromised hosts often have atypical presentations of infection. For example, patients with severe immunocompromise may lack fever or abscess formation.
   - Understanding of the host's immune defect: Recognizing the deficient pathway (cell mediated vs. humoral) enables the physician to expand the differential diagnosis and has implications for empiric therapy.
   - Aggressive diagnostics: Blood work and cultures, imaging, bronchoscopy, and tissue biopsy, if indicated, are all essential in the initial work-up of a suspected infection.
   - Early appropriate antimicrobial therapy: This is key when dealing with infections in the immunocompromised patient.

2. **What is the "net state of immunosuppression," and why is it important?**
   The concept of a net state of immunosuppression describes the infection potential in immunocompromised hosts. For example, a patient who underwent splenectomy 10 years ago after traumatic injury has a very different infection risk than does a patient with HIV/AIDS. This is important in understanding a patient's susceptibility to, and risk for, infection. The net state of immunosuppression is determined by the following characteristics:
   - Immunosuppressive medications. The degree of immunosuppression conferred by these medications will be influenced by their type, dose, and duration of therapy.
   - Presence of leukopenia. Long-standing neutropenia carries a different risk of infection as compared with acute-onset neutropenia. For example, acute neutropenia conveys an increased risk of infections with gram-negative and enteric organisms. As the duration of neutropenia continues, these patients are at increasing risk for invasive fungal infections.
   - Metabolic factors. Poor nutrition, hyperglycemia, and uremia all confer an increased risk for infection.
   - Concurrent infection with immunomodulating viruses such as cytomegalovirus (CMV), Epstein-Barr virus (EBV), hepatitis B and C, human herpes virus 6 (HHV-6), and HIV. These infections can weaken the host's defenses either by a low level of viral replication or by reducing the function of infected white blood cells. This leads to an increased risk for bacterial or fungal infection.
   - Anatomic factors. The presence of obstructing tumors, stents, central venous catheters, and endotracheal tubes can affect a host's risk for infection.

3. **How is immunosuppression measured?**
   Assessment can be based on the following:
   - Duration and level of neutropenia in those undergoing cytotoxic chemotherapy are used to determine the risk of infection and need for empiric antibiotic therapy. For example, patients with a longer duration of absolute neutropenia have a greater risk for invasive fungal infection compared with patients with acute neutropenia.

- CD4 cell count in patients with HIV is an accurate measure of their immune function. A patient with HIV who has an absolute CD4 count of 700/mm^3 has a very different infection risk compared with someone whose CD4 counts are under 100/mm^3.
- Treatment, type, and duration of therapy in patients receiving immunosuppression after solid organ, stem cell, or bone marrow transplantation (BMT). Also, the type of transplant (matched or unmatched donor) may be important. Patients who undergo stem cell transplantation or BMT from an allogeneic human leukocyte antigen–identical sibling or matched unrelated donor are at greatest risk for infection because they may require more immunosuppression.

4. **Do certain immunosuppressive therapies carry a specific risk of infection?**
See Table 40-1.

5. **How does the timing of solid organ transplantation affect a patient's risk for infection?**
See Table 40-2.

6. **Describe the timing of infection in hematopoietic stem cell transplant recipients.**
Preengraftment: generally accepted as the first 2 to 4 weeks after transplantation and lasting until the engraftment of the transplant. During this period patients often have profound neutropenia and may have neutropenic fever and the ensuing complications. Patients are at risk for bacterial infections from their own endogenous bowel flora (*Escherichia coli*, *Klebsiella*, and *Pseudomonas*) and from skin flora such as *Staphylococcus* and *Streptococcus* because of invasive intravenous (IV) lines or skin breakdown. The longer the duration of neutropenia, the greater is the risk of invasive fungal infection with opportunistic fungi, such as aspergillus. Reactivation of latent viruses, such as CMV and herpes simplex virus (HSV), can occur during this period as well, leading to systemic infection.

Early postengraftment: the period from the time of neutrophil engraftment until day 100. With the exception of those patients who still have indwelling catheters, bacterial infection is less common during this time period. Patients who have difficulties with engraftment or those in whom graft-versus-host disease (GVHD) may develop, requiring increased doses of steroids, are at risk for invasive fungal infections as well as viral infections (CMV and HSV).

Late postengraftment: ranging from around day 100 until immunity is restored. Patients are generally at risk for encapsulated bacterial infections (*Haemophilus influenzae*, *Streptococcus pneumoniae*, *Neisseria meningitidis*), fungal infections (*Candida* spp. and *Aspergillus* spp.), and late CMV infection.

7. **What is the initial recommended work-up of suspected infection in the immunocompromised host?**
History and physical. Clinical clues regarding unusual exposures can assist in creating a broad differential for suspected infection. Certain physical examination findings can be indicative of certain types of infection, and through physical examination, including visualization of the oropharynx, skin, and perirectal areas, looking for occult abscess is important.

However, it is important to recognize that digital rectal examinations should not be performed in patients with neutropenia, nor should they be allowed to have rectal instillation of contrast for abdominal computed tomography (CT) scans, because of the risk of hematogenous dissemination of the patients' endogenous bowel flora.

Questions that may provide clinical clues to source of infection:
- Type and duration of immunosuppressive medication
- Duration of time since transplantation
- Sick exposures: family members, co-workers
- Recent travel, both in and outside of the country
- Pets or animal exposures
- Eating habits: raw fish, game meat

TABLE 40-1. COMMON IMMUNOSUPPRESSIVE MEDICATIONS

AGENT	MECHANISM OF ACTION	ASSOCIATED RISK OF INFECTION
Corticosteroids	Down-regulates lymphocyte and macrophage function Interferes with inflammatory response	Long-term use—PCP, hepatitis B, bacterial, molds, mycobacterial disease Bolus use—CMV, BK virus nephropathy
Calcineurin inhibitors • Cyclosporine • Tacrolimus	Blocks T-cell activation targeting calcineurin	Viral infections: BK, CMV, VZV Bacterial and fungal infections
Mycophenolate mofetil	Blocks T- and B-cell proliferation	Viral: CMV, BK virus
Sirolimus	Arrests cell replication Decreases IL-2	PCP, CMV, BK virus
T-lymphocyte depletion* • Antithymocyte globulin • OKT3	Depletes lymphocytes	CMV, HSV reactivation late fungal and viral infections
B-lymphocyte depletion • Plasmapheresis • Rituximab	Depletes B cells	Encapsulated bacterial infections
Anti-TNF (TNF-α agents)	Neutralizes the biologic activity of TNF-α	Mycobacterial infections Hepatitis B reactivation Lymphoma

Modified from Fishman JA, Issa NC: Infections in organ transplantation: risk factors and evolving patterns of infection. Infect Dis Clin North Am 24:273-283, 2010, and Danovitch G: Immunosuppressive medications and protocols for kidney transplantation. In Danovitch G (ed): Handbook of Kidney Transplantation. Philadelphia, Lippincott Williams & Wilkins, 2004, pp 72-134.
IL, Interleukin; *TNF*, tumor necrosis factor; *VZV*, varicella-zoster virus.
*Immunosuppression is greater when used as a bolus for antirejection rather than when used as initial induction therapy.

- Hobbies: hunting, fishing, gardening
- History of tuberculosis exposure
- Use of antimicrobial prophylaxis for viral or bacterial infection
- Insect exposures
- Food-borne illnesses
- Recent home renovations
- Recent unprotected sexual intercourse

TABLE 40-2. RISK OF INFECTION AND TIME FROM TRANSPLANTATION	
MONTHS AFTER TRANSPLANTATION	TYPE OF INFECTION
0-1	**Hospital Derived**
	Surgical site infection
	MRSA, VRE
	Catheter infections
	MRSA, VRE
	Candidal infections
	Ventilator-associated
	Aspiration
	C. difficile colitis
	Donor-Derived Infections
	Reactivated HSV
	West Nile virus
	HIV
1-6*	**Opportunistic Infections**
	CMV
	PCP
	Cryptococcus
	L. monocytogenes
	EBV
	Adenovirus
	HHV-6
	Reactivation of Latent Recipient Infections
	Coccidioides immitis
	Mycobacterium tuberculosis
	Histoplasmosis
	Blastomycosis
	Reactivation of Latent Donor Derived
	HIV
	Hepatitis B or C
≥6	**Community Acquired**
	Pneumonia
	Urinary tract infections
	Fungal Infections
	Atypical molds
	Aspergillus
	Atypical Bacterial
	Nocardia
	Listeria
	Cryptococcus

TABLE 40-2. RISK OF INFECTION AND TIME FROM TRANSPLANTATION—*cont'd*

MONTHS AFTER TRANSPLANTATION	TYPE OF INFECTION
	Late Viral Infections
	Polyomavirus infection
	Reactivated VZV
	CMV
	EBV

Modified from Fishman J: Infection in solid organ transplant recipients. N Engl J Med 357:2601-2614, 2007, and Syndman DR: Epidemiology of infections after solid-organ transplantation. Clin Infect Dis 33 (Suppl 1):S5, 2001.
VZV, Varicella-zoster virus.
*Generally thought to be the time of greatest immunosuppression.

Blood cultures. Two sets should be obtained. If a patient has an indwelling central venous catheter a set should be collected from each lumen; at least one peripheral set should be obtained as well.

Complete blood cell count with differential; serum creatinine, blood urea nitrogen, electrolytes, and liver function tests.

Cultures should be obtained from other sites of potential infection: urine, sputum, and stool.

Imaging. A chest radiograph is clinically indicated for those patients complaining of respiratory symptoms or with objective findings such as changes in oxygenation, chest pain, or cough. Abdominal imaging may be indicated for those with abdominal complaints: nausea, vomiting or diarrhea, abnormal liver function testing, or evidence of gram-negative bacteremia.

8. **What infectious causes should be considered in a patient without a spleen who has suspected sepsis?**
   Patients who have undergone splenectomy represent a special subset of the immune-compromised host. The spleen functions to produce opsonizing antibody and facilitates the clearance of encapsulated bacteria, organisms that can otherwise evade antibody and complement binding. Whether from surgical removal or functional asplenia (radiation, Hodgkin disease), these patients are at risk from a fulminant sepsis syndrome, known as postsplenectomy syndrome (PSS) or overwhelming postsplenectomy infection (OPSI), which carries a mortality rate approaching 70%. PSS is characterized as a fulminant sepsis, meningitis, or pneumonia that occurs days to years after splenic removal. Although the risk of severe infection is highest in the first few years after removal, fatal cases of PSS have been well documented even decades after the initial splenectomy. Encapsulated organisms such *N. meningitidis, H. influenzae,* and *S. pneumoniae* are the three most cited etiologic agents. In addition, *Capnocytophaga canimorsus* can lead to fulminant infection after dog bites. *Babesia microti* in North America and *Babesia bovis* in Europe, in those with appropriate travel history, can cause severe disease in hosts without a spleen. *Salmonella* species, although not a prominent pathogen, is a common cause of illness in children with sickle cell disease and splenic dysfunction. A wide variety of other bacteria have also been implicated in anecdotal reports.

9. **What is the initial treatment for a patient without a spleen who is seen with sepsis?**
   In addition to aggressive supportive care, treatment of suspected postsplenectomy sepsis involves appropriate empiric antibiotic therapy directed at encapsulated organisms. Although *S. pneumoniae* is responsible for 50% of cases, oftentimes no etiologic agent is cultured. Empiric

antibiotic choices should include coverage for *Streptococcus*, allowing for concerns of penicillin resistance, β-lactamase–producing organisms, and broad gram negative to include *Neisseria* and *H. influenzae*. Antibiotic allergy and local antibiotic resistance need to be taken into consideration when choosing an initial empiric regimen. However, combinations such as vancomycin and ceftriaxone or moxifloxacin or vancomycin and cefepime plus moxifloxacin would be reasonable starting regimens while awaiting microbiologic results.

10. **What is the differential diagnosis in an immunocompromised patient who is seen with a central nervous system (CNS) infection?**
Infections of the CNS are a medical emergency. Although compromised hosts are more susceptible to certain pathogens on the basis of their underlying immune defect, they are also at risk for the same infections as the general population. The clinical presentation of disease may be more subacute in the immunocompromised patients and can offer clues as to the microbiologic entity, especially when the nature of the immune defect of the host is taken into consideration as well. An understanding of the net state of immunosuppression of the patient can provide insight into creating a differential diagnosis of the nature of CNS infection based on clinical presentation. See Table 40-3.

TABLE 40-3. DIFFERENTIAL DIAGNOSIS OF SUSPECTED CNS INFECTION BASED ON UNDERLYING IMMUNE DEFECT

IMMUNE DEFECT	MENINGITIS	ENCEPHALITIS	MENINGOENCEPHALITIS
Impaired humoral immunity–B-cell dysfunction			
Multiple myeloma	*S. pneumoniae*	Echovirus	*L. monocytogenes*
Hyposplenism	*N. meningitides*	Poliovirus	*Cryptococcus*
Immunoglobulin deficiencies	*H. influenzae*		
B-cell lymphoma			
CLL			
Alcoholic liver disease			
Impaired cell-mediated immunity–T-cell dysfunction			
HIV/AIDS	*S. pneumoniae*	VZV	*L. monocytogenes*
Corticosteroid use	*N. meningitides*	HSV	*Cryptococcus*
Hodgkin lymphoma	*H. influenzae*	CMV	
Solid organ transplantation	*Cryptococcus*	WNV	
Stem cell transplantation	Acute HIV infection	JC virus	
Chronic renal failure			

TABLE 40-3. DIFFERENTIAL DIAGNOSIS OF SUSPECTED CNS INFECTION BASED ON UNDERLYING IMMUNE DEFECT—*cont'd*

IMMUNE DEFECT	MENINGITIS	ENCEPHALITIS	MENINGOENCEPHALITIS
Impaired granulocyte function			
ALL	*S. pneumoniae*	HSV	
BMT	*S. aureus**		
Chemotherapy-induced leukopenia	*P. aeruginosa**		
	N. meningitides		
	H. influenzae		

Modified from Cunha BA: Central nervous system infections in the compromised host: a diagnostic approach. Infect Dis Clin North Am 15:567-590, 2001, and Linden PK: Approach to the immunocompromised host with infection in the intensive care unit. Infect Dis Clin North Am 23:535-556, 2009.
ALL, Acute lymphocytic leukemia; *CLL,* chronic lymphocytic leukemia; *JC,* John Cunningham virus; *VZV,* varicella-zoster virus.
*Especially in those with indwelling devices (i.e., catheters, pumps).

11. **What is the initial diagnostic approach to an immunocompromised patient who is seen with a suspected CNS infection?**
   Work-up should include the following:
   - Imaging study
     □ CT scan can reveal acute hemorrhage, mass effect, bony or subdural lesions.
     □ Magnetic resonance imaging can better evaluate the brain parenchyma, evidence and characteristics of mass lesions, brainstem and spinal cord lesions, edema.
   - Lumbar puncture
     □ Opening pressure
     □ Cerebrospinal fluid (CSF)
   - Cell count and differential
   - Glucose, protein, and lactate
   - Gram stain and bacterial culture
   - Cryptococcal antigen
   - Acid-fast smear and culture
   - Fungal smear and culture
   - Polymerase chain reaction (PCR) for HSV and other viral causes as clinically appropriate and influenced by seasonal and geographic variation: enterovirus, West Nile virus (WNV), eastern equine encephalitis, western equine encephalitis, sick contacts, and degree of immunosuppression
   - Biopsy
     If no definitive answer can be obtained from lumbar puncture, aspiration or biopsy of CNS lesions may be required for definitive diagnosis.

12. **Do special considerations exist for the treatment of meningitis and mass lesions in the immunocompromised host?**
   Although infection of the CNS is life threatening, it is important to recognize that noninfectious mimics of CNS infections exist that should be taken into consideration as well and will not be discussed in detail here.

Bacterial meningitis. Treatment in the immunocompromised host should include coverage for the usual bacterial pathogens (*N. meningitidis, H. influenzae,* and *S. pneumoniae*), with attention to the possibility of penicillin-resistant *S. pneumoniae, Staphylococcus aureus* (especially in those with indwelling lines or shunts), and also *Listeria monocytogenes*. Often compromised patients with *Listeria* meningitis will be seen with subacute meningitis. However, the organism will usually grow in CSF cultures in 24 to 48 hours; thus empiric therapy should be continued until cultures are negative.

Mass lesions. Several viral, fungal, and parasitic pathogens can present as mass lesions in an immunocompromised host and masquerade as tumor or bacterial abscess. Significant efforts should be made to establish a microbiologic or tissue diagnosis of CNS lesions because the differential is quite broad, making empiric therapy challenging and not recommended.

13. **What is the definition of neutropenia?**
Neutropenia is defined as an absolute neutrophil count (ANC) of <500 cells per cubic millimeter. The term may also be applied to those patients in whom an ANC decrease to <500 cells per cubic millimeter is expected within the next 2 days. Some patients will have a relatively normal ANC yet still have profoundly impaired phagocytosis. These patients are said to have *functional neutropenia* and are still at risk for opportunistic infections despite their normal counts.

14. **Describe empiric therapy for the hospitalized patient with febrile neutropenia.**
Patients with febrile neutropenia require empiric IV antibiotic therapy with an antipseudomonal β-lactam agent, such as meropenem, imipenem-cilastatin, piperacillin-tazobactam, or cefepime. Additional antibiotics (quinolones, vancomycin) may be added if concern exists for resistant organisms, vancomycin-resistant enterococcus (VRE), methicillin-resistant *S. aureus* (MRSA), resistant gram-negative rods, presence of hypotension, or suspicion of a pulmonary infection.

15. **Describe the initial antibiotic regimen in a patient with febrile neutropenia who is allergic to penicillin.**
The majority of patients who report an allergy to penicillin will tolerate cephalosporins and carbapenems. However, in those patients with an immunoglobulin (Ig) E–mediated immediate-type hypersensitivity reaction (hives, bronchospasm), these drug classes should be avoided. In this group of patients, alternative therapeutic options include ciprofloxacin and clindamycin or vancomycin and aztreonam.

16. **What are the most common bacterial causes of community-acquired pneumonia in the immunocompromised host?**
S. pneumoniae, H. influenzae, or *Moraxella catarrhalis* are the most common pathogens. In patients with cell-mediated immune defects, legionnaires disease is the most common atypical pathogen. Compared with normal hosts, oral anaerobes as a result of oropharyngeal aspiration, *Mycoplasma*, and *Chlamydia* are less-common causes of infection in the compromised host. *Pseudomonas aeruginosa*, an unusual respiratory pathogen in normal hosts, has been implicated as a cause of community-acquired pneumonia in patients with cystic fibrosis or bronchiectasis and in patients living with AIDS.

17. **What is the differential diagnosis for an immunocompromised patient with fever and pulmonary infiltrates?**
Respiratory compromise in the immunocompromised host carries with it a significant mortality rate with estimates between 30% and 90%. Although the physician must consider noninfectious causes of pulmonary infiltrates (Box 40-1), infectious causes require early recognition and

---

BOX 40-1. NONINFECTIOUS CAUSES OF PULMONARY INFILTRATES IN IMMUNOCOMPROMISED HOST

- Radiation pneumonitis
- Lymphangitic spread of underlying malignancy
- Drug-induced lung toxicity
- Cryptogenic organizing pneumonia (COP) or bronchiolitis obliterans–organizing pneumonia (BOOP)
- Diffuse alveolar hemorrhage
- ARDS
- Pulmonary edema
- Pulmonary embolism or infarction
- Idiopathic pulmonary fibrosis

---

treatment. The differential is based on understanding of the immune defect and characterization of the radiographic pattern of infiltrate, in conjunction with the timing of onset of symptoms. However, it is vital to recognize that no one radiographic appearance is pathognomonic for a specific infection (Table 40-4).

18. **What is the role of bronchoalveolar lavage (BAL) and lung biopsy in the diagnosis of pulmonary infiltrates?**
See Figure 40-1.

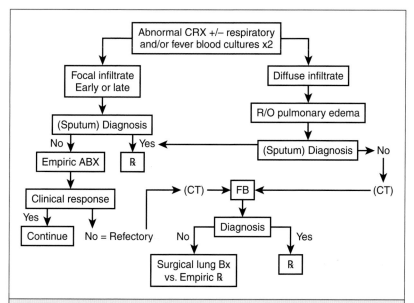

Figure 40-1. Diagnostic algorithm for evaluating pulmonary infiltrates in ill patients with cancer. From White P: Evaluation of pulmonary infiltrates in critically ill patients with cancer and marrow transplant. Crit Care Clin 17:647-670, 2001.

TABLE 40-4. RADIOGRAPHIC PATTERNS OF PULMONARY DISEASE IN THE IMMUNOCOMPROMISED HOST

| | | ONSET OF ILLNESS | |
IMMUNE DEFECT	RADIOGRAPHIC PATTERN	ACUTE	SUBACUTE OR CHRONIC
HIV Long-term steroid use	Consolidation	Bacterial S. pneumoniae H. influenzae Legionella*	Bacterial Rhodococcus equi Cryptococcus
	Reticulonodular		PCP Histoplasmosis Cryptococcus Mycobacterium avium
	Diffuse interstitial	Influenza	PCP CMV
	Discrete nodule		Nocardia Mycobacterium tuberculosis Endemic fungi Coccidioides Histoplasma Cryptococcus
Solid organ transplant recipient	Consolidation	Bacterial S. pneumonia H. influenzae Legionella* RSV Influenza	
	Reticulonodular		Nocardia M. tuberculosis
	Diffuse interstitial	CMV RSV Influenza PCP	Cryptococcus Aspergillosis
	Discrete nodules		Aspergillus M. tuberculosis Nocardia

TABLE 40-4. RADIOGRAPHIC PATTERNS OF PULMONARY DISEASE IN THE IMMUNOCOMPROMISED HOST—*cont'd*

| IMMUNE DEFECT | RADIOGRAPHIC PATTERN | ONSET OF ILLNESS | |
		ACUTE	SUBACUTE OR CHRONIC
HSCT recipients	Consolidation	Bacterial	
		S. pneumoniae	
		H. influenzae	
		*Legionella**	
	Diffuse interstitial	Influenza	
		PCP	
		RSV	
		CMV	
		HSV	
	Reticulonodular		*Nocardia*
			Cryptococcus
			Histoplasmosis
			Aspergillus
	Discrete nodule		*Mycobacterium*
Chemotherapy-induced neutropenia	Lobar consolidation	Bacterial	
		S. pneumoniae	
		H. influenzae	
		*Legionella**	
	Diffuse interstitial	CMV	
		PCP	
	Reticulonodular		*Aspergillus*
			Histoplasmosis
			Coccidiomycosis
	Discrete nodule		*Aspergillus*

Modified from Cunha B: Pneumonias in the compromised host. Infect Dis Clin North Am 15:591-612, 2001, and Linden PK: Approach to the immunocompromised host with infection in the intensive care unit. Infect Dis Clin North Am 23:535-556, 2009.
HSCT, Hematopoietic stem cell transplantation; *RSV*, respiratory syncytial virus.
**Legionella* is usually rapidly progressive asymmetrical infiltrates.

19. Describe the clinical course of *Pneumocystis carinii* pneumonia (PCP) infection and treatment.

This organism was first associated with human disease in 1951 when it was discovered as the cause of severe pneumonitis in severely malnourished infants. Since that time, it has been associated with patients taking long-term steroids and those receiving certain chemotherapeutic regimens. However, it became famous as the major pathogen of patients with HIV infection.

Although this infection was linked with HIV infection, the advent of highly active antiretroviral therapy (HAART) has resulted in effective immune reconstitution, as well as effective prophylactic regimens, thus resulting in a decreased susceptibility to infection. However, we see the incidence of this particular infection increasing among those receiving cytotoxic chemotherapy. Interestingly in patients with HIV the clinical course is usually fairly indolent with complaints of several weeks of cough and increasing dyspnea; at the time of presentation the degree of hypoxemia is usually moderate with little to no peripheral leukocytosis. This is in contrast to the population without HIV, in which the infection can present quite acutely with severe hypoxemia and respiratory failure. Chest radiographs often demonstrate bilateral or asymmetric interstitial infiltrates (more common in the population with HIV). See Table 40-5.

20. How is the diagnosis of PCP made?

- **BAL specimens:** BAL with biopsy can make the diagnosis up to 90% of the time. BAL lavage alone is apt to make the diagnosis approximately 50% of the time in patients without HIV but 90% of the time in those with HIV/AIDS because of the higher burden of organisms in this patient population.
- **Sputum:** Induced (not expectorated) sputum can be useful for diagnosis, especially in patients with AIDS.
- **Biopsy:** Histology will show pathognomonic frothy infiltrate that fills the alveoli; organisms can be seen in tissue sections as well. This infiltrate can be confused with hyaline membranes seen in acute respiratory distress syndrome (ARDS), although often the two disease states coexist.

For all the above, samples should be stained with Giemsa and toluidine blue or silver stain. In addition, **immunohistochemical analysis** using monoclonal antibody directed against the surface epitope of the organism and cytopathologic analysis that reveals foamy eosinophilic material that fills the alveoli and is fairly characteristic may be helpful.

Serum markers:

- **Lactate dehydrogenase:** Often elevated in those with PCP, usually over 300 International Units/mL. Higher levels indicate that a larger amount of lung tissue may be involved.
- **β-D-glucans:** Often positive in the setting of PCP infection, but not diagnostic.

21. When are steroids indicated in the treatment of PCP infection?

Steroids are recommended in addition to antibiotic therapy in patients who have a PaO$_2$ of less than 70 mm Hg on room air arterial blood gas or who have an A − a gradient of >35 mm Hg. Steroids given in the first 72 hours of treatment can lessen the decreases in oxygenation and improve survival. Steroid dosing should consist of prednisone 40 mg daily (or equivalent) orally for 5 days then decreasing to 20 mg daily to complete a total course of 21 days.

22. What are the most common causes of esophageal disease in those undergoing cytotoxic chemotherapy and BMT?

Esophageal disease from both infectious and noninfectious (i.e., GVHD, chemotherapy-induced mucositis) causes is common in this patient population. The normal mucosal barrier is often disrupted by chemotherapeutic agents, and this mucosal disruption can then become a portal of entry for bacteria. Most patients with esophageal disease are initially seen with dysphagia, odynophagia, nausea, or retrosternal pain.

The most common causes of esophageal infection in this patient population are as follows:

HSV: often presents with oropharyngeal ulcers, which can be quite friable and lead to gastrointestinal (GI) bleeding. The infection can have white exudates and is often mistaken for

TABLE 40-5.	TREATMENT OF PCP INFECTION: MODERATE TO SEVERE DISEASE	
DRUGS	**DOSE**	**DURATION AND COMMENTS**
TMP-SMX* IV and PO	15-20 mg/kg per day TMP[†] 75-100 mg/kg per day SMX[†]	Recommended duration 21 days
Alternatives	3-4 mg/kg per day infused over ≥ 60 min	21 days duration
1. Pentamidine	4 mg/kg/day (max 300 mg/day)	
2. Primaquine *plus*	15-30 mg base/day	
Clindamycin	900 mg IV every 8 hr	

Modified from Bartlett JG, Gallant JE, Pham PA: Medical Management of HIV Infection. Durham, N.C., Knowledge Source Solutions, 2009, p 449, and Rubin RH, Young LS: Clinical Approach to Infection in the Compromised Host, 4th ed. New York, Kluwer Academic/Plenum Publishers, 2002, pp 265-289.
PO, Oral; *SMX*, sulfamethoxazole; *TMP*, trimethoprim.
*Some helpful conversions: 16 mg TMP per mL of Bactrim; **Bactrim DS** = 800 mg TMP/160 mg SMX; **Bactrim SS** = 400 mg TMP/160 mg SMX.
[†]Dosing is based on the TMP component.

Candida. The ulcer appearance is not pathognomonic, has similar appearance to that of chemotherapy-induced mucositis, and is best diagnosed by culture or direct fluorescent antibody test of the lesions. Oral trauma from nasogastric (NG) tubes or endotracheal tubes can lead to extension of infection from oral pharynx into lower respiratory tract. This can lead to dissemination and, in certain patients, development of HSV pneumonia.

Candidal esophagitis: most common cause of esophageal infections in compromised hosts. Classic manifestation is thick white plaques adherent to the posterior pharynx and buccal mucosa. Widespread use of azoles for prophylaxis has increased the risk of fluconazole-resistant candidal species.

CMV: can cause infection throughout the entire GI tract. The ulcers do not have a unique appearance and may resemble those of HSV or chemotherapy-induced mucositis. Cultures should be interpreted with caution because trauma and underlying illness may lead to mucosal shedding; biopsy samples of oral and esophageal lesions should be taken for clear diagnosis.

23. **What is typhlitis, and how is it treated?**
Typhlitis, also known as neutropenic enterocolitis, is thought to ensue after a constellation of factors including mucosal injury of the bowel wall due to cytotoxic chemotherapy, impaired host defenses, and neutropenia. It is typically seen in patients with neutrophil counts less than 500/mm^3; those affected often have abdominal pain, fever, nausea, diarrhea, and bloody diarrhea. The diagnosis carries a mortality rate of between 40% and 50%. Concomitant bacteremia, due to normal bowel flora, is common.

The disease has a predilection for the cecum because of its relative lack of vascularization compared with the remainder of the colon; however, other sites of bowel involvement have been described. Radiographs of the abdomen are usually nonspecific, although they may demonstrate evidence of obstruction or free air. CT scans may reveal cecal wall thickening, pneumatosis, free air, or abscess formation. The use of rectal contrast or barium enemas should be avoided in patients with neutropenia because of the high risk of bowel wall perforation. Work-up should include abdominal radiographs, CT scan of abdomen without rectal contrast, blood cultures, stool cultures including stool for *Clostridium difficile* testing, and surgical evaluation.

Treatment includes IV volume resuscitation and broad-spectrum antibiotic therapy (see Box 40-2).

BOX 40-2. EMPIRIC ANTIBIOTIC OPTIONS FOR SUSPECTED TYPHLITIS*

Vancomycin and antipseudomonal carbapenem (meropenem or imipenem)
Or
Vancomycin and ceftazidime and metronidazole
Or
Vancomycin and aztreonam + metronidazole[†]

---

*Regimen will vary according to antibiotic allergies, hospital formulary, and local resistance patterns.
[†]One possibility for patients allergic to penicillin.

24. **Describe some of the common causes of community-acquired bacterial enteritis in the immunocompromised patient.**
    Patients with compromised immune systems are at risk for development of the same community infections as normal hosts, but they may be more severe. In addition, because of low neutrophil counts or loss of mucosal integrity they may be more prone to development of bacteremia from their own endogenous bowel flora. Some of these infections can lead to dissemination outside the GI tract and lead to more severe disease in immunocompromised hosts.
    Listeria. The common food-borne illness caused by this organism leads to outbreaks in immunocompromised and normal hosts alike. However, dissemination outside of the GI tract is increased in those with chronic lymphocytic leukemia, corticosteroid use, allogenic BMT, and pregnancy. Certain chemotherapeutic drugs such as fludarabine will increase this risk as well.
    Salmonella. This is associated with a deficiency in cell-mediated immunity such as corticosteroid use and HIV infection. These hosts are at risk for disseminated *Salmonella* infection.
    C. difficile. *C. difficile* has been associated with a higher mortality risk among BMT recipients compared with a normal host. Increased rates of infection among immunocompromised patients are likely due to frequent antibiotic therapy, increased rates of colonization, and frequent hospital admissions.

25. **Describe the most common causes of viral enteritis in the immunocompromised patient.**
    - **CMV:** one of the more common pathogens in the transplant population. Diagnosis requires colonic biopsy. CT findings are nonspecific, and serologic markers such as antigenemia and viral load are unreliable indicators of disease limited to the GI tract.
    - **Adenovirus:** a common cause in both solid organ recipients and BMT recipients. The clinical picture is often that of diarrhea, although bleeding is not uncommon because the virus can lead to colonic ulceration. Dissemination outside of the GI tract can occur leading to pneumonitis, hepatitis, encephalitis, and cystitis.
    - **Rotavirus:** usually seen in pediatric patients. It can lead to profuse watery diarrhea and is diagnosed by stool PCR testing.
    - **Enterovirus:** presenting with watery diarrhea but can progress to meningoencephalitis. It is diagnosed by stool PCR testing.
    - **HSV:** can lead to ulcerations in the upper and lower GI tract.

26. **What is the best approach to manage HAART therapy for patients with HIV in the ICU?**
    In patients with HIV receiving HAART the therapy should be continued whenever possible to prevent the development of resistance. This may not be possible in some patients when HAART complications such as renal failure and/or liver disease are complicating the patients' clinical course. Administering HAART to patients who take nothing by mouth can be complicated

because some of the medications cannot be crushed for administration through an NG tube, and not all of them are available in liquid form. If HAART medications do need to be stopped it is essential that all HAART be held at the same time. Discontinuation of only part of a patient's HAART regimen can lead to antiviral resistance and ensuing treatment complications down the road.

27. Should antirejection medications be altered for the solid organ transplant recipient with severe sepsis?

In patients with life-threatening infections, withdrawal or reduction of immunosuppressive medications can be an effective treatment modality to assist in the reduction of immunosuppression. However, cessation of antirejection medications can lead to graft rejection and failure, and so changes in medications need to be considered on an individual basis. These decisions regarding medication adjustments should be carried out with the close assistance of the transplant team whenever possible.

Important facts to consider when considering reduction of immunosuppression:

■ Mortality associated with loss of allograft: Graft loss in heart or liver transplant recipients may be very different from graft loss in those who have undergone pancreas or kidney transplantation. If other modalities can be used, that is, insulin or hemodialysis, then, although not ideal, the graft may be able to be sacrificed in the setting of life-threatening infection.

■ Use of steroids: In the setting of acute infection, rapid withdrawal or taper of steroids may lead to adrenal insufficiency complicating the patient's hemodynamics. In addition, the use of steroids may be clinically indicated for treatment of the underlying infection or sequelae thereof (i.e., PCP or cerebral edema associated with toxoplasmosis).

KEY POINTS: IMMUNOCOMPROMISED HOST

1. The *net state of immunosuppression* is critical in assessing a patient's risk for infection.

2. The longer the duration of neutropenia, the greater the risk for invasive fungal disease.

3. Individuals without a spleen are at risk for infection with encapsulated organisms.

4. The greatest degree of immunosuppression in solid organ transplant recipients is 1 to 6 months after transplantation.

5. Early antimicrobial therapy is essential in patients with neutropenic fever.

BIBLIOGRAPHY

1. Baden LR, Maguire JH: Gastrointestinal infections in the immunocompromised host. Infect Dis Clin North Am 15:639-670, xi, 2001.

2. Bartlett JG, Gallant JE, Pham PA: Medical Management of HIV Infection. Durham, N.C., Knowledge Source Solutions, 2009, p 449.

3. Cunha B: Pneumonias in the compromised host. Infect Dis Clin North Am 15:591-612, 2001.

4. Cunha BA: Central nervous system infections in the compromised host: a diagnostic approach. Infect Dis Clin North Am 15:567-590, 2001.

5. Fishman JA: *Pneumocystis carinii* and parasitic infections in the immunocompromised host. In Rubin RH, Young LS (eds): Clinical Approach to Infection in the Compromised Host, 4th ed. New York, Kluwer Academic/Plenum Publishers, 2002, pp 265-325.

6. Fishman JA: Infection in solid-organ transplant recipients. N Engl J Med 357:2601-2614, 2007.

7. Freifeld AG, Bow EJ, Sepkowitz KA, et al. Clinical practice guidelines for the use of antimicrobial agents in neutropenic patients with cancer: 2010 update by the Infectious Diseases Society of America. Clin Infect Dis 52: e56-e93, 2011.

8. Kotloff RM, Ahya VN, Crawford SW: Pulmonary complications of solid organ and hematopoietic stem cell transplantation. Am J Respir Crit Care Med 170:22-48, 2004.

9. Leather HL, Wingard JR: Infections following hematopoietic stem cell transplantation. Infect Dis Clin North Am 15:483-520, 2001.

10. Linden PK: Approach to the immunocompromised host with infection in the intensive care unit. Infect Dis Clin North Am 23:535-556, 2009.

11. Lyons RW: Approach to the immunocompromised host. In Grace C (ed): Medical Management of Infectious Disease. New York, Marcel Dekker, 2003, pp 661-665.

12. Mandell GL, Bennett JE, Dolin R: Principles and Practice of Infectious Diseases, 6th ed. Philadelphia, Elsevier, 2005, pp 3520-3530.

13. Rubin R, Schaffner A, Speich R: Introduction to the Immunocompromised Host Society Consensus Conference on Epidemiology, Prevention, Diagnosis, and Management of Infections in Solid-Organ Transplant Patients. Clin Infect Dis 33(Suppl 1):S1-S4, 2001.

14. Rubin RH, Young LS: Clinical Approach to Infection in the Compromised Host, 4th ed. New York, Kluwer Academic/Plenum Publishers, 2002, pp 265-289.

15. Sumaraju V, Smith LG, Smith SM: Infectious complications in asplenic hosts. Infect Dis Clin North Am 15:551-565, 2001.

16. Syndman DR: Epidemiology of infections after solid-organ transplantation. Clin Infect Dis 33(Suppl 1):S5, 2001.

17. Tasaka S, Hasegawa N, Kobayashi S, et al: Serum indicators for the diagnosis of pneumocystis pneumonia. Chest 131:1173-1180, 2007.

18. White P: Evaluation of pulmonary infiltrates in critically ill patients with cancer and marrow transplant. Crit Care Clin 17:647-670, 2001.

VI. RENAL DISEASE

CHAPTER 41

HYPERTENSION

Stuart L. Linas, MD, and Shailendra Sharma, MD

1. What are the hemodynamic determinants of blood pressure (BP)?
Arterial BP is the product of cardiac output (CO) and systemic vascular resistance (SVR).

$$BP = CO \times SVR \text{ (analogous to Ohm law)}$$

Malignant hypertension is caused by increased SVR.

2. What is hypertensive crisis?
Hypertensive crisis is the turning point in the course of hypertension in which immediate management of the elevated BP has a decisive role in the eventual outcome. It is a condition of severe and uncontrolled increase in the BP. An acute increase in BP can occur in the absence or presence of acute or chronic target organ dysfunction.

3. What are the target organs affected by hypertensive crisis?
Four organs are the usual target of severely elevated BP:
- Kidneys: acute kidney injury caused by proliferative endarteritis and fibrinoid necrosis of afferent artery
- Brain: hypertensive encephalopathy, cerebrovascular accidents (CVA)
- Eye or retina: retinal hemorrhage or exudates or papilledema
- Heart: acute coronary syndrome, decompensated heart failure, aortic dissection, and acute intravascular hemolysis

4. What are malignant hypertension and accelerated hypertension?
Both are syndromes in which a markedly elevated BP is associated with hypertensive neuroretinopathy. In accelerated hypertension, there may be flame hemorrhages or cotton wool exudates. Malignant hypertension is diagnosed when papilledema occurs as well.

5. What are hypertensive urgency (HU) and nonemergent hypertension (NEH)?
When severe hypertension occurs in the absence of any acute end-organ damage, it is classified as HU-NEH. Because the complications from HU are not immediate, this condition can be treated safely outside the intensive care unit and hospital with gentle reduction in BP achieved over hours to days.

6. What is hypertensive encephalopathy?
Hypertensive encephalopathy occurs in the setting of sudden and sustained elevation in BP. It occurs in both benign and malignant hypertension. The clinical presentation is that of altered mental status and/or seizures, but focal neurologic findings are uncommon. This condition can be difficult to distinguish from a primary neurologic event.

7. What are the causes of malignant and accelerated hypertension?
In contrast to ambulatory hypertension (over 90% essential) as many as 50% of patients with malignant or accelerated hypertension have secondary causes. The most important of secondary causes are medications, chronic kidney disease, and renal artery stenosis (RAS).

8. **What is the short-term treatment of hypertension and hypertensive emergency?**
The short-term treatment of choice is intravenous (IV) sodium nitroprusside. The initial dose is 0.5 mcg/kg/min, and this should be increased by 0.5 mcg/kg/min every 2 to 3 minutes until a diastolic BP <110 mm Hg has been attained. Further acute decreases in BP should be avoided to prevent hypoperfusion to vital organ(s) because blood flow autoregulation may have been altered to accommodate chronically elevated BP. Acceptable alternative parenteral drugs for the short-term treatment of malignant hypertension include labetalol, nicardipine, enalaprilat, or fenoldopam. Extreme caution should be taken while using agents known to cause or further worsen intravascular volume status because patients with hypertensive emergency often present with intravascular volume depletion.

9. **Outline the typical long-term antihypertensive regimen after successful treatment of malignant hypertension or hypertensive crisis.**
Because malignant hypertension is mediated by increased SVR, it is recommended that long-term therapy include a vasodilator such as hydralazine or minoxidil. Vasodilators cause reflex tachycardia and sodium retention; therefore it is usually also necessary to include a β-blocker (labetalol) and a diuretic agent. In some cases, long-term BP reduction may be achieved with less potent vasodilators, such as angiotensin-converting enzyme (ACE) inhibitors or calcium channel blockers.

10. **What is the appropriate short-term treatment for hypertension in a patient with pheochromocytoma?**
Hypertension from pheochromocytomas is caused by vascular smooth muscle α_1-receptor activation, which results in vasoconstriction. Thus the best short-term treatment is IV administration of the α_1-blocker phentolamine. Sodium nitroprusside is also a reasonable choice. β-Blockers should initially be avoided because they cause both unopposed peripheral α_1-receptor stimulation and decreased CO.

11. **Describe the short-term treatment of cocaine-induced hypertensive crisis.**
Cocaine-induced hypertensive crisis falls under "catecholamine-associated hypertension." Cocaine causes hypertension by inhibiting catecholamine reuptake at nerve terminals. Therefore drugs that can block α_1-receptors such as labetalol or phentolamine are effective. Selective β-blockers without α_1 blockade such as propranolol are not recommended because of the risk of unopposed α_1 action. If hypertension is severe, sodium nitroprusside is the drug of choice. In the setting of cocaine-related myocardial ischemia, nitroglycerin and benzodiazepines are effective against both cocaine-induced hypertension and vasoconstriction of the coronary arteries. Cocaethylene is a compound formed in vivo when cocaine and ethyl alcohol (EtOH) have been ingested simultaneously. It produces greater increases in heart rate, rate-pressure product, and euphoria compared with the effects of cocaine alone. Therefore the treatment of hypertension tends to pose greater therapeutic challenge in patients consuming EtOH as well as cocaine.
   Cocaine-induced hypertension should be treated with extreme caution and treatment regimens reviewed with passage of time because the condition undergoes spontaneous resolution when cocaine is metabolized.

12. **How is hypertension treated in the short term in patients with aortic dissection?**
Aortic dissection begins with a tear in the intima of the aorta; this is propagated by the aortic pulse wave (dP/dt). Myocardial contractility, heart rate, and BP contribute to the aortic pulse wave. The goal of treatment is to decrease myocardial contractility and heart rate. This goal has traditionally been best achieved with sodium nitroprusside and esmolol. Labetalol alone is also effective in this setting.

13. Why is BP elevated in patients with CVA?

Patients with CVA often have a severe increase in BP potentially resulting from a central mechanism and/or compensatory increase in response to increased intracranial pressure. Stress responses to hospitalization, headache, urinary retention, or concomitant infection may lead to abnormal autonomic activity and raised levels of circulating catecholamines. Greater than 60% of patients with CVA will have an acute hypertensive response.

- Central mechanism

    The primary cause is damage or compression of specific regions in the brain that mediate autonomic control. Increased sympathoadrenal tone and subsequent release of renin, each in isolation or together, can also contribute to high BPs.

- Failure of autoregulation of cerebral blood flow and response to increased intracranial pressure (ICP)

    With acute brain injury, the ability of the brain to autoregulate and maintain cerebral blood flow is impaired. Autoregulation is a mechanism by which the brain can maintain a constant cerebral blood flow despite a wide fluctuation in cerebral perfusion pressure (CPP) (from the range of 60-180 mm Hg).

$$\text{Cerebral blood flow} = \text{CPP}/\text{Cerebral vascular resistance}$$

CPP is the difference between mean arterial pressure (MAP) and ICP. Under physiologic circumstances cerebral venous pressure (backflow in the cerebral venous system) is the primary determinant of ICP. In absence of any pathologic condition, cerebral venous pressure is zero; thus the arterial pressure determines CPP.

When the ICP goes up because of increase in cerebral venous pressure (as in CVA), MAP goes up in an attempt to maintain adequate CPP.

14. How should hypertension be treated in patients with CVA?

- **Hypertensive encephalopathy**

    The goal is gradual and careful reversal of vasogenic subcortical edema. MAP should be cautiously reduced by no more than 15% over a 2- to 3-hour period. Severe neurologic complications have occurred with MAP reductions at 40% or more.

- **Thromboembolic cerebrovascular disease**

    The goal is salvation of ischemic penumbra. For patients thought to be candidates for reperfusion therapy, systolic BP (SBP) >185 mm Hg and diastolic BP (DBP) >110 mm Hg warrant treatment. For the subset of patients who are not candidates for reperfusion therapy, the expert opinion is to treat SBP >220 mm Hg and DBP >120 mm Hg with a goal of 15% to 25% reduction in MAP over the first 24 hours.

- **Subarachnoid hemorrhage**

    Poorly controlled BP increases the risk of rebleeding. The presence of blood in the subarachnoid space induces intense vasospasm and increases the risk of severe ischemia 4 to 12 days after the first bleeding. The goal is 20% to 25% reduction in BP over a 6- to 12-hour period but not less than 160 to 180/100 mm Hg.

- **Intracerebral hemorrhage**

    The consensus guidelines on treatment of intracerebral bleeding:

    □ IV medications should be used to treat SBP >200 mm Hg or MAP >150 mm Hg with BP monitoring done every 5 minutes.

    □ In suspected intracranial hypertension, BP should be lowered with a parenteral agent if SBP is >180 mm Hg or MAP >130 mm Hg while maintaining CPP above 60 to 80 mm Hg.

    □ In the absence of elevated ICP, treat SBP >180 mm Hg and MAP >130 mm Hg with a target BP of 160/90 mm Hg or a MAP of 110 mm Hg.

    □ The rate of BP reduction should be slowed if the patient's neurologic status deteriorates. Oral therapy should be instituted before parenteral treatment is discontinued. Clonidine or α-methyldopa should be avoided because of the risk of impaired cerebral function.

15. **Describe the short-term treatment of hypertension in patients with ischemic heart disease and ongoing angina.**

    Hypertension can precipitate ischemic chest pain in patients with severe coronary artery disease. Alternatively, hypertension can result from chest pain, which results in marked increases in catecholamines and secondary reactive hypertension. In either setting, hypertension is associated with an increase in SVR and increases in myocardial oxygen demand. Nitroglycerin and β-blockers are the initial agents of choice. Because nitroprusside increases heart rate and myocardial oxygen demand in this setting, it is considered a secondary agent.

16. **How should hypertension associated with preeclampsia be treated?**

    The traditional treatments of choice are hydralazine or α-methyldopa. If these drugs are ineffective or poorly tolerated, labetalol is a reasonably safe and effective alternative. Medications to be avoided because of potential teratogenesis include sodium nitroprusside, trimethaphan, diazoxide, ACE inhibitors, β-blockers, and calcium channel blockers. Unfortunately, the safety profile of many antihypertensive drugs during pregnancy is unknown. Because preeclampsia and eclampsia may be life threatening, sometimes it may be necessary to prescribe potent antihypertensive agents (sodium nitroprusside or minoxidil) with unclear fetal toxicity potential.

17. **What are the causes of RAS, and how should it be evaluated?**

    The major causes are fibromuscular dysplasia (especially in young women) and atherosclerosis (in those aged >55 years in association with polycystic kidney disease). Although Doppler ultrasonography of the renal vasculature is an excellent noninvasive test to confirm RAS, it has not been standardized, and magnetic resonance angiography is recommended.

18. **What is reactive hypertension?**

    Patients with stage 1 or 2 hypertension that is poorly controlled with medications can have marked elevation in BP to *stressors* such as pain or shortness of breath. Increases in catecholamines of *stress* lead to severe elevations in BP that should be distinguished from primary hypertension because the approaches to therapy differ. In reactive hypertension it is necessary to treat the cause of BP, for example, chest pain or pancreatitis, rather than the elevated BP.

19. **Why does lowering of BP potentially result in a decline in glomerular filtration rate (GFR) in severe hypertension?**

    Normally, GFR is maintained despite decreases in BP by compensatory increases in efferent arteriolar tone (Fig. 41-1) Two major causes exist of loss of GFR after reduction of BP in the setting of severe hypertension:

    - RAS: In a patient with a fixed atherosclerotic lesion of the main renal artery, a drop in BP can cause a fall in GFR because the fixed lesion limits afferent arteriolar flow to such an extent that even maximal elevation in efferent arteriolar tone cannot compensate and maintain GFR.
    - Long-standing essential hypertension: In this setting, no macrovascular abnormalities are present; the problem is marked sclerosis of the microvasculature of the kidney, including the afferent artery. Because of afferent arteriolar sclerosis, the afferent artery is unable to vasodilate in response to a drop in BP. Hence, GFR falls when BP is lowered even with increases in efferent arteriolar tone that normally would offset, at least partially, decreases in BP.

20. **When should an evaluation for secondary hypertension be considered?**

    - At initial presentation of malignant hypertension (especially if the patient is white, younger than 30 years, or older than 50 years of age)
    - When rapid onset of severe hypertension occurs within less than 5 years
    - When an increase in serum creatinine level occurs after the initiation of ACE inhibitor treatment
    - In compliant patients whose BP is difficult to control after an adequate trial with a combination of diuretic, β-blocker, and potent vasodilator

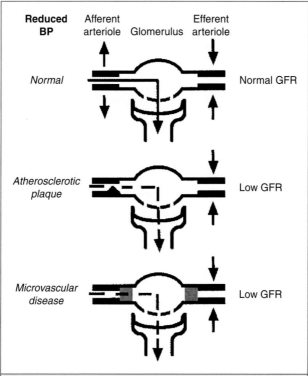

Figure 41-1. Impaired autoregulation of glomerular filtration rate (*GFR*). *BP*, Blood pressure.

21. What are the important causes of secondary hypertension?

Secondary hypertension accounts for 5% of cases of hypertension.

- Renal: renovascular disease, renal parenchymal disease, polycystic kidney disease, Liddle syndrome, syndrome of apparent mineralocorticoid excess, hypercalcemia
- Endocrine: hyperthyroidism, hypothyroidism, primary hyperaldosteronism, Cushing syndrome, pheochromocytoma, congenital adrenal hyperplasia
- Drugs: prescription (e.g., estrogen, cyclosporine, steroids); over-the-counter (e.g., pseudoephedrine, nonsteroidal antiinflammatory drugs); illicit (e.g., tobacco smoking, ethanol, cocaine)
- Neurogenic: increased intracranial pressure, spinal cord section
- Miscellaneous: coarctation of aorta, obstructive sleep apnea, polycythemia vera

22. What are the causes of primary aldosteronism, and how should they be distinguished?

The major causes are unilateral aldosterone-producing adenoma (APA) and bilateral idiopathic adrenal hyperplasia (IAH). Primary aldosteronism should be suspected in a patient with hypokalemia and hypertension with metabolic alkalosis. It is necessary to first demonstrate renal potassium wasting (high urine K^+ in association with low serum K^+) followed by a decrease in renin and an elevated aldosterone level. The plasma aldosterone/renin ratio (>40) is often used. If the ratio is elevated, the aldosterone response to either NaCl infusion or fludrocortisone is used and considered positive if the plasma aldosterone level remains elevated (>10 pg/mL). Treatment of APA is surgical adrenalectomy, whereas mainstays of treatment of IAH are mainly medical. Adrenal imaging can sometimes distinguish between APA and IAH, but it is often necessary to pursue a more definitive study to verify the diagnosis of APA. By far, selective adrenal vein sampling is the most validated technique used to differentiate APA from IAH.

KEY POINTS: HYPERTENSION

1. Hypertensive crisis (or hypertensive emergency) is the turning point in the course of hypertension when the immediate management of elevated BP plays a decisive role in limiting or preventing target organ damage.

2. Hypertensive crises can damage four main target organ systems: eye, brain, heart, and kidney.

3. The short-term treatment of choice for malignant hypertension is IV sodium nitroprusside.

4. Long-term therapy for malignant hypertension should include a vasodilator such as hydralazine or minoxidil, a β-blocker, and a diuretic agent.

5. Nitroglycerin and β-blockers are the initial agents of choice for patients with ischemic heart disease and angina.

BIBLIOGRAPHY

1. Adams HP Jr, del Zoppo G, Alberts MJ, et al: Guidelines for the early management of adults with ischemic stroke. Stroke 5:1655-1711, 2007.

2. Kaplan NM: Pheochromocytoma. In Kaplan NM (ed): Clinical Hypertension, 7th ed. Philadelphia, Lippincott Williams & Wilkins, 1998, pp 345-363.

3. Kelleher CL, Linas SL: Hypertensive crisis: emergency and urgency. In Fink MP, Abraham E, Vincent J-L, et al (eds): Textbook of Critical Care, 5th ed. Philadelphia, Saunders, 2005, pp 879-888.

4. Kitiyakara C, Guzman NJ: Malignant hypertension and hypertensive emergencies. J Am Soc Nephrol 9:133-142, 1998.

5. Lange RA, Hillis LD: Cardiovascular complications of cocaine use. N Engl J Med 345:351-358, 2001.

6. Pohl MA: Renal artery stenosis, renal vascular hypertension, and ischemic nephropathy. In Schrier RW (ed): Diseases of the Kidney, 7th ed. Philadelphia, Lippincott Williams & Wilkins, 2001, pp 1399-1457.

7. Qureshi AI: Acute hypertensive response in patients with stroke: pathophysiology and management. Circulation 118:176-187, 2008.

8. Qureshi AI, Ezzeddine MA, Nasar A, et al: Prevalence of elevated blood pressure in 563,704 adult patients with stroke presenting to the ED in the United States. Am J Emerg Med 25:32-38, 2007.

9. Vaughan CJ, Delanty N: Hypertensive emergencies. Lancet 356:411-417, 2000.

CHAPTER 42

ACUTE RENAL FAILURE

Dinkar Kaw, MD, and Joseph I. Shapiro, MD

1. **How is acute renal failure (ARF) diagnosed?**

   ARF is a rapid loss of glomerular filtration rate (GFR) over a period of hours to a few days. This is usually determined by a sudden rise in plasma creatinine and blood urea nitrogen (BUN) levels. Until the patient achieves a steady state, the level of renal function cannot be assessed by the serum creatinine concentration. If a patient with previously normal renal function suddenly loses all renal function, serum creatinine will rise by only 1 to 2 mg/dL/day. However, patients with muscle wasting who make less creatinine may show smaller increases even with complete cessation of GFR. BUN is another indicator of decreasing glomerular filtration. Although a dramatic rise in BUN compared with creatinine may suggest a prerenal or obstructive (postrenal) cause, one must also consider the possibility that creatinine production by the patient is limited. Measurement of timed creatinine and urea excretion rates allowing for calculation of creatinine and urea clearance is sometimes indicated to clarify this point. In critically ill patients, decrease in urine output can be an indication of decreasing GFR. Increase in serum creatinine or decrease in urine output can be used to assess the risk, injury, and failure stages of ARF.

2. **What features distinguish ARF from chronic renal failure?**

   When a patient is seen some time after the onset of ARF, this distinction may not be easy. Chronic renal failure is more likely than ARF to be associated with anemia, hypocalcemia, normal urine output, and small shrunken kidneys on ultrasound examination. A kidney biopsy may be warranted if the kidneys are of normal size. It has been reported that chronic, but not acute, renal failure may be associated with an increase in the serum osmolal gap (i.e., the difference between measured and calculated serum osmolality).

3. **How is ARF classified?**

   The main categories are prerenal, intrarenal or parenchymal, and postrenal or obstructive (Table 42-1).

TABLE 42-1. DIFFERENTIAL DIAGNOSIS OF ACUTE RENAL FAILURE		
PRERENAL	**POSTRENAL**	**PARENCHYMAL**
Dehydration	Ureter	Glomerular
Impaired cardiac function	Bladder	Interstitial
Vasodilation	Urethra	Allergic interstitial nephritis
Renal vascular obstruction		Vascular
Hepatorenal syndrome		ATN

ATN, Acute tubular necrosis.

4. **How does examination of the urine help in the differential diagnosis of ARF?**
Laboratory evaluation begins with careful examination of the urine. Concentrated urine points more to prerenal causes, whereas isotonic urine suggests parenchymal or obstructive causes. Typically, the urine sediment of patients with prerenal azotemia demonstrates occasional hyaline casts or finely granular casts. In contrast, the presence of renal tubular epithelial cells with muddy and granular casts strongly suggests acute tubular necrosis (ATN), microhematuria and red blood cell casts suggest glomerulonephritis, and white cell casts containing eosinophils suggest acute interstitial nephritis. Benign urine sediment is quite compatible with urinary obstruction.

5. **What are the implications of urinary electrolytes in the differential diagnosis of ARF?**
The determination of urine electrolyte and creatinine concentrations may be helpful in the differential diagnosis of ARF. When used with serum values, urinary diagnostic indexes can be generated. Understanding the concepts behind the interpretation of these indexes is easier and better than trying to remember specific numbers. Quite simply, if the tubule is working well in the setting of decreased GFR, tubular reabsorption of sodium and water is avid, and the relative clearance of sodium to creatinine is low. Conversely, if the tubule is injured and cannot reabsorb sodium well, the relative clearance of sodium to creatinine is not low. Therefore, with prerenal azotemia, the ratio of the clearance of sodium to the clearance of creatinine, which is also called the *fractional excretion of sodium* (FENa) (FENa = [Urinary sodium]/[Urinary creatinine] × [Plasma creatinine]/[Plasma sodium] × 100), is typically less than 1.0, whereas with parenchymal or obstructive causes of ARF, the FENa is generally greater than 2.0 (Fig. 42-1).

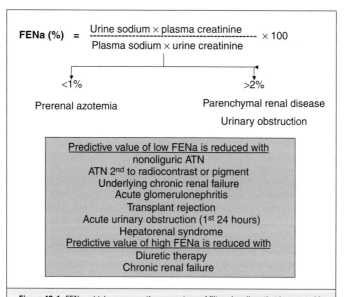

$$\text{FENa (\%)} = \frac{\text{Urine sodium} \times \text{plasma creatinine}}{\text{Plasma sodium} \times \text{urine creatinine}} \times 100$$

<1%

>2%

Prerenal azotemia

Parenchymal renal disease
Urinary obstruction

Predictive value of low FENa is reduced with
nonoliguric ATN
ATN 2nd to radiocontrast or pigment
Underlying chronic renal failure
Acute glomerulonephritis
Transplant rejection
Acute urinary obstruction (1st 24 hours)
Hepatorenal syndrome
Predictive value of high FENa is reduced with
Diuretic therapy
Chronic renal failure

Figure 42-1. FENa, which measures the percentage of filtered sodium that is excreted in the urine, helps to differentiate between prerenal causes of renal failure and both parenchymal renal diseases (e.g., ATN, allergic interstitial nephritis) and urinary obstruction. Under specific conditions, the predictive value of a low FENa (to diagnose prerenal azotemia) or a high FENa (to exclude prerenal azotemia) is limited.

The FENa test is much less useful when patients do not have oliguria. In this setting, the specificity of a low FENa for prerenal azotemia is markedly diminished. In addition to nonoliguria, several causes of ATN, specifically dye-induced ATN or ATN associated with hemolysis or rhabdomyolysis, may typically be associated with a low FENa. Patients who have prerenal azotemia but have either persistent diuretic effect, chronic tubulointerstitial injury, or bicarbonaturia may have a relatively high FENa. In the last case, the fractional excretion of chloride, which is calculated in an analogous way, will be appropriately low ($<1\%$). Finally, the early stages of ARF from glomerulonephritis, transplant allograft rejection, or urinary obstruction may be associated with a low FENa.

6. **What is the pathophysiology of ATN?**
Renal ischemia, toxic injury to the kidney, or a combination of these insults can cause prolonged loss of renal function. Physiologically, decreased GFR must result from an alteration in glomerular hemodynamic factors, such as a decrease in the effective surface area or permeability of the glomerulus (Kf), a decrease in glomerular blood flow, or an abnormality in tubular integrity, including obstruction of tubular flow by cellular debris or back leak of ultrafiltrate through a porous tubule. In fact, each of these pathogenic features can be shown to be operant in some experimental models of ARF.

7. **How does ATN evolve?**
The major mechanism by which renal failure is induced may be different from the primary mechanism by which it is maintained. For example, in ischemic ARF, decreases in renal and glomerular blood flow may cause the initial loss of renal function. However, tubular necrosis, with its attendant obstructing debris and back leak of ultrafiltrate, maintains the low GFR. The tubular mechanisms are usually important in the maintenance of ARF from most causes seen clinically. Therefore pharmacologic efforts to improve renal blood flow are not, by themselves, generally effective in shortening the duration of ARF. Interestingly, modern ATN appears to recover much less quickly than when the syndrome was first described. This slow recovery may be related to repeated bouts of renal ischemia, which can be attributed to altered renal vasodilation related to the initial ATN insult. Therefore even mild degrees of hypotension should be avoided when treating patients with ATN.

8. **How is ARF prevented?**
ATN usually occurs after surgery or preexisting dehydration. In these settings, nephrotoxic drugs, such as radiocontrast dye, aminoglycosides, amphotericin B, nonsteroidal antiinflammatory agents, and some cancer chemotherapeutic agents (e.g., cisplatin, methotrexate), are far more potent in causing ARF. Optimizing volume status and establishing a relatively high rate of urine flow minimize the risk of ARF. In specific situations, such as administration of radiocontrast dye or cisplatin and relatively high-risk surgery (e.g., open heart or biliary tract surgery), mannitol (12.5-25 g administered as an intravenous [IV] infusion) was thought to be a useful adjunct in preventing ARF. However, subsequent studies showed that mannitol actually potentiates ARF after the administration of radiocontrast. Some later studies suggest that administration of *N*-acetylcysteine or sodium bicarbonate infusions may prevent contrast nephropathy in high-risk patients, but the most accepted prophylaxis consists of isosmotic contrast media and cautious hydration before contrast administration.

9. **What are the treatment options in ATN?**
ATN is best treated, as previously discussed, by prevention. Because nonoliguric ATN is associated with lower mortality and morbidity rates than oliguric ATN, some excitement exists about the administration of high-dose loop diuretics (1-3 g/24 h given as an IV infusion or as repeated boluses) in concert with renal doses of dopamine (1-3 mcg/kg/min). This therapy, which converts oliguric ATN in some patients to a nonoliguric state, certainly facilitates management of volume and nutritional status. However, it is not clear whether these

pharmacologic interventions actually improve the prognosis. Optimizations of fluid status and avoidance of and/or therapy for electrolyte disorders are the mainstays of conservative management of ARF.

10. **Which critical electrolyte disorders accompany ARF?**
The most common electrolyte disorders that accompany ARF include hyperkalemia, hypermagnesemia, hyperphosphatemia, hypocalcemia, and acidosis (Table 42-2). Of these disorders, hyperkalemia is the most common and probably the one that is usually most serious.

Hyperkalemia most commonly occurs with oliguric ATN or urinary obstruction. It is truly a medical emergency. A serum potassium level above 6.0 mandates electrocardiography, searching for peaked T waves, diminished P-wave amplitude, or prolonged QRS complex. Any of these findings warrants the use of immediate measures to correct hyperkalemia.

TABLE 42-2. ELECTROLYTE DISTURBANCES IN ACUTE RENAL FAILURE

DISORDER	MECHANISM	FREQUENCY	CLINICAL IMPORTANCE
Hyperkalemia	Decreased K excretion Increased catabolism	Common, especially with oliguric ARF	Life threatening
Hypermagnesemia	Decreased Mg excretion	Common but not usually severe unless Mg is administered	Life threatening only if very severe
Hyperphosphatemia	Decreased phosphate excretion Increased catabolism	Common	Serious only if very severe
Hypocalcemia	Loss of 1,25-vitamin D_3 Calcium phosphate precipitation in tissues	Common but not usually severe	Life threatening if very severe
Acidosis	Decreased acid excretion Increased catabolism	Very common	Not usually life threatening

11. **What immediate measures are used to treat hyperkalemia?**
The quickest-acting parenteral therapy is calcium, administered as chloride or gluconate salts. This therapy does not affect the serum potassium level but does antagonize the effects of hyperkalemia on the membrane potential of the heart and prevents, or reverses, the cardiac effects of hyperkalemia. Another rapidly effective approach is the administration of insulin, which drives potassium into cells and lowers the serum potassium level. In patients who have a normal serum glucose level, insulin (10 units IV) is generally administered with dextrose (one ampule of 50% dextrose in water [$D_{50}W$] or an infusion of $D_{10}W$). The effects of insulin last somewhat longer than those of calcium and can be prolonged by a constant infusion of insulin, usually administered with glucose to prevent hypoglycemia. Bicarbonate may also be used to raise arterial pH and to shift potassium into cells. Complications include potentially adverse hemodynamic effects of IV bicarbonate and volume expansion from sodium load.

12. **What is the uremic syndrome?**

The uremic syndrome is a symptom complex associated with renal failure. It may occur with chronic and acute renal failure and involves virtually all organs of the body. Major manifestations are nausea and vomiting, pruritus, bleeding disorder, encephalopathy, and pericarditis. The syndrome generally mandates initiation of nonconservative therapy for ARF such as hemodialysis, peritoneal dialysis, or continuous arteriovenous hemofiltration. The pathogenesis of the uremic syndrome is still poorly understood; however, neither urea nor creatinine produces any of the known manifestations of uremia.

13. **What are the indications for nonconservative therapy for ARF?**

Indications for nonconservative therapy, such as dialysis, include uremic signs or symptoms, fluid overload, and/or electrolyte abnormalities that are refractory to conservative management. It has become the standard of care to provide nonconservative therapy when the BUN level exceeds 100 mg/dL or the serum creatinine exceeds 10 mg/dL, especially in the setting of oliguric ATN. These latter guidelines are not absolute and must be interpreted in the light of other clinical features.

14. **What are the options for nonconservative therapy of ARF?**

The three main options for nonconservative therapy of ARF are hemodialysis, peritoneal dialysis, and continuous renal replacement therapy (CRRT). Each option has advantages and disadvantages (Box 42-1), and, of course, variations exist of each of these modalities.

Hemodialysis involves the pumping of blood through an artificial kidney that removes solutes primarily by dialysis along a concentration gradient; water is removed by ultrafiltration driven by a pressure gradient. Central venous access, anticoagulation, a skilled technician, and expensive equipment are mandatory for this process.

Peritoneal dialysis involves the repetitive instillation and removal of fluid into and from the peritoneal cavity, respectively. Solute removal again results primarily by dialysis along a concentration gradient, and fluid removal occurs by ultrafiltration driven by an osmotic pressure gradient. Although this method is less efficient and less rapid than hemodialysis, no central venous access, anticoagulation, skilled technician, or expensive equipment is necessary.

The amount of dialysis that needs to be prescribed is still somewhat controversial. Extrapolations from chronic renal failure prescription guidelines may not be sufficient to prevent the signs and symptoms of uremia in patients with ARF. Earlier study suggested that a more intensive regimen of hemodialysis may actually improve survival in this setting. However, later studies did not confirm the benefits of intensive dialysis treatment.

15. **What is CRRT?**

CRRT includes a number of treatments characterized by slow, gradual, continuous removal of fluid and electrolytes. Continuous venovenous hemodialysis (CVVHD) is the most widely used method. It involves solute removal by convection and fluid removal by hydrostatic pressure across high-flux membrane. Like conventional dialysis, CVVHD requires central venous access, anticoagulation, skilled staff, and complex equipment. Continuous arteriovenous hemofiltration and dialysis is a technically simple but less-efficient form of CRRT. Although each of these techniques has advantages and disadvantages, in general, the expertise of the professionals working at the center is probably the most important factor. Because of the difficulty in orienting nursing staff to continuous dialysis methods, slow low-efficiency daily dialysis has been developed that provides dialysis over approximately one half of the hours of the day. Of interest, the biocompatibility of the hemodialysis membrane appears to be an important factor in determining outcome, whereas the intensity of the dialysis prescription (i.e., blood flow, dialysate flow) does not appear to be an important factor in determining patient outcomes.

BOX 42-1. DIALYSIS OPTIONS IN THE TREATMENT OF ACUTE RENAL FAILURE

Intermittent Hemodialysis
Advantages
Efficient and intensive dialysis technique
Dialysis staff required for shorter period of time

Disadvantages
May cause hemodynamic instability
Relative need for anticoagulation
Potential for disequilibrium
Need for expensive machinery
Need for personnel to perform hemodialysis

Requirements
Venous access, anticoagulation, skilled staff, and expensive equipment

Peritoneal Dialysis
Advantages
Slow, gentle form of dialysis
Provides better hemodynamic stability than intermittent hemodialysis
No need for anticoagulation

Disadvantages
Electrolyte disorders and volume corrected slowly
Many nursing units unfamiliar with methodology
Risk for leaks and peritoneal infection

Requirements
Peritoneal catheter, sterile peritoneal dialysis solutions, and trained staff

CRRT
Advantages
Slow, continuous form of dialysis
Provides better hemodynamic stability than intermittent hemodialysis
Efficient solute removal and electrolyte balance
Round-the-clock maintenance of volume status
Nutrition and medications given while volume status is maintained

Disadvantages
Patient immobilization
Systemic anticoagulation
Nursing staff intensive
Expensive machinery

Requirements
Round-the-clock skilled nursing staff, vascular access, anticoagulation, and complex
equipment

KEY POINTS: ACUTE RENAL FAILURE

1. Serum creatinine concentration may be insensitive to the loss of renal function.

2. ARF due to acute tubular necrosis may be initiated by one mechanism and maintained by another different mechanism.

3. Results elicited by measures to prevent ATN are far superior to those yielded by efforts to provide treatment.

4. Urinalysis and urine electrolyte and creatinine estimation can provide important information about the cause of ARF.

5. Hyperkalemia is an important life-threatening complication of ARF requiring urgent management.

6. Renal replacement therapy, in the form of dialysis, may be required for correction of volume status, electrolyte imbalance, and acidosis, if conservative therapy fails.

BIBLIOGRAPHY

1. Asif A, Epstein M: Prevention of radiocontrast induced nephropathy. Am J Kidney Dis 44:12-24, 2004.

2. Bellomo R, Cass A, Cole L, et al: Intensity of continuous renal replacement therapy in critically ill patients. N Engl J Med 361:1627-1638, 2009.

3. Briglia AE: Choosing the best dialysis option in patients with acute renal failure and in intensive care unit. In Henrich WL (ed): Principles and Practice of Dialysis, 4th ed. Philadelphia, Lippincott Williams & Wilkins, 2009, pp 219-240.

4. Conger J: Hemodynamic factors in acute renal failure. Adv Ren Replace Ther 4:25-37, 1997.

5. Esson ML, Schrier RW: Diagnosis and treatment of acute tubular necrosis. Ann Intern Med 137:744-752, 2002.

6. Khosla N, Mehta RL: Continuous dialysis therapeutic techniques. In Henrich WL (ed): Principles and Practice of Dialysis, 4th ed. Philadelphia, Lippincott Williams & Wilkins, 2009, pp 196-218.

7. Lameire N: The pathophysiology of acute renal failure. Crit Care Clin 21:197-210, 2005.

8. Miller TR, Anderson RJ, Linas SL, et al: Urinary diagnostic indices in acute renal failure: a prospective study. Ann Intern Med 89:47-50, 1978.

9. Nowicki M, Zwiech R, Szklarek M: Acute renal failure: the new perspective. Annales Academiae Medicae Bialostocensis 49:145-150, 2004.

10. Palevsky PM: Renal replacement therapy: indications and timing. Crit Care Clin 21:347-356, 2005.

11. Saxena R, Toto RD: Approach to the patient with kidney disease. In Brenner BM (ed): Brenner & Rector's The Kidney, 8th ed. Philadelphia, Saunders, 2008, pp 705-723.

12. Venkataraman R, Kellum JA: Defining Acute Renal Failure: the RIFLE Criteria. J Intensive Care Med 22:187-193, 2007.

13. Wiseman AC, Linas S: Disorders of potassium and acid-base balance. Am J Kidney Dis 45:941-949, 2005.

CHAPTER 43

RENAL REPLACEMENT THERAPY AND RHABDOMYOLYSIS

Brad W. Butcher, MD, and Kathleen D. Liu, MD, PhD, MAS

RENAL REPLACEMENT THERAPY

1. **What are the indications for renal replacement therapy (RRT)?**
   Indications can be grouped by using the AEIOU mnemonic:
   A: (Metabolic) **Acidosis** refractory to bicarbonate administration.
   E: Electrolyte imbalances, of which hyperkalemia is the most life threatening.
   I: Ingestions. Some drugs and toxins (and their toxic metabolites) can be cleared with dialysis, including aspirin, lithium, methanol, or ethylene glycol.
   O: Overload. Ultrafiltration with dialysis can relieve hypoxemia resulting from volume overload, which may be particularly problematic in the setting of oliguria or anuria.
   U: Uremia. Symptoms and signs of uremia can range from mild (anorexia, nausea, pruritus) to severe (encephalopathy, asterixis, pericarditis); patients may also have clinical platelet dysfunction (bleeding) due to uremia.

2. **List the different modes of RRT.**
   Intermittent renal replacement therapies:
   - Peritoneal dialysis (PD)
   - Intermittent hemodialysis (IHD)
   - Pure ultrafiltration (PUF)
   - Hybrid therapies:
     - Sustained low-efficiency dialysis (SLED)
     - Sustained low-efficiency diafiltration (SLEDF)
     - Extended daily dialysis (EDD)
     - Slow continuous dialysis (SCD)

   Continuous renal replacement therapies (CRRT):
   - Slow continuous ultrafiltration (SCUF)
   - Continuous venovenous hemofiltration (CVVH)
   - Continuous venovenous hemodialysis (CVVHD)
   - Continuous venovenous hemodiafiltration (CVVHDF)

3. **What are hybrid therapies?**
   SLED, SLEDF, EDD, and SCD collectively refer to recently developed hybrid modes of dialysis. Dialysis can be delivered through a variety of conventional IHD machines (an advantage over CRRT), usually with some minor modifications to allow for slower dialysate flow rates compared with IHD. Therapy is delivered intermittently but over a longer time period (6-12 hours per session) than conventional IHD (3-4 hours per session) and often on a daily basis. Thus hybrid therapies have many of the benefits of CRRT without some of the disadvantages (see question 5).

4. **In whom should CRRT or hybrid therapy be considered?**
   CRRT or hybrid therapy should be considered in any critically ill patient with an indication for dialysis. CRRT or hybrid modalities tend to be better tolerated hemodynamically than intermittent dialysis because of slower rates of solute flux and fluid removal. CRRT may also allow for increased net daily ultrafiltration compared with IHD because volume removal occurs

continuously, albeit at a slower rate. Furthermore, in highly catabolic, critically ill patients, increased clearance with CRRT or hybrid modalities compared with IHD may allow for better control of azotemia, acidosis, and electrolyte abnormalities, including hyperphosphatemia. Last, patients with elevated intracranial pressure or fulminant hepatic failure may not tolerate IHD because of rapid shifts in solute concentrations. Importantly, IHD is preferable to CRRT in patients with severe, life-threatening hyperkalemia and some types of ingestions because clearance per unit time is slower with CRRT than with IHD.

5. **What are some disadvantages of CRRT?**
Because of its continuous nature, CRRT requires long-term relative immobilization of the patient, which can increase the risk for venous thromboembolism, pressure ulcers, and persistent deconditioning. Continuous anticoagulation is often necessary to prevent filter clotting and subsequent blood loss, and this may increase the bleeding risk. CRRT frequently results in hypothermia as blood is cooled during transit through the extracorporeal circuit; importantly, this can mask the development of a fever. Last, CRRT is highly labor intensive, typically requiring 1:1 nursing, and therefore costly.

6. **Define hemofiltration, hemodialysis, and hemodiafiltration.**
   - **Hemofiltration:** Plasma is forced from the blood space into the effluent via the application of pressure across a highly permeable membrane. This results in *convective* clearance of small and middle-sized molecules through the physical property of solvent drag. This modality does not significantly change the concentration of serum electrolytes and waste products unless a replacement fluid is infused into the blood, effectively diluting out those solutes the physician wishes to remove (e.g., urea nitrogen and potassium) and increasing the concentration of those solutes in which the patient might be deficient (e.g., bicarbonate in a patient with acidemia).
   - **Hemodialysis:** Blood flows on one side of a semipermeable membrane, and the dialysate, which contains various electrolytes and glucose, flows along the other side, usually in the opposite (countercurrent) direction. A concentration gradient drives electrolytes and water-soluble waste products from the plasma compartment into the dialysate. The dialysis machine generates a pressure across the membrane to drive plasma water from the blood side to the dialysate side. Dialysis results in *diffusive* clearance, preferentially of small molecules.
   - **Hemodiafiltration:** This technique makes simultaneous use of hemofiltration and hemodialysis, resulting in both diffusive and convective clearance.

7. **List the basic components of a prescription for IHD and for CRRT.**
   IHD:
   - Dialysis access: Arteriovenous fistula, arteriovenous graft, tunneled dialysis catheter, or temporary dialysis catheter
   - Treatment duration: For most patients with end-stage renal disease, this ranges between 3 and 4 hours. When a patient with acute renal failure or acute kidney injury (AKI) starts hemodialysis, initial sessions may be as short as 1 to 1.5 hours to decrease the risk of dialysis disequilibrium syndrome.
   - Filter size and type: Biocompatible dialysis membranes are now routinely used.
   - Blood flow rate: Blood flow rates of up to 400 to 450 mL/min can be achieved with an arteriovenous fistula or graft and up to 350 mL/min with a tunneled or temporary catheter. Generally, the faster the flow, the more efficient the dialysis.
   - Dialysate flow rate: Typical flow rates range from 500 mL/min to 800 mL/min.
   - Dialysate bath: Concentrations of potassium, sodium, calcium, and bicarbonate can be customized on the basis of the patient's laboratory studies.
   - Ultrafiltration goal: This is the amount of fluid to be removed from the patient over the course of the session; determined by clinical assessment of the patient's volume status.

- Anticoagulation: Clotting within the dialysis circuit can result in significant blood loss; heparin is typically used unless the patient has a contraindication.

CRRT:
- As in IHD, the prescription includes dialysis access, filter size and type, hourly fluid balance, and anticoagulation. An alternative to heparin anticoagulation often used with CRRT is regional citrate anticoagulation, in which citrate is administered to chelate calcium, a critical cofactor in the clotting cascade. Arteriovenous fistular and grafts are not used for CART.
- Blood flow rates are typically slower than in intermittent dialysis (150-200 mL/min).
- Mode of therapy: CVVH, CVVHD, or CVVHDF
- Dialysate or replacement fluid: The specific fluid is based on the metabolic parameters of the patient, including the patient's acid-base status and serum potassium concentration.
- Dialysate or replacement fluid flow rate: Dosing is weight based and is typically prescribed at a dose ranging from 20 mL/kg/hr to 35 mL/kg/hr, based on the patient's weight. Studies have shown no mortality difference between patients with renal replacement therapy administered at these two rates.

8. **What kinds of laboratory tests should be ordered regularly for patients receiving CRRT?**
   Sodium, potassium, bicarbonate, calcium, and phosphate levels can change rapidly during CRRT. Hyperphosphatemia frequently occurs in IHD because of inefficient clearance of phosphate, but hypophosphatemia is more common during CRRT given the continuous clearance of phosphate. Hypocalcemia and hypomagnesemia are also seen, especially when these cations are complexed with citrate (e.g., when citrate is used as an anticoagulant) or when a replacement fluid without these cations is infused into the patient (e.g., during CVVH). Patients with impaired lactate metabolism (e.g., because of severe sepsis or hepatic failure) may have high systemic lactate levels if the dialysate or replacement fluid contains lactate as a base equivalent. In these cases, high lactate levels or worsening acidosis should prompt the use of a bicarbonate-based dialysate or replacement fluid. Blood gas levels should be checked to monitor the patient's acid-base status.

9. **What are nutrition considerations for patients with AKI receiving RRT?**
   - **Amino acids** are lost in both IHD and CRRT. Critically ill patients with AKI are often highly catabolic; many patients receiving CRRT will require at least 1.5 to 2 g/kg/day of protein or amino acids.
   - **Vitamins:**
     □ Water-soluble vitamins are lost in both IHD and CRRT. Replacement of these vitamins can be achieved with the daily administration of a vitamin complex specifically designed for patients receiving RRT.
     □ Fat-soluble vitamins are protein or lipoprotein-bound and are therefore not significantly cleared by CRRT or IHD.
   - **Trace minerals**, such as zinc, may be dialyzed with IHD or CRRT; the benefit of supplementation in this situation remains unproved. Aluminum-containing products, which were used in the past as phosphorus binders, should be avoided because of central nervous system toxicity.

10. **What are the complications of CRRT?**
    Among the most important risks of CRRT are the risks inherent in obtaining central venous access. In general, subclavian venous access should be avoided, given the risk of subclavian stenosis with an indwelling catheter, particularly among patients who might require long-term hemodialysis. Electrolyte abnormalities or hypovolemia may also develop with CRRT. Patients may have hypothermia because of heat loss, which may mask a febrile response to infection.

RHABDOMYOLYSIS

11. **What causes rhabdomyolysis?**
Muscle ischemia, damage, and eventual necrosis lead to rhabdomyolysis. The various causes are grouped into physical and nonphysical causes in Box 43-1. Both groups of causes probably share a common pathway in which increased demand on muscle cells and their mitochondria, because of intrinsic deficiencies or extrinsic forces (i.e., decreased oxygen delivery or increased metabolic demands), leads to ischemia and eventual damage.

BOX 43-1. MAJOR CAUSES OF RHABDOMYOLYSIS

Physical Causes
- Trauma and compression
- Occlusion or hypoperfusion of the muscular vessels
- Excessive muscle strain: exercise, seizure, tetanus, delirium tremens
- Electrical current
- Hyperthermia: exercise, sepsis, neuroleptic malignant syndrome, malignant hyperthermia

Nonphysical Causes
- Metabolic myopathies, including McArdle disease, mitochondrial respiratory chain enzyme deficiencies, carnitine palmitoyl transferase deficiency, phosphofructokinase deficiency
- Endocrinopathies, including hypothyroidism and diabetic ketoacidosis (due to electrolyte abnormalities)
- Drugs and toxins, including medications (antimalarials, colchicine, corticosteroids, fibrates, HMG-CoA reductase inhibitors, isoniazid, zidovudine), drugs of abuse (alcohol, heroin), and toxins (insect and snake venoms)
- Infections (either local or systemic)
- Electrolyte abnormalities: hyperosmotic conditions, hypokalemia, hypophosphatemia, hyponatremia, or hypernatremia
- Autoimmune diseases: polymyositis or dermatomyositis

---

12. **Discuss the symptoms and signs of rhabdomyolysis.**
The classic presentation of rhabdomyolysis, consisting of myalgias, weakness, and dark urine, is rare, and often only one or two of these symptoms are present. A history suggestive of muscle compression, a physical examination demonstrating muscle tenderness, and laboratory tests confirming muscle damage lead to a strong presumptive diagnosis.

13. **What laboratory tests should be ordered to diagnose rhabdomyolysis?**
Creatine phosphokinase activity is the most sensitive indicator of muscle damage; it may continue to increase for several days after the original insult. Hyperkalemia, hyperuricemia, and hyperphosphatemia also occur, as these substances are released from the damaged muscle cells. Hypocalcemia develops as calcium is chelated and deposited in the damaged muscle tissue. Lactic acidosis and an anion gap metabolic acidosis can result from release of other organic acids from cells.

14. **What are the complications of rhabdomyolysis?**
The most immediate concern is hyperkalemia due to cell necrosis, particularly in the setting of AKI, which occurs through several mechanisms. Damaged myocytes release myoglobin and its metabolites, which precipitate with other cellular debris to form pigmented casts in renal tubules, obstructing urinary flow. Third-spacing of fluids, particularly at the site of muscle injury, can lead to both intravascular hypovolemia with impaired renal perfusion and

compartment syndrome. Furthermore, precipitation of myoglobin in the kidney can initiate a cytokine cascade that leads to renal vasoconstriction, further exacerbating acute renal failure.

Although patients usually have hypocalcemia, they rarely have symptoms. Caution should be exercised when treating hypocalcemia because patients often have rebound hypercalcemia during the recovery phase. Symptoms of hypocalcemia, such as tetany, Chvostek or Trousseau signs, or cardiac arrhythmias, should be treated promptly. Other immediate concerns include hypovolemia, particularly in the setting of crush injuries or other causes of compression injury.

15. What treatment options are available?
Supportive care, with intravascular volume repletion and prevention of continued renal insult, is the main strategy. In general, fluids should be instilled at a rate sufficient to result in an hourly urine output of 200 to 300 mL. Although limited clinical evidence supports this strategy, using sodium bicarbonate–based crystalloids to alkalinize the urine is thought to improve the solubility of myoglobin and decrease its direct tubular toxicity. Mannitol can be used to promote an osmotic diuresis, and both thiazide and loop diuretics can also be used to augment urine flow once it is clear that the patient is intravascularly volume replete. Allopurinol, dosed for the degree of renal impairment, reduces the production of uric acid, which can crystallize in the tubules along with myoglobin. Control of hyperkalemia, which may require the provision of dialysis, and treatment of symptomatic hypocalcemia are important parts of the treatment regimen.

16. What kind of prophylactic management options are possible?
Guidelines for the treatment of catastrophic crush injuries (developed in response to natural disasters including earthquakes) recommend the initiation of volume resuscitation with crystalloid even before extrication. In the first 24 hours, up to 10 L of intravascular volume may be lost as sequestrated fluid in the affected limb. Administration of up to 10 to 12 L of fluid may be required during this period, with careful monitoring of urine output.

17. What drugs need to be avoided in patients with rhabdomyolysis?
Succinylcholine, a drug used for rapid muscle paralysis to achieve airway control, causes generalized depolarization of neuromuscular junctions and can cause hyperkalemia if the patient has abnormal proliferations of the motor end plates. Patients with rhabdomyolysis often have hyperkalemia, and therefore succinylcholine should generally be avoided, given the often lethal nature of these hyperkalemic events. In addition, medications that are known to be associated with rhabdomyolysis (e.g., 3-hydroxy-3-methylglutaryl–coenzyme A [HMG-CoA] reductase inhibitors) should be avoided, if possible.

ACID–BASE INTERPRETATION

18. Identify the normal extracellular pH, and define acidosis and alkalosis.
The range for the normal extracellular pH in arterial blood is considered to be 7.37 to 7.43. Of note, the normal pH in venous blood is slightly lower (by 0.05 pH units on average); the lower venous pH results from the uptake of metabolically produced carbon dioxide in the capillary circulation. Acidemia is defined as an increase in the hydrogen ion concentration of the blood, resulting in a decrease in pH, and alkalemia is defined as a decrease in the hydrogen ion concentration in the blood, resulting in an increase in pH. Acidosis and alkalosis refer to processes that lower or raise the pH, respectively. These processes can be either metabolic or respiratory in origin and, occasionally, a combination of both.

19. What information is necessary to properly interpret a patient's acid-base status?
To accurately interpret a patient's acid-base status, an arterial blood gas analysis, serum electrolyte concentrations, and the serum albumin concentration are needed.

20. **What is the anion gap, how is it calculated, and why is it important in understanding a patient's acid-base status?**

The anion gap is defined as the difference between the plasma concentrations of the major cation (sodium) and the major *measured* anions (chloride and bicarbonate), expressed mathematically by the following equation:

$$\text{Anion gap} = [\text{Na}^+] - ([\text{Cl}^-] + [\text{HCO}_3^-])$$

A normal anion gap is generally considered to be 8 to 12 in a patient with a normal serum albumin concentration of 4.0 g/dL. In patients with hypoalbuminemia, the anion gap should be "corrected" by adding 2.5 to the calculated anion gap for every 1 g/dL decrease in albumin concentration. The anion gap is elevated in processes that result in an increase in the plasma concentration of anions that are not routinely measured in conventional chemistry panels, including lactate, phosphates, sulfates, and other organic anions (such as the degradation products of commonly ingested alcohols). Calculating the anion gap is critical when assessing a patient's acid-base status because an elevated anion gap may alert the physician to the presence of a metabolic acidosis that might not be apparent on first glance of the arterial blood gas values. Accordingly, the anion gap should always be calculated when assessing a patient's acid-base status. Furthermore, the different diagnosis of a metabolic acidosis is largely influenced by the presence or absence of an elevated anion gap (see later).

21. **Describe an approach to a comprehensive interpretation of a patient's acid-base status using the arterial blood gas and the serum chemistry values.**
    - Identify whether the patient has acidemia or alkalemia: If the pH is less than 7.37, the patient has acidemia, and, if the pH is greater than 7.43, the patient has alkalemia. Importantly, a pH between 7.37 and 7.43 **does not** imply that the patient does not have an acid-base disturbance; rather it suggests the presence of a mixed acid-base disorder.
    - Determine whether the primary disturbance is respiratory or metabolic: If the patient has acidemia and the PCO_2 is greater than 40 mm Hg, then the primary process is respiratory; if the patient has acidemia and the serum bicarbonate concentration is less than 24 mEq/L, then the primary process is metabolic. If the patient has alkalemia and the PCO_2 is less than 40 mm Hg, then the primary process is respiratory; if the patient has alkalemia and the serum bicarbonate concentration is greater than 24 mEq/L, then the primary process is metabolic.
    - Determine whether appropriate compensation for the primary disorder is present: To determine how the kidneys compensate for a primary respiratory process and vice versa, see Table 43-1. If the compensation is less than or greater than predicted, then another primary acid-base disturbance might be present. For example, in presence of a metabolic acidosis, if the PCO_2 is lower than expected a concomitant primary respiratory alkalosis is present, whereas if the PCO_2 is higher than expected a concomitant primary respiratory acidosis is present.
    - Calculate the anion gap to look for the presence of an anion gap metabolic acidosis.
    - Calculate the *delta-delta*: In the presence of an isolated anion gap metabolic acidosis, the serum bicarbonate concentration should fall by an amount that equals the degree to which the anion gap is raised. If this is not the case, another metabolic disorder (either a non–anion gap metabolic acidosis or a metabolic alkalosis) is present. This can be determined by calculating the delta-delta, which is mathematically expressed as follows:

$$\text{Delta} - \text{delta} = \frac{\text{Calculated anion gap} - \text{Normal anion gap}}{\text{Normal serum bicarbonate} - \text{Measured serum bicarbonate}}$$

Generally, 12 is used as the value of a normal anion gap, and 24 is used as the value for a normal serum bicarbonate. If the delta-delta is between 1 and 2, the disturbance is a pure anion

TABLE 43-1. APPROPRIATE COMPENSATION FOR PRIMARY ACID-BASE DISTURBANCES AND THEIR COMMON CAUSES

PRIMARY ACID-BASE DISTURBANCE	SUBTYPE	EXPECTED COMPENSATION
Metabolic acidosis	Anion gap Non–anion gap	Decrease in $PCO_2 = 1.2 \times \Delta HCO_3$ **or** $PCO_2 = (1.5 \times HCO_3) + 8 \pm 2$
Metabolic alkalosis		Increase in $PCO_2 = 0.7 \times \Delta HCO_3$
Respiratory acidosis	Acute	Increase in $HCO_3 = 0.1 \times \Delta PCO_2$
	Chronic	Increase in $HCO_3 = 0.35 \times \Delta PCO_2$
Respiratory alkalosis	Acute	Decrease in $HCO_3 = 0.2 \times \Delta PCO_2$
	Chronic	Decrease in $HCO_3 = 0.4 \times \Delta PCO_2$

gap metabolic acidosis. If the quotient is less than 1 a non–anion gap metabolic acidosis is also present, whereas if the quotient is greater than 2 a metabolic alkalosis is also present.
- After all of these steps have been completed, the physician should have an assessment of all of the acid-base disorders present and should use the clinical information to determine the underlying cause(s).

22. **List the differential diagnoses of the major acid-base disturbances.**
Each of the primary acid-base disturbances has its own differential diagnosis, and many acronyms have been generated to help the student or physician remember them. Of these, the most popular is the MUDPILERS acronym for the differential diagnosis of an anion-gap metabolic acidosis. If an anion gap acidosis is present, the osmolar gap should be measured and calculated; the presence of an osmolar gap in addition to an anion gap suggests a toxic alcohol ingestion, such as ethylene glycol, methanol, or ethanol. A more comprehensive differential diagnosis for each of the primary disturbances is presented in Box 43-2.

BOX 43-2. DIFFERENTIAL DIAGNOSES OF THE PRIMARY ACID-BASE DISTURBANCES

Anion Gap Metabolic Acidosis
Common causes can be remembered with the *MUDPILERS* mnemonic:
Methanol
Uremia with accumulation of organic anions (phosphates, sulfates, urate)
Diabetic ketoacidosis (and other forms of ketoacidosis: alcoholic, starvation)
Paraldehyde and **p**ropylene glycol (carrier for certain medications, including intravenous lorazepam and diazepam)
Isoniazid
Lactic acidosis: type A, type B, D-lactic acidosis
Ethylene glycol
Rhabdomyolysis
Salicylates
Other ingestions associated with anion gap metabolic acidosis include acetaminophen (from accumulation of 5-oxoproline) and toluene from glue sniffing.

BOX 43-2   DIFFERENTIAL DIAGNOSES OF THE PRIMARY ACID-BASE DISTURBANCES—*cont'd*

Non–Anion Gap Metabolic Acidosis

- Gastrointestinal loss of bicarbonate: diarrhea, intestinal or pancreatic fistulas or drainage
- Renal dysfunction: renal failure (leading to impaired ammoniagenesis) or renal tubular acidosis
- Dilutional: caused by rapid infusion of bicarbonate-free fluids, such as normal saline solution
- Posthypocapnia
- Ureteral diversion

Metabolic Alkalosis

- Gastrointestinal loss of hydrogen ions: removal of gastric secretions (vomiting, nasogastric tube suction)
- Renal loss of hydrogen ions: primary mineralocorticoid excess, administration of thiazide or loop diuretics, posthypercapneic alkalosis, milk-alkali syndrome with associated hypercalcemia, congenital syndromes (Bartter syndrome and Gitelman syndrome)

Respiratory Acidosis

- Neuromuscular diseases: Guillain-Barré syndrome, myasthenia gravis, botulism, hypophosphatemia and hypokalemia, poliomyelitis, diaphragmatic dysfunction
- Central hypoventilation: congenital central hypoventilation syndrome (Ondine curse), obesity hypoventilation syndrome, Cheyne-Stokes breathing
- Medications that depress respiratory drive: narcotics, benzodiazepines, barbiturates, heroin
- Endocrine causes: hypothyroidism
- Airway obstruction: epiglottis, chronic obstructive pulmonary disease, severe and late phase asthma
- Trauma leading to chest wall abnormalities or restrictive lung disease from severe kyphoscoliosis

Respiratory Alkalosis

- Central nervous system process: stroke, infection, trauma, tumor
- Hypoxemia
- Hyperthermia
- Sepsis
- Liver disease
- Pain or anxiety (a diagnosis of exclusion)
- Medications: medroxyprogesterone, theophylline, salicylates
- Pregnancy

KEY POINTS: MANAGEMENT OF RHABDOMYOLYSIS

1. Volume resuscitation

2. Vigilance for hyperkalemia and treatment with dialysis or other supportive measures, if necessary

3. Treatment of symptomatic hypocalcemia

4. Alkalinization of urine with sodium bicarbonate (limited data)

KEY POINTS: POTENTIAL ADVANTAGES OF CONTINUOUS RENAL REPLACEMENT THERAPIES OR HYBRID THERAPIES OVER INTERMITTENT HEMODIALYSIS

1. Hemodynamic stability

2. Increased volume removal

3. Increased clearance of nitrogenous wastes

4. Improved control of acidosis

5. Fewer fluctuations in intracranial pressure

KEY POINTS: ACID-BASE DISORDERS

1. An organized approach to the analysis of acid-base disorders is key.

2. The approach starts by determining whether the patient has acidemia or alkalemia; note that the presence of a normal serum pH does not imply that an acid-base disorder is not present.

3. Determine whether the primary process is metabolic or respiratory.

4. Determine whether there is appropriate compensation for the primary process.

5. Calculate the anion gap and the "delta-delta" to determine whether unrecognized metabolic disturbances exist, including gap and non-gap metabolic acidosis and metabolic alkalosis.

BIBLIOGRAPHY

1. Bellomo R, Cass A, Cole L, et al: Intensity of continuous renal-replacement therapy in critically ill patients. N Engl J Med 361:1627-1638, 2009.

2. Huerta-Alardin AL, Varon J, Marik PE: Bench-to-bedside review: rhabdomyolysis—an overview for clinicians. Crit Care 9:158-169, 2005.

3. Malinoski DJ, Slater MS, Mullins RJ: Crush injury and rhabdomyolysis. Crit Care Clin 20:171-192, 2004.

4. Marshall MR, Golper TA: Sustained low efficiency or extended daily dialysis: www.uptodate.com. Accessed March 27, 2012.

5. McClave SA, Martindale RG, Vanek VW, et al: Guidelines for the provision and assessment of nutrition support therapy in the adult critically ill patient. J Parenter Enteral Nutr 33:277-316, 2009.

6. Palevsky PM: Renal replacement therapy (dialysis) in acute kidney injury (acute renal failure) in adults: indications, timing, and dialysis dose: www.uptodate.com. Accessed March 27, 2012.

7. Palevsky PM, Zhang JH, O'Connor TZ, et al: Intensity of renal support in critically ill patients with acute kidney injury. N Engl J Med 359:7-20, 2008.

8. Seifter J: Acid-base disorders. In Goldman L, Schafer A: Goldman's Cecil Medicine, 24th ed. St. Louis, Saunders, 2011.

9. Vanholder R, Sever MS, Erek E, et al: Rhabdomyolysis. J Am Soc Nephrol 11:1553-1561, 2000.

CHAPTER 44

HYPOKALEMIA AND HYPERKALEMIA

Stuart L. Linas, MD, and Shailendra Sharma, MD

HYPOKALEMIA

1. **Is serum potassium level an accurate estimate of total body potassium?**
   No. The majority of potassium is distributed in the intracellular fluid (ICF) compartment, with only approximately 2% of the total body potassium in the extracellular fluid (ECF) compartment. Alterations in serum potassium can result from transcellular potassium shift between ECF and ICF compartments or from actual changes in total body potassium.

2. **When does serum potassium level falsely estimate total body potassium?**
   Transcellular potassium shifts between ECF and ICF compartments can have profound effects on serum potassium. Buffering of the ECF compartment, with reciprocal movement of potassium and hydrogen across the cell membrane, can result in a rise in serum potassium in the case of acidemia and a fall in serum potassium in the case of alkalemia. Two important hormones that are known to drive potassium into the ICF compartment are insulin and catecholamines.

   The classic example of how serum potassium falsely estimates total body potassium is a patient with diabetic ketoacidosis. Insulin deficiency and acidemia cause potassium to shift to the ECF compartment so that serum potassium may be normal or high despite profound total body potassium depletion (due to osmotic diuresis and hyperaldosteronemic state). Only after proper treatment of insulin deficiency and acidosis does the total body potassium depletion become apparent.

3. **Why is tight regulation of serum potassium concentrations so critical?**
   Although a small fraction of total body potassium is in the ECF compartment, changes in ECF potassium, either by compartmental shifts or by net gain or loss, significantly alter the ratio of ECF to ICF potassium, which determines the cellular resting membrane potential. As a consequence, small fluctuations in ECF potassium can have profound effects on cardiac and neuromuscular excitability.

4. **How do you estimate the total body potassium deficit?**
   It is difficult to predict accurately the total body potassium deficit on the basis of serum potassium, but in uncomplicated potassium depletion a useful rule of thumb is as follows: For each 100 mEq potassium deficit, the fall in serum potassium level is 0.27 mEq/L. Thus, for a 70-kg patient, serum potassium of 3 mEq/L reflects a 300- to 400-mEq deficit, whereas potassium of 2 mEq/L reflects a 500- to 700-mEq deficit. In patients with acid-base disorders, this rule of thumb is not accurate because of shifts in compartmental potassium.

5. **What is the relationship between potassium and magnesium?**
   Magnesium depletion typically occurs after diuretic use, sustained alcohol consumption, or diabetic ketoacidosis. Magnesium depletion can cause hypokalemia that is refractory to oral or intravenous (IV) potassium chloride therapy because severe magnesium depletion causes renal potassium wasting through undefined mechanisms. In the setting of severe magnesium and potassium depletion, magnesium and potassium must be replaced simultaneously.

Magnesium regulates activity of the renal outer medullary potassium (ROMK) channel. Intracellular magnesium is inversely proportional to the open ROMK channel pore. Therefore low intracellular magnesium causes more ROMK channels to open, allowing more K^+ efflux into the urine.

Magnesium is also closely related to sodium-potassium–adenosine triphosphatase (Na^+,K^+-ATPase), possibly explaining failure to retain intracellular potassium in hypomagnesemia.

6. **What factors are important in K^+ balance?**
   K^+ is mostly intracellular cation. Of 3500 mEq of total body potassium only approximately 60 mEq is in the extracellular compartment. Dietary K^+ must be rapidly shifted from the vascular space into cells (internal K^+ balance) before excretion by kidneys and GI tract (external balance). Internal balance is primarily regulated by insulin, whereas external balance is regulated by kidneys (85%) and gastrointestinal (GI) tract (15%).

7. **What are the factors that dictate urine potassium excretion?**
   Key factors influencing potassium secretion include adequate sodium delivery to the distal nephron and increased aldosterone action.

8. **What are the causes of hypokalemia?**
   - Redistribution: Intracellular potassium redistribution or shift can be caused by metabolic alkalosis, increased insulin availability, increased β_2-adrenergic activity, and periodic paralysis (classically associated with thyrotoxicosis).
   - GI loss: Diarrhea or poor K^+ intake.
   - Renal loss: Diuretics, vomiting, and states of mineralocorticoid excess (e.g., primary hyperaldosteronism, Cushing disease, European licorice ingestion, and hyperreninemia). Increases in distal sodium delivery in the setting of high plasma aldosterone levels (due to lower blood volume) result in increases in urinary potassium and subsequent hypokalemia. Other causes include hypomagnesemia and familial hypokalemic alkalosis syndromes (Bartter and Gitelman syndromes)
   - Low intake: Poor oral intake or total parenteral nutrition with inadequate potassium supplement.

9. **What are the clinical manifestations of hypokalemia?**
   By depressing neuromuscular excitability, hypokalemia leads to muscle weakness, which can include quadriplegia and hypoventilation. Severe hypokalemia disrupts cell integrity, leading to rhabdomyolysis. Among the most important manifestations of hypokalemia are cardiac arrhythmias, including paroxysmal atrial tachycardia with block, atrioventricular dissociation, first- and second-degree atrioventricular block with Wenckebach periods, and even ventricular tachycardia or fibrillation. Typical electrocardiographic (ECG) findings include ST-segment depression, flattened T waves, and prominent U waves.

10. **Which drugs can cause hypokalemia?**
    The most common drugs are diuretics: loop diuretics, thiazides, and acetazolamide. Penicillin and penicillin analogs (e.g., carbenicillin, ticarcillin, piperacillin) also cause renal potassium wasting that is mediated by various mechanisms, including delivery of nonreabsorbable anions to the distal nephron, which results in potassium trapping in the urine. Drugs that damage renal tubular membranes such as amphotericin, cisplatin, and aminoglycosides cause renal potassium wasting even in the absence of decreases in glomerular filtration rate (GFR).

11. **What is the diagnostic approach to a patient with hypokalemia?**
    After eliminating spurious causes (such as leukocytosis), the diagnosis of true hypokalemia can be approached on the basis of urine potassium concentration, systemic acid-base status, urine chloride level, and blood pressure (Fig. 44-1).

    Urine potassium excretion is best measured by a 24-hour urine collection. A spot urine potassium concentration can also be measured (less accurate, but easier to obtain thus most commonly obtained) with a value of < 15 mEq/L indicating extrarenal loss (poor oral intake,

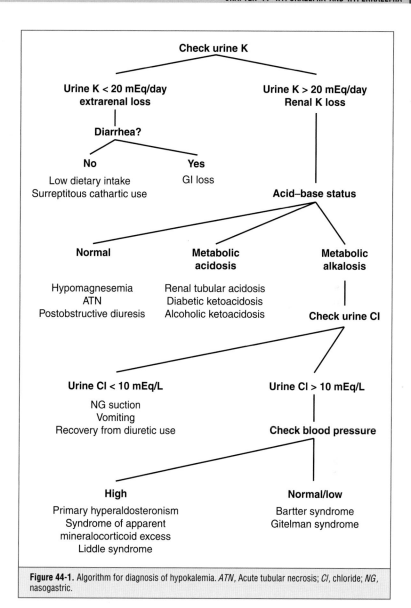

Figure 44-1. Algorithm for diagnosis of hypokalemia. *ATN,* Acute tubular necrosis; *Cl,* chloride; *NG,* nasogastric.

GI loss, intracellular shift) and a value of >15 mEq/L indicating renal potassium wasting. Low urine osmolality can interfere with interpretation of isolated urine potassium by diluting the urinary K^+ concentration.

12. **Why is serum K^+ often low in patients with myocardial infarction or acute asthma?**
Both conditions are associated with activation of the sympathetic nervous system. β_2-Adrenergic activation results in transcellular shift of K^+.

13. **How do you treat hypokalemia in the setting of K$^+$ depletion?**
Oral replacement is the safest route, and administration of doses of up to 40 mEq multiple times daily is allowed. In most cases, potassium chloride is used because metabolic alkalosis and chloride depletion often accompany hypokalemia, such as in patients who are taking diuretics or who are vomiting. In these settings, coadministration of chloride is important for correction of both the metabolic alkalosis and hypokalemia. In other settings, potassium should be administered with other salt preparations. For example, in metabolic acidosis, replacement with potassium bicarbonate or bicarbonate equivalent (e.g., potassium citrate, acetate, or gluconate) is recommended to help alleviate the acidosis. Persons who abuse alcohol or who have diabetes with ketoacidosis often have concomitant phosphate deficiency and should receive some of the potassium in the form of potassium phosphate.

14. **How do you treat hypokalemia in patients requiring loop diuretics?**
Positive K$^+$ balance is important in patients requiring loop diuretics because hypokalemia is arrhythmogenic. Increases in dietary K$^+$ and or K$^+$ supplements are often inadequate. Amiloride (Na$^+$ channel inhibitor) and spironolactone or eplerenone (mineralocorticoid receptor antagonist) are used. Consider measuring 24-hour K$^+$ excretion, then adjusting the dose of these agents to account for intake. The usual K$^+$ intake is 40 to 80 mEq/day.

15. **How do you treat hypokalemia in the setting of periodic paralysis?**
In both familial and nonfamilial periodic paralysis (e.g., from thyrotoxicosis), hypokalemia can be life threatening. Oral propranolol (nonselective β-blocker) at the dose of 1-2 mg/kg is an effective treatment to treat an acute attack of thyrotoxic periodic paralysis.

16. **When is IV potassium replacement necessary? What are the risks?**
In life-threatening situations such as severe weakness, respiratory distress, cardiac arrhythmias, and rhabdomyolysis, or in situations when oral administration is not possible, potassium must be replaced intravenously. Infusion rates in the intensive care unit should be limited to 20 mEq/hr to prevent the potentially catastrophic effect of a potassium bolus to the heart.

17. **What are the circumstances requiring special care in monitoring potassium replacement?**
    - Patients with defects in potassium excretion (e.g., renal failure, use of potassium-sparing diuretics or angiotensin-converting enzyme [ACE] inhibitors) must have their serum potassium concentrations monitored frequently when potassium is being replaced to prevent overcorrection.
    - Patients who are receiving digitalis therapy and have hypokalemia are prone to having serious cardiac arrhythmias (especially in overdose situations) and must be treated urgently.
    - Patients with significant magnesium deficiency have renal potassium wasting and often must have their magnesium levels corrected before therapy for hypokalemia is initiated.

KEY POINTS: CIRCUMSTANCES REQUIRING SPECIAL CARE IN MONITORING POTASSIUM REPLACEMENT

1. Patients with defects in potassium excretion (e.g., renal failure, use of potassium-sparing diuretics or ACE inhibitors) must have their serum potassium concentration monitored (i.e., daily laboratory checks) when potassium is being replaced to prevent overcorrection.

2. Patients who are receiving digitalis therapy and have hypokalemia are prone to having serious cardiac arrhythmias (especially in overdose situations) and must be treated urgently.

3. Patients with significant magnesium deficiency have renal potassium wasting and often must have their magnesium level corrected before therapy for hypokalemia is initiated.

HYPERKALEMIA

18. **What are the causes of hyperkalemia?**
    - *High potassium intake* (e.g., oral potassium replacement, total parenteral nutrition, and high-dose potassium penicillin) can cause hyperkalemia, usually in the setting of low renal potassium excretion.
    - *Extracellular potassium redistribution* can be caused by metabolic acidosis, insulin deficiency, β-adrenergic blockade, rhabdomyolysis, massive hemolysis, tumor lysis syndrome, periodic paralysis (hyperkalemic form), and heavily catabolic states such as severe sepsis.
    - *Low renal potassium excretion* can be caused by renal failure, decreased effective circulating volume (e.g., severe sepsis, congestive heart failure, cirrhosis), and states of hypoaldosteronism. States of hypoaldosteronism include decreased renin-angiotensin system activity (e.g., hyporeninemic hypoaldosteronism in diabetes, interstitial nephritis, ACE inhibitors, nonsteroidal antiinflammatory drugs [NSAIDs], cyclosporine), decreased adrenal synthesis (e.g., Addison disease, heparin), and aldosterone resistance (e.g., high-dose trimethoprim, potassium-sparing diuretic agents).

19. **Which drugs can cause hyperkalemia?**
    Drugs that cause release of intracellular potassium include succinylcholine and, rarely, β-blockers. Drugs that block the renin-angiotensin-aldosterone axis will result in decreased renal potassium excretion; these include spironolactone, ACE inhibitors, cyclosporine, heparin (low molecular weight and unfractionated), and NSAIDs. Drugs that impair the process of sodium and potassium exchange include digitalis; drugs that block sodium and potassium exchange in the distal nephron include amiloride and trimethoprim.

20. **How do states of decreased circulatory volume cause hyperkalemia?**
    Urinary K^+ is primarily dependent on aldosterone action mediated through activation of the epithelial Na^+ channel (ENaC). In states of volume deficiency, there is enhanced proximal nephron Na^+ reabsorption, hence decreased Na^+ availability to ENaC. Even in the setting of high aldosterone (e.g., congestive heart failure), insufficient Na^+ reabsorption occurs to cause electrogenic K^+ secretion.

21. **What are the clinical manifestations of hyperkalemia?**
    Clinical manifestations of hyperkalemia are dependent on many other variables such as calcium, acid-base status, and chronicity.
    The most serious manifestation of hyperkalemia involves the electrical conduction system of the heart. Profound hyperkalemia can lead to heart block and asystole. Initially, the ECG shows peaked T waves and decreased amplitude of P waves followed by prolongation of QRS waves. With severe hyperkalemia, QRS and T waves blend together into what appears to be a sine-wave pattern consistent with ventricular fibrillation. A good way to think about ECG changes in hyperkalemia is to imagine lifting the T wave, in which the T gets taller first followed by flattening of P and QRS. Other effects of hyperkalemia include weakness, neuromuscular paralysis (without central nervous system disturbances), and suppression of renal ammoniagenesis, which may result in metabolic acidosis.

22. **What degree of chronic kidney disease causes hyperkalemia?**
    Chronic kidney disease per se is not associated with hyperkalemia until the GFR is reduced to approximately 75% of normal levels (serum creatinine level >3 mg/dL). Although more than 85% of filtered potassium is reabsorbed in the proximal tubule, urinary excretion of potassium is determined primarily by potassium secretion along the cortical collecting tubule. Hyperkalemia disproportionate to reductions in GFR usually results from decreases in potassium secretion (due either to decreases in aldosterone, as may occur in Addison disease, or to diabetes with hyporeninemic hypoaldosteronism) or from marked decreases in sodium delivery to the distal nephron, as may occur in severe prerenal states.

23. **What is the transtubular potassium gradient (TTKG)? When should it be used?**
TTKG was developed to account for the potentially confounding effect of urine concentration on the interpretation of the urine potassium concentration. The TTKG provides a better clinical approach to uncover defects in urinary potassium (U_K) excretion as compared with U_K alone because the latter fails to account for plasma potassium concentration and for medullary water abstraction. TTKG is calculated as follows:

$$\text{Urine K} \times \text{Serum osm} / \text{Serum K} \times \text{Urine osm}$$

It is most commonly used in patients with hyperkalemia, where a TTKG <6 indicates an inappropriate renal response to hyperkalemia, that is, reduced renal potassium excretion. Two limitations exist to using the TTKG:
- Urinary sodium must be >25 mEq/L (so that sodium delivery is not the limiting factor for K^+ secretion). Na^+ is reabsorbed by the cortical collecting tubule (epithelial Na channel), then removed from the cell (Na^+,K^+-ATPase), resulting in an increase in cellular K^+ that then moves through a K^+ channel into the urine.
- Urine must be hypertonic (because vasopressin is required for optimal potassium conductance in the distal nephron).
  TTKG is of limited use in patients with a varying K^+ diet or after acute diuretic use.

24. **What is the diagnostic approach to hyperkalemia?**
The cause is often apparent after a careful history and review of medications and basic laboratory values, including a chemistry panel with blood urea nitrogen and creatinine concentrations. Additional laboratory tests can be performed if clinical suspicion exists for any of the following:
- Pseudohyperkalemia (look for high white blood cell and platelet counts)
- Rhabdomyolysis (look for high creatinine kinase concentration)
- Tumor lysis syndrome (look for high lactate dehydrogenase, uric acid, and phosphorus and low calcium levels)
- Hypoaldosteronemic state (look for a TTKG <5 in the setting of hyperkalemia)

25. **What is the effect of heparin on K^+?**
Heparin can cause hyperkalemia by blocking aldosterone biosynthesis. Both low-molecular-weight heparin and unfractionated heparin can cause hyperkalemia.

26. **What is pseudohyperkalemia?**
Serum potassium measurements can be falsely elevated when potassium is released during the process of blood collection from the patient or during the process of clot formation in the specimen tube. These situations do not reflect true hyperkalemia. Potassium release from muscles distal to a tight tourniquet can artifactually elevate potassium level by as much as 2.7 mEq/L. Potassium release during the process of clot formation in the specimen tube from leukocytes (white blood cell counts $>70,000/mm^3$) or platelets (platelet count $>1,000,000/mm^3$) can also become quite significant and distort serum potassium measurement results. In these circumstances, an unclotted blood sample (i.e., plasma potassium determination) should be obtained.

27. **What are the indications for emergent therapy?**
- ECG changes. Because cardiac arrest can occur at any point during ECG progression, hyperkalemia with ECG changes constitutes a medical emergency.
- Severe weakness.
- Serum potassium level above 6 mEq/L. ECG changes may not always be present, although this level of hyperkalemia predisposes to rhythm abnormalities.

28. **How do you treat hyperkalemia?**
The general approach is to use therapy involving each of the following:

- **Membrane stabilization:** Calcium antagonizes the cardiac effects of hyperkalemia. It raises the cell depolarization threshold and reduces myocardial irritability. Calcium is given regardless of serum calcium levels. One or two ampules of IV calcium chloride result in improvement in ECG changes within seconds, but the beneficial effect lasts only approximately 30 minutes. The dose can be repeated in absence of obvious change in ECG or with recurrence of ECG changes after initial resolution.
- **Shifting potassium into cells:** IV insulin with glucose administration begins to lower serum potassium levels in approximately 2 to 5 minutes and lasts a few hours. Correction of acidosis with IV sodium bicarbonate has a similar duration and time of onset. Nebulized β-adrenergic agonists such as albuterol can lower serum potassium level by 0.5 to 1.5 mEq/L with an onset within 30 minutes and an effect lasting 2 to 4 hours. Albuterol, however, may be ineffective in a subset of patients with end-stage renal disease (from 20%-40%).
- **Removal of potassium:** Loop diuretics can sometimes cause enough renal potassium loss in patients with intact renal function, but usually a potassium-binding resin must be used (e.g., Kayexalate, 30 gm taken orally or 50 gm administered by retention enema). The effect of resin on potassium is slow, and the full effect may take up to 4 to 24 hours. Acute hemodialysis is quick and effective at removing potassium and must be used when the GI tract is nonfunctional or when serious fluid overload is already present. Rarely, when chronic hyperkalemia is secondary to hypoaldosteronism, mineralocorticoids can be of use.

29. **Should glucose always be given with insulin?**
Glucose elevation in the extravascular space (e.g., with administration of 50% dextrose) results in K^+ movement from the intracellular to extracellular space. Thus hyperglycemia in diabetes may cause hyperkalemia, especially in the absence of insulin. After insulin therapy for hyperkalemia, glucose should not be administered if the serum glucose concentration is over 175 mg/dL.

BIBLIOGRAPHY

1. Choi MJ, Ziyadeh FN: The utility of the transtubular potassium gradient in the evaluation of hyperkalemia. J Am Soc Nephrol 19:424-426, 2008.
2. Chou TC: Electrolyte imbalance. In Chou TC, Knilans K (eds): Electrocardiography in Clinical Practice, 4th ed. Philadelphia, Saunders, 1996, pp 535-540.
3. Chou-Long H, Kuo E: Mechanism of hypokalemia in magnesium deficiency. J Am Soc Nephrol 18:2649-2652, 2007.
4. Hartman RC, Auditore JV, Jackson DP: Studies on thrombocytosis: 1 Hyperkalemia due to release of potassium from platelets during coagulation. J Clin Invest 37:699-707, 1958.
5. Hyman D, Kaplan NM: The difference between serum and plasma potassium. N Engl J Med 313:642, 1985.
6. Malnic G, Muto S, Giebisch G: Regulation of potassium excretion. In Seldin DW, Giebisch G (eds): The Kidney, 3rd ed. New York, Lippincott Williams & Wilkins, 2000, pp 1592-1601.
7. Rosa RM, Epstein FH: Extrarenal potassium metabolism. In Seldin DW, Giebisch G (eds): The Kidney, New York, Lippincott Williams & Wilkins, 2000, pp 1551-1552.
8. Rose B, Post TW: Hypokalemia. In Rose B, Post TW (eds): Clinical Physiology of Acid–Base and Electrolyte Disorders, New York, McGraw-Hill, 2001, pp 871-872.
9. Sevastos N, Theodossiades G, Archimandritis AJ: Pseudohyperkalemia in serum: a new insight into an old phenomenon. Clin Med Res 6:30-32, 2008.
10. Weiner ID, Wingo CS: Hypokalemia: consequences, causes, and correction. J Am Soc Nephrol 8:1183, 1997.

CHAPTER 45

HYPONATREMIA AND HYPERNATREMIA

Brad W. Butcher, MD, and Kathleen D. Liu, MD, PhD, MAS

1. **Why is sodium balance critical to volume control?**

   Sodium and its corresponding anions represent almost all of the osmotically active solutes in the extracellular fluid under normal conditions. Therefore the serum concentration of sodium reflects the tonicity of body fluids. Small changes in osmolality are counteracted by thirst regulation, antidiuretic hormone (ADH) secretion, and renal concentrating or diluting mechanisms. Preservation of normal serum osmolality (i.e., 285-295 mOsm/L) guarantees cellular integrity by regulating net movement of water across cellular membranes.

2. **What is another name for ADH? What is its mechanism of action?**

   ADH is also called *arginine vasopressin* or simply *vasopressin*. ADH is a small peptide hormone produced by the hypothalamus that binds to the vasopressin 1 and 2 receptors (V1 and V2). Vasopressin release is regulated by osmoreceptors in the hypothalamus, which are sensitive to changes in plasma osmolality of as little as 1% to 2%. Under hyperosmolar conditions, osmoreceptor stimulation leads to stimulation of thirst and vasopressin release. These two mechanisms result in increased water intake and retention, respectively. Vasopressin release is also regulated by baroreceptors in the carotid sinus and aortic arch; under conditions of hypovolemia, these receptors stimulate vasopressin release to increase water retention by the kidney. At very high concentrations, vasopressin also causes vascular smooth muscle constriction through the V1 receptor, increasing vascular tone and therefore the blood pressure. Accordingly, vasopressin is often administered parenterally as a vasopressor agent in patients with hypotension that is refractory to volume resuscitation.

3. **Does hyponatremia simply mean there is too little sodium in the body?**

   No. The serum sodium concentration is not a reflection of the total body sodium content; instead, it is more representative of changes in the total body water. With hyponatremia, defined as serum sodium level less than 135 mEq/L, there is too much total body water relative to the amount of total body sodium, thereby lowering its concentration. Despite this key observation, the serum sodium concentration is *not* a reflection of volume status, and it is possible for hyponatremia to develop in states of volume depletion, euvolemia, and volume excess. Assessing a patient's volume status is therefore the key step in identifying the underlying cause of hyponatremia (Fig. 45-1). Helpful physical findings include tachycardia, dry mucous membranes, orthostatic hypotension, increased skin turgor (associated with hypovolemia) or edema, an S_3 gallop, jugular venous distention, and ascites (present in hypervolemic states).

4. **Are *hyponatremia* and *hypoosmolality* synonymous?**

   No. Hyponatremia can occur without a change in total body sodium or total body water in two settings. The first is pseudohyponatremia, which is a laboratory artifact in patients with severe hyperlipidemia or hyperproteinemia. This laboratory abnormality has been essentially eliminated by the use of ion-specific electrodes (rather than flame photometry) to determine the serum sodium concentration. The second setting occurs when large quantities of osmotically active substances (such as glucose or mannitol) cause hyponatremia but not hypoosmolality, a condition known as *translocational hyponatremia*. In such states, water is drawn out of cells into the extracellular space, diluting the plasma solutes and equilibrating osmolar differences. In addition,

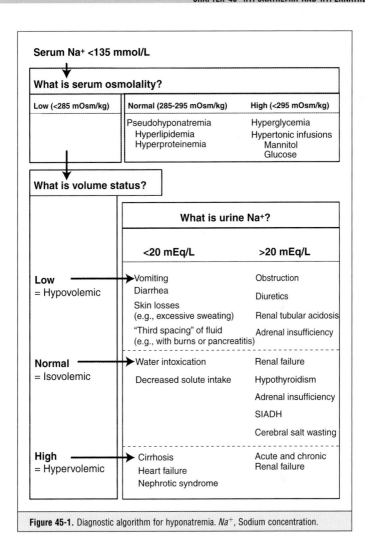

Figure 45-1. Diagnostic algorithm for hyponatremia. Na^+, Sodium concentration.

use of large quantities of irrigant solutions that do not contain sodium (but instead contain glycine, sorbitol, or mannitol) during gynecologic or urologic surgeries can also cause severe hyponatremia.

5. **How can hyponatremia develop in a patient with hypovolemia?**
   Hypovolemic hyponatremia represents a decrease in total body sodium in excess of a decrease in total body water. Simultaneous sodium and water loss can be due to renal (such as diuretic use) or extrarenal causes. Hypovolemia results in a decrease in renal perfusion, a decrement in the glomerular filtration rate, and an increase in proximal tubule reabsorption of sodium and water; all three mechanisms contribute to decreased water excretion. Furthermore, hypovolemia supersedes the expected inhibition of vasopressin release by hypoosmolality and maintains the secretion of the hormone. In other words, the body protects volume at the expense of osmolality.

6. **How does hypervolemic hyponatremia differ from hypovolemic hyponatremia?**
   In hypervolemic hyponatremia, the kidneys are at the center of the problem because of either intrinsic renal disease or the renal response to extrarenal pathophysiology. Physical examination reveals edema and no evidence of volume depletion. Intrinsic renal disease with a compromised glomerular filtration rate (acute or chronic) prevents adequate excretion of sodium and water. Intake of sodium in excess of what can be excreted leads to hypervolemia (edema), whereas excessive intake of water leads to hyponatremia. In contrast, in congestive heart failure, hepatic cirrhosis, and nephrotic syndrome, the intrinsically normal kidney is stimulated to retain sodium and water in response to perceived decrements in intravascular volume and renal perfusion; as a result, hypervolemia and hyponatremia develop. In general, hypervolemic hyponatremia due to an extrarenal cause is characterized by a low urine sodium concentration ($\leq$10-20 mEq/L); this distinguishes it from hypervolemic hyponatremia due to intrinsic renal causes, where the urine sodium is >20 mEq/L.

7. **What is the syndrome of inappropriate secretion of antidiuretic hormone (SIADH)?**
   SIADH is a common cause of euvolemic hyponatremia and is associated with malignancies, pulmonary disease, central nervous system disorders, pain, nausea, and many drugs. Common offending medications include hypoglycemic agents, psychotropics (including antipsychotics and antidepressants), narcotics, and chemotherapeutic agents. Other causes of euvolemic hyponatremia include psychogenic polydipsia, a low-solute diet (beer potomania or the *tea and toast* diet), hypothyroidism, and adrenal insufficiency.

8. **What diagnostic tests are useful in the evaluation of hyponatremia?**
   The physical examination is critical to the determination of volume status, as previously described. Serum electrolyte and serum and urine osmolality measurements are useful. High urine osmolality despite low serum osmolality suggests either hypovolemic hyponatremia or SIADH if the patient is in a euvolemic state. Very low urine osmolality suggests excessive water intake, as in psychogenic polydipsia or a low-solute diet. Measurements of thyroid-stimulating hormone and cortisol can be used to assess endocrine causes of hyponatremia. As mentioned above, the urine sodium concentration can help distinguish renal and extrarenal causes of hypervolemic hyponatremia.

9. **Why do patients with diabetic ketoacidosis frequently have hyponatremia?**
   Diabetic ketoacidosis is an example of hyperosmotic hyponatremia. In general, serum sodium decreases by approximately 2.4 mEq/L for every increase of 100 mg/dL over normal glucose levels. In this setting, the serum sodium level should not be interpreted without an accompanying serum glucose measurement, and the appropriate correction should be made if the glucose exceeds 200 mg/dL.

10. **What is the difference between acute and chronic hyponatremia?**
    - **Acute hyponatremia:** A distinct entity in terms of morbidity, mortality, and treatment strategies. Acute hyponatremia most commonly occurs in the hospital (frequently in the postoperative setting), in psychogenic polydipsia, and in elderly women taking thiazide diuretic agents.
    - **Chronic hyponatremia:** Chronic hyponatremia is defined as hyponatremia lasting longer than 48 hours. The majority of patients who are seen by physicians or emergency departments with hyponatremia should be assumed to have chronic hyponatremia.

11. **What are the signs and symptoms of hyponatremia?**
    Hyponatremia is the most common electrolyte disorder in hospitalized patients, with a prevalence of approximately 2.5%. Although the majority of patients have no symptoms, symptoms often develop in patients with a serum sodium concentration <125 mEq/L or in whom the

sodium has decreased rapidly. Gastrointestinal symptoms of nausea, vomiting, and anorexia occur early, but neuropsychiatric symptoms such as lethargy, confusion, agitation, psychosis, seizure, and coma are more common. Clinical symptoms roughly correlate with the amount and rate of decrease in serum sodium levels.

12. **What drugs, if any, are associated with hyponatremia?**
Many drugs are associated with hyponatremia, but several warrant special note. Thiazide diuretics frequently cause hyponatremia by promoting sodium excretion in excess of water. Of note, because loop diuretics directly impair the creation and maintenance of the medullary osmotic gradient, they are far less likely to cause hyponatremia, as little stimulus for water reabsorption occurs as urine passes through the collecting duct. Selective serotonin reuptake inhibitors and several chemotherapeutic agents cause hyponatremia, and this is thought to occur through the inappropriate release of ADH. Nonsteroidal antiinflammatory drugs block the production of renal prostaglandins and allow vasopressin to act unopposed in the kidney, which can lead to water retention. Tricyclic antidepressants and a number of anticonvulsants are also associated with hyponatremia. Last, use of 3,4-methylenedioxymethamphetamine, or Ectasy, particularly in combination with consumption of large volumes of water, is associated with severe, life-threatening hyponatremia.

13. **Is there a standard therapy for hyponatremia?**
Although controversy exists regarding treatment strategies, there is a consensus that not all patients with hyponatremia should be treated alike. Duration (acute vs. chronic) and the presence or absence of neurologic symptoms are the most critical factors in determining the therapeutic strategy. The prescribed therapy must take into consideration the patient's current symptoms and the risk of provoking a demyelinating syndrome with overly rapid correction. The first priority is circulatory stabilization with normal saline solution in patients with significant volume depletion. In patients with acute symptomatic hyponatremia, the risks of delaying treatment, which could lead to cerebral edema, subsequent seizures, and respiratory arrest, clearly outweigh any risk of treatment. Hypertonic (3%) saline solution, with or without furosemide (which promotes free water excretion), should be given until symptoms subside. It is possible to calculate the expected change in serum sodium concentration on the basis of the volume of and rate at which hypertonic saline solution is infused, and this should be done before its administration. In contrast, the patient with asymptomatic chronic hyponatremia in high-risk categories (e.g., alcoholism, malnutrition, and liver disease) is at greatest risk for complications of the correction of hyponatremia, namely central pontine myelinolysis. Such patients are best treated with water restriction. Vasopressin V2 receptor antagonists are newer agents (also known as *aquaretics* or *vaptans*) that are available in the United States for treatment of hypervolemic and euvolemic hyponatremia; these agents promote free water excretion and are useful in selected patients.

14. **What are some helpful guidelines for treatment of hyponatremia?**
In patients with chronic asymptomatic hyponatremia, simple free water restriction (e.g., 1000 mL/day) allows a slow and relatively safe correction of the serum sodium concentration. This strategy, however, requires patient compliance, which may be particularly challenging in the outpatient setting. In selected patients who are behaviorally or physiologically resistant to free water restriction, administration of salt tablets, an ADH antagonist (e.g., demeclocycline, 600-1200 mg/day), or a maneuver to increase urinary solute excretion, such as the ingestion of a high-solute diet, may be necessary.

A difficult therapeutic dilemma is posed by patients with neurologic symptoms and hyponatremia of unknown duration. Such patients are at risk for development of a demyelinating disorder if treated too aggressively, yet the presence of symptoms is reflective of central nervous system dysfunction. These patients should be given treatment with hypertonic saline solution (and furosemide if necessary), and their serum sodium level should be monitored every

1 to 2 hours initially. The rate of increase should not exceed 8 to 10 mEq/L in a 24-hour period. Acute therapy can be slowed once symptoms have improved or a *safe* serum sodium level (typically 120-125 mEq/L) is stably attained (note that if the serum sodium level is extremely low, this may be too aggressive a correction for the first 24 hours).

15. **What is central pontine myelinolysis?**

Central pontine myelinolysis is a rare neurologic disorder of unclear cause characterized by symmetric midline demyelination of the central pons. Extrapontine lesions can occur in the basal ganglia, internal capsule, lateral geniculate body, and cortex. Symptoms include motor abnormalities that can progress to flaccid quadriplegia, respiratory paralysis, pseudobulbar palsy, mental status changes, and coma. Central pontine myelinolysis is often fatal in 3 to 5 weeks; of the patients who survive, many have significant residual deficits. Alterations in the white matter are best visualized by magnetic resonance imaging. Central pontine myelinolysis is one of the most feared complications of therapy for hyponatremia. Risk factors include a change in serum sodium level of >12 mEq/L in 24 hours, correction of serum sodium level to a normal or hypernatremic range, symptomatic and coexistent alcoholism, malnutrition, and liver disease.

16. **Can hypernatremia also occur in hypovolemic, euvolemic, and hypervolemic states?**

Yes, and these categories, based on physical examination, provide a useful framework for understanding and treating patients. Hypernatremia, defined as a serum sodium concentration greater than 145 mEq/L, occurs when too little total body water exists relative to the amount of total body sodium, thereby raising the sodium concentration. Given that even small rises in the serum osmolality trigger the thirst mechanism, hypernatremia is relatively uncommon unless the thirst mechanism is impaired or access to free water is restricted. As a result, hypovolemic hypernatremia tends to occur in the very young, the very old, and the debilitated. It is typically due to extracellular fluid losses accompanied by inability to take in adequate amounts of free water. Febrile illnesses, vomiting, diarrhea, and renal losses are common causes.

Euvolemic hypernatremia can also be due to extracellular loss of fluid without adequate access to water or from impaired water hemostasis. Diabetes insipidus, either central (i.e., inadequate ADH secretion) or nephrogenic (i.e., renal insensitivity to ADH), results in the inability to reabsorb filtered water, which causes systemic hyperosmolality but hypoosmolar (dilute) urine. Hypervolemic hypernatremia, although uncommon, is iatrogenic. Sodium bicarbonate injection during cardiac arrest, administration of hypertonic saline solution, saline abortions, and inappropriately prepared infant formulas are several examples of induced hypernatremia.

17. **What are the causes of diabetes insipidus?**

Central diabetes insipidus can result from trauma, tumors, strokes, granulomatous disease, and central nervous system infections, and it commonly occurs after neurosurgical procedures. Nephrogenic diabetes insipidus can be congenital or it can occur in acute or chronic renal failure, hypercalcemia, hypokalemia, and sickle cell disease, or after treatment with certain drugs (e.g., lithium, demeclocycline).

18. **What are the signs and symptoms of hypernatremia?**

In awake and alert patients, thirst is a prominent symptom. Anorexia, nausea, vomiting, altered mental status, agitation, irritability, lethargy, stupor, coma, and neuromuscular hyperactivity are also common symptoms.

19. **What is the best therapy for hypernatremia?**

The first priority is circulatory stabilization with normal saline solution in patients with significant volume depletion. Once normotensive, patients can be rehydrated with oral water, intravenous 5% dextrose in water (D_5W), or even one-half normal saline solution. Overly rapid correction of long-standing hypernatremia can result in cerebral edema. Water deficit can be calculated with the formula in question 20. Some investigators have suggested that in patients with long-standing hypernatremia, the water deficit should be corrected by no more than 10 mEq/L/day or 0.5 mEq/L/hr. If the hypernatremia has occurred over a short period (hours), it can be corrected more rapidly, with the goal of correcting half of the water deficit in the first 24 hours. In addition to correcting the already established free water deficit, daily ongoing losses of free water in the urine and stool and from the respiratory tract and skin (particularly in patients with fever) should be replaced. In patients with central diabetes insipidus, a synthetic analog of ADH (i.e., 1-deamino-8-D-arginine vasopressin) can be administered, preferably by the intranasal route.

20. **What are some helpful formulas for assessing sodium abnormalities?**
   - **Serum osmolality =** $2 [Na^+] + Glucose/18 + Blood\ urea\ nitrogen/2.8 + Ethyl\ alcohol/4.6$
   - **Total body water (TBW) =** Body weight $\times$ 0.6 (for men)
     TBW = Body weight $\times$ 0.5 (for women and the elderly)
   - **TBW excess in hyponatremia =** TBW $(1 - [Serum\ Na^+]/140)$
     Expected change in serum sodium level after 1 L 3% saline solution = $(513\ mEq/L - Serum [Na^+])/(TBW + 1)$
   - **TBW deficit in hypernatremia =** TBW $(Serum\ [Na^+]/140 - 1)$
     Expected change in serum sodium level after 1 L D5W = $(Serum\ [Na^+])/(TBW + 1)$

Acknowledgment

The authors acknowledge the contributions of Stuart Senkfor, MD, and Tomas Berl, MD.

KEY POINTS: USEFUL DIAGNOSTIC TESTS IN HYPONATREMIA

1. Serum osmolality measurement is useful in the diagnosis of hyponatremia.

2. Determination of volume status is necessary.

3. If urine osmolality is inappropriately high, it is easier to differentiate causes of euvolemic hyponatremia. High urine osmolality implies inappropriate levels of ADH or ADH-like hormones.

4. Urine sodium concentration needs to be interpreted with caution in cases of renal failure.

BIBLIOGRAPHY

1. Adrogue HJ, Madias NE: Hyponatremia. N Engl J Med 342:1581-1589, 2000.
2. Anderson RJ, Chung HM, Kluge R, et al: Hyponatremia: a prospective analysis of its epidemiology and the pathogenetic role of vasopressin. Ann Intern Med 102:164-168, 1985.
3. Budisavljevic MN, Stewart L, Sahn SA, et al: Hyponatremia associated with 3-4-methylenedioxymethylamphetamine ("Ectasy") abuse. Am J Med Sci 326:89-93, 2003.
4. Elhassan EA, Schrier RW: Hyponatremia: diagnosis, complications and management including V2 receptor antagonists. Curr Opin Nephrol Hypertens 20:161-168, 2011.
5. Ellison DH, Berl T: The syndrome of inappropriate antidiuresis. N Engl J Med 356:2064-2072, 2007.
6. Hillier TA, Abbott RD, Barrett EJ: Hyponatremia: evaluating the correction factor for hyperglycemia. Am J Med 106:399-403, 1999.

7. Lin M, Liu SJ, Lim IT: Disorders of water imbalance. Emerg Med Clin North Am 23:749-770, 2005.

8. Milionis HJ, Liamis GL, Elisaf MS: The hyponatremic patient: a systematic approach to laboratory diagnosis. Can Med Assoc J 166:1056-1062, 2002.

9. Moritz ML, Ayus JC: The pathophysiology and treatment of hyponatremic encephalopathy: an update. Nephrol Dial Transplant 18:2486-2491, 2003.

10. Sterns RH: Osmotic demyelination syndrome and overly rapid correction of hyponatremia: www.uptodate.com. Accessed February 23, 2011.

11. Verbalis J: Disorders of body water homeostasis. Best Pract Res Clin Endocrinol Metab 17:471-503, 2003.

12. Verbalis JG, Berl T: Disorders of water balance. In Brenner BM (ed): Brenner and Rector's The Kidney, 8th ed. Philadelphia, Saunders, 2007, pp 460-504.

GASTROINTESTINAL BLEEDING IN THE CRITICALLY ILL PATIENT

George Kasotakis, MD, and George C. Velmahos, MD, PhD, MSEd

1. **What are the anatomic definitions of upper versus lower gastrointestinal (GI) bleeding?**

   The GI tract is anatomically divided into upper and lower by the ligament of Treitz. Although this classification has little physiologic significance, it is important to bear in mind that bleeding originating distal to the ligament of Treitz cannot travel backward to the upper GI tract because of the acute angle of the small bowel at this site. Bleeding from the upper GI tract is far more common than in the lower, and this is particularly true in the critically ill.

2. **What are *hematemesis, coffee-ground emesis, hematochezia,* and *melena*? Are these features helpful in determining the site and rate of bleeding?**

   - *Hematemesis* is vomiting of fresh, red blood and indicates bleeding in the upper GI tract. Approximately 50% of patients with upper GI bleeding (UGIB) will present with hematemesis.
   - If the blood is older, it can appear like *coffee grounds*. The return of bright red blood or coffee grounds through a nasogastric tube (NGT) is highly specific for hemorrhage proximal to the ligament of Treitz.
   - *Hematochezia* is used to describe passage of bright red or maroon-colored blood through the rectum and typically indicates a lower tract source. Less commonly ($< 15\%$) it may indicate the rapid transit of torrential hemorrhage from the upper tract.
   - *Melena* is the passage of black, tarry, and usually foul-smelling stool because of degradation of blood components as they traverse the GI tract. It typically signifies upper GI tract bleeding (70%) or, less often, hemorrhage from the proximal lower tract (30%).

3. **Do all patients with GI bleeding need to be monitored in the intensive care unit (ICU)?**

   No, but patients with evidence of active bleeding (ongoing transfusion requirement, hemodynamic instability) or other significant comorbidities should be closely monitored in a high-acuity setting, such as an ICU.

4. **What are the most common causes of upper and lower GI bleeding?**

   See Tables 46-1 and 46-2.

TABLE 46-1. CAUSES OF UPPER GASTROINTESTINAL BLEEDING	
CAUSE	**PREVALENCE (%)**
Peptic ulcer disease	55
Gastritis-duodenitis	20
Esophageal varices	12
Mallory-Weiss tears	8
Neoplasm	3
Angiodysplasia	2

TABLE 46-2. CAUSES OF LOWER GASTROINTESTINAL BLEEDING

CAUSE	PREVALENCE (%)
Diverticular disease	40
Angiodysplasia	20
Colitis	20
Anorectal bleeding (hemorrhoids, anal fissures)	7
Neoplasm	7
Small bowel bleeding	6

5. **What risk factors are associated with higher mortality in patients with upper GI tract hemorrhage?**
   - Shock
   - Melena
   - Anemia at presentation
   - Significant fresh blood in vomit, gastric aspirate, or rectum
   - Concurrent sepsis
   - Poor general health
   - Comorbidities (liver, renal, cardiac disease)
   - Large ulcer size
   - Persistent bleeding despite endoscopic therapy
   - Recurrent bleeding

6. **What are the most common causes of GI tract bleeding in critically ill patients?**
   Although critically ill patients can have any of the usual causes of GI bleeding, they are at particular risk for development of stress-related mucosal disease (SRMD) in the upper GI tract and hypotension-induced colonic ischemia. In addition, the increasing use of rectal tubes for the management of antibiotic- and enteral feeding–associated diarrhea is associated with a rise in incidence of lower GI bleeding (LGIB) due to iatrogenic rectal fissures and ulcers.

7. **What are the immediate actions that need to be taken in an acute GI tract hemorrhage in the ICU?**
   - Ensure patient has at least two large-bore (at least 18 gauge) intravenous catheters.
   - Insert Foley and nasogastric catheter (if not already in place), and initiate resuscitation (with crystalloids or blood products) per the local guidelines and policies.
   - Consider obtaining a definitive airway in the uncooperative, agitated, or encephalopathic patient at risk for aspiration.
   - Aspirate sample from nasogastric tube and perform rectal examination (attempt to localize the source of bleeding).
   - If UGIB, initiate medical therapy with intravenous proton pump inhibitors.
   - If suspicious of bleeding varices, start an octreotide infusion.
   - Consult the endoscopy and/or radiology and surgical services as needed.
   - For more details on managing acute GI tract bleeding, see algorithms in Figures 46-1 to 46-3.

8. **Does a nonbloody NGT aspirate rule out UGIB?**
   A bloody nasogastric aspirate indicates an upper source of bleeding. Lavage may also be used to quantify the active bleeding: Bright blood suggests active hemorrhage, whereas darker coffee grounds suggest recent or slower bleeding. However, a negative NGT aspirate is not helpful, as it may miss up to 50% of patients with recent duodenal bleeding. Therefore a nonbloody nasogastric aspirate may indicate bleeding originating in the lower GI tract or one in the upper GI tract that has ceased.

9. **What medical therapies are available for the management of GI bleeding?**
   - Somatostatin analogs: Octreotide is a long-acting somatostatin analog that inhibits glucagon-induced mesenteric vasodilation and has been shown to decrease the risk for persistent bleeding and rebleeding in patients with both variceal and nonvariceal upper tract bleeding. Although somatostatin analogs do not improve mortality rates, they are helpful in reducing bleeding and minimizing transfusion requirements. The recommended dose for octreotide is 250 mcg IV bolus followed by a 250 mcg/hr infusion.
   - Proton pump inhibitors (PPI): They have been shown to reduce risk of rebleeding, transfusion requirements, and need for surgical intervention. Their effect on mortality is questionable. They are recommended before endoscopy, as they decrease the likelihood of bleeding or need for intervention during endoscopy. Continuous PPI infusion does not appear to be better than intermittent administration and is less cost-effective. H_2-receptor blockers have not proved to be valuable in the management of acute UGIB, as they lack benefit in duodenal ulcers and afford only a weak benefit in bleeding gastric ulcers.

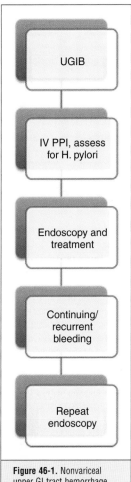

Figure 46-1. Nonvariceal upper GI tract hemorrhage management algorithm.

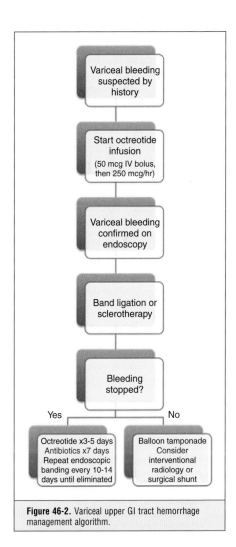

Figure 46-2. Variceal upper GI tract hemorrhage management algorithm.

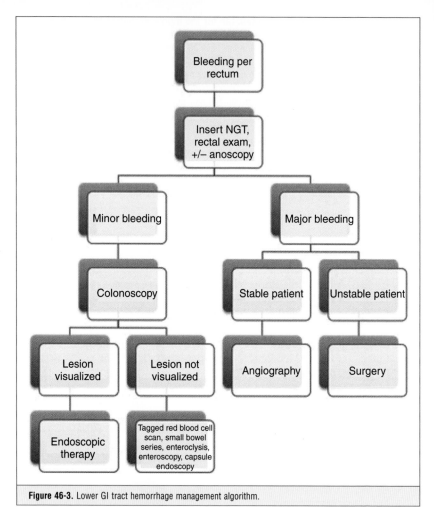

Figure 46-3. Lower GI tract hemorrhage management algorithm.

- Vasopressin: This is a potent vasoconstrictor that has been used extensively for UGIB, most commonly for variceal bleeding. However, its unfavorable safety profile has led to its progressively diminishing use. Common adverse events include a significant rebleeding rate when the infusion is stopped and a high rate of complications (myocardial and peripheral tissue ischemia, dysrhythmias, hypertension, and decreased cardiac output).

10. **What is the role of endoscopy in the management of UGIB?**
Endoscopic assessment constitutes a risk-assessing tool for ongoing or recurrent bleeding by visualizing the offending lesions: Actively bleeding ulcers, nonbleeding visible vessels, and adherent clots require aggressive intervention, as rebleeding is associated with a fivefold to 16-fold increase in mortality. On the contrary, the rebleeding rate of ulcers with a clean base or red or blue spots is low, and endoscopic intervention is not warranted. Newer methods of assessment (combining Doppler evaluation with endoscopy) may provide a more accurate assessment of the bleeding risk.

Endoscopic intervention is beneficial in high-risk patients with UGIB, as it reduces the rate of rebleeding, need for surgical intervention, length of stay, and mortality. Injection of dilute

(1:10,000) epinephrine around the bleeding points, laser and argon plasma coagulation, bipolar electrocoagulation and heater probe thermocoagulation, as well as Endoloops and clips, appear to be very effective at achieving hemostasis. Varices may be band ligated or injected with sclerosing agents. Endoscopic suturing and cryotherapy hold promise for even better bleeding control endoscopically.

11. **How does ulcer appearance help predict rebleeding or mortality risk?**
See Table 46-3.

12. **What is SRMD? Who is at risk?**
SRMD represents a continuum of conditions ranging from stress-related injury (superficial mucosal damage) to stress ulcers (focal deep mucosal injuries). Frequently, the terms *stress ulcers, stress gastritis,* or *erosions* are used interchangeably. The etiology of SRMD is multifactorial, with a common end pathway being the breakdown of mucosal defenses, typically because of ischemia (decreased prostaglandin and alkaline mucus production). SRMD is typically seen in the acid-producing areas of the stomach (corpus and fundus), unlike peptic ulcer disease (PUD), which is more common in the antrum and duodenal bulb and typically affects the critically ill. Risk factors for SRMD include coagulopathy and respiratory failure requiring mechanical ventilation. Mortality is high, ranging between 20% and 40%.

13. **What are the indications for stress ulcer prophylaxis?**
   - Respiratory failure requiring mechanical ventilation
   - Coagulopathy
   - Traumatic brain injury
   - Burns >30%
   - Patients already taking acid-suppression medications
   - Diagnosis of PUD or UGIB in the last 6 weeks

14. **What agents are typically used?**
PPIs, H_2-receptor antagonists, sucralfate (mucosal protective), and misoprostol (a prostaglandin E_1 analog) are the agents most frequently used.

15. **What are Curling ulcers?**
A Curling ulcer is an acute peptic ulcer resulting as a complication from severe burns, when reduced plasma volume leads to sloughing off of the gastric mucosa. They appear to be more prevalent in pediatric patients with burns compared with adults.

TABLE 46-3. PREVALENCE AND OUTCOMES OF PEPTIC ULCER DISEASE BASED ON ENDOSCOPIC FINDINGS

ENDOSCOPIC FINDING	PREVALENCE (%)	REBLEEDING (%)	SURGICAL INTERVENTION (%)	MORTALITY (%)
Clean base	42	5	0.5	2
Pigmented flat spot	20	10	6	3
Adherent clot	17	22	10	7
Visible vessel	17	43	34	11
Active bleeding	18	55	35	11

16. **What are Cushing ulcers?**
    Cushing ulcers are peptic ulcers (usually in the stomach, or less commonly in the duodenum or distal esophagus) that develop in patients with brain injury. They are thought to arise from gastric acid oversecretion, as a result of intracranial hypertension.

17. **What is the role of endoscopy in the management of LGIB?**
    Urgent colonoscopy for acute LGIB is less established than urgent endoscopy is for acute UGIB. Bowel preparation is generally recommended, as it improves the efficacy of endoscopy to identify the offending lesion and decreases perforation risk. Hemostatic therapy can also be applied endoscopically, by means of epinephrine injection, heater probe and polar electrocoagulation, argon plasma coagulation, hemoclips, and band ligation. Attempts to visualize the entire colon should ideally be made, as more than one source of bleeding may be identified in up to 40% of cases.

18. **What is the role of angiography in the management of GI tract bleeding?**
    Angiography can identify and localize bleeding accurately, but this requires a bleeding rate of at least 0.5 to 1 mL/min to be positive. This can be problematic because of the intermittent nature of bleeding. However, it has the advantage of not requiring bowel preparation. When the bleeding site is identified, it may be treated with intraarterial infusion of vasopressin or super-selective embolization.

19. **What is the role of a tagged red blood cell scan in the workup of LGIB?**
    If bleeding is clinically significant, yet too slow or intermittent to be picked up by colonoscopy, a tagged red blood count scan can be performed. Typically, 20 mL of the patient's own red blood cells are tagged with technetium and subsequently reinjected into the patient. Then scintigraphy identifies the bleeding in 15% to 70% of cases, as an area of increased uptake. This study is more sensitive than angiography in detecting bleeding, as it requires a rate of only 0.1 mL/min of bleeding. However, it cannot localize the precise area of hemorrhage and has no therapeutic role.

20. **What is the role of surgery in the management of LGIB?**
    Surgery is typically employed for hemorrhage in the setting of massive or recurrent bleeding not amenable to endoscopic intervention. It is required in 20% of patients with diverticular bleeding and usually reserved for patients with high transfusion requirements. Efforts should be made to accurately identify and mark the bleeding site before surgery, so that selective, rather than subtotal, colectomy can be performed.

21. **What is ischemic colitis (IC)? What are the risk factors?**
    IC constitutes a wide spectrum of clinical diseases of the large bowel, ranging from superficial mucosal ischemia to bowel gangrene and perforation, and the more severe forms carry a high mortality. Nonocclusive IC usually results from low cardiac output, whereas occlusive disease can be due to arterial embolism or thrombosis, or venous thrombosis. Risk factors for development of IC include cardiovascular surgery or disease, cardiac arrhythmias, hypovolemia, and medications with vasoconstrictive properties.

22. **How does IC manifest, and how is the diagnosis made?**
    The clinical features of IC are protean and nonspecific: Diffuse or localized crampy abdominal pain and passage of bright red or maroon blood per rectum are very common. As superficial ischemic changes progress to transmural ischemia, bowel gangrene, and perforation, patients may present with peritonitis. Plain abdominal radiographs may demonstrate *thumbprinting*, indicating submucosal edema. Computed tomography may reveal thickened colonic wall or *pneumatosis* (air in the wall of the colon). No laboratory tests exist to aid in early diagnosis of IC, but in advanced disease lactic acidosis and elevated lactate dehydrogenase, creatine

phosphokinase, and amylase levels may be present. Definitive diagnosis is made by colonoscopy, which can also provide information about the degree and extent of involvement, but it is contraindicated in the presence of peritoneal signs.

23. **What is the treatment of IC?**
For the least severe forms of IC, treatment is largely supportive and revolves around resuscitation, cardiac function optimization, and prophylactic broad-spectrum antibiotics. In patients with IC of thrombotic etiology, systemic anticoagulation or catheter-directed thrombolysis may be considered. In patients with severe physiologic derangements and viable bowel, surgical revascularization may be attempted. If bowel necrosis or perforation has occurred, surgical intervention is warranted for resection of the affected part of the colon.

KEY POINTS: GI BLEEDING

1. Always insert a nasogastric tube to rule out UGIB, even in cases that present with copious fresh blood from the rectum.

2. Early endoscopy is key in both upper and lower GI tract bleeding for diagnosing, risk-stratifying, localizing, and treating bleeding.

3. Do not forget about stress ulcer prophylaxis in critically ill patients with the appropriate indications. Remember to discontinue it when the indications cease to exist.

4. A systematic approach is key in managing all patients with GI bleeding.

BIBLIOGRAPHY

1. Barnert J, Messmann H: Diagnosis and management of lower gastrointestinal bleeding. Nat Rev Gastroenterol Hepatol 6:637-646, 2009.
2. Cappell M, Friedel D: Initial management of acute upper gastrointestinal bleeding: from initial evaluation up to gastrointestinal endoscopy. Med Clin North Am 92:491-509, 2008.
3. Ferguson CB, Mitchell RM: Nonvariceal upper gastrointestinal bleeding: standard and new treatment. Gastroenterol Clin North Am 34:607-621, 2005.
4. Green BT, Rockey DC: Lower gastrointestinal bleeding-management. Gastroenterol Clin North Am 34:665-678, 2005.
5. Laine L, Peterson WL: Bleeding peptic ulcer. N Engl J Med 331:717-727, 1994.
6. Reissfelder C, Sweiti H, Antolovic D, et al: Ischemic colitis: Who will survive? Surgery 149:585-592, 2011.
7. Rockey DC: Gastrointestinal bleeding. Gastroenterol Clin North Am 34:581-588, 2005.
8. Spirt MJ: Stress-related mucosal disease: risk factors and prophylactic therapy. Clin Ther 26:197-213, 2004.
9. Yüksel I, Ataseven H, Köklü S, et al: Intermittent versus continuous pantoprazole infusion in peptic ulcer bleeding: a prospective randomized study. Digestion 78:39-43, 2008.
10. Zaman A, Chalasani N: Bleeding caused by portal hypertension. Gastroenterol Clin North Am 34:623-642, 2005.

CHAPTER 47

ACUTE PANCREATITIS

Neeraj K. Sardana, MD, Jon (Kai) Yamaguchi, MD, FACS,
and David W. McFadden, MD, FACS

1. **What is acute pancreatitis (AP)?**

   AP is an inflammatory condition of the pancreas that has a broad spectrum of severity ranging from mild and self-limited to severe and associated with multiorgan failure. Clinically it is associated with the acute onset of abdominal pain and elevation of serum biochemical markers. The underlying pathophysiology is early and inappropriate activation of digestive enzymes within acinar cells.

2. **What are the different degrees of AP, and how are they defined?**

   Mild AP is defined as pancreatic inflammation (of any cause) without persistent organ failure or local complications. Severe acute pancreatitis (SAP) is associated with systemic complications, including multiple-organ failure, and local complications, such as necrosis, abscess, and/or pseudocyst. This degree of pancreatitis requires aggressive therapy in an intensive care setting to prevent significant morbidity or mortality.

3. **What are the causes of AP?**

   Gallstone-related disease and excessive alcohol intake are the two most common causes of AP in the developed world, comprising 70% of all cases. Beyond these, a number of independent factors are thought to cause pancreatitis, including hypertriglyceridemia (serum triglyceride level above 1500 mg/dL), trauma, and hypercalcemia. Evidence is growing that smoking is a risk factor for AP in a time- and dose-dependent manner. A large number of medications have been implicated in causing AP, including angiotensin-converting enzyme inhibitors, furosemide, tetracycline, aminosalicylic acid, corticosteroids, procainamide, thiazides, metronidazole, and ranitidine. Because of the varied duration between exposure and development of symptoms, and the usual lack of a clear mechanism, it is often difficult to identify a drug as the sole cause of AP. True idiopathic cases of AP are diminishing as more genetic causes of the disease are discovered. Endoscopic retrograde cholangiopancreatography (ERCP) causes pancreatitis in approximately 5% of individuals who undergo this procedure.

4. **What are the presenting signs and symptoms of AP?**

   AP is characterized by the sudden onset of abdominal pain, classically located in the epigastrium and usually associated with nausea and/or vomiting. Radiation of pain from the epigastrium through to the back that is alleviated with the patient leaning forward is a typical but not a necessary feature. Tachycardia related to pain or volume depletion and low-grade fever may be present. Two additional findings associated with severe pancreatitis may be present, the Grey Turner and Cullen signs. The Grey Turner sign is an ecchymosis of the flank due to retroperitoneal hemorrhage. When present, it usually occurs 3 to 7 days after the onset of pain and is indicative of severe pancreatitis. The Cullen sign is periumbilical ecchymosis associated with both severe necrotizing pancreatitis and retroperitoneal hemorrhage of various causes.

5. **Are amylase and/or lipase measurements helpful in the diagnosis?**

   The most commonly used diagnostic markers are serum amylase and lipase. Although serum amylase levels have a high sensitivity in the first 24 hours the specificity is very low.

In addition to pancreatitis, elevated amylase levels are seen with many other conditions including bowel infarction, renal failure, perforated peptic ulcer, trauma to the salivary glands, and macroamylasemia. In contrast, serum lipase levels are both more specific and more sensitive than amylase measurements. Of note, no correlation exists between the absolute levels of amylase and lipase and the severity of pancreatitis.

6. **What is the role of imaging in the diagnosis of AP?**
Abdominal plain radiographs may be nonspecific or reveal an ileus if the pancreatitis is severe. Ultrasound evaluation of the pancreas itself is often limited by overlying bowel gas and/or patient discomfort. This test may, however, detect signs of biliary abnormalities in cases where this cause is suspected.
   Computed tomography (CT) with oral and intravenous (IV) contrast can offer information regarding severity of disease (see question 9) and development of complications. Features that may be identified on CT include evidence of inflammation (pancreatic parenchymal edema or peripancreatic fat stranding), peripancreatic or intrapancreatic fluid collections, pancreas perfusion, and presence and extent of pancreatic necrosis.

7. **Should all patients have imaging studies done at the time of presentation?**
The timing of performing CT in the evaluation of AP has been frequently debated and studied. Obtaining CT early in the course of illness has not been shown to establish alternative diagnoses or change clinical management. The need for cross-sectional imaging should be evaluated on a case-by-case basis and reserved for those who do not improve clinically after several days of supportive therapy and/or in whom worrisome symptoms such as fever or leukocytosis develop. Advanced imaging should be considered early in a patient's course of illness if the diagnosis itself is uncertain or if suspicion exists of a complication from AP that, if identified, would significantly alter management, or if alternative diagnoses requiring surgical management are considered.

8. **What if the patient cannot receive contrast for imaging?**
Magnetic resonance imaging (MRI) has a growing role in the diagnosis and management of AP and is a reasonable option in patients who cannot receive iodinated contrast for CT. Enhanced MRI requires the administration of gadolinium, which has been implicated in severe toxic side effects (nephrogenic systemic fibrosis) in patients with compromised renal function. Good correlation has been noted, however, when comparing magnetic resonance cholangiopancreatography (MRCP), with or without gadolinium contrast, with CT in the evaluation AP. MRCP also has the added benefit of being able to better define the pancreatic and biliary ductal system in cases where this cause is suspected but the pretest probability is too low to proceed directly to ERCP.

9. **How do you determine the severity and prognosis of AP?**
Recognizing and differentiating mild AP from SAP is important so that patients can be triaged to the appropriate setting and treatment plan. Over decades, several clinical predictors have emerged. Although all are imperfect, they are considered superior to clinical judgment alone.
   Ranson criteria (Table 47-1) were one of the earliest and widely used scoring systems. Their major disadvantage was that they required 48 hours to complete. The Acute Physiology and Chronic Health Evaluation (APACHE) II system, developed to evaluate critically ill patients, has also been used to differentiate mild AP from SAP. The major disadvantage of this system is that many find it cumbersome as it requires 12 physiologic measures to calculate. A CT severity index (Balthazar score, Table 47-2), has been developed and often used to predict severity of pancreatitis on the basis of radiographic features. The bedside index of severity in AP (BISAP) score (Table 47-3) integrates the systemic inflammatory response syndrome (SIRS) criteria and can be calculated relatively quickly on admission.

TABLE 47-1.   RANSON PROGNOSTIC SIGNS

	ETIOLOGY OF PANCREATITIS	
	NONGALLSTONE	GALLSTONE
At initial presentation		
Age (yr)	>55	>70
White blood cell count (k/mm^3)	>16	>18
Glucose (mg/dL)	>200	>220
Lactate dehydrogenase (U/L)	>350	>400
Aspartate (AST) (U/L)	>250	>250
During first 48 hours		
Decrease in hematocrit (%)	≥10	>10
Elevation in blood urea nitrogen (mg/dL)	>5	>2
Serum total calcium (mg/dL)	<8	<8
Partial pressure of oxygen (mm Hg)	<60	NA
Base deficit (mmol/L)	>4	>5
Fluid sequestration (L)	>6	>4
PROGNOSIS	**NO. OF CRITERIA MET**	**PREDICTED MORTALITY**
	≤2	0.9%
	3-4	16%
	5-6	40%
	7-8	100%

Modified from Ranson JH, Rifkind KM, Roses DF, et al: Prognostic signs and the role of operative management in acute pancreatitis. Surg Gynecol Obstet 139:69-81, 1974; and Ranson JH: Etiological and prognostic factors in human acute pancreatitis: a review. Am J Gastroenterol 77:633-638, 1982. *NA*, Not applicable.

10. **What is the treatment for AP?**

    The mainstay of treatment in AP is aggressive supportive and symptomatic therapy that includes volume repletion, pain control, nutritional support, correction of electrolyte abnormalities, treatment of infection (if present), and treatment of associated or causative conditions.

    Adequate volume repletion and restoration of perfusion to pancreatic microcirculation is imperative to stave off progression of disease and development of local complications. Inadequate volume repletion is associated with higher rates of pancreatic necrosis. No randomized trials exist to guide rate or volume of fluid administration. Most experts recommend isotonic crystalloid infusion rates of 250 to 300 mL/hr or greater for the first 48 hours or enough to maintain urine output at 0.5 mL/kg/hr. Narcotics are usually necessary to establish pain control. IV morphine or hydromorphone at 2- to 4-hour intervals should be considered. Occasionally, continuous infusion with additional patient-administered boluses is necessary.

    Antisecretory agents have been considered for use in pancreatitis. The inhibitory effect of octreotide, a pharmaceutical analog of somatostatin, on pancreatic enzyme secretion has led to its study in the treatment of AP. The largest randomized trial comparing placebo with octreotide in the treatment of moderate or severe pancreatitis found no significant difference with regard to mortality, rate of new complications, rate of surgical intervention, duration of pain, or length of hospital stay.

TABLE 47-2. BALTHAZAR CT GRADING OF AP AND CT SEVERITY INDEX

GRADE	DESCRIPTION OF CT FINDINGS
A	Normal pancreas
B	Enlarged pancreas
C	Inflammation of pancreas or peripancreatic fat
D	One peripancreatic fluid collection
E	More than one peripancreatic fluid collection and/or air in retroperitoneum

		NECROSIS FACTOR	
CT GRADE	POINTS	% NECROSIS	POINTS
A	0		
B	1	0	0
C	2	<30	2
D	3	30-50	4
E	4	>50	6

SEVERITY INDEX*	% MORBIDITY	% MORTALITY
0-3	8	3
4-6	35	6
7-10	92	17

Modified from Balthazar EJ: Acute pancreatitis: assessment of severity with clinical and CT evaluation. Radiology 223:603-613, 2002.
*CT grade points + necrosis points.

11. **How should patients with pancreatitis be fed?**
Enteral feeding is the preferred method of nutritional support for all patients who are seen with pancreatitis. It is thought to help maintain the intestinal mucosal barrier, thereby preventing translocation, which is thought to be a major source of infection. No strong evidence exists that nasojejunal feeding is advantageous over nasogastric feeding. Still, many experts recommend fluoroscopic or endoscopic placement of a jejunal, or postpyloric, feeding tube if possible. Parenteral nutrition should be initiated in patients unable to tolerate oral feeding because of pain, ileus, and/or nausea. Opinion with regard to the timing of initiation of parenteral nutrition ranges from 2 to 5 days after presentation.

12. **Should all patients with AP receive antibiotics?**
No. The use of prophylactic antibiotics to prevent infection of pancreatic necrosis has been controversial but is not currently recommended. No significant benefit has been found with regard to mortality, rates of infected necrosis, need for operative treatment, or overall infections when administering prophylactic antibiotics.

Broad-spectrum antibiotics should be administered if objective evidence exists of infected necrosis on the basis of clinical status (i.e., fever) or cultured aspirate. Some experts believe antibiotics are warranted when evidence is seen on CT of necrosis in >30% of the pancreas. In such cases, the use of antibiotics should be limited to 7 to 14 days because of the risk of fungal superinfection. If the patient's condition continues to deteriorate, he or she should be evaluated for minimally invasive and/or surgical debridement or necrosectomy (see question 14).

TABLE 47-3. BISAP SCORE

1 point for each of the following if present, 0 points if absent

BUN >25 mg/dL (8.9 mmol/L)

Impaired mental status

SIRS (two or more of the following)

- Pulse >90 beats/min
- Respiratory rate >20/min or $PaCO_2$ >32 mm Hg
- Temperature >38° C or <36° C
- WBC >12,000 or <4000 cells/mm^3 or >10% immature neutrophils (bands)
  Age >60 yr

Pleural effusion

BISAP interpretation

BISAP SCORE	MORTALITY (%)
0-2	<1
2	2
3-5	5-20

Modified from Wu BU, Johannes RS, Sun X, et al: The early prediction of mortality in acute pancreatitis: a large population-based study. Gut 57:1698-1703, 2008.
BUN, Blood urea nitrogen; *WBC*, white blood cells.

---

13. **What are the most common bacteria responsible for infected pancreatic necrosis?**

    Culprit infective agents are usually gut derived, including *Escherichia coli, Bacteroides,* and *Enterococcus. Staphylococcus* and *Pseudomonas* are also potential pathogens and should be considered. Fungal infection of necrosis is rare but more common when prophylactic antibiotics are given. It is unclear whether fungal superinfection has any impact on mortality.

14. **What is the role of surgery for AP?**

    Surgery may be necessary for delayed complications of AP (i.e., pancreatic pseudocysts, persistent sterile necrosis) or for cholecystectomy to prevent future episodes of biliary pancreatitis. Surgical necrosectomy is the gold standard treatment for infected pancreatic necrosis resulting from severe AP. Retrospective reviews addressing timing of intervention found that postponing surgery until 4 or 6 weeks after admission correlated with decreased mortality compared with earlier intervention. Expert panels recommend delaying necrosectomy at least 3 to 4 weeks after hospitalization if possible, while administering antibiotics and allowing the necrosis to organize.

    Principles of surgical management of infected pancreatic necrosis include debridement of all infected necrotic material and drainage of the remaining pancreatic bed. Debridement is done bluntly and gently, with hydrosonic irrigation frequently used, to avoid vascular injury. Adequate debridement may require multiple trips to the operating room. The current favored drainage option includes closure of the abdomen over multiple large closed sump drains with or without irrigation. These patients are usually critically ill and require vigorous supportive care.

15. **When should minimally invasive or image-guided therapy be considered?**

    Although surgical necrosectomy remains the gold standard for definitive management of pancreatic necrosis, percutaneous and endoscopic therapies have a growing role in at least adjunctive management. Percutaneous drainage (followed by surgery if necessary) has been associated with fewer major complications than open necrosectomy alone but did not offer any mortality benefit. One third to one half of patients who undergo percutaneous drainage have no need for surgical necrosectomy. CT-guided percutaneous drainage of necrotizing pancreatic collections may be considered as a bridge to necrosectomy in patients with sepsis who are too ill to proceed directly to surgery. Drainage of a walled-off necrotic cavity by endoscopic ultrasonography (EUS) via transgastric or transduodenal approach has been shown to be effective; however, this modality should be considered only in a carefully selected patient population and is dependent on local expertise.

16. **Are there additional treatment options for acute biliary pancreatitis?**
Early ERCP has previously been the standard of care for patients with AP suspected to be due to gallstones. All patients who have signs or symptoms of cholangitis should have early ERCP to relieve biliary obstruction. Other patients with AP in which cholangitis is not present should be evaluated on a case-by-case basis with the understanding that investigations have shown that early ERCP in patients with predicted mild or severe pancreatitis does not significantly reduce the risk for overall complications or mortality.

17. **What are pancreatic pseudocysts?**
Pancreatic pseudocysts are localized fluid collections rich in amylase and other pancreatic enzymes surrounded by a wall of fibrous tissue that are not lined by epithelium. Pseudocysts can form as a result of pancreatic necrosis during an episode of pancreatitis or because of disruption in the normal duct anatomy due to stenosis, calculus, or trauma. Pancreatic pseudocysts may be asymptomatic, present with pain alone, or present with a variety of other clinical complications including bleeding, infection, or rupture. Rare complications include gastric outlet and/or biliary obstruction and thrombosis of splenic or portal veins with development of gastric varices. Diagnosis is usually made on the basis of clinical and radiographic evidence.

18. **What is the best approach to the management of pseudocysts?**
Pancreatic pseudocysts require treatment if they become symptomatic or develop a complication (see question 17). Surgical, percutaneous, and endoscopic approaches have all been used to manage these collections. No randomized trials have been performed to compare these modalities. Endoscopic drainage has advantages of being less invasive, more cost-effective, and associated with lower lengths of stay than surgery, but its use may be limited on the basis of anatomy. Modality of treatment for pancreatic pseudocysts should be based on a combination of factors including patient comorbidities and clinical status, site and characteristics of the lesion, and available local expertise.

KEY POINTS: COMMON CAUSES OF AP

B: Biliary—gallstones, parasites, or malignancy
A: Alcohol
D: Drugs
T: Trauma, toxins
I: Idiopathic, ischemic, infectious, inherited
M: Metabolic—hyperlipidemia, hypercalcemia
E: ERCP
S: Smoking

BIBLIOGRAPHY

1. Cheung MT, Li WH, Kwok PC, et al: Surgical management of pancreatic necrosis: towards lesser and later. J Hepatobiliary Pancreat Sci 17:338-344, 2010.

2. Lindkvist B, Appelros S, Manjer J, et al: A prospective cohort study of smoking in acute pancreatitis. Pancreatology 8:63-70, 2008.

3. McClave SA, Chang WK, Dhaliwal R, et al: Nutrition support in acute pancreatitis: a systematic review of the literature. JPEN J Parenter Enteral Nutr 30:143-156, 2006.

4. Moretti A, Papi C, Aratari A, et al: Is early endoscopic retrograde cholangiopancreatography useful in the management of acute biliary pancreatitis? A meta-analysis of randomized controlled trials. Dig Liver Dis 40:379-385, 2008.

5. Spanier BW, Nio Y, van der Hulst RW, et al: Practice and yield of early CT scan in acute pancreatitis: a Dutch Observational Multicenter Study. Pancreatology 10:222-228, 2010.

6. Talukdar R, Swaroop Vege S: Early management of severe acute pancreatitis. Curr Gastroenterol Rep 13:123-130, 2011.

7. Thrower EC, Gorelick FS, Husain SZ: Molecular and cellular mechanisms of pancreatic injury. Curr Opin Gastroenterol 26:484-489, 2010.

8. Uhl W, Buchler MW, Malfertheiner P, et al: A randomised, double blind, multicentre trial of octreotide in moderate to severe acute pancreatitis. Gut 45:97-104, 1999.

9. van Baal MC, van Santvoort HC, Bollen TL, et al: Systematic review of percutaneous catheter drainage as primary treatment for necrotizing pancreatitis. Br J Surg 98:18-27, 2011.

10. Villatoro E, Mulla M, Larvin M: Antibiotic therapy for prophylaxis against infection of pancreatic necrosis in acute pancreatitis. Cochrane Database Syst Rev 5:CD002941, 2010.

11. Warndorf MG, Kurtzman JT, Bartel MJ, et al: Early fluid resuscitation reduces morbidity among patients with acute pancreatitis. Clin Gastroenterol Hepatol 9:705-709, 2011.

12. Wittau M, Mayer B, Scheele J, et al: Systematic review and meta-analysis of antibiotic prophylaxis in severe acute pancreatitis. Scand J Gastroenterol 46:261-270, 2011.

CHAPTER 48

HEPATITIS AND CIRRHOSIS

Zechariah S. Gardner, MD, and Jaina Clough, MD

1. **What is hepatitis?**
   Hepatitis is defined as inflammation of the liver. It can be divided into infectious and noninfectious causes.

2. **What are liver function tests?**
   The term *liver function tests* (LFTs) commonly refers to alkaline aminotransferase (ALT), aspartate aminotransferase (AST), alkaline phosphatase, bilirubin, albumin, and protein. ALT and AST (transaminases) are enzymes found in hepatocytes whereas alkaline phosphatase is found in cells in the bile ducts. Gamma-glutamyl transpeptidase is an additional test that is used to determine whether alkaline phosphatase elevations originate from hepatobiliary sources. Prothrombin time is used to assess liver synthetic function.

3. **Elevations of which LFTs are associated with hepatitis?**
   Hepatitis is a process of hepatocellular inflammation and damage that causes spillage of cellular elements into the blood. Hepatitis therefore results primarily in elevations in ALT and AST. Elevations can be modest in some forms of hepatitis (alcoholic) or extreme in others (acute viral hepatitis). Alkaline phosphatase levels can also be elevated in hepatitis, but elevations are generally less significant than those of the transaminases. Bilirubin can reach very high levels in hepatitis but usually lags behind the transaminases.

4. **What are the types of infectious hepatitis?**
   Hepatitis viruses primarily infect the liver and include hepatitis A, B, C, D, and E. Other nonhepatitis viruses can cause hepatitis including cytomegalovirus, Epstein-Barr virus, and human immunodeficiency virus (HIV).

5. **What is hepatitis A, how is it diagnosed, and what are the disease course and management?**
   Hepatitis A is a disease caused by an RNA virus that is transmitted by the fecal-oral route, is endemic in the developing world, and occurs sporadically in the United States. Most childhood infections are asymptomatic. Adults are more likely to have acute symptoms. The incubation period is 2 to 6 weeks, after which patients have fatigue, malaise, fever, and abdominal pain followed by jaundice. Transaminase levels are markedly elevated.

   Diagnosis is by a positive anti–hepatitis A virus (HAV) immunoglobulin (Ig) M antibody that denotes active infection and remains elevated for 3 to 6 months. HAV anti-IgG antibody positivity occurs later, remains elevated for decades, and indicates past infection.

   Treatment is supportive. Significant morbidity and mortality are uncommon, but development of fulminant hepatic failure (FHF) can occur (<1%) and carries significant mortality (see question 20). HAV vaccine is effective and widely available. It is recommended for individuals with chronic liver disease, child-care workers, and those traveling to endemic areas.

6. **What is hepatitis E?**
   Like HAV, hepatitis E virus (HEV) is an RNA virus that is transmitted by the fecal-oral route. It is endemic to Southeast Asia, Africa, India, and Central America. Infection in the United States is uncommon and is almost always associated with individuals who have

recently traveled to endemic areas. It causes a self-limiting hepatitis similar to HAV infection but has a significantly higher tendency to progress to FHF in pregnant women. Laboratory tests for diagnosis include HEV IgG and IgM antibody testing, as well as HEV RNA polymerase chain reaction (PCR).

7. **What is hepatitis B?**
   Hepatitis B is a disease caused by a DNA virus that is transmitted through blood and body fluids. Risk factors include intravenous (IV) and intranasal drug use, unprotected sex with multiple partners, men who have sex with men, health care workers exposed to blood, children born to infected mothers, incarceration, and spouses of infected individuals. Acute infection is most commonly asymptomatic but can cause constitutional symptoms including fatigue, malaise, nausea, vomiting, headache, arthralgias, myalgias, and low-grade fever, as well as jaundice, dark urine, clay-colored stools, and tender hepatomegaly. FHF occurs in 1% of infections. Other complications include a serum sickness–like syndrome (5%-10% of cases), glomerular nephritis with nephrotic syndrome, systemic vasculitis, and progression to chronic hepatitis B infection, which occurs in approximately 5% of cases. Some individuals go on to a carrier state in which they have persistent hepatitis B virus (HBV) in the liver without any significant inflammation. These individuals can be infectious and are termed inactive carriers.

8. **How is hepatitis B diagnosed?**
   Serologic testing for hepatitis B is complicated by the fact that there are multiple blood tests routinely used to assess infection.
   - Hepatitis B surface antigen (HBsAg) is the lipid and protein layer that forms the outer shell of HBV. It is not infectious and is produced in excess during viral replication. It is the first viral antigen to become positive in the serum with acute infection, and its presence indicates active infection. It may be negative early in the acute infection, and it is also the first serum marker to be cleared by the host immune system, becoming undetectable 6 to 12 weeks after infection.
   - Hepatitis B surface antibody (HBsAb) is the antibody to HBsAg. It develops to detectible levels 6 to 8 weeks after infection and remains detectible for life. Positive HBsAb indicates past or resolving infection. Hepatitis B vaccine uses the surface particle, and vaccinated individuals will also be HBsAb positive.
   - Hepatitis B core antibody (HBcAb) is an antibody to a core viral protein. HBcAb can be measured as IgG or IgM and can also be reported as total, which includes both. IgM makes up the immune system's early response and is later replaced by IgG. Positive HBcAb IgM indicates early or chronic infection. Positive HBcAb IgG indicates past or chronic infection.
   - Hepatitis B early antigen (HBeAg) is a protein produced during viral replication, and detectible levels of this antigen indicate high levels of viral replication, increased infectivity, and higher risk of progression to fibrosis. It is positive during both acute infection and active viral phases of chronic infection.
   - HBV DNA can also be measured and is one of the diagnostic criteria for chronic HBV infection.

9. **What is hepatitis C?**
   Hepatitis C is caused by a blood-borne RNA virus. It is transmitted primarily through contact with blood products from infected individuals. Risk factors include current or past IV drug use, health care workers exposed to blood, or transfusion of infected blood products (rare since routine screening was introduced in 1992). Sexual transmission can occur but is uncommon with hepatitis C virus (HCV). Most acute infections are asymptomatic, but 20% to 30% of infected individuals will have a self-limiting illness similar to other acute viral hepatitis infections. A majority (70%-85%) of those infected with HCV will go on to have chronic infection. It is currently estimated that more than 3 million individuals have chronic HCV in the United States, where it is the leading indication for liver transplantation.

10. **How is HCV infection diagnosed?**
    Screening for infection is by serum testing for anti-HCV antibody. Antibody positivity occurs at 4 to 10 weeks and remains positive for life regardless of whether chronic infection develops. All positive antibody tests should be followed up with an HCV RNA PCR to determine whether active infection exists. Of those infected, 15% to 25% will spontaneously clear the virus and are not at risk for complications of chronic infection. If virus is detected viral genotyping should be done.

11. **What are HCV genotypes, and how do they affect management?**
    At least six genotypes and more than 50 subtypes of HCV have been identified. Genotype 1 is the most common genotype, accounting for 60% to 80% of all hepatitis C. Genotype 1 is more difficult to eradicate with treatment than other common genotypes. Treatment for chronic hepatitis C infection is with pegylated interferon-α and ribavirin. Treatment length is dependent on genotype and viral response. Genotype 1 traditionally requires a longer treatment course (48 weeks) and has lower response rates (50%). Recent data have shown that the addition of telaprevir or boceprevir to interferon and ribavirin for treatment of genotype 1 hepatitis C infection significantly improves achievement of sustained viral response to levels similar to those of other common hepatitis C genotypes. The Food and Drug Administration approved their use for treatment of genotype 1 hepatitis C infection in early 2011.

12. **What other extrahepatic conditions can be caused by hepatitis C infection?**
    Some individuals with chronic hepatitis C infection can have other medical conditions that are thought to be due to the body's immune response to the HCV infection. These conditions are uncommon but are noted to occur at increased frequency in those infected with hepatitis C. They include diabetes mellitus, glomerulonephritis, mixed cryoglobulinemia, porphyria cutanea tarda, and non-Hodgkin lymphoma.

13. **What is hepatitis D?**
    Hepatitis D virus (HDV) or hepatitis delta virus is a small RNA viral particle that can cause infection only in the presence of hepatitis B virus. It is blood borne, and IV drug use is the most common route of infection. Infection can occur either as coinfection when both HBV and HDV viruses are acquired together or as superinfection when HDV infection occurs in a patient with chronic hepatitis B infection. Concomitant infection with hepatitis B and D results in a higher likelihood of development of FHF, more rapid progression to cirrhosis, and higher rates of hepatocellular carcinoma.

14. **What viral serologies should be tested in a patient with acute hepatitis?**
    All patients with acute hepatitis should undergo testing for anti-HAV IgM, anti-HCV antibody, HBsAg, and HBcAb.

15. **Who should be screened for HCV infection?**
    Because chronic hepatitis C infection is prevalent and treatment can reduce the morbidity and mortality associated with infection, screening is recommended for anyone who has used injection drugs, people who received clotting factors before 1987 or other blood products before 1992, patients undergoing hemodialysis, those with unexplained abnormal LFTs, health care workers with needle-stick injuries, individuals positive for HIV, and babies born to women positive for HCV. Patients with similar risk factors should be screened for HBV as well.

16. **What are the risks associated with chronic hepatitis?**
    Chronic hepatitis can develop with HBV, HCV, and HDV infections, as well as many nonviral causes of hepatitis. It is characterized by persistent liver inflammation. Chronic hepatitis is associated with the development of liver fibrosis and cirrhosis and with increased risk for the development of hepatocellular carcinoma.

17. **What are nonviral causes of hepatitis?**

    There are many nonviral causes of hepatitis, which can be broken down into several broad categories including toxic or drug induced, autoimmune, and metabolic. The list of drugs and toxins that can cause liver injury is extensive. The two most common causes of drug- or toxin-induced liver injury are alcohol and acetaminophen. Metabolic causes of hepatitis include hemochromatosis, Wilson disease, and nonalcoholic fatty liver disease. Hepatitis can also develop as a result of other organ system dysfunction. An example of this is liver hypoperfusion in shock states, known as shock liver.

18. **What is autoimmune hepatitis (AIH)?**

    AIH is a chronic inflammatory liver disease caused by a host immune response to portions of the hepatocyte. This chronic inflammation can lead to progressive fibrosis and cirrhosis if left untreated. AIH can occur at any age but occurs most often in young women and is commonly associated with other autoimmune disorders. Circulating autoantibodies associated with AIH are antinuclear antibody, anti–smooth muscle antibody, and liver kidney microsomal antibody. Elevated immunoglobulin levels are also common. Liver biopsy is necessary for diagnosis of AIH. Treatment is with steroids alone or in combination with azathioprine, and remission can be achieved in 60% to 80% of cases.

19. **How is alcoholic hepatitis managed?**

    Alcoholic hepatitis can have a 1-month mortality rate as high as 30% to 50%. The Maddrey discriminant function score is a validated mechanism to score disease severity. It uses prothrombin time and total bilirubin to calculate a disease severity score with scores ≥ 32 indicating severe disease. Data suggest that patients with severe disease benefit from treatment with a 4-week course of steroids or pentoxifylline if steroids are contraindicated. Additionally all patients with alcoholic hepatitis should be counseled to abstain from alcohol and should undergo nutritional assessment and receive aggressive nutritional therapy.

20. **What is FHF?**

    FHF or acute liver failure is a gastrointestinal emergency characterized by the rapid arrest of normal hepatic function. A defining feature of FHF is the rapid onset of hepatic encephalopathy. FHF can result from the most severe forms of most of the causes of hepatitis. This includes the viral hepatitides, drugs, toxins, autoimmune hepatitis, and metabolic conditions affecting the liver. In addition to encephalopathy, FHF can result in coagulopathy, increased risk for infection, metabolic derangements including acute renal failure, electrolyte abnormalities, hypoglycemia, and pancreatitis. Significant cardiorespiratory and hemodynamic sequelae of FHF also occur that are characterized by hypotension resulting from low systemic vascular resistance, increased cardiac output, and tissue hypoxia.

21. **What is the treatment and prognosis of FHF?**

    Treatment for patients with FHF is supportive while allowing the liver time to regenerate. Mortality rates are high, and the only intervention with proved benefit is liver transplantation. Early referral to a transplant center should be considered when FHF is suspected. Some causes of FHF can be reversed with immediate treatment and should be assessed for rapidly. These include acetaminophen, amanita mushroom poisoning, herpes simplex virus, acute fatty liver disease of pregnancy, and Wilson disease.

22. **What is cirrhosis?**

    Cirrhosis is a progressive process of hepatic injury, subsequent fibrosis, and destruction of normal liver architecture. It may result from any chronic liver disease but is most commonly associated with viral hepatitis and alcoholic liver disease. Cirrhosis was the 12th leading cause of death in the United States in 2007.

23. **What are the causes of cirrhosis?**
The most common causes of cirrhosis are alcoholic liver disease and hepatitis C. Cryptogenic cirrhosis accounts for up to 18% of cases. Many cryptogenic cases may be due to nonalcoholic fatty liver disease. Other causes include hepatitis B, autoimmune hepatobiliary disease, hemochromatosis, extrahepatic biliary obstruction, Wilson disease, α_1-antitrypsin deficiency, and drug toxicity.

24. **Describe the clinical presentation of cirrhosis.**
Cirrhosis is often asymptomatic and discovered incidentally. Well-compensated cirrhosis can manifest as anorexia and weight loss, weakness, and fatigue. More progressive disease may present with the following signs: jaundice, pruritus, coagulopathy, increasing abdominal girth, splenomegaly, abdominal wall vascular collaterals (caput medusae), spider telangiectasia, palmar erythema, mental status changes, and asterixis. Advanced cirrhosis may present with severe complications such as upper gastrointestinal tract bleeding or hepatic encephalopathy.

25. **How is cirrhosis diagnosed?**
Liver biopsy provides the definitive diagnosis of cirrhosis and may be indicated when the clinical diagnosis is uncertain. Abdominal ultrasound findings of liver nodularity, irregularity, increased echogenicity, and atrophy are consistent with cirrhosis. LFTs (including prothrombin time and albumin), hepatitis serologies, autoantibodies, and a complete blood cell count may reveal the underlying causes of cirrhosis and the extent of liver dysfunction.

26. **What are the major complications of cirrhosis?**
The most common complication of cirrhosis is ascites, followed by gastroesophageal variceal hemorrhage and hepatic encephalopathy. Ascites and variceal hemorrhage are direct consequences of portal hypertension.

27. **What is portal hypertension?**
Portal hypertension is defined as a portal pressure of greater than 12 mm Hg or a hepatic venous wedge pressure that exceeds the pressure of the inferior vena cava by >5 mm Hg. The portal hypertension of cirrhosis is caused by the disruption of hepatic sinusoids, leading to increased resistance in the portal venous system. A compounding effect is increased portal flow due to vasodilation and increased cardiac output associated with cirrhosis. This leads to an imbalance of Starling forces, which results in fluid accumulation in the peritoneal cavity (ascites), as well as gastroesophageal varices.

28. **What are other complications of cirrhosis?**
Other complications of cirrhosis include altered hemodynamics, hyponatremia, immune compromise, and coagulopathy.

29. **How is cirrhotic ascites diagnosed?**
New-onset ascites should be assessed with diagnostic paracentesis to confirm cirrhosis as the cause and rule out spontaneous bacterial peritonitis (SBP). The serum-ascites albumin gradient (SAAG) is the most important diagnostic parameter in determining the cause of ascites. A SAAG of ≥ 1.1 g/dL indicates ascites from portal hypertension with a specificity of 97%. Ascitic fluid cell count, differential, and total protein should also be performed. Ascitic fluid culture should be obtained if any suspicion of SBP exists.

30. **How is cirrhotic ascites managed?**
Initial management focuses on dietary sodium restriction and abstinence from alcohol in alcohol-related liver disease. Diuretic therapy is the mainstay of medical management of ascites. Dual therapy with furosemide and spironolactone is the recommended starting regimen if renal function is stable. Large-volume paracentesis is used to relieve the discomfort of tense ascites.

Serial paracentesis may be indicated for ascites refractory to medical therapy. Transjugular intrahepatic portosystemic shunt (TIPS) and liver transplantation should be considered in refractory cases. Surgically placed peritoneovenous shunts may be an option in patients who are not candidates for paracentesis, TIPS, or transplantation.

31. What is TIPS?

TIPS is a treatment for portal hypertension. It is reserved for patients with severe ascites and variceal bleeding who do not respond to medical therapy. Reduced portal pressure is achieved by a stent placed through the liver between the portal and hepatic circulation.

32. What are the complications of cirrhotic ascites?

Ascites is associated with the complications of SBP and the hepatorenal syndrome (HRS).

33. What is the mortality of cirrhotic ascites?

Cirrhotic ascites carries a 3-year mortality rate of 50%.

34. How is SBP diagnosed and managed?

A positive ascitic fluid culture and absolute polymorphonuclear leukocyte (PMN) count of ≥ 250 cells/mm^3 are diagnostic of SBP in the absence of an intraabdominal, surgically treatable source of infection.

Empirical antibiotics should be initiated for SBP in any hospitalized patient with an ascitic fluid PMN count of ≥ 250 cells/mm^3 or an ascitic protein level of less than 1 g/dL or in a patient with clinical suspicion of SBP (i.e., fever, abdominal pain) regardless of PMN count. A third-generation cephalosporin is the initial antibiotic choice, ideally cefotaxime. Oral ofloxacin is an acceptable substitute in patients who are quinolone naïve and are clinically stable.

35. What are risk factors for SBP, and how is it prevented?

Risk factors for SBP include prior SBP, variceal hemorrhage, and low-protein ascites. Prevention of SBP may be achieved with use of quinolones or a third-generation cephalosporin in patients with variceal hemorrhage. Oral quinolones may be used in patients who have had prior episodes of SBP. Antibiotic prophylaxis may be considered in those with low-protein ascites.

36. What is HRS, and how is it managed?

HRS is renal dysfunction (creatinine level > 1.5 mg/dL) that persists after 2 days of diuretic withdrawal and volume expansion in patients with cirrhosis and ascites. Type I HRS is rapidly progressive and fatal without treatment. Type II HRS progresses over months with a median survival of 3 to 6 months.

Type I HRS warrants an expedited referral for liver transplantation. Dialysis may be needed to bridge patients to transplantation. Medical therapies such as octreotide and midodrine may be used as temporizing measures as well.

37. What is variceal bleeding?

Variceal bleeding is upper gastrointestinal tract bleeding due to rupture of gastroesophageal varices. It is the most common life-threatening complication of cirrhosis and occurs at a rate of 5% to 15% per year in patients with cirrhosis. Size of varices and severity of liver disease are the most important predictors of bleeding.

38. How is variceal bleeding prevented?

At the time cirrhosis is diagnosed, esophagogastroduodenoscopy (EGD) should be performed to screen for varices. If medium to large varices are present with a high risk of bleeding, nonselective β-blocker therapy or endoscopic variceal ligation (EVL) is recommended. For medium varices or small varices with a high risk of bleeding, nonselective β-blocker therapy is preferred with EVL reserved for patients intolerant to β-blocker therapy.

39. **What are other sources of upper gastrointestinal tract bleeding in patients with cirrhosis?**
   Sources include portal hypertensive gastropathy and gastric antral vascular ectasia.

40. **How is variceal bleeding managed?**
   Acute management consists of volume resuscitation, blood transfusion to maintain a hemoglobin level of ≥ 8 g/dL, and EGD within 12 hours to diagnose variceal bleeding and treat with EVL or sclerotherapy.

   Medications that promote splanchnic vasoconstriction are also used (octreotide, a somatostatin analog, and terlipressin). Balloon tamponade is an effective short-term strategy to control bleeding, but it carries a 20% mortality rate due to complications. It should be reserved for patients with uncontrolled bleeding within 24 hours of a more definitive therapy, such as TIPS.

   Short-term antibiotic treatment is indicated in patients with variceal bleeding and ascites because of their high risk for SBP, other infections, and subsequent risk of rebleeding. A 7-day course of norfloxacin (400 mg twice daily) is recommended. IV ciprofloxacin may be used in patients unable to tolerate the oral route. Ceftriaxone is an alternative in areas with high quinolone resistance.

41. **What is hepatic encephalopathy?**
   Hepatic encephalopathy is a syndrome of altered mental status in the setting of portosystemic shunting, either through collateral vessels or through surgically placed shunts. The mechanism is uncertain but may relate to changes in the blood-brain barrier that allow passage of neurotoxic substances, including ammonia and manganese, into the brain. Another theory suggests that accumulation of circulating ammonia due to decreased hepatocyte function leads to encephalopathy.

42. **How is hepatic encephalopathy diagnosed and managed?**
   Elevated serum ammonia levels indicate hepatic encephalopathy in patients with cirrhosis and altered mental status that cannot be explained by any other cause. Precipitating factors include gastrointestinal bleeding, infection, constipation, and metabolic disturbances. Treatment focuses on reducing intestinal production of ammonia, typically through the use of cathartics (such as lactulose) and antibiotics (such as neomycin and rifaximin). Low-protein diets are no longer recommended as they do not appear to be effective at reducing encephalopathy and may contribute to malnutrition.

43. **Describe the pulmonary syndromes associated with chronic liver disease.**
   Hepatopulmonary syndrome is a mismatch of ventilation and perfusion that results primarily from vasodilation of pulmonary capillaries. Arteriovenous communication in the lungs and pleura may occur as well. It is characterized by hypoxia and dyspnea that worsen with upright position (orthodeoxia and platypnea, respectively).

   Portopulmonary hypertension is the development of pulmonary hypertension in the presence of portal hypertension.

44. **When should patients with cirrhosis be referred for liver transplantation?**
   Patients with cirrhosis should be referred for transplantation when they have their first major complication (ascites, variceal bleeding, hepatic encephalopathy) or evidence of significant hepatic dysfunction (Model for End-Stage Liver Disease [MELD] score ≥ 10, Child-Turcotte-Pugh [CTP] score ≥ 7. MELD score calculator: http://optn.transplant.hrsa.gov/resources/allocationcalculators.asp). Type 1 HRS is an indication for expedited referral for liver transplantation.

KEY POINTS: HEPATITIS

1. Pregnant women are at significant risk for FHF with hepatitis E infection.

2. End-stage liver disease from HCV is the leading indication for liver transplantation in the United States.

3. Steroids should be considered for the treatment of severe alcoholic hepatitis.

4. Some causes of FHF can be reversed with immediate treatment, including acetaminophen, amanita mushroom poisoning, herpes simplex virus, acute fatty liver disease of pregnancy, and Wilson disease.

KEY POINTS: CIRRHOSIS

1. Critical complications of cirrhosis include ascites, SBP, HRS, hepatic encephalopathy, and upper gastrointestinal tract bleeding due to gastroesophageal varices.

2. Management of variceal bleeding involves volume resuscitation, use of somatostatin or analogs, endoscopic treatment with sclerotherapy or EVL, and antibiotics to prevent SBP.

3. TIPS is reserved for refractory ascites or uncontrolled variceal bleeding. TIPS carries a high risk for encephalopathy.

4. Referral for liver transplantation is indicated in FHF when the MELD score is ≥ 10 or when major complications of cirrhosis develop. Type 1 HRS is an indication for expedited liver transplantation referral.

BIBLIOGRAPHY

1. Centers for Disease Control and Prevention: Hepatitis C information for health professionals: www.cdc.gov/hepatitis/HCV/HCVfaq.htm#section2. Accessed July 15, 2011.

2. Cordoba J, Lopez-Hellin J, Planas M, et al: Normal protein diet for episodic hepatic encephalopathy: results of a randomized study. J Hepatol 41:38-43, 2004.

3. Dienstag JL: Acute viral hepatitis. In Fauci AS, Braunwald E, Kasper DL, et al: Harrison's Principles of Internal Medicine, 17th ed. New York, McGraw-Hill, 2008.

4. Garcia-Tsao G, Sanyal AJ, Grace ND, et al: Practice Guidelines Committee of American Association for Study of Liver Diseases; Practice Parameters Committee of American College of Gastroenterology: Prevention and management of gastroesophageal varices and variceal hemorrhage in cirrhosis. Am J Gastroenterol 102:2086-2102, 2007.

5. Ghany MG, Strader DB, Thomas DL, et al: Diagnosis, management and treatment of hepatitis C: an update. AASLD Practice Guidelines. Hepatology 49:1335-1374, 2009.

6. Gines P, Quintero E, Arroyo V, et al: Compensated cirrhosis: natural history and prognostic factors. Hepatology 7:122-128, 1987.

7. Heidelbaugh J, Bruderly M: Cirrhosis and chronic liver failure: part I. Diagnosis and evaluation. Am Fam Physician 74:756-762, 2006.

8. Hézode C, Forestier N, Dusheiko G, et al: Telaprevir and peginterferon with or without ribavirin for chronic HCV infection. N Engl J Med 360:1839-1850, 2009.

9. Krajden M, McNabb G, Petric M: The laboratory diagnosis of hepatitis B virus. Can J Infect Dis Med Microbiol 16:65-72, 2005.

10. Lok AS, McMahon BJ: Chronic hepatitis B. AASLD Practice Guidelines. Hepatology 45:507-539, 2007.

11. Manns MP, Czaja AJ, Gorham JD, et al: Diagnosis and management of autoimmune hepatitis. Hepatology 51:2193-2213, 2010.

12. Murray K, Carithers R: Practice Guidelines Committee of American Association for Study of Liver Diseases; Practice Parameters Committee of American College of Gastroenterology: Evaluation of the patient for liver transplantation. Hepatology 41:1-26, 2005.

13. O'Shea RS, Dasarathy S, McCullough AJ: Alcoholic liver disease. AASLD Practice Guidelines. Hepatology 51:307-328, 2010.

14. Poordad F, McCone J Jr, Bacon BR, et al: Boceprevir for untreated chronic HCV genotype 1 infection. N Engl J Med 364:1195-1206, 2011.

15. Rodríguez-Roisin R, Krowka M: Hepatopulmonary syndrome—a liver-induced lung vascular disorder. N Engl J Med 358:2378-2387, 2008.

16. Runyon BA: AASLD Practice Guidelines Committee: Management of adult patients with ascites due to cirrhosis: an update. Hepatology 49:2087-2107, 2009.

17. Rutherford A, Dienstag JL: Viral hepatitis. In Greenberger NJ, Blumberg RS, Burakoff R (eds): Current Diagnosis & Treatment: Gastroenterology, Hepatology, & Endoscopy, New York, McGraw-Hill, 2009.

18. Sass DA, Shakil AO: Fulminant hepatic failure. Liver Transpl 11:594-605, 2005.

19. Xu J, Kochanek KD, Murphy SL, et al: Deaths: final data for 2007. Natl Vital Stat Rep 58:1-135, 2010.

CHAPTER 49

ACUTE ABDOMEN AND PERITONITIS

William E. Charash, MD, PhD, and Sarah Pesek, MD

1. **What is an acute abdomen?**
   Any abdominal process that requires urgent (often surgical) intervention. Peritonitis (see question 7) is commonly but not necessarily present. Trauma is generally excluded from discussions of the acute abdomen.

2. **What are some causes of acute abdomen that require invasive intervention?**
   - Perforated hollow viscus (e.g., perforated ulcer, appendicitis, diverticulitis). Perforations that are walled off by the host and not associated with diffuse peritonitis may in certain cases be managed noninvasively.
   - Gangrenous hollow viscus, even in the absence of perforation (e.g., mesenteric ischemia, volvulus, complete large bowel obstruction, closed-loop small bowel obstruction, severe acalculous cholecystitis)
   - Occlusive mesenteric ischemia, even in the absence of necrosis
   - Intraabdominal abscess
   - Uncontrolled hemorrhage
   - Infected pancreatic necrosis

3. **Name some causes of the acute abdomen that are initially treated medically but may ultimately require surgery.**
   - *Clostridium difficile* colitis (see questions 11-13)
   - Abdominal compartment syndrome (see questions 14-17)
   - Ogilvie syndrome (see questions 19-20)
   - Pancreatitis (see question 28)
   - Diverticulitis, small bowel obstruction, inflammatory bowel disease, pelvic inflammatory disease
   - Ischemic colitis
   - Nonocclusive mesenteric ischemia

4. **Which causes of acute abdomen should not require surgery?**
   Spontaneous bacterial peritonitis (see question 7), gastroenteritis.

5. **List thoracic conditions that can cause abdominal pain.**
   Lower lobe pneumonia, pulmonary embolism, pleuritis, empyema, ruptured esophagus, lower rib fractures, pericarditis, and myocardial infarction.

6. **How does the initial evaluation of abdominal pain differ in critically ill patients?**
   The history and physical examination, the mainstay of abdominal evaluation, are often limited because of the patient's depressed level of consciousness. Nonspecific findings such as unexplained sepsis, hypovolemia, and abdominal distention may suggest an acute abdomen.

7. **What is peritonitis?**
   Inflammation of the peritoneum (visceral and/or parietal). Peritonitis is often accompanied by systemic sepsis. When it occurs spontaneously without any known source of contamination it is

termed primary bacterial peritonitis. Secondary bacterial peritonitis originates from visceral pathology or from external sources, such as iatrogenic introduction or penetrating injury.

8. **How does peritonitis manifest itself clinically?**
As an acute abdomen. Abdominal findings include pain, tenderness, distention, involuntary guarding, or rigidity. Bowel sounds are not typically helpful in this diagnosis but are generally diminished. Other findings are those of systemic infection and may include fever, chills, tachycardia, diaphoresis, tachypnea, oliguria, disorientation, and circulatory collapse. The surface area of the peritoneum is large, roughly the same as the human body (approximately 1.7 m^2 for a typical adult). Peritoneal inflammation will generate significant third-space fluid losses and resultant hypovolemia.

9. **What laboratory tests are helpful in the setting of abdominal pain?**
   - A complete blood cell count. An elevated hemoglobin or hematocrit level may suggest third-space fluid losses with hemoconcentration. A low hematocrit may indicate preexisting anemia or active hemorrhage. Elevated white blood cell (WBC) count, especially with left shift, suggests an inflammatory process. A low WBC count may be present if a viral process or gastroenteritis exists, or in the case of overwhelming sepsis.
   - Metabolic acidosis on an arterial blood gas level determination, or an elevated lactate level, may indicate an ischemic abdominal process.
   - Elevated amylase and/or lipase level may suggest pancreatitis. Amylase may also be elevated with gastric or intestinal pathologic condition.
   - Liver function tests may also be helpful.

10. **What imaging studies can aid in the diagnosis?**
   - Oral and intravenous (IV), contrast-enhanced abdominal-pelvic computed tomography (CT) scanning provides the greatest yield. However, this requires a potentially high-risk patient transport. Further, IV contrast might result in contrast-induced nephropathy in a patient already at risk for acute kidney injury. Renal protection with sodium bicarbonate is recommended for high-risk patients.
   - Upright (or semiupright) chest radiograph and two-position abdominal radiographs can demonstrate free air (hollow viscus perforation), bowel distention with air, and fluid levels (obstruction).
   - Abdominal ultrasound can demonstrate peritoneal fluid collections and acute cholecystitis.
   - Angiography or CT-angiography can reveal occlusive vascular disease or active hemorrhage.

11. **What causes *C. difficile* colitis?**
Elaboration of toxin A and toxin B by living *C. difficile* organisms in the colon of the patient. Two conditions are necessary for this to happen. *C. difficile,* not a component of normal colonic flora, must be iatrogenically introduced into the host. Second, the host's protective flora must be altered, most typically through the prior use of antibiotics. Both of these factors are within the control of the health care system. Risk factors for severe colitis include age greater than 60 years, residence in a long-term-care facility, gastric acid suppression, severe underlying disease, recent surgery, and immunosuppression.

12. **How can *C. difficile* colitis be prevented?**
The two primary approaches to preventing *C. difficile* infection are preventing exposure and decreasing risk of colitis once exposure has occurred. Clostridia species are spore-forming organisms. These spores are difficult to eradicate. Health care institutions must take great care to reduce the prevalence of these spores in their environment. Contact precautions should be used with patients with clinical symptoms consistent with *C. difficile* infection even before the results of diagnostic testing are known. Health care workers must wash their hands with soap and water after contact with patients and contaminated surfaces. Healthy gut flora

decreases the risk of colitis if exposure occurs. Antibiotics alter this flora and should always be used judiciously.

13. How is *C. difficile* colitis treated?

The first step is discontinuation of the inciting antibiotic(s) as soon as possible. Antibiotic therapy directed at *C. difficile* consists of either metronidazole (oral preferred, or IV) or vancomycin (orally and/or rectally). Antimotility agents should not be used. Other therapies that might have benefit include probiotics, fecal transplantation, and IV immunoglobulin. Surgical treatment with colectomy (subtotal colectomy with ileostomy) is indicated for patients with fulminant colitis. Peritoneal signs, failure of improvement with antibiotic therapy, and signs of multiorgan failure all indicate the need for surgery.

14. What is intraabdominal hypertension (IAH)?

Sustained intraabdominal pressure of 12 mm Hg or higher.

15. How is intraabdominal pressure monitored?

Most commonly by transducing the pressure in the urinary bladder via a Foley catheter. Twenty to 50 mL saline solution is instilled into the urinary bladder to ensure a continuous column of fluid. A needle (connected to a pressure transducer) is aseptically placed into the sampling port of the drainage tubing, which is clamped downstream from the port. The pubic symphysis is used as a zero reference. Alternatively, the drainage tubing itself can be used as a manometer. Because urinary specific gravity is approximately 1, the height of the fluid column in centimeters needs to be multiplied by 0.74 to convert to millimeters of mercury. Respiratory variation should be observed in the measured pressure to confirm that pressure is being transduced in the abdomen.

16. What is abdominal compartment syndrome?

Intraabdominal hypertension (typically sustained above 20 mm Hg) with end-organ dysfunction (renal dysfunction, ventilator failure, or intestinal ischemia).

Risk factors include acute abdomen, peritonitis, abdominal surgery, trauma, burns, retroperitoneal bleeding, the systemic inflammatory response syndrome, and overresuscitation with fluids.

17. How is abdominal compartment syndrome managed?

Optimize sedation and analgesia. Avoid overresuscitation with fluids. Neuromuscular blockade may be used, if necessary. Prolonged requirement for neuromuscular blockade should prompt invasive intervention. Percutaneous catheter drainage of intraabdominal fluid may be effective. When a patient's end-organ dysfunction is refractory to nonoperative management, surgical decompression is warranted. The open abdomen that is created is then typically managed with some form of negative pressure dressing.

18. What is Ogilvie syndrome?

Ogilvie syndrome, also known as acute colonic pseudoobstruction, is a massive dilation of the colon (cecum and right colon, potentially extending to the rectum) in the absence of mechanical obstruction. Although it can occur at any age, it is most prevalent in patients over 60 years of age. Ogilvie syndrome is seen in association with a wide spectrum of illnesses including abdominal or orthopedic surgery, trauma, severe infection, myocardial infarction, heart failure, neurologic disorders, metabolic derangements, and opiate administration.

19. How is Ogilvie syndrome treated?

Treat the underlying medical conditions. Correct fluid and electrolyte imbalances. Minimize use of narcotics and anticholinergics. Administer nothing by mouth (NPO) with nasogastric tube decompression. A rectal tube may also be helpful. Patients should be ambulated, if possible. If no resolution occurs in 48 hours, or if cecal diameter exceeds 10 to 12 cm (see question 27), IV administration of 2.5 mg neostigmine over a 3-minute period may be therapeutic. Repeat once after 30 minutes if necessary. Profound bradycardia and heart block may result. Alternatively, colonoscopic decompression may be performed. Air insufflation must be avoided. Surgery is indicated in cases of actual or imminent perforation or in patients who are unresponsive to maximal nonsurgical measures.

20. How is acalculous cholecystitis managed?
Percutaneous cholecystostomy is appropriate for most critically ill patients. Cholecystectomy (open) should rarely be necessary in the critically ill patient.

21. When should an abdominal abscess be suspected?
When medical management for bacterial peritonitis fails. Also consider abdominal abscess in patients with fever, leukocytosis, and/or sepsis who have had blunt abdominal trauma, are recovering from abdominal surgery, or have unexplained abdominal findings.

22. Describe the management of nonocclusive mesenteric ischemia.
The strategy is to increase mesenteric blood flow. This is done by ensuring adequate intravascular volume replacement. Vasopressin and α-adrenergic drugs should be avoided. β-Adrenergic agonism might be required. Surgery is reserved for patients with transmural necrosis or perforation.

23. How is occlusive mesenteric ischemia managed?
Time is of the essence. During the work-up of this diagnosis, the strategy described above for nonocclusive mesenteric ischemia should be employed. Once occlusive mesenteric ischemia is confirmed, emergent intervention is necessary. If bowel gangrene or perforation is suspected, emergent laparotomy with resection of necrotic bowel and restoration of blood flow via embolectomy or mesenteric revascularization should be performed. A second-look laparotomy is often planned at the conclusion of the initial surgery. Percutaneous catheter embolectomy or thrombolysis may be an option when perforation and necrosis are not suspected.

24. Which antibiotics should be used for intraabdominal infections?
Antibiotics with broad-spectrum activity against gram-negative organisms in combination with metronidazole should be used for patients with severe community-acquired intraabdominal infection. It is not generally necessary to cover methicillin-resistant *Staphylococcus aureus* (MRSA) in these patients. Enterococcus coverage should be reserved for high-risk patients. For infections that are hospital acquired, the regimen should be based on local microbiologic susceptibilities. MRSA and enterococcus coverage is often appropriate. Antifungal therapy might be appropriate. Broad-spectrum regimens should be tailored as culture and sensitivity results become known.

25. What should the duration of antibiotic treatment be?
Discontinue antibiotics once signs of abdominal infection have resolved (e.g., afebrile, benign abdominal examination results, normal WBC count, tolerating enteral feeding). Continued requirement beyond 7 days implies inadequate source control. Imaging to identify intraabdominal abscess should then be performed. Antibiotic treatment for uncomplicated acute appendicitis or gastric or small intestinal perforation should generally be limited to 24 hours.

26. How does the management of small bowel obstruction differ from that of large bowel obstruction?
Partial small bowel obstruction may be managed expectantly with a nasogastric (NG) tube, NPO, and IV fluids. Surgery is indicated if there is a failure to resolve or in the setting of complete or closed-loop obstruction. Large bowel obstruction usually requires more urgent intervention. A competent ileocecal valve will not allow for relief of colonic pressure. The increase in pressure may result in gangrene and/or perforation, particularly of the cecum.

27. **What cecal diameter is worrisome for impending perforation?**

Acute distention to 12 to 14 cm puts a patient at risk for ischemic necrosis and perforation. According to Laplace's law, wall tension is proportional to diameter. If the diameter increases acutely, wall tension rises. The increase in wall tension results in a decrease in tissue perfusion. This can result in necrosis and perforation. Chronic distention does not generally result in increased wall tension and is not associated with ischemic necrosis.

28. **When should surgery be considered for acute pancreatitis?**

Surgical intervention may be required for certain complications of acute pancreatitis such as hemorrhage (from erosion into a blood vessel, or splenic vein thrombosis with spontaneous rupture of the spleen) or necrosis of an adjacent viscus (such as the transverse colon). Open debridement is indicated in the setting of infected pancreatic necrosis. Debridement for necrotizing pancreatitis in the absence of infection is rarely undertaken because of the high morbidity and mortality of operative intervention without compelling evidence of benefit. Abdominal decompression through midline laparotomy or catheter drainage of significant fluid collections may be required if abdominal compartment syndrome develops.

29. **How does diagnosis of the acute abdomen differ in immunocompromised patients?**

Immunocompromised patients may have the same diseases as immunocompetent patients. However, they may be seen initially only with nonspecific symptoms such as altered mental status and tachycardia. They may lack the classic signs of an acute abdomen because of their blunted immune response. In addition, the differential diagnosis in this patient population should be expanded to include cytomegalovirus infection, opportunistic infections, neutropenic enterocolitis (typhlitis), and drug toxicity.

30. **What is the significance of bloody diarrhea after abdominal aortic aneurysm (AAA) repair?**

Evacuation of the colon (with or without bloody mucus) in the immediate postoperative period is highly concerning for ischemic colitis. Bedside proctosigmoidoscopy should be immediately performed. Ideally, the surgeon who would intervene operatively should be present. Melena or hematochezia in a patient with a more distant history of AAA repair could signify aortoenteric fistula.

31. **When is early surgical consultation warranted?**

If reasonable suspicion exists that a patient's condition will ultimately require surgical management, the surgical service should be consulted, even if surgical intervention is not yet required. A worsening abdominal examination result may signal the need for surgical involvement. An open collaborative relationship between consulting services should be fostered.

KEY POINTS: ACUTE ABDOMEN AND PERITONITIS

1. **Peritonitis is associated with hypovolemia.** This is due to (third space) fluid losses into the inflamed peritoneal membranes, visceral walls, and the free peritoneal space. Circulatory shock may ensue.

2. **Prevention of *C. difficile* infection.** Every one of us must take ownership of this nosocomial epidemic! Wash your hands with soap and water!

3. **Abdominal compartment syndrome.** Consider this diagnosis in all patients with organ failure and abdominal distention.

4. **Be sure no mechanical obstruction exists before administering neostigmine in Ogilvie syndrome.** Obtain a water-soluble contrast enema first.

5. **Cecal diameter in large bowel obstruction or pseudoobstruction.** Monitor cecal diameter with serial abdominal radiographs. Acute cecal distention to 12 cm or greater may demand immediate intervention.

BIBLIOGRAPHY

1. Bobo LD, Dubberke ER: Recognition and prevention of hospital-associated enteric infections in the intensive care unit. Crit Care Med 38(8 Suppl):S324-S334, 2010.

2. Cheatham ML: Abdominal compartment syndrome. Curr Opin Crit Care 15:154-162, 2009.

3. Chen EH, Mills AM: Abdominal pain in special populations. Emerg Med Clin North Am 29:449-458, 2011.

4. De Giorgio R, Knowles CH: Acute colonic pseudo-obstruction. Br J Surg 96:229-239, 2009.

5. Frossard JL, Steer ML, Pastor CM: Acute pancreatitis. Lancet 371:143-152, 2008.

6. Heinlen L, Ballard JD: *Clostridium difficile* infection. Am J Med Sci 340:247-252, 2010.

7. Kolkman JJ, Mensink PB: Non-occlusive mesenteric ischaemia: a common disorder in gastroenterology and intensive care. Best Pract Res Clin Gastroenterol 17:457-473, 2003.

8. Renner P, Kienle K, Dahlke MH, et al: Intestinal ischemia: current treatment concepts. Langenbecks Arch Surg 396:3-11, 2011.

9. Solomkin JS, Mazuski JE, Bradley JS, et al: Diagnosis and management of complicated intra-abdominal infection in adults and children: guidelines by the Surgical Infection Society and the Infectious Diseases Society of America. Surg Infect (Larchmt) 11:79-109, 2010.

10. Stoker J, van Randen A, Laméris W, et al: Imaging patients with acute abdominal pain. Radiology 253:31-46, 2009.

11. Trevisani GT, Hyman NH, Church JM: Neostigmine: safe and effective treatment for acute colonic pseudo-obstruction. Dis Colon Rectum 43:599-603, 2000.

DIABETIC KETOACIDOSIS AND HYPEROSMOLAR HYPERGLYCEMIC STATE

Joel J. Schnure, MD, and Jack L. Leahy, MD

CHAPTER 50

1. What is diabetic ketoacidosis (DKA)?

DKA is a serious acute metabolic decompensation in persons with known or newly presenting diabetes. It is a consequence of a relative or an absolute insulin deficiency in combination with an excess of counterregulatory hormones (primarily glucagon and catecholamines, but also cortisol and growth hormone). The classic triad of features is hyperglycemia (typically >250 mg/dL), anion gap metabolic acidosis, and ketosis.

2. Describe the tissue actions of insulin.

The major action of endogenously secreted or injected insulin is to lower blood glucose level by increasing glucose uptake into peripheral tissues such as skeletal muscle and adipose and by promoting glycogen production and stopping gluconeogenesis in the liver. Additionally its anabolic effects inhibit adipose breakdown to free fatty acids and muscle breakdown to amino acids. The sensitivity of these actions differs in the various target tissues, with small amounts of insulin fully preventing triglyceride metabolism and release of free fatty acids from adipose tissue whereas larger amounts are needed for suppression of hepatic glucose production and to promote glucose clearance into peripheral tissues.

3. What is the pathogenesis of DKA?

DKA starts with *absolute insulin deficiency* because of a broken or clogged insulin pump, missed injections, or progression of an unknown illness to overt insulin deficiency or with *relative insulin deficiency* from a rise in tissue insulin requirements from infection, trauma, or other stresses. Glucose production from the liver increases, and glucose clearance into peripheral tissues is impaired, causing the blood glucose level to rise. Stress-related increases in counterregulatory hormones exacerbate these effects. As the renal glucose threshold is passed, an osmotic diuresis occurs causing urinary losses of water and electrolytes. The ensuing dehydration further increases the level of catecholamines. Also, because glucagon and insulin levels are normally inversely related, the insulin deficiency causes hyperglucagonemia. The increased catecholamines and glucagon and the insulin deficiency promote excess release of fatty acids from the adipose tissue that further impairs insulin-mediated glucose uptake into peripheral tissues. The capacity of the liver for β-oxidation of the fatty acids is exceeded, resulting in ketone production. This ketonemia and the resulting acidosis often cause nausea and vomiting; the patient's polydipsia therefore stops, worsening the dehydration. The patient is now in DKA with this whole process occurring over a 12- to 48-hour period. This sequence of events is depicted in Figure 50-1.

4. How does DKA cause an anion gap metabolic acidosis?

The insulin deficiency and increased glucagon and catecholamines cause excess release of fatty acids from the adipose tissue and activation of metabolic pathways in the liver for conversion to ketoacids: acetoacetate, acetone, and β-hydroxybutyrate. Their accumulation results in the anion gap metabolic acidosis that is characteristic of DKA. The *anion gap* is calculated by subtracting the serum concentration of the major anions (chloride and bicarbonate)

359

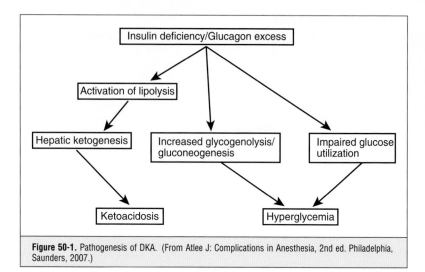

Figure 50-1. Pathogenesis of DKA. (From Atlee J: Complications in Anesthesia, 2nd ed. Philadelphia, Saunders, 2007.)

from the main cation (sodium). A difference of greater than 12 mEq/L along with a lowered bicarbonate level (<15 mEq/L) shows the presence of anions that are not identified in this calculation, thus the anion gap (in this case the ketoacids).

5. **How is type 1 diabetes diagnosed?**
   Type 1 diabetes results from autoimmune-mediated destruction of islet beta cells. Most patients therefore present with signs and symptoms of insulin deficiency: exhaustion, weight loss, nocturia, the *polys* (polyuria and polydipsia), and sometimes DKA. It is usually diagnosed because of a typical clinical presentation and can be confirmed with use of specific markers for the autoimmune beta cell destruction. The best known is glutamic acid decarboxylase-65 (GAD-65) antibody, which is directed against a beta cell enzyme called glutamic acid decarboxylase. A positive test confirms type 1 diabetes, but a negative test does not rule it out. It is not necessary to perform GAD-65 antibody testing in all patients with newly identified type 1 diabetes, but it is most useful in those with elements of both type 1 and type 2 diabetes. In contrast, insulin or C peptide testing is not recommended, because insulin secretion is driven by glycemia, and the patient's hyperglycemia and short duration of diabetes mean that these measures are rarely absent in patients with new-onset type 1 diabetes.

6. **Does DKA develop in persons with type 2 diabetes?**
   Most series of persons with DKA show a 10% to 30% incidence of type 2 diabetes usually in association with an accompanying severe medical illness. The concept is that the added stress of the associated illness allows ketoacidosis to occur, in part because catecholamines are potent inhibitors of insulin secretion from the beta cell. This accompanying illness also impacts the course. Mortality rates are much higher in persons with DKA who are older than 50 years of age versus younger patients, with the older group dying of sepsis, adult respiratory distress syndrome, shock, or cardiovascular collapse.
   A form of type 2 diabetes also exists that is ketosis prone, so-called *Flatbush diabetes* or *ketosis-prone type 2 diabetes*. These patients are mostly from minority populations (most studied are black and Latino) who have ketosis and sometimes DKA, often with obesity, but test negative for markers of type 1 diabetes. The defining clinical feature is being able to stop insulin months later, sometimes permanently. The pathogenesis is thought to be a heightened sensitivity for suppression of insulin secretion during stress that partially reverses with time.

7. **What are the common precipitating events for DKA?**
The most frequent initiating events for DKA are infection, insulin underdelivery, and newly presenting type 1 diabetes. Cardiovascular events and cerebrovascular accidents also occur, mostly in older patients. Insulin omission used to be most common in teenagers and young adults, although the growing use of insulin pumps in all ages means DKA from pump failure or catheter occlusion is age independent. Among infections pneumonias, gastrointestinal tract viral infections, and urinary tract infections are most common. Other causes are pancreatitis, drug abuse, or severe medical illness of any type. Even with all of the known causes, failure to identify a precipitating event is relatively common.

8. **Describe the common signs and symptoms of DKA.**
Patients typically describe 1 to 3 days of polyuria, nocturia, and thirst. Fatigue also occurs, and often a rapid weight loss reflects the catabolic effect of the insulin deficiency and volume depletion. As the ketonemia and metabolic acidosis progress, nausea and repeated vomiting may occur, exacerbating the dehydration. Abdominal pain is also common related to gastric distention from the metabolic acidosis or irritation from repeated vomiting. Patients may report shortness of breath from their Kussmaul respirations that can be mistaken for a pulmonary infection or cardiac event. What is not usually reported is confusion or coma; fewer than 20% of patients are stuporous or show any confusion.

On examination, patients often show the Kussmaul breathing pattern of deep, sighing breaths as they attempt to compensate for the metabolic acidosis by lowering their PCO_2. Tachycardia is common. In contrast the systolic blood pressure is rarely less than 100 mm Hg because of the osmotic effect of the hyperglycemia keeping fluid in the vascular space. Body temperature is usually normal even when an infection is present because the metabolic acidosis blunts the fever response. A distinguishing feature of DKA is the fruity sweet smell of the patient's breath from their exhaling the ketone acetone. The remainder of the physical examination is typically unremarkable except for a generalized abdominal tenderness.

9. **How does the hyperosmolar hyperglycemic state (HHS) differ from DKA?**
HHS also is characterized by profound hyperglycemia but without ketoacidosis.
The distinguishing clinical features of HHS are as follows:
- Occurs most often in the elderly and those with known type 2 diabetes
- Very high blood glucose levels of 600 mg/dL or greater
- Markedly elevated serum osmolarity of 320 mOsm/kg or greater
- Frequent occurrence of altered mental state or coma
- More serious hypotension and overt dehydration including substantially larger electrolyte losses than DKA
- High mortality rate that averages 15% versus less than 2% in uncomplicated DKA

10. **What is the pathogenesis of HHS?**
The major difference from DKA is a modestly higher circulating insulin level that prevents much of a rise in free fatty acids and thus blocks ketone production from the liver but is not enough to suppress hepatic glucose production or promote glucose clearance into peripheral tissues. Therefore the main feature is hyperglycemia without ketoacidosis, although small amounts of urinary ketones and a modest widening of the anion gap can be seen. As such the metabolic acidosis–induced vomiting and abdominal pain that are common in DKA, and often are what gets the patient to seek medical help, are lacking. Instead the worsening hyperglycemia and osmotic diuresis go on for much longer, typically many days or a couple of weeks, and the presentation is often insidious, manifesting in symptoms such as bed-wetting or modest confusion that may be unnoticed in the elderly. Thus the dehydration and urinary electrolyte losses are considerably worse than in DKA, and it is this dehydration that is the key feature leading to HHS by causing a fall in urine output and with it glycosuria. The blood glucose level now rises above the renal threshold to values that can exceed 1000 mg/dL. Serum osmolarity

rises in parallel, and the resulting confusion or coma is usually why the patient is brought for medical attention.

11. **What are the common precipitating events in HHS?**

HHS occurs most often in patients with known type 2 diabetes although it is the first evidence of diabetes in 30% to 40% of patients. The most common cause is a medical crisis such as infection or sepsis, cardiovascular event, cerebrovascular accident, pancreatitis, or acute abdomen. Pharmaceuticals that raise glycemia also are sometimes at fault, with the best known high-dose thiazides, corticosteroids, sympathomimetic agents, atypical antipsychotics, and β-blockers. Another common feature is caregivers having restricted the patient's access to water because of incontinence or bed-wetting.

12. **Describe the common signs and symptoms of HHS.**

Patients are usually brought for medical evaluation because of a mood change, fall-off in appetite, confusion, or coma. Particularly common are subtle behavior changes over several weeks such as lethargy or less interaction with the family. Also hints to the precipitating cause or illness may be elicited. Useful history is a worsening of bed-wetting or incontinence to gauge the duration of the osmotic diuresis.

On examination, patients typically show some mental alteration from slow answers to questions or searching for words to obtundation or coma. Because of the advanced age of many of these patients and the potential for underlying central nervous system (CNS) pathologic conditions, they may have focal findings that mimic a stroke. In addition, these patients usually are seen with signs of severe volume depletion such as marked hypotension, dry mucous membranes, and skin tenting. As with DKA, the absence of a fever does not exclude infection especially because of the blunted fever response in elderly patients.

13. **Which initial laboratory tests are obtained in DKA and HHS?**

Laboratory testing at presentation includes a complete blood cell count, serum electrolytes, arterial blood gases, serum creatinine, serum ketones including β-hydroxybutyrate when available, a Chem 12 panel, and urinalysis for signs of infection. In DKA, radiographs or scans, pan-cultures, drug screens, and serum brain natriuretic peptide, lactate, lipase, or markers of ischemic cardiac damage are not usually obtained without suggestive history or physical findings. In HHS because of the advanced age of many patients and the insidious nature of the presentation, pan-testing is common particularly in patients who are confused or comatose: urine and blood cultures, electrocardiogram, cardiac enzymes, and CNS imaging, especially if there are focal neurologic findings. Hemoglobin A_{1c} testing is very helpful to determine the patient's diabetes control before the acute hyperglycemic event or the chronicity of hyperglycemia in patients with new-onset diabetes.

14. **How and when to test for ketones?**

Testing for ketones in the serum or urine is done with the nitroprusside reaction that gives a semiquantitative estimate of acetoacetate and acetone levels. However, it does not recognize β-hydroxybutyrate. Therefore the severity of DKA may be underestimated if the ratio of β-hydroxybutyrate to the others is increased as can occur with lactic acidosis or alcohol. The common observation of the ketone reaction becoming more positive during therapy when the patient is clinically improving represents conversion of β-hydroxybutyrate to acetoacetate during metabolic breakdown of that ketone body. As such, it is recommended to test serum ketones only at presentation. Direct measures of serum β-hydroxybutyrate are increasingly available and have been advocated as a better diagnostic test for DKA than urine ketones but also not for repeated monitoring. However, the Joint British Diabetes Societies have recently recommended bedside monitoring of blood ketones during therapy because of the availability of reliable handheld meters.

15. **How to interpret the complete blood cell count results in DKA and HHS?**
The white blood cell (WBC) count is usually elevated in DKA, sometimes to 20,000 or 25,000/mm^3, with a leftward shift from stress hormone–induced demargination. The WBC count typically returns to the normal range in several hours to a day of treatment of the DKA. In contrast, hemoglobin and hematocrit values are typically normal unless a prior abnormality such as chronic renal impairment exists. Therefore a large decrease from the patient's pre-DKA baseline hemoglobin level should be evaluated for gastrointestinal bleeding or another source of internal or external hemorrhage.
   The findings in HHS are more varied because of the older age of many of the patients and the presence of preexisting comorbidities or severe precipitating illnesses. A stress-induced leukocytosis is common but unlike in DKA may persist for a few days from the prolonged course of treatment in many patients. Dehydration is also more severe than in DKA, and a fall in hemoglobin level by 1 to 3 g with rehydration is often seen.

16. **What changes in serum sodium level occur in DKA and HHS?**
The osmotic diuresis in DKA and HHS results in large total-body reductions in volume and electrolytes. Impaired water intake is also a common feature both from the nausea and/or vomiting in DKA and the blunted thirst response of the elderly in HHS. Still, serum sodium is usually below normal in DKA because of the osmotic effect of the hyperglycemia drawing cellular and interstitial fluid into the vascular space. The sodium concentration of this fluid is less than in blood (intracellular fluid is only 3-5 mEq), diluting the serum sodium concentration, an effect termed *pseudohyponatremia*. One can correct for this effect by adding 1.6 mEq/L of sodium to the measured value for every 100 mg/dL of glucose above the normal 100 mg/dL.
   The sodium concentration in HHS is a major contributor to the hyperosmolarity as it is often normal or above the normal range despite the marked hyperglycemia. This is because of the protracted diuresis of hypotonic urine that is a key pathogenic factor in HHS resulting in a greater whole-body water deficit versus DKA. An additional feature in many patients is continued use of diuretics that exacerbate the urinary water losses.

17. **What are the changes in serum potassium level in DKA and HHS?**
In DKA, serum potassium level is altered by an adaptation to the metabolic acidosis of an electroneutral shift of H$^+$ out of blood into cells in exchange for K$^+$ from cells back to blood. A formula to estimate the serum potassium at physiologic pH is 0.8 mEq of potassium for every 0.1 pH from 7.4. This shift explains the high level of concern over *normal* potassium levels in patients with acidosis and how treatment with bicarbonate could cause a hypokalemic crisis. In addition, serum potassium losses persist during early DKA therapy related to the effect of insulin to drive potassium into cells and additional urinary losses from the osmotic diuresis until the hyperglycemia is controlled. Thus DKA is characterized by large reductions in total-body potassium that are not accurately reflected in the initial serum potassium level.
   In HHS, the lack of significant acidosis means there is little K$^+$-H$^+$ exchange effect. Still, whole-body potassium losses typically exceed those seen with DKA, and there are the ongoing losses during treatment; therefore the concern over low or low-normal potassium levels is equal to that of DKA.

18. **How is the anion gap calculated and interpreted?**
The anion gap is calculated by subtracting the serum concentrations of chloride and bicarbonate from the sodium concentration. A difference of greater than 12 mEq/L along with a lowered bicarbonate level (<15 mEq/L) shows the presence of an anion gap metabolic acidosis and is a defining feature of DKA. Other causes of anion gap metabolic acidosis are lactic acidosis, advanced renal failure, and ingestion of high-dose salicylates, methanol, or ethylene glycol. Some patients with DKA have a complex acid–base disorder that can include a metabolic

alkalosis from protracted vomiting or the marked dehydration, and/or a respiratory alkalosis from fever, pain, or an accompanying pulmonary or CNS illness.

In HHS, the anion gap is often modestly increased from increased lactate because of the marked dehydration, but the bicarbonate level is greater than 15 mEq/L and pH is greater than 7.3.

19. **How is hyperosmolarity calculated in HHS?**
The defining clinical feature of HHS is hyperosmolarity. The normal serum osmolarity is 275 to 295 mOsm/L. It is made up of the osmotic effects of serum sodium, potassium, glucose, and urea. However, urea traverses membranes relatively freely and thus does not contribute to the serum tonicity that is also called the *effective osmolarity,* which is calculated by using the following formula:

$$2 \times [Na(mEq/L) + K(mEq/L)] + \text{Plasma glucose}(mg/dL)/18$$

A relatively linear relationship exists between the effective osmolarity and mental state in HHS, with deficits beginning to occur at values above 320 mOsm/L and coma above 340 mOsm/L. As such, stupor or coma in a patient with hyperglycemia with values below 320 mOsm/L warrants a careful work-up for other causes of the mental status change.

Mortality also rises substantially with levels above 350 mOsm/L.

20. **What are the goals of therapy in DKA?**
The main pathogenic features of DKA are dehydration, insulin deficiency, and an excess of stress hormones that collectively cause the hyperglycemia and metabolic acidosis. Treatment goals are as follows:
- Reverse the ketogenesis and return the pH to normal.
- Restore blood glucose control.
- Correct the hypovolemia.
- Replete the whole-body electrolyte stores.
- Identify and reverse any precipitating illness.
- Prevent the complications that can occur during DKA therapy.

21. **Describe insulin therapy for DKA.**
DKA is usually treated with a continuous intravenous (IV) infusion of regular insulin at 0.1 unit/kg per hour. Hourly intramuscular injections or 2-hour subcutaneous injections of a rapid-acting insulin at the same amounts as the IV insulin can be used when IV insulin is not possible. Once insulin is started, blood glucose level should fall 50 to 70 mg/dL per hour. If it does not, the recommendation after 2 hours is to double the insulin dose hourly until that occurs. The insulin infusion is continued until the blood glucose level falls below 200 mg/dL and then is lowered by 50% along with switching the IV fluids to contain 5% dextrose (D_5) or 10% dextrose to keep the blood glucose level between 100 and 200 mg/dL. The insulin infusion is also continued for another 6 to 12 hours to prevent recurrence of the ketoacidosis. A controversial issue is whether to give a bolus of insulin before starting the infusion because studies have failed to show a benefit of the bolus approach. Still it is commonly used because many believe it gets therapy started while the patient is being fully evaluated, and they give 10 units of regular insulin rapidly IV, believing that gives an hour before the infusion must be started.

22. **What is appropriate fluid therapy in DKA?**
The osmotic effect of the hyperglycemia keeps the vascular space relatively fluid replete as the DKA develops. Administering insulin without fluid can reverse this effect and cause cardiovascular collapse. Unless an illness prevents aggressive fluid replacement such as chronic renal failure with anuria or congestive heart failure, 1 L of normal saline solution is usually given quickly followed by isotonic saline solution or half-normal saline solution at 300 to 500 mL

per hour depending on the patient's sodium level. Potassium is added to the IV fluids as described below. Glucose is also added to the IV fluids once blood glucose is brought below 200 mg/dL to prevent hypoglycemia while the insulin infusion is continued for full reversal of the ketogenesis. The fluid deficit in DKA is up to 100 mL/kg, but larger volumes are often needed to restore euvolemia, because much of the infused volume over the first 5 to 6 hours is lost in the urine until glycemia is below the renal threshold. A common finding after closure of the anion gap is a subnormal serum bicarbonate and raised chloride level. This hyperchloremic metabolic acidosis occurs because of the large amount of NaCl in the administered IV fluids, plus the loss of ketones in the urine that equates to a loss of "bicarbonate equivalents," because bicarbonate is regenerated as the ketones are metabolized during the DKA therapy. However, it is harmless and reverts to normal over a few days without therapy.

23. **Describe potassium replacement in DKA.**
Whole body potassium stores are lowered 150 to 250 mEq in DKA. This depletion is usually not apparent in the initial serum potassium because of the H^+-K^+ cellular shift, with the potential for severe hypokalemia and life-threatening arrhythmias with low or normal potassium levels at presentation without adequate replacement. Usually 20 to 40 mEq of KCl is included in all IV bags after the initial liter of run in saline solution, except if the potassium level exceeds 5.5 mEq/L. In that case, potassium is added to the IV fluids as soon as the potassium level falls below 5.5 mEq/L. In addition, oral potassium supplements can be given to patients with a high risk of treatment-associated hypokalemia in the absence of severe nausea or vomiting. After the first few liters of IV fluids, some clinicians replace the KCl with potassium phosphate in 1 or 2 L of IV fluid, because insulin drives phosphorus intracellularly so that a common finding in DKA 12 to 24 hours after starting therapy is hypophosphatemia. However, this is not supported by evidence-based outcomes, because trials of phosphate replacement in DKA have not shown a benefit. Many authors recommend phosphate replacement only for phosphate levels below 1 mmol/L.

24. **How are patients' conditions monitored during DKA therapy?**
Bedside fingerstick glucose, inputs and outputs, and vital signs are monitored hourly. Every-2-hour measures are serum glucose and electrolytes to monitor the K^+, Na^+, and anion gap. Once the anion gap is closed and the blood glucose falls below 200 mg/dL, a bedside glucose level is monitored every 1 to 2 hours and electrolytes every 4 to 6 hours to confirm reversal of the ketoacidosis as indicated by continued normalization of the anion gap.

25. **When is bicarbonate given?**
Studies have failed to show any benefit of bicarbonate in patients with DKA. Concerns also exist that the rapid rise in pH could acutely lower the serum potassium. It is recommended that bicarbonate be given only with life-threatening acidosis, with most authors advocating a pH threshold of below 6.9. Then up to 100 mmol of sodium bicarbonate diluted in 400 mL sterile water plus 20 mEq KCl can be administered over a 2-hour period.

26. **How is the patient transitioned from the insulin infusion?**
Closure of the anion gap, along with clinical stability in terms of volume status and resolution of the marked hyperglycemia and symptoms such as nausea or vomiting, signifies cessation of the DKA. The insulin and fluid-electrolyte infusions are continued for another 12 hours if possible as recurrence of ketoacidosis from turning off the infusion too fast is a common occurrence. The patient's usual therapy is then restarted—pump or injections—at the prior doses or adjusted as needed on the basis of the hemoglobin A_{1c} level at presentation and reported home blood glucose values. It is necessary to wait 2 to 3 hours after restarting the subcutaneous insulin before turning off the insulin infusion.

27. **Is the treatment of DKA in children different than in adults?**

The general recommendations for diagnosis, therapy, and monitoring in children with DKA are similar to those for an older population. One difference is that children are treated in acute-care settings whereas, increasingly, uncomplicated DKA in adults is treated in emergency departments or monitored noncritical beds. The fluid and electrolyte replacement is also appropriate to the size and age of the child. Insulin infusion rates in preschool children are often started at 0.05 units/kg per hour, but in older children it is 0.1 unit/kg per hour as in adults. One issue of great concern in children is cerebral edema during the DKA treatment. Although uncommon, DKA-related cerebral edema occurs almost exclusively in children and is often fatal. Studies have shown some degree of brain swelling in virtually all children during DKA therapy although the clinical syndrome of acute onset of altered mental state or frank coma is rare.

28. **Is the treatment of DKA in pregnancy different?**

Elements of the adaptive physiology of pregnancy have the potential to increase the risk of marked hyperglycemia and DKA in women with type 1 diabetes. Human placental lactogen, along with growth hormone and prolactin, markedly impairs insulin sensitivity. There is also an accelerated lipolytic rate during normal pregnancy. In addition, the expanding abdominal girth causes rapid shallow breathing and a respiratory alkalosis that leads to a compensatory wasting of bicarbonate in the urine, lowering the patient's buffering capacity. Still, DKA is uncommon in pregnant patients, in part reflecting today's intensive diabetes management in pregnancy. When seen, DKA in a pregnant patient may be the first sign of diabetes or occur because of a broken pump or from an infection. The treatment is similar to that in nonpregnant patients, with mortality rates that are similarly low. On the other hand, older statistics that are still quoted suggest a high fetal loss rate: one review reported 9%.

29. **What are the goals of therapy in HHS?**

The main feature of HHS is extreme dehydration that results in marked hyperglycemia and hyperosmolarity-induced mental status changes. These patients frequently present with a precipitating illness that may be the main medical focus. As such, the primary goal is restoration of the vascular volume and electrolytes. Although insulin is usually needed for full blood glucose control, volume replacement will improve most of the metabolic derangements including inducing a marked fall in glycemia. The other major goal is to identify and start therapy for the precipitating illness. Because of the advanced age and comorbidities of many of these patients, plus their altered mental state and frequency of a serious accompanying illness, these patients are almost always treated in an intensive care unit (ICU) setting. The goals are as follows:
- Correct the hypovolemia for hemodynamic stability, and restore renal perfusion and glycosuria.
- Identify and reverse any precipitating illness.
- Recover blood glucose control.
- Slowly reverse the hyperosmolarity with return to the patient's baseline mental state.
- Replete whole-body electrolyte stores.
- Prevent the complications that can occur with HHS therapy.

30. **What is appropriate fluid therapy in HHS?**

Because the fluid and electrolyte losses in HHS are typically greater than in DKA, patients often have hypotension or are in shock. The first priority is to restore adequate intravascular volume and renal perfusion followed by a gradual return to euvolemia and normal electrolyte stores. A liter or more of 0.9% saline solution is given quickly, especially to patients who have hypotension or are in shock unless a complicating issue exists such as renal failure with anuria or congestive heart failure. Several methods are then used to determine whether to continue with 0.9% saline solution or reduce the osmotic load by switching to half-normal saline, with the more dilute fluid recommended when the corrected sodium is at or above the normal range, or for an effective osmolarity of greater than 330 mOsm/L. Because the rate of the fluid replacement is individualized, the serum osmolarity is lowered no more than 3 mOsm hourly to minimize risk of cerebral edema. Another common guideline is to replace half of the patient's fluid deficit in the first 12 hours and the remainder over the next 12 to 24 hours, again to prevent rapid changes in tonicity that could precipitate cerebral edema. This is particularly important in pediatric patients with HHS who are at highest risk for cerebral edema; it is recommended they receive no more than 50 mL/kg of saline solution over the first 4 hours, with correction of the remaining fluid deficit over 48 hours versus the 24 hours in adults. As in DKA, 20 to 40 mEq of potassium is added to each liter of IV fluids after the initial run in saline solution. Glucose-containing IV fluids are started earlier than in DKA, once the blood glucose falls below 250 to 300 mg/dL, along with titration of the insulin infusion to keep the blood glucose level between 100 and 200 mg/dL.

31. **How is a patient's water deficit calculated?**
The average fluid deficit in HHS is 100 to 200 mL/kg or 8 to 12 L. A patient's total body water deficit can be calculated with use of the following assumptions and formula. Body water is 60% of the body weight in men and 50% in women. The patient's corrected sodium is calculated by adding 1.6 mEq/L of sodium to the measured value for every 100 mg/dL of glucose above 100 mg/dL. This value minus a normal sodium concentration of 140 mEq/L divided by 140 gives the percent deviation from the normal sodium concentration. Multiplying it by the patient's calculated total body water gives the fluid deficit. For instance, a 100 kg man with a glucose level of 800 mg/dL and measured sodium concentration of 145 mEq/L:

$$\text{Total body water} = 100 \times 60\% = 60 \text{ L}$$
$$\text{Corrected sodium} = 145 + (7 \times 1.6 \text{ mEq/L}) = 156 \text{ mEq/L}$$
$$\text{Fluid deficit} = (156 - 140)/140 = 11.6\% \times 60 \text{ L} = 6.9 \text{ L}$$

32. **Describe insulin therapy for HHS.**
Unlike in DKA where immediate insulin replacement is required to reverse the ketoacidosis, in HHS insulin therapy is secondary to restoration of the intravascular volume. Only after fluid support has been established and the patient is hemodynamically stable is insulin begun. It is administered as an IV infusion at 0.1 unit/kg, with or without an initial bolus as preferred by the caregivers. The goal is to lower the glucose level by 50 to 70 mg/dL per hour after the large drop from the initial fluid push. Thus the insulin infusion rate is adjusted hourly up or down until the blood glucose falls below 250 to 300 mg/dL, and then it is lowered by 50% along with switching the IV fluids to contain D_5, with continued hourly titration to keep the blood glucose level between 100 and 200 mg/dL. The clinical course of these patients often entails a lengthy ICU admission related to comorbidities, with maintenance of the insulin infusion until the patient is medically stable. The patient's usual therapy is then restarted or changed as deemed appropriate. Unlike in DKA, some patients do not require long-term insulin therapy after HHS.

33. **What complications can occur in DKA and HHS?**
Today's aggressive fluid and potassium replacement along with close monitoring of patients during treatment of DKA and HHS has markedly reduced the risks of hypotension and shock related to correction of hyperglycemia without adequate volume replacement, hypoglycemia, and severe hypokalemia. A key principle in comatose patients is protection of the airway and prevention of aspiration. Severe and at times life-threatening complications still can occur, sometimes in patients who have responded well to therapy but whose conditions then rapidly deteriorate, often with no identifiable cause: disseminated intravascular coagulation, acute respiratory distress syndrome, rhabdomyolysis, cerebral edema, and various thromboembolic events such as pulmonary embolus, stroke, bowel infarction, or myocardial infarction. Some authors recommend prophylaxis against thromboembolic events especially in severely dehydrated patients with HHS.

KEY POINTS: GOALS OF THERAPY FOR HYPERGLYCEMIC CRISES

1. Restore hemodynamic stability, and replete whole-body electrolyte stores with fluid replacement.

2. Recover blood glucose control with insulin therapy.

3. Identify and start therapy for any precipitating illness.

4. Prevent hypophosphatemia and hypoglycemia.

5. Closely monitor for the complications that can occur during therapy.

BIBLIOGRAPHY

1. Arora S, Henderson SO, Long T, et al: Diagnostic accuracy of point-of-care testing for diabetic ketoacidosis at emergency-department triage: β-hydroxybutyrate versus the urine dipstick. Diabetes Care 34:852-854, 2011.

2. Canarie MF, Bogue CW, Banasiak KJ, et al: Decompensated hyperglycemic hyperosmolarity without significant ketoacidosis in the adolescent and young adult population. J Pediatr Endocrinol Metab 20:1115-1124, 2007.

3. Ennis ED, Kreisberg RA: Diabetic ketoacidosis and the hyperglycemic hyperosmolar syndrome. In LeRoith D, Taylor SL, Olesfsky JM, (eds): Diabetes Mellitus: A Fundamental and Clinical Text, 3rd ed. Philadelphia, Lippincott Williams & Wilkins, 2004, pp 627-642.

4. Kitabchi AE, Murphy MB, Spencer J, et al: Is a priming dose of insulin necessary in a low-dose insulin protocol for the treatment of diabetic ketoacidosis? Diabetes Care 31:2081-2085, 2008.

5. Kitabchi AE, Nyenwe AE: Hyperglycemic crisis in diabetes mellitus: diabetic ketoacidosis and hyperglycemic hyperosmolar state. Endocrinol Metab Clin North Am 35:225-251, 2006.

6. Kitabchi AE, Umpierrez GE, Fisher JN, et al: Thirty years of personal experience in hyperglycemic crisis: diabetic ketoacidosis and hyperglycemic hyperosmolar state. J Clin Endocrinol Metab 93:1541-1552, 2008.

7. Kitabchi AE, Umpierrez GE, Murphy MB, et al: Hyperglycemic crises in adult patients with diabetes: a consensus statement from the American Diabetes Association. Diabetes Care 29:2739-2748, 2006.

8. Krane EJ, Rockoff MA, Wallman JK, et al: Subclinical brain swelling in children during treatment of diabetes ketoacidosis. N Engl J Med 312:1147-1151, 1985.

9. Morris LR, Murphy MB, Kitabchi AE, et al: Bicarbonate therapy in severe diabetic ketoacidosis. Ann Intern Med 105:836-840, 1986.

10. Nugent BW: Hyperosmolar hyperglycemic state. Emerg Med Clin North Am 23:629-648, 2005.

11. Orlowski JP, Cramer CL, Fiallos MR: Diabetic ketoacidosis in the pediatric ICU. Pediatr Clin North Am 55:577-587, 2008.

12. Parker JA, Conway DL: Diabetic ketoacidosis in pregnancy. Obstet Gynecol Clin North Am 34:533-543, 2007.

13. Rosenbloom AL: Hyperglycemic hyperosmolar state: an emerging pediatric problem. J Pediatr 156:180-184, 2010.

14. Savage MW, Dhatariya KK, Kilvert A, et al: Joint British Diabetes Societies guideline for the management of diabetic ketoacidosis. Diabet Med 28:508-511, 2011.

15. Umpierrez G: Narrative review: ketosis-prone type 2 diabetes mellitus. Ann Intern Med 144:350-357, 2006.

16. Usher-Smith JA, Thompson MJ, Sharp SJ, et al: Factors associated with the presence of diabetic ketoacidosis at diagnosis of diabetes in children and young adults: a systematic review. BMJ 343:d4092, 2011.

17. Westphal SA: The occurrence of diabetic ketoacidosis in non-insulin-dependent diabetes and newly diagnosed diabetic adults. Am J Med 101:19-24, 1996.

18. Wilson JF: In the clinic. Diabetic ketoacidosis. Ann Intern Med 152:ITC1-ITC16, 2010.

19. Wolfsdorf J, Craig ME, Daneman D, et al: Diabetic ketoacidosis in children and adolescents with diabetes. Pediatr Diabetes 10 Suppl 12:118-133, 2009.

20. Wyckoff J, Abrahamson MJ: Diabetic ketoacidosis and hyperosmolar hyperglycemic state. In Kahn CR, Weir GC, King GL, et al (eds): Joslin's Diabetes Mellitus, 14th ed. Philadelphia, Lippincott Williams & Wilkins, 2005, pp 887-899.

CHAPTER 51

MANAGEMENT OF HYPERGLYCEMIA IN THE CRITICALLY ILL

Matthew P. Gilbert, DO, MPH, and Alison Schneider, MD

1. **Who is at risk for development of hyperglycemia?**

   Hyperglycemia can occur in patients with known or undiagnosed diabetes mellitus. Hyperglycemia during acute illness can also occur in patients with previously normal glucose tolerance, a condition called *stress hyperglycemia.*

2. **How common is hyperglycemia in critically ill patients?**

   Acute hyperglycemia is common in critically ill patients. It is estimated that in 90% of all patients blood glucose concentrations >110 mg/dL develop during critical illness. Stress-induced hyperglycemia has been associated with adverse clinical outcomes in patients with trauma, acute myocardial infarction, and subarachnoid hemorrhage.

3. **What causes hyperglycemia in critically ill patients?**

   In healthy individuals, blood glucose concentrations are tightly regulated within a narrow range. The cause of hyperglycemia in critically ill patients is multifactorial. Physiologic and emotional stress leads to intense activation of counterregulatory hormones such as cortisol and epinephrine. The release of inflammatory cytokines causes an increase in peripheral insulin resistance and hepatic glucose production. The use of glucocorticoids and parenteral and enteral nutrition is an important contributor to hyperglycemia.

4. **What is the relationship between hyperglycemia and acute illness?**

   The relationship between hyperglycemia and acute illness is complex. Severe hyperglycemia (>250 mg/dL) has been shown to have a negative impact on the vascular, hemodynamic, and immune systems. Hyperglycemia can also lead to electrolyte imbalance, mitochondrial injury, and both neutrophil and endothelial dysfunction. Acute illness increases the risk for hyperglycemia through the release of counterregulatory hormones, increased insulin resistance, and immobility. Figure 51-1 illustrates the relationship between acute illness and hyperglycemia.

5. **Should oral medications used to treat diabetes be continued in the intensive care unit (ICU)?**

   Given the high incidence of renal and hepatic impairment, oral medication to treat diabetes should not be continued in the ICU. Medications such as metformin are contraindicated in patients with renal or hepatic dysfunction and congestive heart failure. Long-acting formulations of sulfonylureas have been associated with episodes of prolonged severe hypoglycemia in hospitalized patients. Oral medications are not easily titrated to meet glycemic targets and may take weeks to effectively lower blood glucose levels.

6. **Should injectable, noninsulin medications be used in the ICU?**

   Noninsulin, injectable medications such as exenatide, liraglutide, and pramlintide have similar limitations as oral agents and should not be used in the ICU setting.

7. **What is the most effective way to treat hyperglycemia in the ICU?**

   An intravenous insulin infusion is the safest and most effective way to treat hyperglycemia in critically ill patients. Because of the short half-life of circulating insulin (minutes), an insulin

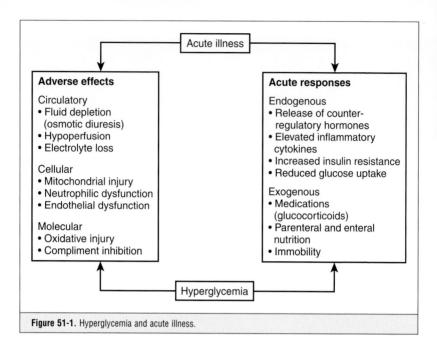

Figure 51-1. Hyperglycemia and acute illness.

infusion can be frequently adjusted to match the often-variable insulin requirements of critically ill patients. Intravenous insulin therapy should be administered by validated written or computerized protocols that outline predefined adjustments in the insulin dose based on frequent measurement of blood glucose concentrations.

8. **When should treatment with an intravenous insulin infusion be initiated?**
   Intravenous insulin therapy should be initiated for the treatment of persistent hyperglycemia starting at a blood glucose concentration of no greater than 180 mg/dL.

9. **What is the appropriate glycemic target for critically ill patients?**
   Recognizing the importance of glycemic control in critically ill patients, a number of professional societies have developed treatment guidelines and/or consensus statements that provide evidence-based glycemic targets. Although the glycemic targets are not identical, all of the groups advocate for good glycemic control while avoiding hypoglycemia (see Table 51-1).

10. **What is the evidence supporting the current glycemic targets?**
    The first randomized controlled trial (RCT) comparing tight glycemic control (target blood glucose concentration of 80-110 mg/dL) with conventional insulin therapy (target blood glucose concentration of 180-200 mg/dL) was conducted by Van den Berghe and colleagues (2001) in a population of surgical ICU patients. The single-center trial enrolled more than 1500 patients and showed a 34% reduction in mortality associated with tight glycemic control. However, subsequent studies in both medical and surgical ICU populations have not shown consistent reductions in mortality with tight glycemic control. A recent meta-analysis of RCTs that included 8432 critically ill adult patients did not show a significant difference in mortality between tight glycemic control and control groups.

TABLE 51-1. SUMMARY OF GLYCEMIC TARGETS FROM THE MEDICAL LITERATURE

PROFESSIONAL SOCIETY/CONSENSUS STATEMENT	GLYCEMIC TARGET FOR CRITICALLY ILL PATIENTS
American Diabetes Association	140-180 mg/dL
American Association of Clinical Endocrinologists	140-180 mg/dL
Surviving Sepsis Campaign	150-180 mg/dL
American College of Physicians	140-200 mg/dL
American Thoracic Society	<180 mg/dL (in patients undergoing cardiac surgery)

11. What was the NICE-SUGAR study?

The Normoglycemia in Intensive Care Evaluation–Survival Using Glucose Algorithm Regulation (NICE-SUGAR) was a multicenter, multinational RCT that evaluated the effect of tight glycemic control (target glucose level of 81-108 mg/dL) on a number of clinical outcomes in 6104 critically ill adults. Greater than 95% of the patients in the trial required mechanical ventilation. The 90-day mortality was significantly higher in the tight glycemic control group (78 more deaths; 27.5% vs. 24.9%; $P = 0.02$). Cardiovascular mortality and severe hypoglycemic events were also more common in the tight glycemic control group.

It is important to note that studies have not evaluated tight glycemic control versus poor glycemic control but rather have compared tight control versus good control. Given the limitations of current technology in the monitoring of blood glucose levels, tight glycemic control with intensive insulin therapy cannot be achieved safely. Advances in technology, particularly continuous glucose monitoring systems, will be needed to better evaluate the risks and benefits of tight glycemic control in critically ill adults.

12. How should patients be transitioned from an intravenous insulin infusion to subcutaneous insulin therapy?

Patients should be transitioned from an insulin infusion to a subcutaneous insulin program when clinically stable. In patients who are eating, the use of once- or twice-daily administered basal insulin in combination with scheduled mealtime rapid-acting insulin and a supplemental (correction) component has been shown to maintain adequate glycemic control without clinically significant hypoglycemia. Subcutaneous insulin therapy should be initiated at least 2 hours before the discontinuation of the insulin infusion to reduce the risk of hyperglycemia. The use of a sliding-scale insulin regimen as the sole means of treatment of hyperglycemia is ineffective and should be avoided.

13. How is hypoglycemia defined?

Hypoglycemia is defined as any blood glucose level <70 mg/dL. This level correlates with the initial release of counterregulatory hormones. Cognitive impairment begins at a blood glucose concentration of approximately 50 mg/dL, and severe hypoglycemia occurs when blood glucose concentrations are <40 mg/dL.

14. What is the clinical impact of hypoglycemia?

The incidence of severe hypoglycemia in the tight glycemic arm of the NICE-SUGAR trial was significantly higher (relative risk of 13.7). However, a clear link between the increased 90-day mortality rate and incidence of severe hypoglycemia in the tight glycemic control group has not yet been established. Recent observational studies illustrate a relationship between mild to severe hypoglycemia and death. Hypoglycemia has been associated with increased risk for cardiovascular death and death due to infectious disease after adjustment for insulin therapy. In addition, hypoglycemia has also been shown to prolong hospital stay for various patient populations. Some have hypothesized that hypoglycemia may be a marker of the severity of illness, rather than a mediator of poor clinical outcomes.

15. How do we prevent severe hypoglycemic events in the ICU?

Critically ill patients are not likely able to report symptoms of hypoglycemia; thus it is important that patients be closely monitored. Early recognition and treatment of mild hypoglycemia can prevent the adverse outcomes associated with severe hypoglycemia. The establishment of a system for documenting the frequency and severity of hypoglycemic events and the implementation of policies that standardize the treatment of hypoglycemia are essential components of an effective glycemic management program.

16. Is intensive treatment of hyperglycemia cost-effective?

Intensive treatment of hyperglycemia not only reduces morbidity and mortality but is also cost-effective. The cost savings have been attributed to reductions in laboratory and radiology cost, decreased ventilator days, and reductions in ICU and hospital length of stay.

KEY POINTS: MANAGEMENT OF HYPERGLYCEMIA IN CRITICALLY ILL PATIENTS

1. Hyperglycemia is common in critically ill patients and has been independently associated with increased ICU mortality.

2. Oral medications and noninsulin injectable therapies should not be used to treat hyperglycemia in critically ill patients.

3. An intravenous insulin infusion is the safest and most effective way to treat hyperglycemia in critically ill patients.

4. A glycemic target of 140 to 180 mg/dL is recommended for critically ill patients.

5. Early recognition and treatment of mild hypoglycemia can prevent the adverse outcomes associated with severe hypoglycemia.

BIBLIOGRAPHY

1. Clement S, Braithwaite S, Magee M, et al: Management of diabetes and hyperglycemia in hospitals. Diabetes Care 27:856, 2004.
2. Cryer P, Davis S, Shamoon H: Hypoglycemia in diabetes. Diabetes Care 26:1902-1912, 2003.
3. Dellinger R, Levy M, Carlet J, et al: Surviving Sepsis Campaign: international guidelines for management of severe sepsis and septic shock. Crit Care Med 36:1394-1396, 2008.
4. Egi M, Bellomo R, Stachowski E, et al: Hypoglycemia and outcomes in critically ill patients. Mayo Clin Proc 85:217-224, 2010.
5. Egi M, Finfer S, Bellomo R: Glycemic control in the ICU. Chest 140:212-220, 2011.
6. NICE-SUGAR Study Investigators; Finfer S, Chittock D, Su S, et al: Intensive versus conventional glucose control in critically ill patients. N Engl J Med 360:1283-1297, 2009.
7. Insucchi S: Management of hyperglycemia in the hospital setting. N Engl J Med 355:1903-1911, 2006.

8. Lazar H, McDonnnell M, Chipkin S, et al: The Society of Thoracic Surgeons practice guideline series: blood glucose management during adult cardiac surgery. Ann Thorac Surg 87:663-669, 2009.

9. Levetan C, Salas J, Wilets I, et al: Impact of endocrine and diabetes team consultation on hospital length of stay for patients with diabetes. Am J Med 99:22-28, 1995.

10. McCowen K, Malhotra A, Bistrian B: Stress-induced hyperglycemia. Crit Care Clin 17:107-124, 2001.

11. Moghissi E, Korytkowski M, DiNardo M, et al: AACE/ADA consensus statement on inpatient glycemic control. Endocr Pract 15(4):1-17, 2009.

12. Qaseem A, Humphrey LL, Chou R, et al: Use of intensive insulin therapy for the management of glycemic control in hospitalized patients: a clinical practice guideline from the American College of Physicians. Ann Intern Med 154:260-267, 2011.

13. Umpierrez G, Smiley M, Zisman A, et al: Randomized study of basal-bolus insulin therapy in the inpatient management of patients with type 2 diabetes (RABBIT 2 Trial). Diabetes Care 30:2181-2186, 2007.

14. Van den Berghe G, Wouters P, Weekers F, et al: Intensive insulin therapy in the critically ill patients. N Engl J Med 345:1359-1367, 2001.

15. Wiener R, Wiener D, Larson R: Benefits and risk of tight glucose control in critically ill adults: a meta-analysis. JAMA 300:933-944, 2008.

ADRENAL INSUFFICIENCY IN THE INTENSIVE CARE UNIT

Michael Young, MD

1. **Is adrenal insufficiency common among patients in the intensive care unit (ICU)?**
   The incidence of adrenal insufficiency in the ICU population is 1% to 6% and may be as high as 74% for patients with septic shock. However, no gold standard is agreed on for confirming adrenal insufficiency among ICU patients, and, in many cases, uncertainty exists on how to respond to this diagnosis.

2. **Describe the main types of adrenal insufficiency seen in patients in the ICU.**
   - **Relative adrenal insufficiency:** This is the most common and perplexing type of adrenal insufficiency seen in patients in the ICU. Patients with relative adrenal insufficiency may present with vasopressor dependency, acute multiple organ dysfunction, hypothermia, or an inability to wean from mechanical ventilation. These patients can be identified by their limited response to adrenal stimulation tests or lower-than-expected basal cortisol levels despite critical illness.
   - **Acute adrenal crisis or insufficiency:** The acute clinical presentation typically includes profound hypotension, fever, and hypovolemia. These patients will have very low cortisol levels (<3 mcg/dL).
   - **Chronic adrenal insufficiency**
     - □ **Primary adrenal insufficiency (Addison disease):** The most common causes are autoimmune diseases (70%) and tuberculosis (10%). Rare causes include adrenal hemorrhage, adrenal metastasis, cytomegalovirus, human immunodeficiency virus (HIV) disease, amyloidosis, and sarcoidosis.
     - □ **Secondary adrenal insufficiency:** This condition is caused by inadequate production of adrenocorticotropic hormone (ACTH) due to long-term use of exogenous steroids (most common cause), hypopituitary state, or isolated ACTH deficiency.

   Controversy: Etomidate, an anesthetic agent often used for rapid-sequence intubation in critically ill patients, increases the relative risk of adrenal insufficiency by more than 60%. Whether this increased risk of adrenal insufficiency increases the risk of mortality for adult ICU patients remains controversial.

3. **What are the clinical markers of acute adrenal insufficiency?**
   Acute adrenal insufficiency presents with various combinations of hypotension, tachycardia, severe hypovolemia, respiratory failure, nausea, vomiting, diarrhea, lethargy, and weakness. Patients with acute adrenal insufficiency due to chronic exogenous replacement may not initially exhibit hypotension because mineralocorticoid secretion can be intact until late-stage illness.

4. **List the laboratory abnormalities associated with adrenal insufficiency.**
   - Hyponatremia is most common.
   - Low levels of chloride and bicarbonate and high levels of potassium occur frequently.
   - Also seen are moderate eosinophilia, lymphocytosis, hypercalcemia, and hypoglycemia.

5. **How is adrenal insufficiency diagnosed?**
   - **In ICU patients:** The use of provocative adrenal stimulation tests in critically ill patients remains controversial. Perhaps the most widely used protocol (from Annane et al.) identifies

patients with septic shock as having relative adrenal insufficiency if their baseline cortisol level is <35 mcg/dL and they respond to an ACTH stimulation test (250 mcg corticotropin) with a bump in cortisol of <10 mcg/dL (see Fig. 52-1). The patients identified as nonresponders appeared to have a reduction in mortality when given stress-dose steroids. However, in a large subsequent study, no mortality benefit with stress-dose steroids was observed for patients with or without evidence of *relative adrenal insufficiency*.

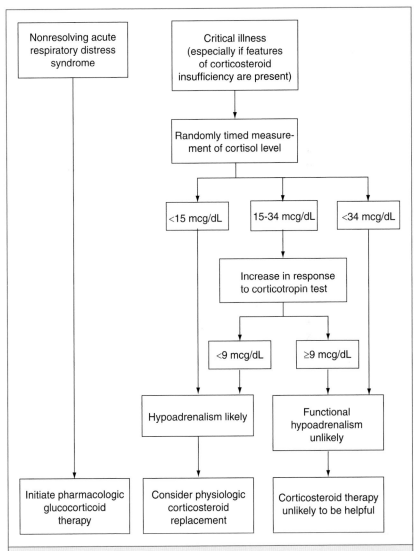

Figure 52-1. Steroid replacement in severe sepsis and septic shock. Steroid use for "late acute respiratory distress syndrome" is controversial (see www.ardsnet.org). (From Cooper MS, Stewart PM: Corticosteroid insufficiency in acutely ill patients. N Engl J Med 348:727–734, 2003.)

■ **In non-ICU patients:** In a nonstressed patient, a random cortisol level >20 mcg/dL may rule out the diagnosis of adrenal insufficiency. A random cortisol level <3 mcg/dL confirms the diagnosis of adrenal insufficiency.

6. **How should one use the ACTH stimulation test?**
Cortisol levels are measured before and 30 to 60 minutes after a supraphysiologic dose of ACTH (250 mcg corticotropin given intravenously). In patients who are not critically ill, a normal response generates a poststimulation cortisol level of ≥20 mcg/dL. However, for patients with septic shock, on the basis of the results of the Corticosteroid Therapy of Septic Shock (CORTICUS) study and the 2008 Surviving Sepsis Campaign International Guidelines, it is recommended that ACTH stimulation tests should *not* be used to determine whether adult patients with septic shock should receive steroids.

7. **What about corticotropin-releasing hormone (CHR) stimulation?**
CHR is given to stimulate cortisol levels. Unlike the ACTH stimulation test, CHR stimulation can rule out central adrenal insufficiency. A normal response generates a poststimulation cortisol level ≥20 mcg/dL or a 30- to 60-minute rise in cortisol ≥7 mcg/dL.

8. **Should the low-dose ACTH (1 mcg) stimulation test be used?**
This test may detect adrenal atrophy associated with adrenal insufficiency. No consensus exists on how to determine the lower level that equates with a normal cortisol response.

9. **How does one distinguish between acute adrenal insufficiency and other illness states in the ICU?**
The clinical findings and laboratory findings among patients with acute adrenal insufficiency are also common in the ICU population. Distinguishing between adrenal insufficiency and other illnesses in critically ill patients requires clinical suspicion and at least one of the following:
■ Failure to respond adequately to an adrenal stimulation test
■ Inappropriately low basal cortisol levels
■ An unequivocal clinical response to empiric exogenous steroids

10. **Should steroids be administered to ICU patients with a history of long-term steroid use?**
Patients' adrenals may become insufficient after taking the equivalent of 20 mg/day of prednisone for just 5 days, but adrenal insufficiency is rare among patients taking steroids for <7 days. Patients' adrenals may become insufficient after taking very-low-dose steroids for months to years (>5 mg/day prednisone equivalent). Fearing life-threatening adrenal impairment, many physicians give *stress doses* (hydrocortisone 300-400 mg/day or equivalent) to critically ill ICU patients who have received a course of steroids in the weeks or months before their admission to the ICU.

11. **What ICU patient groups are at high risk for adrenal insufficiency?**
■ Patients with septic shock
■ Patients taking chronic steroids: See question 10.
■ Patients with HIV disease: The adrenal gland may be involved in >50% of patients infected with HIV. However, because adrenal function requires <20% of the gland to function, adrenal insufficiency in this population is uncommon (3%).
■ Patients with cancer: Even when cancers metastasize to the adrenal gland, adrenal dysfunction is uncommon.
■ High-risk postoperative patients: Patients >55 years old, patients undergoing major operations (e.g., coronary artery bypass grafting, abdominal aortic aneurysm repair, Whipple procedure), patients with multiple trauma, and postoperative patients requiring vasopressors or failing to wean from mechanical ventilation appear to be at higher risk for adrenal insufficiency.

12. **Do neurotrauma patients have special problems with adrenal insufficiency?**
Fifty percent of patients with moderate to severe traumatic head injury have cortisol levels
≤15 mcg/dL. This is especially true among patients receiving pentobarbital or propofol.
These patients often require vasopressors. Thus monitoring cortisol levels in patients with
moderate to severe head injury may be warranted. Steroid supplementation can be considered in
patients with head trauma who have relative adrenal insufficiency and sustained hypotension.

13. **Should every critically ill ICU patient with relative adrenal insufficiency receive
stress-dose steroids?**
The evidence for steroid use among ICU patients with septic shock is controversial. On the basis
of the conflicting evidence, the 2008 Surviving Sepsis Campaign International Guidelines
recommend that stress-dose steroids be used only among patients with septic shock whose
blood pressure is poorly responsive to both fluid resuscitation and vasopressor therapy. No
randomized trials have been done to guide clinicians when confronted with critically ill patients
without septic shock who show evidence of relative adrenal insufficiency, such as postoperative
surgical patients, patients with severe pancreatitis, and patients with moderate to severe
traumatic head injury.

14. **What are the indicated therapies for ICU patients with septic shock who may or
may not have adrenal insufficiency?**
   - **Fluid resuscitation:** Patients with septic shock typically require multiple large boluses of
intravenous fluids and often vasopressors to maintain effective arterial circulation. If the
patient's blood pressure responds poorly to fluids and vasopressors, the administration of
stress-dose steroids should be initiated.
   - **Steroid dosing:** Administration of hydrocortisone, 300 to 400 mg/day given intravenously in
three or four divided doses with or without fludrocortisone (50 mcg enterally every day), is
accepted practice.
   - **Steroid duration:** For adult patients with septic shock whose blood pressure is poorly
responsive to multiple intravenous fluid boluses *and* vasopressor for >1 to 2 hours, the author
recommends administration of stress-dose hydrocortisone (300 mg/day) for 4 days. If the
patient shows rapid clinical improvement, the steroids may be stopped or tapered over 1 to
2 days. If significant hypotension recurs, steroid dosing should return to the initial dose, and a
rapid taper can be undertaken after 7 days.

15. **Should stress-dose steroid supplementation be strongly considered in all
patients with septic shock?**
Because of conflicting studies, opinions on this point differ.
   - **Yes, of course:** A majority of patients with septic shock have relative adrenal insufficiency. The
mortality rate for such patients is 30% to 60%. A landmark randomized control trial found an
absolute mortality reduction of 10% among patients with severe sepsis or septic shock
and relative adrenal insufficiency who received stress-dose steroids versus placebo. This
finding is supported by a recent systematic review that concluded that prolonged low-dose
steroid use reduces all-cause mortality among adult patients with septic shock. Steroid
supplementation for most ICU patients with septic shock makes sense given the modest risk of
a short course of low-dose steroids.
   - **No, the data are too mixed:** The Annane trial did not demonstrate across-the-board mortality
reduction in the steroid group with severe sepsis and septic shock. The subsequent CORTICUS
study showed no mortality benefit after hydrocortisone therapy in patients with septic
shock. No mortality benefit of steroids was seen even among patients who met criteria for
relative adrenal insufficiency. In addition, the steroid arm of the CORTICUS trial had
significantly more superinfections. Early, smaller studies indicated a survival benefit from
using steroids in septic shock. However, this benefit was not seen in meta-analysis of later and
larger studies. The Surviving Sepsis Campaign International Guidelines recommend using

steroids for patients with septic shock unresponsive to fluids and vasopressors. This is largely a consensus-based recommendation rather than an evidence-based conclusion. The scientific evidence to support even this limited use of steroids in patients with septic shock is modest.

KEY POINTS: ADRENAL INSUFFICIENCY

1. Relative adrenal insufficiency is common in ICU patients with septic shock, but its clinical importance remains controversial.

2. To decide if and when a patient should receive hydrocortisone therapy for septic shock, there is no need to evaluate the patient for relative adrenal insufficiency.

3. ICU patients with septic shock whose blood pressure does not respond to fluid boluses *and* vasopressors should receive stress-dose steroids.

4. Critically ill ICU patients who recently received a prednisone equivalent to ≥ 5 mg/day for ≥ 7 days should probably receive stress-dose steroid coverage.

BIBLIOGRAPHY

1. Albert SG, Ariyan S, Rather A: The effect of etomidate on adrenal function in critical illness: a systematic review. Intensive Care Med 37:901-910, 2011.

2. Annane D, Bellissant E, Bollaert P, et al: Corticosteroids in the treatment of severe sepsis and septic shock in adults. JAMA 301:2362-2375, 2009.

3. Annane D, Sebille V, Charpentier C, et al: Effect of treatment with low doses of hydrocortisone and fludrocortisone on mortality in patients with septic shock. JAMA 288:862-871, 2005.

4. Brown CJ, Buie WD: Perioperative stress dose steroids: do they make a difference? J Am Coll Surg 193:678-686, 2001.

5. Cohan C, Wang C, McArthur D, et al: Acute secondary adrenal insufficiency after traumatic brain injury: a prospective study. Crit Care Med 22:2358-2366, 2005.

6. Cooper MS, Stewart PM: Corticosteroid insufficiency in acutely ill patients. N Engl J Med 348:727-734, 2003.

7. Dellinger RP, Levy MM, Carlet JM, et al: Surviving Sepsis Campaign: international guidelines for management of severe sepsis and septic shock. Crit Care Med 36:296-327, 2008.

8. Ehrman R, Wira C, Lomax A, et al: Etomidate use in severe sepsis and septic shock patients does not contribute to mortality. Intern Emerg Med 6:253-257, 2011.

9. Hamrahian AH, Oseni TS, Arafah BM: Measurements of serum free cortisol in critically ill patients. N Engl J Med 50:1629-1638, 2004.

10. Krasner AS: Glucocorticoid-induced adrenal insufficiency. JAMA 282:671-676, 1999.

11. Mayo J, Collazos J, Martinez E, et al: Adrenal function in the human immunodeficiency virus–infected patient. Arch Intern Med 162:1095-1098, 2002.

12. Rivers EP, Gaspari M, Saad GA, et al: Adrenal insufficiency in high-risk surgical ICU patients. Chest 119:889-896, 2001.

13. Sligl WI, Milner DA, Sundar S, et al: Safety and efficacy of corticosteroids for the treatment of septic shock: a systematic review and meta-analysis. Clin Infect Dis 49:93-101, 2009.

14. Sprung CL, Annane D, Key D, et al: The CORTICUS randomized, double-blind, placebo-controlled study of hydrocortisone therapy in patients with septic shock. N Engl J Med 358:111-124, 2008.

15. Sprung CL, Brezis M, Goodman S, et al: Corticosteroid therapy for patients in septic shock: some progress in a difficult decision. Crit Care Med 39:571-574, 2011.

16. Zaloga GP, Marik P: Hypothalamic-pituitary-adrenal insufficiency. Crit Care Clin 17:25-41, 2001.

CHAPTER 53

THYROID DISEASE IN THE INTENSIVE CARE UNIT

Annis Marney, MD, MSCI

1. **What thyroid conditions require intensive care?**
   - **Thyroid storm:** Life-threatening thyrotoxicosis (accounts for 1%-2% of admissions for thyrotoxicosis and carries 20%-30% mortality)
   - **Myxedema coma:** Life-threatening hypothyroidism (approximately 20% mortality)

   Note: Nonthyroidal illness syndrome (NTIS), formerly known as euthyroid sick syndrome, is not life threatening.

2. **How do you diagnose thyroid storm?**

   Thyroid storm often occurs in people with Graves disease who have stopped medication or whose condition is undiagnosed. In addition, a precipitating factor often exists such as severe infection, diabetic ketoacidosis, myocardial infarction (MI), cerebrovascular accident (CVA), heart failure, trauma, amiodarone therapy (short or long term), or a recent test involving iodinated contrast load (less than 6 weeks before presentation). It shares laboratory findings with thyrotoxicosis but is different from simple thyrotoxicosis in that it involves **fever**.

   Clinical symptoms include the following:
   - Fever $>102°$ F $(38.9°$ C) (hallmark): most consider this the sine qua non of thyroid storm
   - Tachycardia
   - Tachypnea
   - Blood pressure not necessarily high or low
   - Cardiac arrhythmias, heart failure, and/or ischemia: common
   - Nausea, vomiting, diarrhea
   - Agitation, tremulousness, delirium
   - Jaundice: a particularly worrisome sign

   Laboratory findings include suppressed (undetectable, not just low) thyroid-stimulating hormone (TSH) and elevated serum total thyroxine (T_4) (TT_4), free T_4 (FT_4), total triiodothyronine (T_3) (TT_3), and free T_3 (FT_3).

3. **How do you treat thyroid storm?**

   Use common sense. First, support the patient as you would any critically ill patient and be sure to initiate cardiac monitoring. Next, reduce thyroid hormone production with thioureas. Finally, stop release of preformed hormone by adding iodide. Simultaneously with these measures give β-blockade to slow heart rate and reduce conversion of T_4 to T_3 (see Table 53-1).

4. **How do you diagnose myxedema coma?**

   Myxedema coma often occurs in people with undiagnosed or untreated hypothyroidism and is the end stage of a process that takes days to weeks. Often these people have had a precipitating event such as MI, CVA, acute infection, trauma, or hemorrhage. There may be a history of previous thyroid surgery or radioactive iodine ablation for hyperthyroidism, but because of mental status changes you may not get that history. Always look for an anterior neck scar for previous thyroid surgery.

   Clinical symptoms include the following:
   - Altered mental status (coma not strictly necessary, but altered mental status is)
   - Hypothermia (as low as $75°$ F [$23.9°$ C] has been reported)

TABLE 53-1. SUPPORTIVE CARE AND SPECIFIC MEDICATIONS FOR THYROID STORM

INTERVENTION AND MECHANISM OF ACTION	DOSE	ROUTE
Supportive care		
Isotonic fluids	Patient specific	IV
Oxygen	Patient specific	Nasal cannula if stable enough
Cooling blanket		Topical
Acetaminophen or other antipyretics	Adult dosing	Oral, rectal, or NG
Thioureas: reduce thyroid hormone production		
Propylthiouracil	150 mg every 6 hr	Oral, rectal, or NG
Methimazole (Tapazole)	20 mg every 8 hr	Oral, rectal, or NG
Iodide: reduce hormone production and T_4 to T_3 conversion 2-4 hr after starting thioamide (above)		
Saturated solution of potassium iodide	5 drops (250 mg) twice daily	Oral
Iopanoic acid	0.5 g twice daily	Oral or IV
Iohexol	0.6 g (2 mL of Omnipaque 300) twice daily	IV
β-Blockade: reduce heart rate and reduce conversion of T_4 to T_3		
Propranolol	40-80 mg every 6 hr	Oral
Propranolol	0.5-1.0 mg over 10 min every 3 hr	IV
Esmolol (especially if patient has asthma and needs β_1-selective agent)	0.25-0.5 mg/kg bolus followed by 0.05-0.1 mg/kg/min infusion	IV
Glucocorticoids: support circulation, supplement glucocorticoid reserve because of increased metabolism and reduced half-life with thyrotoxicosis, and reduce T_4 to T_3 conversion		
Dexamethasone	2 mg every 6 hr × 48 hr, then taper dose rapidly	Oral or IV
Hydrocortisone	100 mg every 8 hr × 48 hr, then taper dose rapidly	IV
Resin binders: remove T_4 in the gut to reduce enterohepatic circulation of free T_4		
Cholestyramine or colestipol	20-30 g daily	Oral or NG

IV, Intravenous; *NG*, nasogastric.

- Dry, coarse skin
- Gravelly, hoarse voice
- Thick tongue
- Thin scalp and eyebrow hair
- Pleural and cardiac effusions
- Delayed relaxation time of reflexes (Achilles = most sensitive)
  Laboratory findings include elevated TSH with low or low-normal serum TT_4, FT_4, TT_3, and FT_3.

5. **How do you treat myxedema coma?**

Again, use common sense. First, support the patient as you would any critically ill patient and be sure to initiate cardiac monitoring and ventilatory support and secure intravenous access (avoid oral or nasogastric medications because of possible ileus, which is common in myxedema coma). Next, administer glucocorticoids. Thyroid hormone speeds metabolism throughout the body, including metabolism of glucocorticoids. If the patient has underlying or undiagnosed adrenal insufficiency (autoimmune, typically), administration of thyroid hormone with a backdrop of adrenal insufficiency can precipitate adrenal crisis and is avoidable. Not every patient requires this, but it is impossible to differentiate acutely who does and who does not; therefore everyone should get it. You can taper quickly once you determine who needs steroids. Finally, give a parenteral thyroid hormone (see Table 53-2).

Different schools of thought exist about T_3 therapy. It increases cardiac metabolic demands acutely and so can be unwise in elderly patients already acutely ill. Many practitioners believe that patients can convert T_4 to T_3 on their own and thus administering T_3 is unnecessary and potentially dangerous.

TABLE 53-2. SUPPORTIVE CARE AND SPECIFIC MEDICATIONS FOR MYXEDEMA COMA		
INTERVENTION	**DOSE**	**ROUTE**
Supportive care		
Isotonic fluids but avoid overloading because of hyponatremia	Patient specific	IV
Oxygen	Patient specific	Nasal cannula if stable enough
Thyroid hormone replacement therapy		
Levothyroxine (T_4)	300-400 mcg loading dose then 50-100 mcg daily (based on weight)	IV
Liothyronine (T_3) (controversial)	10 mcg every 8 hr × 48 hr	IV
Glucocorticoid therapy: support circulation, supplement glucocorticoid reserve because of possible adrenal insufficiency		
Dexamethasone	2 mg every 6 hr × 48 hr, then taper dose rapidly	IV
Hydrocortisone	100 mg every 8 hr × 48 hr, then taper dose rapidly	IV

IV, Intravenous.

6. **How do you diagnose NTIS?**
   NTIS, formerly known as *euthyroid sick syndrome*, often occurs in patients who have severe, prolonged critical illness and is essentially a laboratory abnormality to be monitored. It is not a primary thyroid disorder but instead results from a resetting of the hypothalamic-pituitary-thyroid axis, as well as changes in peripheral thyroid hormone metabolism and transport induced by nonthyroidal illness. The laboratory abnormalities occur sequentially as follows:
   - Serum TT_3 and FT_3 levels are low (decreased conversion of T_4 to T_3 in peripheral tissues).
   - TT_3 and FT_3 levels are even lower. FT_4 level may be normal, decreased, or increased. TSH level is normal or slightly decreased.
   - FT_4 level is low and TSH is high (may transiently be significantly elevated in the teens and 20s). This is the recovery phase and can be prolonged. Normalization of laboratory values can take weeks to months.

7. **Could these laboratory values be confused with central hypothyroidism or pituitary dysfunction, and how can you tell the difference?**
   The laboratory results can be confusing, and you do have to take a careful history to be sure the patient has not had pituitary surgery or radiation therapy. Also, pituitary apoplexy could present with similar laboratory values, but the patient would have symptoms of severe headache and adrenal insufficiency as well. Only in cases where patients have symptoms concerning for apoplexy or a mass do you need to do magnetic resonance imaging (e.g., visual disturbance). Yes, sex hormones and insulin-like growth factor–1 levels may also be low, but this is likely the body's adaptive function and does not require therapy (also therapy with sex steroids and growth hormone have been proved not to help). Adrenal insufficiency that is clinically significant will cause symptoms, and testing for it can be tricky but may be necessary (see Chapter 52 on the adrenal gland).

8. **How do you treat NTIS?**
   Most often, you do not. There is a great deal of controversy in this area, however. The few studies that have been done show no benefit to giving T_4 in these patients. The recommendation is to recheck thyroid laboratory results in 4 to 6 weeks. It is possible that in cases of severely low T_4 and T_3 some patients may benefit from levothyroxine therapy, especially those with cardiac failure, but the evidence is far from conclusive.

KEY POINTS: THYROID DISORDERS

1. Thyroid storm is life-threatening thyrotoxicosis that often presents with a precipitating factor and carries a high mortality rate if not treated promptly and appropriately.

2. When thyroid storm is diagnosed or suspected, give appropriate supportive care and treat with antithyroid drugs, cold iodine, β-blockers, and stress doses of glucocorticoids, along with management of any precipitating factors.

3. Myxedema coma is life-threatening hypothyroidism that often has an identifiable precipitating cause and has a high mortality rate if not promptly and adequately treated.

4. When myxedema coma is diagnosed or suspected, first treat with stress doses of glucocorticoids followed by rapid repletion of the thyroid hormone and treatment of any precipitating causes.

5. NTIS is not a thyroid disorder but rather laboratory changes in serum TSH, T_4, and T_3 resulting from cytokines and inflammatory mediators produced in patients with nonthyroidal illnesses and generally does not require treatment.

BIBLIOGRAPHY

1. DeGroot L: "Non-thyroidal illness syndrome" is functional central hypothyroidism, and if severe, hormone replacement is appropriate in light of present knowledge. J Endocrinol Invest 26:1162, 2003.

2. Farwell AP: Thyroid hormone therapy is not indicated in the majority of patient with sick euthyroid syndrome. Endocr Pract 14:1180-1187, 2008.

3. Goldberg PA, Inzucchi SE: Critical issues in endocrinology. Clin Chest Med 24:583-606, 2003.

4. Kwaku MP, Burman KD: Myxedema coma. J Intensive Care Med 22:224-231, 2007.

5. Warner MH, Beckett GJ: Mechanisms behind the non-thyroidal illness syndrome: an update. J Endocrinol 205:1-13, 2010.

BLOOD PRODUCTS AND COAGULATION

George Kasotakis, MD, and Hasan B. Alam, MD, FACS

CHAPTER 54

1. **What components of blood are available for transfusion?**

   Components available for transfusion include whole blood, packed red blood cells (PRBCs), fresh frozen plasma (FFP), platelets, factor concentrates, cryoprecipitate, and white cell preparations. Fresh whole blood is sometimes used by the military but is not typically available for civilian use.

2. **What are PRBCs?**

   Red blood cells contain hemoglobin and serve as the primary oxygen-transporting agent to tissues. Red blood cells are obtained by centrifugation of whole blood to remove much of the plasma, or by apheresis (a procedure in which blood is drawn and separated into its components, with the unwanted ones being returned by transfusion to the donor). The resulting product is called PRBCs, because of its high hematocrit (65%-80%) concentration. The usual volume of 1 unit of PRBCs ranges between 225 and 350 mL, and its shelf life ranges from 21 to 42 days, depending on the type of anticoagulant-preservatives added. When transfused, 1 unit of PRBCs typically raises the hemoglobin by 1 mg/dL or the hematocrit by an average of three points.

3. **What are the main red blood cell surface antigen systems?**

   An individual's red cells may express A, B, both, or no surface antigens, which determine that individual's blood type. Those who do not express an antigen will eventually develop antibodies against it. People carrying anti-A or anti-B antibodies cannot receive red blood cells with the corresponding surface antigens, or immunologic destruction of the transfused red cells may occur. Consequently, type O individuals are considered *universal donors*, whereas AB individuals may donate only to other AB recipients. Similar to the ABO system, a separate Rh surface antigen exists that may be either present (Rh+) or absent (Rh−) from the red cell plasma membrane. Individuals who are Rh negative will develop antibodies to the Rh factor when exposed to Rh+ blood. This is not a problem with the initial exposure, but hemolysis may occur with subsequent transfusions (Table 54-1).

TABLE 54-1.	COMPATIBLE PACKED RED BLOOD CELLS DONOR–RECIPIENT COMBINATIONS					
	DONOR					
PRBC	A	B	O	AB	RH+	RH−
Recipient						
A	×		×			
B		×	×			
O			×			
AB	×	×	×	×		
Rh+					×	×
Rh−						×

4. **What are blood typing, screening, and crossmatching?**
Donor and recipient blood **typing** is a process that determines what ABO and Rh antigens are expressed on the red cell surface. **Screening** is a process that detects circulating antibodies to various other antigens that might interact with the donor blood components. **Cross-matching** involves directly mixing the recipient's plasma with the donor's red cells to ensure that hemolysis does not occur from undetected antibodies.

5. **What are potential transfusion hazards?**
The adverse events of blood component transfusions can be generally grouped into immunologic and nonimmunologic complications.
   Immunologic complications include the following:
- Hemolytic (immediate or delayed) and immune-mediated platelet destruction transfusion reactions
- Febrile nonhemolytic reactions
- Allergic and anaphylactic reactions
- Transfusion-related acute lung injury (TRALI)
- Transfusion-associated graft-versus-host disease (TA-GVHD)
   Non–immune-mediated complications include the following:
- Transmission of infectious agents
- Transfusion-associated circulatory overload (TACO)
- Hypothermia
- Metabolic complications, such as citrate toxicity (transient manifestations of hypocalcemia until citrate gets cleared in the liver) and hyperkalemia or hypokalemia

6. **What is a febrile nonhemolytic reaction?**
A febrile nonhemolytic reaction manifests as a mild to moderate temperature elevation (typically $\leq 2°$ F or $< 1.1°$ C) during or shortly after a transfusion and in the absence of any other pyretic stimuli. Febrile reactions occur in fewer than 1% of all transfusions and are thought to arise from circulating molecules or cells either in the transfused product or generated by the recipient. Routine pretreatment with antihistamines and antipyretics may ameliorate symptoms. Patients having recurrent severe febrile reactions may benefit from leukocyte-reduced blood products.

7. **What is a hemolytic reaction?**
It is the immunologic destruction of the transfused cells due to incompatibility of the antigen on their surface with preexisting circulating antibodies in the recipient's plasma. It may occur when as little as 10 mL of blood is infused and is associated with significant morbidity. Associated mortality may be as high as 35%. The most common cause of acute hemolytic reactions is transfusion of ABO- or Rh-incompatible blood, resulting from identification errors. Serologic incompatibility undetected during pretransfusion testing is much less common. *Delayed hemolytic reactions* can also occur in previously alloimmunized patients in whom antigens on the transfused product provoke anamnestic antibody production. This anamnestic response is usually most evident within 2 to 14 days after the transfusion.

8. **What are the classic findings in a hemolytic transfusion reaction?**
Fever (with or without chills), tachycardia, back or flank pain, chest pain, dyspnea, hypotension, and oliguria are frequently present. *Disseminated intravascular coagulopathy* (DIC) may become clinically evident in severe cases. Laboratory findings include hemoglobinuria and elevation of the indirect serum bilirubin and lactate dehydrogenase levels. The direct antiglobulin test is also positive.

9. **How should a hemolytic transfusion reaction be managed?**
When an acute hemolytic reaction is recognized, the transfusion must be stopped immediately. The blood bank should be notified and transfusion forms and labels rechecked. Postreaction

blood samples need to be sent along with the remaining blood component. Treatment is supportive and includes administration of intravenous fluids, diuretics, inotropes, and close monitoring as needed. Delayed reactions are typically benign and require no treatment.

10. **What are the infectious risks of transfusion?**
    - The incidence of transmission of hepatitis C, human T-lymphotropic virus, and human immunodeficiency virus in the United States through a blood component transfusion is approximately 1:2,000,000 units transfused.
    - Hepatitis B is transmitted in 1:270,000 transfusions.
    - The risk of transfusion-related bacterial infections is much higher at 1:2000 units of platelets transfused (platelets carry a higher risk of contamination because they are stored at room temperature).
    - Transmission of other infectious agents (e.g., *Babesia* spp, variant Creutzfeldt-Jakob disease agent, West Nile virus) for which blood products are not routinely tested is possible, yet even rarer.

11. **What is TRALI?**
    TRALI describes the acute onset of hypoxemia (within 6 hours) after a blood component transfusion and is the most common cause of transfusion-related death in the United States. In addition to hypoxemia, criteria for diagnosis include bilateral infiltrates on chest radiograph and exclusion of preexisting lung injury or circulatory overload. Postulated mechanisms include *second-hit* injuries to the lungs from lipid products in stored blood products, human neutrophil antibodies, and human leukocyte antigen antibodies. Treatment consists of aggressive pulmonary support, frequently requiring mechanical ventilation.

12. **When should red cells be transfused to critically ill adults?**
    This has been one of the most hotly debated topics in critical care for the last decade. It appears that a restrictive transfusion strategy (hemoglobin level of 7 g/dL as transfusion trigger) is at least as effective as, and possibly superior to, a liberal transfusion strategy (hemoglobin trigger of 10 g/dL) with regard to overall mortality. It is also known from studies in populations with anemia who decline transfusions for religious reasons that perioperative mortality increases from zero to 9% as the hemoglobin levels drop below 7 g/dL. Patients with acute myocardial infarction and unstable angina are an exception, and higher transfusion triggers should be maintained for them. Other parameters, including patient age, chronic anemia or acute blood loss, and vasoocclusive disease should also be taken into consideration when individualizing transfusion triggers.

13. **What are the most commonly used techniques of autologous transfusion?**
    - **Preoperative autologous blood donation (PABD).** Blood is donated at frequent intervals (as often as every 3 days) starting 4 to 6 weeks before surgery and transfused after surgery as needed. Benefits include freedom from hemolytic, allergic, and febrile reactions, as well as alloimmunization and transfusion-related infections.
    - **Acute normovolemic intraoperative hemodilution (ANH).** This blood conservation technique entails the removal of blood (typically 500-1500 mL) from a patient immediately before surgery, with maintenance of normovolemia with crystalloids and/or colloids. Intraoperative blood loss leads to smaller hemoglobin losses due to hemodilution. The removed blood, which is anticoagulated and stored for up to 8 hours, is reinfused during or after surgery as needed.
    - **Intraoperative blood salvage (*Cell Saver*) (IBS).** Blood is aspirated from the surgical field, anticoagulated, and collected for centrifuging. Salvaged red cells are washed and reinfused to the patient as needed. Contraindications include bacteremia, gross operative field contamination, and cancer.

14. **What else can be done to minimize blood loss and transfusion requirements?**
    - **Antifibrinolytic agents** (*ε-aminocaproic acid* and *tranexamic acid* [TXA]) are synthetic lysine analogs that have been used extensively, mainly in cardiac surgery, to minimize blood loss and decrease transfusion requirements. They also appear to minimize blood loss and improve survival in trauma patients, and their use has been increasing in the field. (Aprotinin, an older-generation antifibrinolytic, was withdrawn from the market in 2008 when it was found to be associated with a higher risk for cardiovascular complications and death). A recent multiinstitutional large prospective randomized clinical trial has shown survival advantage in trauma patients treated early with TXA.
    - Recombinant **erythropoietin**, a normally endogenously produced hormone that stimulates erythropoiesis, was previously thought to decrease tranfusion requirements and possibly improve survival in the critically ill. However, recent evidence suggests that the benefit may be too small to outweigh risks (thrombotic events). This finding, in addition to the fact that it does not work quickly enough to have a role in the management of acute blood loss, has led to the abandonment of its routine use in modern intensive care units.
    - **Recombinant human factor VIIa** is licensed for use in patients with hemophilia but has gained momentum in recent years as a potent agent in controlling life-threatening hemorrhage, usually after trauma. However, significant complications (thromboembolic episodes), along with two prospective randomized trials in trauma patients that failed to show any clear benefits, have dampened enthusiasm for its use.
    - **Desmopressin** increases plasma levels of von Willebrand factor (vWF) and factor VIII and is licensed for use in von Willebrand disease and hemophilia A. It can also be used to control bleeding in patients with uremia.
    - Factor concentrates (**fibrinogen concentrate** [FC], **prothrombin complex concentrate** [PCC]) have emerged recently as potential adjuvant therapies in the management of the acute, massive bleeding with associated hypofibrinogenemia (the former) and emergent reversal of warfarin anticoagulation (the latter). FC contains fibrinogen at very high concentrations (even higher than cryoprecipitate), and PCCs are preparations containing near-physiologic concentrations of factors II, IX, and X and proteins C and S and variable levels of factor VII. FC has been approved for management of acute bleeding episodes in patients with congenital fibrinogen deficiency, but PCC, although its use in Europe and Canada is on the rise, is still undergoing phase III testing in the United States.

15. **What are the characteristics of an ideal oxygen carrier?**
    - Effective O_2 carrying capacity and delivery to the peripheral tissues
    - Favorable interaction with nitric oxide
    - Universal compatibility (crossmatching elimination)
    - Minimal side effects
    - Easy storage, long shelf life, immediate availability
    - Cost-effective

16. **What alternative oxygen carriers are available for use in the critically ill?**
    Two types of oxygen carriers are available as alternatives to PRBC transfusion: *hemoglobin-based oxygen carrier* and *perfluorocarbons*, but neither of them is currently commercially available. The former has been associated with adverse outcomes in human studies, whereas the latter is currently undergoing phase III testing in Europe.

17. **What is FFP?**
    FFP is plasma obtained from single units of whole blood collected by apheresis. It is frozen and maintained at $-18°$ to $-30°$ C to preserve the labile coagulation factors. FFP contains all of the coagulation factors present in blood, along with antithrombin III and proteins C and S, at near-physiologic concentrations. It has a half life of approximately 1 year and has to be thawed before administration. It has to be matched for ABO system compatibility (Table 54-2) but not Rh compatibility.

TABLE 54-2. COMPATIBLE FRESH FROZEN PLASMA DONOR–RECIPIENT COMBINATIONS

FFP	DONOR			
	A	B	O	AB
Recipient				
A	×			×
B		×		×
O	×	×	×	×
AB				×

18. **List the indications for FFP.**
   - Coagulopathy due to a congenital or acquired deficiency of multiple factors (severe liver disease, DIC, dilutional or consumption coagulopathy)
   - Emergent reversal of warfarin effect or vitamin K deficiency
   - Massive transfusion protocol
   - Treatment of antithrombin III deficiency

19. **What is cryoprecipitate?**
   Cryoprecipitate is the precipitate that remains when FFP is thawed slowly at 4° C. It is a concentrated preparation (10-15 mL) that contains virtually all of the factor VIII, XIII, fibrinogen, and vWF that are in the FFP (without the additional volume).

20. **List the indications for cryoprecipitate.**
   - Fibrinogen repletion (levels <100 mg/dL) and a clinical need to avoid excessive transfusion volume (unable to give FFP)
   - Von Willebrand disease
   - Factor XIII deficiency

21. **What is measured by prothrombin time (PT)? What is international normalized ratio (INR)?**
   - PT is used to assess the extrinsic pathway of clotting, namely the activity of factor VII and the common pathway factors (fibrinogen and factors II, V, and X). It is prolonged in patients with liver disease, vitamin K deficiency, or circulating lupus anticoagulants or receiving warfarin therapy.
   - INR is a standardized method of reporting the PT, so that values from various laboratories can be directly comparable. It is most commonly used to monitor patients receiving oral warfarin therapy.

22. **What is measured by partial thromboplastin time (PTT)?**
   PTT assesses the intrinsic coagulation pathway, which includes factors XII, XI, IX, and VIII, along with the common pathway factors (fibrinogen and factors II, V, and X). It is used to monitor heparin therapy.

23. **How does warfarin work?**
   Warfarin (Coumadin) inhibits the conversion of vitamin K to its active form. This inhibition interferes with the hepatic synthesis of the vitamin K–dependent clotting factors (II, VII, IX, and X and proteins C and S). Warfarin therapy is routinely monitored by following the INR.

24. How does dabigatran work?

Dabigatran is an orally active direct thrombin inhibitor that has been recently approved for use in patients with nonvalvular atrial fibrillation. It has also been shown that it is at least as effective as warfarin for the treatment of acute venous thromboembolism and with a similar safety profile. Its main benefit is that it does not require laboratory monitoring, but its high cost is likely to prevent mass adoption.

25. How does heparin work?

Heparin binds to and activates antithrombin III, which in turn inhibits several coagulation enzymes, including thrombin and activated factors X, XII, XI, and IX. The biologic half-life of heparin is 30 to 60 minutes, and its effects are reversed within 2 to 4 hours after an infusion is stopped. If urgent reversal is required, protamine can be given intravenously. Heparin therapy is monitored by serial PTT measurements.

26. What is low-molecular-weight heparin (LMWH)?

LMWH is a fragment produced by the chemical breakdown of heparin. It exerts its anticoagulant effect by binding with antithrombin III and inhibiting several coagulation enzymes. LMWH principally inhibits activated factor X.

27. What are the major differences between standard heparin and LMWH?

- LMWH has a longer half-life and thus can be administered once daily.
- LMWH provides a more predictable anticoagulant response and thus can be administered without monitoring.
- LMWH is as effective as heparin but produces fewer bleeding complications at equivalent antithrombotic doses.

28. What is *damage control resuscitation*?

The basic tenets of damage control resuscitation are as follows:
- Avoid crystalloid resuscitation.
- Aim for permissive hypotension whenever possible.
- Prevent coagulopathy through early use of blood products.
- Aggressively break the vicious cycle of acidosis, coagulopathy, and hypothermia.

A key component of this damage control approach is early hemorrhage control. Another core concept is that resuscitation fluids should resemble what the trauma patient loses—*warm fresh whole blood*. In civilian settings, fresh whole blood is not available for transfusion, and blood components in appropriate ratios should be used toward this goal. A number of studies suggest that FFP and platelets should be given early and in high ratios (e.g., PRBCs/FFP/platelets in a ratio of 1:1:1) in patients who require *massive transfusion* (>10 units PRBCs). A randomized trial is about to begin to identify the optimal ratio of component therapy.

KEY POINTS: BLOOD PRODUCTS AND COAGULATION

1. Controlling the bleeding is more important than replacing the losses.

2. Blood products carry significant risks. Transfuse only when necessary.

3. Know the mechanism of warfarin and heparin anticoagulants and how they can be reversed.

4. Early use of blood component therapy can prevent development of coagulopathy in massively bleeding patients.

5. Excessive crystalloid resuscitation can worsen coagulopathy.

BIBLIOGRAPHY

1. Alter HJ, Stramer SL, Dodd RY: Emerging infectious diseases that threaten the blood supply. Semin Hematol 44:32-41, 2007.

2. Brown CV, Foulkrod KH, Sadler HT, et al: Autologous blood transfusion during emergency trauma operations. Arch Surg 145:690-694, 2010.

3. Carless PA, Henry DA, Carson JL, et al: Transfusion thresholds and other strategies for guiding allogeneic red blood cell transfusion. Cochrane Database Syst Rev 10: CD002042, 2010.

4. Carson JL, Noveck H, Berlin JA, et al: Mortality and morbidity in patients with very low postoperative hemoglobin levels who decline blood transfusion. Transfusion 42:812-818, 2002.

5. CRASH-2 trial collaborators : Effects of tranexamic acid on death, vascular occlusive events, and blood transfusion in trauma patients with significant haemorrhage (CRASH-2): a randomised, placebo-controlled trial. Lancet 376:23-32, 2010.

6. Duchesne JC, Hunt JP, Wahl G, et al: Review of current blood transfusions strategies in a mature level I trauma center: were we wrong for the last 60 years? J Trauma 65:272-276, 2008.

7. Hauser CJ, Boffard K, Dutton R, et al: Results of the CONTROL trial: efficacy and safety of recombinant activated factor VII in the management of refractory traumatic hemorrhage. J Trauma 69:489-500, 2010.

8. Henry DA, Carless PA, Moxey AJ, et al: Anti-fibrinolytic use for minimising perioperative allogeneic blood transfusion. Cochrane Database Syst Rev 3: CD001886, 2011.

9. Holcomb JB, Wade CE, Michalek JE, et al: Increased plasma and platelet to red blood cell ratios improves outcome in 466 massively transfused civilian trauma patients. Ann Surg 248:447-458, 2008.

10. Inaba K, Lustenberger T, Rhee P, et al: The impact of platelet transfusion in massively transfused trauma patients. J Am Coll Surg 211:573-579, 2010.

11. Kennedy LD, Case LD, Hurd DD, et al: A prospective, randomized, double-blind controlled trial of acetaminophen and diphenhydramine pretransfusion medication versus placebo for the prevention of transfusion reactions. Transfusion 48:2285-2291, 2008.

12. Levi M, Levy JH, Andersen HF, et al: Safety of recombinant activated factor VII in randomized clinical trials. N Engl J Med 363:1791-1800, 2010.

13. Martí-Carvajal AJ, Solà I, González LE, et al: Pharmacological interventions for the prevention of allergic and febrile non-haemolytic transfusion reactions. Cochrane Database Syst Rev 6: CD007539, 2010.

14. Roberts I, Shakur H, Ker K, et al: Antifibrinolytic drugs for acute traumatic injury. Cochrane Database Syst Rev 1: CD004896, 2010.

15. Schulman S, Kearon C, Kakkar AK, et al: Dabigatran versus warfarin in the treatment of acute venous thromboembolism. N Engl J Med 361:2342-2352, 2009.

16. Vanderlinde ES, Heal JM, Blumberg N: Autologous transfusion. BMJ 324:772-775, 2002.

CHAPTER 55

THROMBOCYTOPENIA AND PLATELETS

Chad T. Wilson, MD, MPH, and Hasan B. Alam, MD, FACS

1. **What are two principal functions of platelets in effecting hemostasis?**
   Platelets function to effect hemostasis by the following:
   - Formation of an initial platelet plug
   - Degranulation and secretion of proteins and catalysts for the clotting cascade
     The initial platelet plug is due to loose aggregation of platelets in an area of injury and requires the presence of von Willebrand factor. Heparin does not affect this primary hemostasis, which explains why hemostasis can still occur in heparinized patients.

2. **What is the most common congenital platelet deficiency?**
   von Willebrand disease. The absence of von Willebrand factor disrupts the formation of platelet aggregates (see question 1).

3. **Define thrombocytopenia.**
   No single value for platelet count universally defines thrombocytopenia; however, conventionally, platelet count of less than $100,000/mm^3$ is considered to constitute thrombocytopenia.

4. **What are the basic mechanisms of thrombocytopenia?**
   Thrombocytopenia can be caused by decreased platelet production (marrow failure or replacement by cancerous cells or fibrosis), disordered platelet distribution or sequestration (hypersplenism), or increased platelet destruction (antibody mediated, prosthetic valves, extracorporeal bypass, disseminated intravascular coagulation [DIC]). These mechanisms can occur in isolation or in combination.

5. **How prevalent is thrombocytopenia in critically ill patients, and what are the most common causes of thrombocytopenia in the intensive care unit (ICU)?**
   Thrombocytopenia has a prevalence of 30% to 50% of patients in the ICU. Some of the most common causes of thrombocytopenia in the ICU are recent surgery and hemorrhage, blood transfusions, drug-induced thrombocytopenia, intravascular catheters or aortic balloon pumps and vascular grafts, sepsis, renal replacement therapy, DIC, and myelodysplastic and metastatic disease. Most patients who have thrombocytopenia in the ICU have multifactorial causes or idiopathic thrombocytopenia.

6. **What are the most common agents used in the ICU that cause drug-induced thrombocytopenia?**
   - Antibiotics: for example, linezolid, vancomycin, β-lactams
   - Glycoprotein (GP) IIb/IIIa inhibitors: abciximab, eptifibatide, lotrifiban
   - Histamine 2 (H_2) blockers: cimetidine, famotidine, ranitidine
   - Antiseizure: valproic acid, phenytoin
   - Heparin: unfractionated heparin and low-molecular-weight heparin

7. **What is heparin-induced thrombocytopenia (HIT)?**
   HIT is a life- and limb-threatening prothrombotic complication of heparin administration (risk of 0.6% with unfractionated heparin and 0.3% with low-molecular-weight heparin in a recent large

multicenter trial of ICU patients). It results from an immune response triggered by the interaction of heparin with a specific platelet protein, platelet factor 4 (PF4). Certain patient populations are at higher risk than others for development of HIT, with patients after cardiac surgery having a risk of HIT that can be greater than 2%. HIT with thrombotic complication has a mortality rate of 20%, with approximately 20% to 30% having permanent disability (i.e., amputations, stroke).

8. **When should a patient have a work-up for HIT?**
   The diagnosis must be considered in any patient in whom thrombocytopenia develops, who has an unexplained fall in platelet count of 50%, or who has thrombotic complication 5 to 10 days (may be as late as 20 days) after heparin exposure.

9. **How is HIT diagnosed?**
   Almost all the patients with HIT have circulating antibodies to complexes between PF4 and heparin. However, in most of the patients who have circulating antibodies, HIT does not develop clinically. Therefore it is currently not indicated to screen patients without symptoms for these antibodies. Two different types of assays are available:
   - The *functional assays* measure heparin-dependent platelet activation by PF4-heparin antibody in vitro. One of the functional assays, ^{14}C-serotonin release assay (SRA), is considered the *gold standard* in diagnosis with a positive predictive value of almost 100% (but a negative predictive value of approximately 20%).
   - *Immunoassays* (such as enzyme-linked immunosorbent assay [ELISA]) measure the levels of antibodies in circulation (sensitivity 93%-97%, positive predictive value 93%-100%, specificity 86%-100%, and negative predictive value 88%-95%). ELISA is easy and rapid to obtain, but only 25% of the ELISA-positive specimens are SRA positive.

10. **Is repeating HIT testing useful?**
    Testing should be repeated for negative but borderline ELISA results. The chances of a negative test turning positive 3 days later depends on the titer levels. Approximately 45% of high-titer negative (almost positive) may turn positive, whereas approximately 15% and 5% of the medium- and low-titer results respectively are likely to turn positive.

11. **How is HIT treated?**
    Diagnosis of HIT requires immediate withdrawal of all heparin and treatment with anticoagulation agents. The Warkentin criteria may be used to determine the patient's pretest probability of HIT (Table 55-1). All patients (with or without thrombosis) with HIT must be anticoagulated, as the risk of thrombosis is >50% without anticoagulation. Do not transfuse platelets unless clearly indicated, as platelet transfusion actually increases the amount of PF4 and may exaggerate the antigen response. If continued anticoagulation is required, a vitamin K antagonist (warfarin) should be initiated *after* the patient is fully treated with one of the following agents:
    - Danaparoid (low-molecular-weight glycosaminoglycan composed of heparan sulfate, dermatan sulfate, and chondroitin sulfate). This drug has mostly anti-factor Xa activity with a limited antithrombin action. Dose is titrated to keep anti-Xa levels between 0.5 and 0.8 units/mL. There is no antidote for bleeding.
    - Recombinant hirudin (lepirudin [Refludan]) is a 7-kDa peptide that acts directly on circulating and clot-bound thrombin. Anticoagulant effects last about 40 minutes. It is given as a slow bolus (0.4 mg/kg) followed by continuous infusion at 0.15 mg/kg to maintain activated partial thromboplastin time (aPTT) between 1.5 and 2.5 times baseline. This is a good choice for patients who will need to get transitioned to warfarin. Lepirudin does not alter the interpretation of international normalized ratio (INR) as significantly as argatroban.
    - Argatroban is a 509-Da arginine-based direct thrombin inhibitor that inhibits both soluble and clot-bound thrombin. Half-life is 46.2 ± 10.2 minutes, and steady-state activity is achieved

TABLE 55-1.	WARKENTIN CRITERIA TO DETERMINE THE PROBABILITY OF HEPARIN-INDUCED THROMBOCYTOPENIA		
CRITERIA	2 POINTS	1 POINT	0 POINT
Thrombocytopenia	>50% fall or platelet nadir of 20-100 × 10^9/L	30%-50% fall or platelet nadir of 10-19 × 10^9/L	<30% fall or platelet nadir of <10 × 10^9/L
Timing of platelet drop	Clear onset day 5-10 or <1 day (if heparin exposure within past 100 days)	Consistent with immune activation but not clear (e.g., missing data) or onset after day 10	Platelet count fall too early (without recent heparin exposure)
Thrombosis or other sequelae	New thrombosis, skin necrosis, post-heparin bolus acute reaction	Progressive or recurrent thrombosis, erythematous skin lesions, suspected thrombosis (not yet proved)	None
Other causes for thrombocytopenia	No other cause for platelet count drop evident	Possible other causes	Definite other cause present

Pretest probability score 6-8 = high; 4-5 = intermediate; 0-3 = low.

within 1 to 2 hours of continuous infusion. Dose is 2.0 mcg/kg per minute and adjusted to keep aPTT between 1.5 and 3 times baseline (maximum 10 mcg/kg per minute).
- Fondaparinux is a newer drug that is given via the subcutaneous route. Dose is 7.5 mg once a day.

12. **How should you monitor warfarin effect when it is coadministered with argatroban?**
Chromogenic factor X assay can be helpful in determining when the patient is therapeutically anticoagulated with warfarin while receiving argatroban (which in itself elevates the INR value). Switch to the measurement of INR 3 hours after discontinuation of argatroban to be certain that a therapeutic level is maintained after discontinuation of argatroban.

13. **What are different treatment options for patients with immune thrombocytopenic purpura (ITP)?**
ITP is caused by immunoglobulin G antibodies against the platelet GPs (GPIIb/IIIa and GP Ib/IX). Corticosteroids have been the mainstay of therapy for a long time, but alternative therapies are

now commonly prescribed. These include intravenous gamma globulins (IVIG) and intravenous anti-D (IV anti-D). Both cause *Fc receptor blockade* as an important mechanism of acute platelet increase. IVIG works fast (24 hours) and can be used in Rh-negative patients and patients after splenectomy, whereas IV anti-D causes a slower rate of platelet increase (72 hours) and is relatively ineffective in Rh-negative patients and patients after splenectomy. It is, however, effective in patients positive for the human immunodeficiency virus. Patients who initially respond to medical management but have a relapse within 1 to 3 months may be considered candidates for splenectomy. For refractory ITP, combination chemotherapies are used (cyclophosphamide, hydroxydaunomycin, Oncovin, and prednisone [CHOP]-like; vincristine–IVIG–Solu-Medrol) followed by maintenance therapy (using combinations of steroids, danazol, Imuran, CellCept, cyclosporin among others).

14. **How do you differentiate between thrombotic thrombocytopenic purpura (TTP) and hemolytic uremic syndrome (HUS)?**
    TTP and HUS share thrombocytopenia, hemolytic anemia, and thrombotic occlusions in terminal arterioles and capillaries. Differentiating clinical features are the presence of focal neurologic symptoms in TTP and renal impairment in HUS. In addition, levels of plasma von Willebrand factor–cleaving protease are low in TTP and normal in HUS.

15. **What are some causes of platelet dysfunction in the ICU?**
    The principal causes of platelet dysfunction and thrombocytopenia in the ICU are due to drug side effects (e.g., aspirin, clopidogrel), uremia, and sepsis. Antibiotics, nitrates, local anesthetics, α- and β-adrenergic blockers, xanthine derivatives, diuretics, H_2 receptor blockers, and dextran are some examples of drugs that can impair platelet activity.

16. **What are the indications for platelet transfusion?**
    The platelet counts that should serve as a trigger for platelet transfusion continue to evolve. Although somewhat controversial, the following threshold levels have been proposed in the literature:
    - Bleeding prophylaxis in a stable oncology patient: 10,000/mm^3 (previously <20,000/mm^3)
    - Lumbar puncture in a patient with leukemia: 10,000/mm^3
    - Stable HIT: 10,000/mm^3
    - Bone marrow aspiration: 20,000/mm^3
    - Gastrointestinal endoscopy in cancer: 20,000-40,000/mm^3
    - DIC: 20,000 to 50,000/mm^3
    - Fiberoptic bronchoscopy: 20,000 to 50,000/mm^3
    - Major surgery: 50,000/mm^3
    - Thrombocytopenia resulting from massive transfusion: 50,000/mm^3
    - Invasive procedures in cirrhosis: 50,000/mm^3
    - Cardiopulmonary bypass: 50,000 to 60,000/mm^3
    - Neurosurgical procedures: 100,000/mm^3
    - Thrombocytopenia and bleeding (intracerebral, gastrointestinal, genitourinary, or retinal hemorrhage): 100,000/mm^3

    There is no specific count at which bleeding is completely prevented. In addition to the count, the quality and function of the platelets are also important. However, life-threatening bleeding can occur with platelet counts less than 5000/mm^3 and spontaneous bleeding with counts less than 10,000 to 20,000/mm^3.

17. **How does aspirin affect platelet function?**
    Aspirin irreversibly inhibits platelet cyclooxygenase, resulting in a functional defect that lasts the duration of the platelet's life span (8-9 days).

18. What laboratory test measures platelet function?
Bleeding time is a sensitive indicator of overall platelet function.

19. How are platelet disorders managed?
The patient's drug regimen should be carefully scrutinized, eliminating or substituting medications implicated in thrombocytopenia. Platelet transfusion may be required (see answer to question 16). Uremia-associated thrombocytopenia can be treated with hemodialysis. Cryoprecipitate, 1-desamino-8-D-arginine vasopressin, and conjugated estrogens have also been used with good results.

KEY POINTS: THROMBOCYTOPENIA AND PLATELETS

1. Thrombocytopenia is a common finding in intensive care unit patients, and the basic rule for management is to treat the underlying cause.

2. Transfuse platelets only if needed (question 16) or if the platelet count is less than $10,000/mm^3$.

3. HIT is a relatively uncommon but potentially serious complication of heparin administration.

4. Platelet counts should be followed in all patients that are receiving heparin (unfractionated or low molecular weight). A drop in platelet count ($>50\%$ from baseline or below $100,000/mm^3$) is a reason to suspect HIT.

5. Most of the patients who have circulating antibodies to PF4 do not have clinical development of HIT. Therefore screen patients for these antibodies only when clinically indicated.

6. All patients (with or without thrombosis) with HIT (type II) must be anticoagulated, as the risk of thrombosis is $>50\%$ without anticoagulation.

BIBLIOGRAPHY

1. AuBuchon JP: Platelet transfusion therapy. Clin Lab Med 16:797-816, 1996.
2. Chong BH, Eisbacher M: Pathophysiology and laboratory testing of heparin-induced thrombocytopenia. Semin Hematol 35:3-8, 1998.
3. Fuse I: Disorders of platelet function. Crit Rev Oncol Hematol 22:1-25, 1996.
4. Lipsett PA, Perler BA: The use of blood products for surgical bleeding. Semin Vasc Surg 9:347-353, 1996.
5. Martel N, Lee J, Wells PS: Risk for heparin-induced thrombocytopenia with unfractionated and low molecular weight heparin thromboprophylaxis: a meta-analysis. Blood 106:2710-2715, 2005.
6. McCrae KR, Bussel JB, Mannucci PM, et al: Platelets: an update on diagnosis and management of thrombocytopenic disorders. Hematology Am Soc Hematol Educ Program 2001:282-305, 2001.
7. Platelet transfusion therapy. Natl Inst Health Consens Dev Conf Consens Statement 6:1-6, 1986.
8. Priziola JL, Smythe MA, Dager WE: Drug induced thrombocytopenia in critically ill patients. Crit Care Med 38 (6 Suppl):S145-S152, 2010.
9. PROTECT Investigators for the Canadian Critical Care Trials Group and the Australian and New Zealand Intensive Care Society Clinical Trials Group, et al: Dalteparin versus unfractionated heparin in critically ill patients. N Engl J Med 364:1305-1314, 2011.
10. Rebulla P: Platelet transfusion trigger in difficult patients. Transfus Clin Biol 8:249-254, 2001.
11. Selleng K, Warkentin TE, Greinacher A: Heparin induced thrombocytopenia in intensive care patients. Crit Care Med 35:1165-1176, 2007.

CHAPTER 56

DISSEMINATED INTRAVASCULAR COAGULATION

Pavan K. Bendapudi, MD, and David J. Kuter, MD, DPhil

1. **What is disseminated intravascular coagulation (DIC)?**

   DIC is caused by aberrant activation of the clotting cascade, leading to fibrin deposition in small vessels, combined with activation of fibrinolytic mechanisms, leading to bleeding. DIC is usually a common final hemostatic disorder caused by other conditions such as sepsis, pancreatitis, or trauma. Because they are consumed by the ongoing prothrombotic and fibrinolytic processes, coagulation proteins and platelets can become depleted, leading to bleeding. Thus, in DIC, hemorrhage and thrombosis can occur simultaneously. DIC can be an acute or a chronic disorder, and the latter is seen mostly in obstetric and oncology patients. Hereafter, the discussion will focus primarily on acute DIC, the form most likely to be encountered in the critical care setting.

2. **Why is DIC important?**

   DIC is a common cause of concurrent thrombocytopenia and prolonged clotting times (activated partial thromboplastin time [aPTT] and prothrombin time [PT]) in hospitalized patients. It can also be an independent predictor of mortality. DIC leads to fibrin and platelet deposition in small vessels, which can cause tissue ischemia and result in organ dysfunction (Figure 56-1). The consumptive coagulopathy can also lead to clinically significant bleeding.

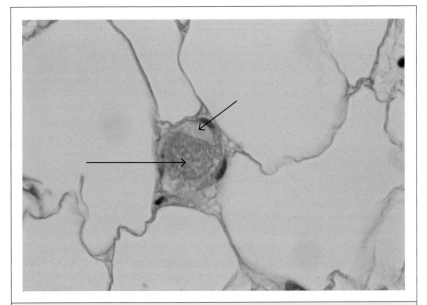

Figure 56-1. Microvascular thrombosis in skin of patient with severe disseminated intravascular coagulation. Lumen (*short arrow*) of blood vessel is partly occluded by fibrin-platelet thrombosis (*long arrow*).

3. **What is the pathophysiology of acute DIC?**

Although the pathophysiology of DIC remains incompletely understood, it is thought to begin at the level of the microvasculature. As a result of widespread endothelial damage due to an underlying illness (i.e., sepsis, trauma, or pancreatitis), tissue factor is released into the circulation, where it combines with factor VIIa to produce thrombin via the extrinsic pathway. Thrombin then activates platelets and cleaves fibrinogen such that platelets and fibrin are deposited in the microvasculature. Concurrently, fibrinolytic pathways are activated. As platelets and coagulation proteins are consumed, bleeding can occur as the result of a consumptive coagulopathy. Thus DIC is characterized by simultaneous clotting and hemorrhage.

4. **In critical care patients, what conditions are associated with DIC?**
   - Sepsis
   - Trauma
   - Malignancy: adenocarcinoma, acute promyelocytic leukemia (incidence approaches 100%)
   - Obstetric: **h**emolysis, **e**levated **l**iver enzymes, and **l**ow **p**latelet count (HELLP) syndrome; retained uterine placental or fetal tissue; placental abruption or previa; amniotic fluid embolus
   - Vascular: vasculitis, abdominal aortic aneurysm, cavernous hemangiomas
   - Miscellaneous: burns, anaphylaxis, transfusion reaction, snake bite, acute pancreatitis, transplant rejection, intravenous anti-D immunoglobulin

5. **How does DIC present clinically?**

In acutely ill hospitalized patients, DIC usually presents with prolongation of the PT and aPTT along with decreased fibrinogen and platelets; systemic bleeding may or may not be present. Typically, bleeding manifests as ecchymoses, purpura, and petechiae; it also occurs at surgical incisions or insertion sites of vascular access catheters. Mucosal and urinary bleeding are common, whereas pulmonary, gastrointestinal, and central nervous system bleeding occur less frequently. Because of widespread intravascular coagulation, tissue ischemia can occur, resulting in cyanosis, delirium, oliguria, hypoxia, and frank tissue necrosis (Figure 56-2).

6. **What laboratory abnormalities are typical of acute DIC?**

Thrombocytopenia; prolongation of the PT, aPTT, and thrombin time; and hypofibrinogenemia are characteristic. Early in the course of DIC, the platelet count may be in the normal range but is often decreased from baseline. Platelet counts are rarely less than $20,000/mm^3$. D-dimer and fibrin degradation product (FDP) levels are almost always markedly elevated. The haptoglobin level is variably affected and is not helpful in confirming the diagnosis of DIC.

7. **Is the peripheral blood smear useful in the diagnosis of DIC?**

The peripheral blood smear from a patient typically shows mild to moderate thrombocytopenia. The finding of schistocytes (red blood cell fragments created by intravascular hemolysis) (Figure 56-3) is neither sensitive nor specific, and schistocytes are present in only 10% to 50% of cases of acute DIC. If present in DIC, there are usually only one to four per high-power field, in contrast to thrombotic thrombocytopenic purpura where they are much more abundant.

8. **What conditions make interpretation of laboratory abnormalities in DIC more difficult?**

Fibrinogen is an acute-phase reactant. As such, it can be within the normal range in occasional patients with acute DIC, especially if an underlying inflammatory disorder exists; comparison with a baseline value would therefore be useful. In addition, the D-dimer can be chronically elevated in patients with cancer and in those with recent clots or liver disease (see later).

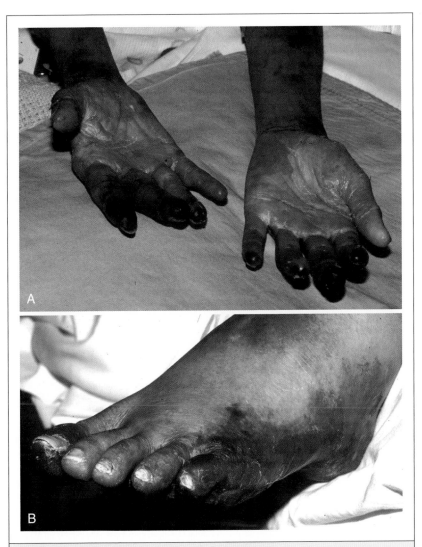

Figure 56-2. Ischemic necrosis of fingers (**A**) and feet (**B**) of patient with disseminated intravascular coagulation as a result of bacterial sepsis.

9. **Why is it difficult to make the diagnosis of DIC in patients with advanced liver disease?**

The liver produces most coagulation proteins, and most cases of advanced liver disease are characterized by a prolonged PT and aPTT with decreased fibrinogen. The liver is also responsible for clearing D-dimers, which are therefore often elevated in liver disease. Additionally, the platelet count may be reduced in patients with cirrhosis due to hypersplenism and reduced production of thrombopoietin by the liver.

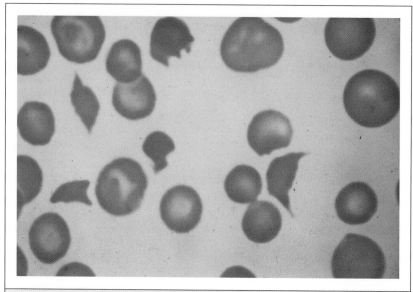

Figure 56-3. Schistocytes in peripheral blood smear of patient with severe acute disseminated intravascular coagulation. Note also the absence of platelets.

10. **When and how is DIC treated?**

Because DIC tends to be secondary to other disorders, addressing the underlying disorder is the mainstay of treatment. Therapy is otherwise supportive. Blood products should be administered in cases of DIC complicated by clinically significant bleeding or a significantly elevated risk of bleeding (e.g., a patient with recent vascular surgery) and are not routinely required. Blood components should not be given solely in response to laboratory abnormalities.

11. **How should blood products be administered in cases of acute DIC?**

Platelet transfusions should be reserved for patients with signs of clinical bleeding; a platelet goal of $>30,000/mm^3$ with minor bleeding or $>50,000/mm^3$ with major bleeding is reasonable in DIC, except in patients with recent major neurosurgical procedures where platelet counts of $>100,000/mm^3$ may be required. Cryoprecipitate may be administered to keep the fibrinogen level >80 to 100 mg/dL. Fresh frozen plasma should be given only if clinically significant bleeding is present or if a significant risk for bleeding exists (e.g., for invasive procedures); it should not be used solely to *correct* a prolonged PT or aPTT. It should also be noted that international normalized ratio values of up to 1.7 are not associated with an increased risk for bleeding. Paradoxically, blood products are not associated with a worsening of DIC. See Figure 56-4 for additional details.

12. **Are there special causes of DIC that require specific treatment?**

HELLP syndrome is a peripartum form of DIC, resulting in clinically significant hepatic injury and hemolytic anemia. In addition to supportive care, treatment for HELLP includes either delivery of the fetus or dilatation and curettage to remove retained fetal or placental fragments. Acute promyelocytic leukemia is almost always associated with DIC. In addition to appropriate transfusions for the treatment of DIC, urgent initiation of chemotherapy, which should include all-*trans*retinoic acid, is indicated.

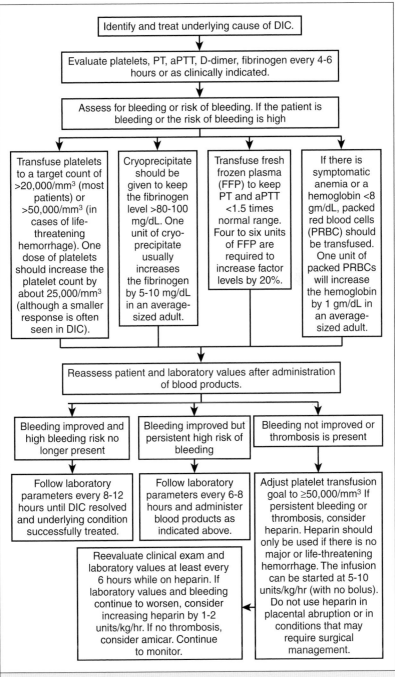

Figure 56-4. Treatment algorithm for disseminated intravascular coagulation.

13. **In what scenarios should heparin be considered for the treatment of DIC?**
In cases of acute DIC characterized by clinically significant bleeding despite administration of blood products or in thrombotic DIC with digital ischemia, heparin may be considered. Heparin should be used with caution, as it can exacerbate bleeding. The rationale for using heparin is to limit microvascular clotting in DIC and thus correct the resultant consumptive coagulopathy. Use of heparin requires that the platelet count be maintained at $>50,000/mm^3$ and that there be no concurrent gastrointestinal or central nervous system bleeding. Heparin is contraindicated in conditions that require surgical management, such as retained uterine placental tissue. In addition, its use should be avoided in patients with placental abruption.

14. **How should heparin be administered?**
No bolus dose should be given. A continuous infusion of unfractionated heparin, 5 to 10 units/kg per hour, is reasonable, until the bleeding has lessened or stopped and/or the underlying clinical condition has been effectively treated. Low-molecular-weight heparin has not been adequately studied for the treatment of acute DIC complicated by bleeding, and its use cannot currently be recommended.

15. **What other agents have been considered for use in DIC?**
Fibrinolysis inhibitors, such as ε-aminocaproic acid (Amicar) and tranexamic acid, can be used to treat DIC-associated refractory bleeding by preventing systemic fibrinolysis. However, these inhibitors should be administered with caution in DIC as they can worsen systemic fibrin deposition. Combining their use with low-dose heparin infusion is one way to avoid converting a patient with hemorrhage into one with life-threatening thrombosis. In addition, no role exists for recombinant VIIa or activated plasma-derived clotting factors in the treatment of DIC.

16. **How is the efficacy of DIC treatment evaluated?**
Laboratory parameters, including the PT, aPTT, fibrinogen, and platelet count, should be followed and should return to baseline levels as the disorder is effectively treated. In addition, clinical bleeding should improve. The D-dimer should also decline with treatment but may remain persistently elevated from other causes (unresolved clot, liver failure). The time course of recovery from DIC is usually linked to recovery from the underlying illness.

17. **What treatments are controversial in DIC?**
Randomized trials in patients with DIC are lacking. Because DIC is associated with mortality in sepsis, recombinant activated protein C (drotrecogin alfa) was approved in 2001 for use in severe sepsis with organ failure. However, use of drotrecogin alfa is associated with an increased risk of bleeding, and the agent was withdrawn from the market in 2011 after follow-up studies failed to demonstrate efficacy.

18. **What new treatments may be available in the future for DIC?**
A number of treatments directed against either the aberrant coagulation or fibrinolysis seen in DIC have been proposed. Recently, recombinant thrombomodulin (which operates in the same pathway as protein C) has shown promising results in an unrandomized trial using historical controls. Antithrombin concentrate has also been evaluated in small uncontrolled trials but has not demonstrated benefit. Other agents that have been proposed for the treatment of DIC include recombinant tissue factor pathway inhibitor (failed to demonstrate efficacy in a phase III trial), recombinant factor VIIa (yet to undergo large randomized trials), recombinant hirudin (animal studies only), and recombinant nematode anticoagulant c2 (animal studies only).

KEY POINTS: DISSEMINATED INTRAVASCULAR COAGULATION

1. Definition: DIC is a syndrome involving the activation of both coagulation and fibrinolysis, resulting in the intravascular deposition of fibrin and the consumption of coagulation proteins and platelets, which commonly leads to bleeding.

2. Importance: DIC can lead to organ dysfunction and is associated with high mortality.

3. Diagnosis: No single laboratory test can be used to diagnose DIC. Instead, a combination of a prolonged aPTT and PT, decreased fibrinogen, decreased platelets, increased D-dimer or FDPs, and schistocytes on a blood smear in an appropriate clinical context may suggest the diagnosis.

4. Treatment: Management of DIC should focus primarily on treatment of the underlying disorder.

BIBLIOGRAPHY

1. Abraham E, Reinhart K, Opal S, et al: Efficacy and safety of tifacogin (recombinant tissue factor pathway inhibitor) in severe sepsis: a randomized controlled trial. JAMA 290:238-247, 2003.

2. Abraham E, Reinhart K, Svoboda P, et al: Assessment of the safety of recombinant tissue factor pathway inhibitor in patients with severe sepsis: a multicenter, randomized, placebo-controlled, single-blind, dose escalation study. Crit Care Med 29:2081-2089, 2001.

3. Asakura H, Ontachi Y, Mizutani T, et al: An enhanced fibrinolysis prevents the development of multiple organ failure in disseminated intravascular coagulation in spite of much activation of blood coagulation. Crit Care Med 29:1164-1168, 2001.

4. Bick RL: Disseminated intravascular coagulation: objective clinical and laboratory diagnosis, treatment, and assessment of therapeutic response. Semin Thromb Hemost 22:69-88, 1996.

5. Hermida J, Montes R, Paramo JA, et al: Endotoxin-induced disseminated intravascular coagulation in rabbits: effect of recombinant hirudin on hemostatic parameters, fibrin deposits, and mortality. J Lab Clin Med 131:77-83, 1998.

6. Kitchens CS: Thrombocytopenia and thrombosis in disseminated intravascular coagulation (DIC). Hematology Am Soc Hematol Educ Program 2009:240-246, 2009.

7. Levi M, Ten Cate H: Disseminated intravascular coagulation. N Engl J Med 341:586-592, 1999.

8. Manios SG, Kanakoudi F, Maniati E: Fulminant meningococcemia. Heparin therapy and survival rate. Scand J Infect Disease 3:127-133, 1971.

9. Schmaier AH: Disseminated intravascular coagulation. N Engl J Med 341:1937-1938, 1999.

10. Segal J, Dzik W: Paucity of studies to support that abnormal coagulation test results predict bleeding in the setting of invasive procedures: an evidence-based review. Transfusion 45:1413, 2005.

11. Stouthard JM, Levi M, Hack CE, et al: Interleukin-6 stimulates coagulation, not fibrinolysis, in humans. Thromb Haemost 76:738-742, 1996.

12. Toussaint S, Gerlach H: Activated protein C for sepsis. N Engl J Med 361:2646-2652, 2009.

13. Yamakawa K, Fujimi S, Mohri T, et al: Treatment effects of recombinant human soluble thrombomodulin in patients with severe sepsis: a historical control study. Crit Care 15:R123, 2011.

CHAPTER 57

ONCOLOGIC EMERGENCIES (INCLUDING HYPERCALCEMIA)

Marie E. Wood, MD

1. **Define oncologic emergency.**
   A unique set of complications associated with patients with cancer requiring emergent evaluation and treatment.

2. **List the four types of oncologic emergencies, and give examples of each.**
   - **Metabolic:** Tumor lysis syndrome, hypercalcemia, syndrome of inappropriate antidiuretic hormone, lactic acidosis
   - **Structural or mechanical:** Spinal cord compression, superior vena cava (SVC) syndrome, malignant pericardial effusion
   - **Hematologic:** Neutropenic fever, leukostasis, disseminated intravascular coagulation, thrombosis, hyperviscosity
   - **Side effects of chemotherapy:** Extravasation, hemorrhagic cystitis, typhlitis

METABOLIC EMERGENCIES

3. **What are the symptoms of hypercalcemia?**
   Symptoms can be vague but most classically include lethargy, confusion, anorexia, nausea, constipation, polyuria, and polydipsia. Hypercalcemia occurs in 10% to 30% of individuals with advanced or metastatic cancer.

4. **What are the important treatments for hypercalcemia?**
   - Hydration: Use normal saline solution, watching for congestive heart failure.
   - Bisphosphonate therapy: The most common choices of therapy include either pamidronate 60 to 90 mg intravenously (IV) over a 2- to 4-hour period or zoledronic acid 4 mg IV over a 15-minute period (the latter must be adjusted for renal insufficiency).
   - Stop medications that contribute to hypercalcemia: calcium, vitamin D, thiazide diuretics.

5. **Discuss reasons for not using furosemide (Lasix), calcitonin glucocorticoids, and other older therapies.**
   The easy answer is that bisphosphonates work much better. However, furosemide can be helpful but only if the patient is hydrated. Calcitonin works but only for a short time. Glucocorticoids are really only a temporizing measure.

6. **Which patients with cancer are at risk for lactic acidosis?**
   Lactic acidosis is a rare complication of malignancy and is seen in patients who have cancer with a high proliferative rate such as lymphoma, leukemia, and small cell carcinoma.

7. **How does lactic acidosis present, and how should it be treated?**
   Common symptoms include tachypnea, tachycardia, abdominal pain, and hepatomegaly. Mortality is very high and institution of chemotherapy the most effective treatment.

8. **Can tumor lysis syndrome be prevented?**
   Absolutely yes, with early initiation of allopurinol or rasburicase, close monitoring of laboratory values, and aggressive hydration.

9. **Which patients are at risk for tumor lysis syndrome?**
   Patients with large tumor burden and tumors with a high proliferative rate that are highly sensitive to chemotherapy (acute myelogenous leukemia, acute lymphocytic leukemia, Burkitt lymphoma, multiple myeloma, small cell carcinoma) are at risk for tumor lysis. Dehydration, renal insufficiency or obstruction, or elevated lactate dehydrogenase (LDH) or uric acid level before initiation of chemotherapy may increase the risk for complications from tumor lysis.

10. **Can tumor lysis happen before administering therapy?**
    Yes, tumor lysis can be seen in very actively growing tumors with a high proliferative rate.

11. **Discuss the features of tumor lysis syndrome.**
    Tumor lysis is caused by release of cell contents into the bloodstream. Therefore patients have elevated levels of LDH, uric acid, potassium, urea nitrogen, creatinine, and phosphate, and low calcium.

12. **How should tumor lysis be treated?**
    Patients at risk should start taking allopurinol (300-600 mg/day for 2 days) and be aggressively hydrated before initiation of chemotherapy. If tumor lysis develops despite these measures patients should have alkalinization of urine with forced diuresis with furosemide and frequent monitoring of urine volume, cardiac and volume status, and laboratory values (blood urea nitrogen, creatinine, uric acid, calcium, phosphate, and potassium levels).

13. **When should rasburicase be used?**
    Rasburicase promotes the degradation of uric acid whereas allopurinol decreases the formation of uric acid. One study shows improved control of uric acid compared with allopurinol. Rasburicase can be considered in patients with very high uric acid level in need of urgent treatment.

STRUCTURAL EMERGENCIES

14. **What is the single most important predictor of functional status for a patient with cord compression?**
    The neurologic status at presentation predicts functional status after treatment. Patients presenting with pain only are far more likely to be ambulatory after treatment than patients presenting with neurologic dysfunction.

15. **Because back pain is common, how can you distinguish pain due to cord compression from other back pain?**
    The cardinal features of cord compression include pain that worsens when supine and that can be reproduced with vertebral percussion. Additional findings of cord compression include constipation and incontinence (usually due to overflow incontinence) and sensory loss.

16. **Should a patient with suspected cord compression receive steroids before imaging studies?**
    Therapy for cord compression should be initiated as soon as possible after imaging studies have been done. However, it is not wrong to give steroids (dexamethasone 10-20 mg IV) before imaging for a patient with symptoms.

17. **How important is a tissue biopsy in a patient with cord compression?**
A tissue biopsy is critical for a patient without a cancer diagnosis or with cancer that uncommonly metastasized to bone (as a second malignancy may exist). Biopsy is less important for patients with known metastatic malignancy.

18. **Should patients with cord compromise be evaluated for surgery?**
Absolutely, yes. Although the mainstay of treatment had been steroids and radiation therapy a seminal paper published in 2005 demonstrated that patients treated with surgery (compared with radiation) were more likely to walk after treatment (84% vs. 57%), retained the ability to walk significantly longer, and required fewer steroids and less narcotic analgesia.

19. **Are there any patients with cord compression who should receive chemotherapy?**
Chemotherapy should be considered for patients with very chemosensitive tumors such as myeloma, small cell carcinoma, and lymphoma.

20. **How do patients with brain metastasis commonly present?**
Patients may present with headache, and classically this is a headache that worsens at night, may wake the patient from sleep, and may be associated with nausea and/or vomiting. Patients may have seizures or isolated neurologic findings. A careful neurologic examination in a patient with cancer is required to determine whether the lesion is central or in the spinal cord. The most common primary tumors with metastasis to the brain include lung cancer, breast cancer, and melanoma, although any cancer can metastasize to the brain.

21. **What is the best test for identifying central nervous system (CNS) metastasis?**
The gold standard is magnetic resonance imaging with gadolinium. Computed tomography scanning is less sensitive and may miss multiple small metastases.

22. **How should a patient with brain metastasis be treated?**
Patients with symptomatic brain metastasis should be given steroids. Resection can be considered for a solitary lesion in an accessible area. This should be followed by whole brain radiation. Stereotactic radiosurgery may be an option for individuals with one to three lesions and lesions less than 2 to 3 cm. Whole brain radiation would be the treatment of choice for individuals with multiple lesions. Chemotherapy is almost never used for control of brain metastasis.

23. **What about anticonvulsant therapy?**
Anticonvulsant therapy should not be started empirically.

24. **Patients with what tumor types are most likely to present with SVC syndrome?**
SVC syndrome is caused by invasion or compression of the SVC. Invasion of the SVC is seen in thrombosis, which can develop in any patient with cancer and a central line. Compression of the SVC is most commonly associated with lung cancer (both small and non–small cell types), lymphoma, and germ cell tumors. SVC syndrome can also occur as a result of radiation-induced fibrosis.

25. **Discuss the signs and symptoms of SVC syndrome.**
The most common symptom is dyspnea. Patients may also complain of facial and/or arm swelling, head fullness, and/or headache. Symptoms may worsen with bending over or lying down. Rarely patients may present with confusion and coma related to SVC compression or invasion.

26. **How should SVC syndrome be treated?**
    The urgency of treatment should be guided by symptoms. Occasionally patients will present with stridor (due to airway obstruction or laryngeal edema), respiratory distress, or even coma. In this case stent placement and/or radiation should be considered. In less urgent situations care should be directed at obtaining a diagnosis as this may direct therapy. Options may include the following:
    - Stent placement: Percutaneous endovascular stents have been shown to provide effective symptom relief.
    - Steroids: Steroids are used to reduce edema or treat lymphoma.
    - Chemotherapy: Chemotherapy should be considered for very chemosensitive tumors such as germ cell, lymphoma, and small cell carcinomas.
    - Radiation: Radiation is used less commonly now but is still an important palliative modality.
    - Anticoagulation and/or thrombolytics: These can be helpful and considered for patients with thrombosis.
    - Support: Elevation of the head and/or diuretics can provide relief of symptoms.

27. **Who is at risk for a malignant pericardial effusion?**
    Any and all cancers have been associated with pericardial effusions. Effusions are most commonly seen in association with lung cancer and less commonly seen with breast and esophageal cancer, melanoma, lymphoma, and leukemia. Rarely pericardial effusions have been seen with radiation fibrosis.

28. **How should a malignant pericardial effusion be treated?**
    The fluid should be drained and sent for cytologic analysis. This is important for patients without a diagnosed malignancy. The effusion can recur, and a pericardial window may be necessary.

HEMATOLOGIC EMERGENCIES

29. **What is leukostasis, and who gets it?**
    Leukostasis is seen in patients with elevated blast counts (usually over 30,000). Although hyperleukocytosis (white blood cell count over 50,000) is commonly seen with acute and chronic leukemia, leukostasis is seen with acute myeloid and lymphoid leukemia and chronic myeloid leukemia in blast crisis. Symptoms relate to decreased tissue perfusion due to microvascular changes. The most common symptoms are dyspnea, hypoxia, and those affecting the central nervous system (CNS): visual changes, headache, dizziness, tinnitus, gait instability, confusion, somnolence, and, occasionally, coma.

30. **How is leukostasis treated?**
    The goal of treatment is to reduce the blast count. This can be done quickly with hydroxyurea (50-100 mg/kg) and leukapheresis. These are temporizing measures, and definitive treatment should be initiated as soon as possible.

31. **Should a blood transfusion be avoided in patients with leukostasis?**
    Yes, as transfusion can increase blood viscosity and potentially worsen symptoms.

32. **Define neutropenic fever.**
    A neutropenic fever is defined as a single temperature over 38.3° C (101° F) or sustained temperature (over a 1-hour period) of 38° C (100.5° F) in a patient with an absolute neutrophil count of less than 500 cells/mm^3.

33. **Is a neutropenic fever ever fatal?**
    Yes, but prompt evaluation and treatment essentially eliminate this risk.

34. **What should be included in the evaluation of a patient with neutropenia?**
Patients suspected of having a neutropenic fever should have a thorough examination looking for potential sources of infection. A laboratory evaluation, including a complete blood cell count and differential, at least two blood cultures (one being from central venous access if present), chest radiograph, and culture of appropriate sites, is indicated.

35. **Should the preceding evaluation be complete before the institution of antibiotics?**
Absolutely not; antibiotics should be started immediately after the blood cultures are obtained.

36. **What would be considered appropriate antibiotic coverage for a neutropenic fever?**
Broad-spectrum IV therapy covering serious gram-negative bacteria and *Pseudomonas aeruginosa* is appropriate. Monotherapy with cefepime, ceftazidime, carbapenem, or piperacillin-tazobactam are all appropriate choices.

37. **Does empirical vancomycin improve survival for neutropenic fever?**
No, but vancomycin should be started if concern exists for a catheter-related skin or soft tissue infection, pneumonia, or hemodynamic instability.

38. **How long should a neutropenic fever be treated?**
The short answer is until both the neutropenia and fever resolve. Antibiotic coverage appropriate for the identified organism may be continued for the appropriate duration (i.e., for fungal sepsis). Coverage may be modified on the basis of cultures and sensitivities; however, a broad spectrum of coverage should be maintained until the neutropenia resolves.

39. **Venous thromboembolism is common in patients with cancer; when is it considered an emergency?**
Patients with massive clot burden and/or limb-threatening disease (i.e., phlegmasia cerulea dolens) would be considered in need of emergent interventions. These patients may be considered for thrombectomy or thrombolysis.

SIDE EFFECTS OF CHEMOTHERAPY

40. **What is typhlitis?**
Typhlitis or neutropenic enterocolitis is often a diagnosis of exclusion. The pathophysiology is not well understood but seems to be a combination of mucosal injury and neutropenia. The cecum is almost always involved, commonly with extension to the ascending colon and terminal ileum. Typhlitis is seen more commonly in patients with hematologic malignancy although it can be seen in any patients with severe mucosal injury from chemotherapy (such as capecitabine).

41. **How should typhlitis be managed?**
Patients should initially be evaluated by a surgeon because typhlitis is often a diagnosis of exclusion, and other abdominal catastrophes should be excluded. Patients with perforation, peritonitis, or bleeding should be taken to the operating room. If not going to the operating room, patients' conditions should be conservatively managed with the following:
- Bowel rest with nasogastric suction.
- Hydration and nutritional support.
- Blood product (packed red blood cells and platelets) support as needed.
- Antibiotic coverage is reasonable, and antifungal coverage may be considered for patients with persistent fever.

Avoid anticholinergic, antidiarrheal, or opioid agents as their use may create or aggravate ileus. Granulocyte colony-stimulating factor may be considered for patients expected to have a prolonged and/or profound neutropenia.

KEY POINTS: CHARACTERISTICS OF TUMOR LYSIS

1. Increased LDH level

2. Increased uric acid level

3. Increased phosphorus level

4. Increased potassium level

5. Increased blood urea nitrogen and creatinine levels

6. Decreased calcium level

BIBLIOGRAPHY

1. Cairo M, Bishop M: Tumour lysis syndrome: new therapeutic strategies and classification. Br J Haematol 127:3-11, 2004.

2. Cortes J, Moore JO, Maziarz RT, et al: Control of plasma uric acid in adults at risk for tumor lysis syndrome: efficacy and safety of rasburicase alone and rasburicase followed by allopurinol compared with allopurinol alone—results of a multicenter phase III study. J Clin Oncol 28:4207-4213, 2010.

3. Freifeld AG, Bow EJ, Sepkowitz KA, et al: Clinical practice guideline for the use of antimicrobial agents in neutropenic patients with cancer: 2010 update by the Infectious Diseases Society of America. Clin Infect Dis 52: e56-e93, 2011.

4. Jabr FI: Lactic acidosis in patients with neoplasms: an oncologic emergency. Mayo Clin Proc 81:1505-1506, author reply 1506, 2006.

5. Jenkinson MD, Haylock B, Shenoy A, et al: Management of cerebral metastasis: evidence-based approach for surgery, stereotactic radiosurgery and radiotherapy. Eur J Cancer 47:649-655, 2011.

6. Lepper PM, Ott SR, Hoppe H, et al: Superior vena cava syndrome in thoracic malignancies. Respir Care 56:653-666, 2011.

7. Lewis MA, Hendrickson AW, Moynihan TJ: Oncologic emergencies: pathophysiology, presentation, diagnosis, and treatment. CA Cancer J Clin 61:287-314, 2011.

8. Patchell RA, Tibbs PA, Regine WF, et al: Direct decompressive surgical resection in the treatment of spinal cord compression caused by metastatic cancer: a randomised trial. Lancet 366:643-648, 2005.

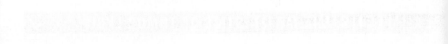

RHEUMATOLOGIC DISEASE IN THE INTENSIVE CARE UNIT

Lynda S. Tilluckdharry, MB, BCh, BAO, LRCP&SI, and Christine Haas Jones, MD

CHAPTER 58

1. **A critically ill patient is seen with an acute hot, swollen joint. What is the next step in management? What are the most common organisms found in a septic joint?**

   Aspiration of the joint should be performed immediately to rule out a septic joint, crystalline disease, or other inflammatory forms of arthritis. The synovial fluid should be sent for cell count and differential, Gram stain, culture, and crystalline analysis. High fevers and elevated inflammatory markers: erythrocyte sedimentation rate (ESR), C-reactive protein, and white cell counts, may be found in both infection and crystalline arthropathy. It is important to remember that septic arthritis and crystal-induced arthropathy can occur concurrently in a joint.

   In all age and risk groups, the most common causative organisms of septic arthritis are *Staphylococcus aureus* and *Streptococci* strains. In nursing home patients, intravenous abusers, elderly people, and patients with recent orthopedic procedures, consider *methicillin-resistant S. aureus*. These populations are also susceptible to mixed bacterial infections, gram-negative organisms, fungal infections, and unusual organisms. In young adults, consider *Neisseria gonorrhoeae* as a cause of septic arthritis. Treatment includes prompt removal of purulent material from the joint space and initiation of appropriate intravenous antibiotics targeting suspected organisms. Serial arthrocentesis or open surgical drainage may be necessary.

2. **List the risk factors for the development of septic arthritis.**
   - Diabetes
   - Alcoholism
   - Joint prosthesis
   - Intravenous drug abuse
   - Skin infections or cutaneous ulcers
   - Recent joint surgery or intraarticular corticosteroid injection
   - Age: elderly or young
   - Previous joint pathologic condition, for example, rheumatoid arthritis (RA), osteoarthritis, or crystal-induced arthropathy

3. **Name the common risk factors for gout.**
   - Surgery
   - Dehydration
   - Drugs such as diuretics
   - High purine intake in diet
   - Trauma
   - Infections
   - Renal insufficiency
   - Excess alcohol intake

TABLE 58-1. SYNOVIAL FLUID ANALYSIS

TOTAL WHITE CELL COUNT (/MM³)	PMN CELLS (%)	APPEARANCE	FLUID TYPE	COMMONLY ASSOCIATED CONDITIONS
0-200	<10	Pale yellow, clear	Normal	
200-2000	<20	Clear or slightly cloudy	Noninflammatory	Osteoarthritis, joint trauma, avascular necrosis
2000-50,000	20-70	Slightly cloudy	Inflammatory	Crystalline arthropathy— gout or pseudogout, RA, psoriatic arthritis, sarcoidosis, infectious arthritis, vasculitis, HLA B27–related arthritis (e.g., reactive arthritis, ankylosing spondylitis)
>50,000	>70	Cloudy or opaque	Pyarthrosis	Septic arthritis, pseudosepsis— gout, reactive arthritis, and RA

HLA, Human leukocyte antigen; *PMN*, polymorphonuclear; *RA*, rheumatoid arthritis.

4. **How do you interpret synovial fluid analysis?**
   See Table 58-1.

5. **What specific precautions should be taken when performing intubation in a patient with RA?**
   Cervical spine disorders occur in 30% to 50% of patients with RA. The most common presentation of cervical spine arthritis is C1-C2 subluxation or atlantoaxial subluxation (AAS). Vertical and subaxial subluxation occurs less commonly. It is prudent for providers to use caution when performing any manipulations of the cervical spine, particularly endotracheal intubation in patients with RA. Spinal cord compression due to C1 and C2 instability may lead to neurologic deficits or death. Lateral and flexion cervical spine radiographs or magnetic resonance imaging should be obtained before intubation in the following situations:
   - RA duration >3 years
   - Long-term use of corticosteroid
   - Severe peripheral joint deformities from RA
   - Male sex
   - Neck pain

- Risk factors for osteoporosis
- Prior cervical spine subluxation
- Clinical evidence of cervical myelopathy
  If clinical or radiographic evidence of subluxation exists and intubation is required, an anesthesiologist should be present during the procedure. In patients with AAS, subluxation is

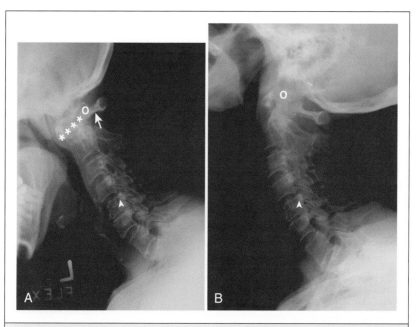

Figure 58-1. Rheumatoid arthritis of the cervical spine. (From Firestein GS, Budd RC, Harris ED, et al: Kelley's Textbook of Rheumatology, 8th ed, vol 1. Philadelphia, Saunders, 2008, p 810.)

worsened with cervical flexion and reduced by cervical extension. Cricoarytenoid arthritis may also complicate endotracheal intubation. These patients may present with symptoms of tracheal pain, stridor, dysphonia, and shortness of breath (see Fig. 58-1).

6. **What is scleroderma renal crisis (SRC)? When should this diagnosis be considered, and how is it confirmed?**
   SRC will occur in 15% of patients with systemic sclerosis (SSc). SRC is a medical emergency and presents with an abrupt onset of hypertension (>150/85 mm Hg) and acute renal failure (>30% reduction of glomerular filtration rate). SRC can precede the diagnosis of SSc, and patients can initially be seen with normal blood pressures.
   - *Clinical symptoms* include headaches, visual disturbances from hypertensive retinopathy, seizures, encephalopathy, fever, general malaise, pulmonary edema. Less commonly, patients may have arrhythmias, myocarditis, and pericarditis.
   - *Laboratory tests* typically show an elevated creatinine level, microangiopathic hemolytic anemia, and thrombocytopenia. Urinalysis may show mild proteinuria, hematuria, and granular casts.

7. **Who is at risk for SRC, and what are risk factors indicating poor prognosis? What treatment should be initiated in SRC?**

The major risk factors for the development of SRC are early diffuse cutaneous systemic sclerosis, positive antinuclear antibody (ANA) with a diffuse speckled pattern, rapidly progressive skin disease, and recent corticosteroid use. Patients with positive anti-fibrillarin, anti-U1RNP, and RNA polymerase I and II antibodies are at a higher risk for SRC.

Poor prognosis for recovery from SRC is associated with the following:

- Male sex
- Age >50 years
- Persistent renal failure
- Initial presentation with normal blood pressure

Treatment should include early therapy with angiotensin-converting enzyme inhibitors (ACEi) such as captopril and lisinopril. To avoid hypoperfusion, ensure gradual decrease in blood pressure with other antihypertensives such as calcium channel blockers, nitrates, and β-blockers. Transient mild increases in creatinine level are common and are not an indication to stop the ACEi. Many patients will require supportive care with dialysis, and kidney function may take up to 3 years to improve. Plasma exchange can be considered in patients with microscopic angiopathy.

8. **What conditions can be associated with a positive ANA test in a critical care patient?**

- Systemic lupus erythematosus (SLE) or drug-induced lupus
- Mixed connective tissue disease
- Autoimmune liver disease
- Systemic sclerosis
- Sjögren syndrome
- RA
- Polymyositis (PM)
- Malignancy
- Thyroid disease
- Miscellaneous: normal population (5%-10%), elderly (20%), medications

9. **How do you interpret a positive ANA test? What additional investigations should be ordered if there is a positive ANA test?**

In isolation, a positive ANA test should not be used to make a specific diagnosis, and a negative ANA does not exclude an autoimmune condition. In most laboratories an ANA titer of >1:40 is considered positive, and clinically significant titers are usually >1:160.

Additional investigations that should be obtained include double-stranded DNA (dsDNA), SS-A (Ro) and SS-B (La) antibodies, Smith antigen (Sm), ribonuclear protein (RNP), centromere antibody, urinalysis, complement levels (C3 and C4), and a complete blood cell count with differential, which may show leucopenia and lymphopenia.

10. **What clinical findings in a patient whose condition is deteriorating would prompt the consideration of SLE?**

- Unexplained fevers
- Unexplained neurologic symptoms such as altered mental status, seizures, psychosis (lupus cerebritis)
- Renal abnormalities with proteinuria and cellular casts (lupus nephritis)
- Hematologic disorders such as hemolytic anemia
- Serositis such as pericardial effusion and pleural effusion
- Multiorgan failure

TABLE 58-2. CLINICAL FEATURES AND INVESTIGATIONS OF ANTIPHOSPHOLIPID SYNDROME

CLINICAL FEATURES	INVESTIGATIONS
Hematologic: recurrent venous or arterial thromboses, thrombocytopenia, hemolytic anemia, renal thrombotic microangiopathy **Neurologic:** stroke, transient ischemic attacks, seizures, transverse myelitis, migraines, chorea, multiinfarct dementia **Cutaneous:** livedo reticularis, distal gangrene, thrombophlebitis **Pulmonary:** embolism, intraalveolar hemorrhage, hypertension **Cardiac:** valvular disease (vegetations), myocardial infarction **Musculoskeletal:** osteonecrosis **Obstetric:** recurrent miscarriages, placental insufficiency, preeclampsia, or severe eclampsia	• False-positive serologic test for syphilis: VDRL test or rapid plasma reagin • Prolonged activated partial thromboplastin time • Prolonged Russell viper venom time (lupus anticoagulant) • Positive anti-cardiolipin antibody • Positive $\beta2$ glycoprotein 1 antibody

VDRL, Venereal Disease Research Laboratory.

MD SOAP 'N HAIR: Malar rash, **D**iscoid rash, **S**erositis, **O**ral ulcer, **A**rthritis, **P**hotosensitivity, **N**eurologic abnormality, **H**ematologic abnormality, **A**NA (positive), **I**mmunologic abnormality, **R**enal involvement.

TABLE 58-3. AUTOANTIBODIES AND ASSOCIATED DISORDERS

AUTOANTIBODY	DISORDER
Rheumatoid factor	RA (80%); SLE (10%); MCTD (50%-60%); Sjögren syndrome (80%-90%); infections; chronic liver and pulmonary disease and cryoglobulinemia (>40%)
Anti–cyclic citrulline peptide antibody	RA
ANA profile	
• Anti-dsDNA	SLE
• Anti-Sm (Smith antigen)	SLE
• Anti-SS-A	Sjögren syndrome (70%); SLE (30%); RA; scleroderma and MCTD (rare)

(Continued)

TABLE 58-3. AUTOANTIBODIES AND ASSOCIATED DISORDERS—*cont'd*

AUTOANTIBODY	DISORDER
Anti-SS-B	Sjögren syndrome (60%); SLE (15%); RA; scleroderma; MCTD (rare)
Anti-RNP	MCTD (95%); SLE (30%)
Anti–Scl-70	Diffuse scleroderma (20%-40%)
Anti-centromere	Limited scleroderma (60%-90%); diffuse scleroderma (30%)
Anti-histone	Drug-induced lupus erythematosus
Anti–Jo-1	Polymyositis
Anti–neutrophilic cytoplasmic antibody	Vasculitis

MCTD, Mixed connective tissue disease; *RA*, rheumatoid arthritis; *RNP*, ribonuclear protein; *SLE*, systemic lupus erythematosus.

11. **Describe antiphospholipid syndrome (APS).**

APS is an acquired cause of hypercoagulability. Fifty percent of patients with APS have SLE. Recurrent venous and arterial thromboses and embolism are the hallmark of this syndrome. See Table 58-2.

Catastrophic APS is a rare presentation with 50% mortality and usually is characterized by widespread small vessel thrombosis with multiorgan failure.

12. **What other laboratory evaluations may be useful in the diagnosis of other connective tissue disorders?**

See Table 58-3.

BOX 58-1. CONDITIONS ASSOCIATED WITH POSITIVE ANTINEUTROPHIL CYTOPLASMIC ANTIBODY

P-ANCA

MPO positive:
Microscopic polyarteritis
Churg-Strauss vasculitis
Pauci immune glomerulonephritis
Drug-induced ANCA vasculitis
    (minocycline, hydralazine,
    propylthiouracil)
Wegener granulomatosis (10%)
Goodpasture disease

MPO negative:
Autoimmune disease (RA, SLE, Sjögren)
Ulcerative colitis
Cystic fibrosis
Infections (HIV, subacute bacterial
    endocarditis, parvovirus, EBV)
Malignancy

> ### BOX 58-1. CONDITIONS ASSOCIATED WITH POSITIVE ANTINEUTROPHIL CYTOPLASMIC ANTIBODY—cont'd
>
> #### C-ANCA
>
> **PR3 positive:**
>
> Wegener granulomatosis (80%-90%) Churg-Strauss vasculitis (rare)
> Microscopic polyarteritis Goodpasture disease (rare) Drug-induced ANCA
> vasculitis (rare)
>
> *ANCA,* Antineutrophil cytoplasmic antibody; *EBV,* Epstein-Barr virus; *MPO,* myeloperoxidase; *PR3,* serine proteinase-3; *RA,* rheumatoid arthritis; *SLE,* systemic lupus erythematosus.

13. **Patients with antineutrophil cytoplasmic antibody (ANCA)–associated vasculitis frequently are seen in the intensive care unit (ICU). What diseases are associated with a positive ANCA test?**

    Systemic vasculitis is categorized into small, medium, and large vessel involvement. It should be considered in any patient with rapidly progressive multisystemic organ dysfunction, pulmonary-renal syndromes, or unexplained stroke or in young persons with ischemic signs, fever of unknown origin, unexplained constitutional symptoms, purpuric skin lesions, and/or mononeuritis multiplex.

    There are two forms of ANCA: cytoplasmic (c-ANCA) and perinuclear (p-ANCA). If the ANCA is positive, two target antigens should also be checked: myeloperoxidase (MPO) and serine proteinase-3 (PR3). See Box 58-1.

14. **Diffuse alveolar hemorrhage (DAH) is a common presentation to the ICU. What are the clinical features? What are the common autoimmune conditions associated with DAH?**

    DAH is a catastrophic clinical syndrome caused by the accumulation of intraalveolar red blood cells from the alveolar capillaries. Patients may present with hemoptysis, anemia, radiographic findings of diffuse pulmonary infiltrates, and respiratory failure. In up to a third of cases, hemoptysis may be initially absent and patients may only describe symptoms of fever, chest pain, shortness of breath, or cough. High clinical suspicion is essential to make the diagnosis. Serial bronchoalveolar lavage is the gold standard and confirms this clinical diagnosis when lavage aliquots are progressively more hemorrhagic.

    The common autoimmune diseases presenting with DAH include the following:
    - ANCA-associated vasculitis: Wegener granulomatosis and microscopic polyangiitis
    - SLE
    - Goodpasture syndrome
    - Mixed connective tissue disease
    - APS
    - RA
    - Scleroderma
    - PM

15. **A patient with RA comes to the ICU with severe shortness of breath. Describe the different pulmonary causes.**
Pulmonary complications from RA account for 10% to 20% of all mortality.
   - **Parenchymal involvement:** interstitial lung disease, bronchiolitis obliterans with organizing pneumonia, rheumatoid nodules
   - **Airway involvement:** upper airway obstruction, obstructive sleep apnea, bronchiolitis (obliterative), bronchiectasis, Caplan syndrome, cricoarytenoid arthritis
   - **Vascular involvement:** pulmonary hypertension, pulmonary vasculitis
   - **Pleural involvement:** pleural effusion, empyema, bronchopleural fistula or pyopneumothorax, chyliform effusions, lung entrapment
   - **Drug-related lung toxicity:** methotrexate, leflunomide, tumor necrosis factor (TNF) inhibitors, gold salts, and D-penicillamine
   - **Infections:** pneumonia, bronchiectasis, empyema, infected nodules
   Remember: Patients with RA are predisposed to atypical and fungal infections, in addition to common bacterial and viral infections. Fever and leucocytosis may be absent.
   - **Cardiovascular disease:** pericardial effusion, myocardial infarction, angina
   - **Thoracic cage immobility**
   - **Coexisting medical conditions:** asthma, emphysema, congestive heart failure

16. **An elderly woman comes to the ICU with fever of unknown origin, an elevated ESR, headaches, disorientation, and weakness. What rheumatologic condition should not be missed?**
Giant cell arteritis (GCA) or temporal arteritis is a large-vessel vasculitis that occurs more commonly in elderly patients >50 years old and women. It can present with the following:
   - Cranial symptoms: headaches, scalp tenderness, jaw claudication, diplopia, blindness, diminished temporal artery pulse, and stroke
   - Polymyalgia rheumatica (PMR): gradual or acute onset of symmetric stiffness and pain in proximal muscle groups such as shoulders, hips, thighs, and neck
   - Combination of PMR and cranial symptoms
   - Abdominal symptoms: upper back pain, chest pain, dysphagia, dyspnea, superior vena cava syndrome due to thoracic aorta aneurysm or dissection; mesenteric ischemia
   - Systemic symptoms: weight loss, fevers, fatigue, and malaise
   High-dose corticosteroids (prednisone 1 mg/kg) should be started urgently to prevent visual loss from ischemic optic neuritis. ESR is usually elevated and can be helpful but if normal does not exclude GCA. A 3- to 6-cm temporal biopsy should be performed to confirm diagnosis, but steroid therapy should not be delayed while awaiting the biopsy results. The patient can still have GCA with a negative biopsy because patchy arterial involvement usually exists and therefore the right clinical context must be considered.

17. **Describe important side effects of biologic agents, such as TNF-α antagonists (e.g., etanercept, infliximab, adalimumab, certolizumab, and golimumab) that should be considered in an acutely ill ICU patient.**
A higher occurrence of both typical and atypical infections is documented in patients taking TNF inhibitors. These include the following:
   - Typical bacterial infections
   - Reactivation of latent and miliary tuberculosis (TB)
   - Listeriosis with symptoms of meningoencephalitis or septicemia
   - Disseminated fungal diseases such as histoplasmosis and coccidioidomycosis
   - *Pneumocystis carinii (jirovecii)* pneumonia (PCP)

BOX 58-2. COMMON ACUTE AND CHRONIC ADVERSE EFFECTS OF GLUCOCORTICOIDS

ACUTE	CHRONIC
■ Hyperglycemia ■ Hypertension ■ Infections ■ Behavioral changes including steroid psychosis, insomnia, and emotional instability ■ Fluid retention ■ Peptic ulcer disease and pancreatitis ■ Impaired wound healing and ecchymoses	■ Atypical presentations of community-acquired and opportunistic infections ■ Osteoporosis-associated fractures occurring with minor trauma ■ Osteonecrosis of large joints especially the hips, knees, ankles, and shoulders ■ Proximal muscle weakness due to steroid-induced myopathy ■ Higher risk of adverse cardiovascular and cerebrovascular disease ■ Adrenal insufficiency

---

■ Reactivation of hepatitis B virus and herpes zoster infection

Risk factors such as occupational exposure, living in nursing homes, and living in areas where TB is endemic should be evaluated because tuberculin skin testing may be negative in immunocompromised patients.

Controversial data also exist about patients receiving biologic agents being at a higher risk for malignancy because of their immunogenic nature and demyelinating disease.

Remember: Live vaccinations should not be administered to patients taking biologic agents.

18. **What adverse events associated with short- and long-term steroid use can be present in patients in the ICU?**
See Box 58-2.

19. **What precautions should be undertaken when admitting a patient taking long-term low-dose steroids to the ICU for an acute illness?**
Patients taking long-term low-dose steroid therapy (prednisone >5 mg/day) for many years or taking higher doses of steroids (prednisone >20 mg) for more than several weeks may have adrenal insufficiency that may present during an acute illness or high metabolic state.

Symptoms may include fevers, severe hypotension, electrolyte disturbances, fatigue, nausea, and vomiting. Long-term steroid therapy leads to suppression of the hypothalamic-pituitary-adrenal axis. If this diagnosis is suspected, treatment with stress-dose steroids (hydrocortisone 300 mg IV in three divided doses daily) should be initiated.

20. **What are the sinister signs of back pain? What causes of back pain should not be missed in a critically ill patient?**
Red flags:
■ Age <18 or >50 years
■ Back pain >6 weeks
■ History of cancer
■ Unexplained weight loss, night sweats, fevers, chills
■ Recent bacterial infection

- Back pain that wakes patient from sleep
- Increasing or persistent back pain despite analgesia and rest
- Immunocompromised patient or intravenous drug abuse
- Trauma
- Bowel or bladder incontinence or saddle anesthesia
- Severe or progressive neurologic deficits or motor weakness
- Prolonged corticosteroid use

A detailed history and physical examination, with emphasis on localizing the involved nerve distribution, should always be performed. In cases where this is not possible or there is suspicion of involvement, consider performing magnetic resonance imaging (MRI) or computed tomography of the spine.

Spinal epidural abscess, epidural spinal cord compression, malignancy, septic discitis, and osteomyelitis should not be missed as they could lead to neurologic deficits or death.

21. **What are the causes of central nervous system (CNS) vasculitis? What specific investigations should be performed?**

There are two categories of CNS vasculitis. Primary angiitis of the CNS (PACNS) is confined to the CNS without any other identifiable cause. It occurs in the fourth or fifth decade of life, in men, and rarely presents acutely. PACNS lacks systemic symptoms, and patients have normal inflammatory markers in comparison with secondary vasculitis.

Secondary CNS vasculitis usually presents with symptoms typical for the specific systemic vasculitis. Autoimmune causes include Wegener granulomatosis, Behçet disease, SLE, and, less commonly, Sjögren syndrome, RA, mixed connective tissue disease, Hashimoto thyroiditis, and multiple sclerosis.

Patients may have symptoms of severe headaches, seizures, strokelike episodes, ataxia, cognitive impairment, encephalopathy, movement disorders, and neurologic deficits.

Infections and malignancy should be ruled out. Inflammatory and autoimmune laboratory tests, lumbar puncture, MRI and angiogram, and cerebral angiogram should be performed. Leptomeningeal brain biopsy is the gold standard for diagnosis.

22. **What is macrophage activation syndrome (MAS)? What investigation should be performed?**

MAS is an autoimmune illness that is a form of hemophagocytic lymphohistiocytosis syndrome and is due to uncontrolled macrophage activation. It usually occurs in children or adults with autoimmune disease, especially systemic-onset juvenile idiopathic arthritis, adult-onset Still disease, or more rarely SLE.

These patients are critically ill and have fever, splenomegaly, cytopenias, hypertriglyceridemia, hypofibrinogenemia, coagulopathies, high ferritin (usually ferritin >500 mcg/L). One of the hallmarks of this disease is that they will present with decreasing cell counts and inflammatory markers. Malignancy and infection can occur concurrently or mimic MAS and therefore should be ruled out. Patients suspected to have this condition should have a bone marrow test performed, which will usually show normal or increased cellularity.

23. **In the ICU, patients are seen acutely with an elevated creatine kinase (CK) level. What is the differential of an elevated CK level?**

- **Drug and toxin induced:** statins, colchicine, ethanol, cocaine, antimalarials, corticosteroid-induced myopathy, barbiturates, zidovudine
- **Infectious myositis:** bacterial, viral, fungal, mycobacterial, or parasitic
- **Endocrine disorders:** hypothyroidism, hyperthyroidism, acromegaly, Cushing or Addison disease
- **Myocardial injury**
- **Trauma**
- **Metabolic myopathies:** glycogen storage or lipid metabolism disorders, electrolyte disorders

- **Miscellaneous:** seizures, malignant hyperthermia, motor neuron disease, rhabdomyolysis, organ failure
- **Autoimmune or rheumatologic disorders:** PM or dermatomyositis (DM), PMR, systemic vasculitis, sarcoidosis, inflammatory arthritides

24. **What are the clinical signs and symptoms that suggest an inflammatory myopathy? What other investigations may be helpful in diagnosing an inflammatory myopathy?**

    In a critical setting it may be difficult to differentiate the cause of an elevated CK level. The symptoms of gradual, progressive, symmetric proximal muscle weakness or neck muscle weakness are usually suggestive of PM or PMR. In addition, if certain rashes such as a heliotrope rash, Gottron papules, shawl sign, V sign, or mechanic's hands are present consider DM or mixed connective tissue disease.

    Aldolase, aspartate transaminase, lactate dehydrogenase, and ESR may be elevated in an inflammatory myopathy. Myositis-specific autoantibodies may be present in PM and DM. An electromyogram and muscle biopsy should be performed if PM or DM is suspected. There is a 10% to 15% association with malignancy over the next 3 years in PM and DM.

KEY POINTS: RHEUMATOLOGIC EMERGENCIES IN THE INTENSIVE CARE UNIT

1. An acute swollen joint indicates septic arthritis until proved otherwise. Crystal-induced arthropathy and septic arthritis can occur simultaneously in a joint.

2. Patients with severe peripheral RA are at higher risk for spinal cord compression from AAS during intubation. Beware of cricoarytenoid obstruction also occurring in these patients.

3. Prompt treatment with an ACEi should be initiated in patients with SRC.

4. Patients taking biologic medications are at a higher risk for typical bacterial infections and atypical infections such as reactivation of TB, hepatitis B, herpes zoster, PCP, listeriosis, and disseminated fungal infections.

5. In a patient in the ICU who is seen with multiorgan failure or a clinical picture resembling fulminant sepsis, consider the diagnosis of SLE or vasculitis.

BIBLIOGRAPHY

1. Corwell BN: The emergency department evaluation, management and treatment of back pain. Emerg Med Clin N Am 28:811-839, 2010.

2. Denton CP, Lapadula G, Mouthon L, et al: Renal complications and scleroderma renal crisis. Rheumatology 48: iii32-iii35, 2009.

3. Hajj-Ali RA: Primary angiitis of the central nervous system: differential diagnosis and treatment. Best Pract Res Clin Rheumatol 24:413-426, 2010.

4. Hoffman GS, Specks U: Antineutrophil cytoplasmic antibodies (ANCA). Arthritis Rheum 41:1521-1537, 1998.

5. Jacobs JWG, Bijlsma JWJ: Glucocorticoid therapy. In Firestein GS, Budd RC, Harris ED, et al (eds): Kelley's Textbook of Rheumatology, 8th ed. vol 1. Philadelphia, Saunders, 2009, pp 863-881.

6. Janka G: Hemophagocytic syndromes. Blood Rev 21:245-253, 2007.

7. Lara AR, Schwarz MI: Diffuse alveolar hemorrhage. Chest 137:1164-1171, 2010.

8. Mathews CJ, Weston VC, Jones A, et al: Bacterial septic arthritis in adults. Lancet 375:846-855, 2010.

9. Rendt K: Inflammatory myopathies: narrowing the differential diagnosis. Cleve Clin J Med 68:505-519, 2001.

10. Ruiz-Irastorza G, Crowther M, et al: Antiphospholipid syndrome. Lancet 376:1498-1509, 2010.

11. Sorokin R: Management of the patient with rheumatic disease going to surgery. Med Clin North Am 77:453-464, 1993.

12. Tassiulas IO, Boumpas DT: Clinical features and treatment of systemic lupus erythematosus. In Firestein GS, Budd RC, Harris ED, et al (eds): Kelley's Textbook of Rheumatology, 8th ed, vol 1. Philadelphia, Saunders, 2009, pp 1263-1300.

13. Tokunaga D, Hase H, Mikami Y, et al: Atlantoaxial subluxation in different intraoperative head position in patients with rheumatoid arthritis. Anesthesiology 104:675-679, 2006.

COMA

Ala Nozari, MD, PhD, Corey R. Fehnel, MD, and Lee H. Schwamm, MD, FAHA

1. **What is coma, and how is it different from persistent vegetative state (PVS), minimally conscious state (MCS), or locked-in syndrome?**
   - *Coma* is a state of profound unresponsiveness caused by structural, metabolic, physiologic, or psychogenic brain dysfunction. The comatose patient is unaware of self and environment and cannot be roused to respond to vigorous stimulation.
   - In contrast to coma, patients with *PVS* are in a state of partial arousal and may briefly alert to sound or visual stimuli. They withdraw to noxious stimuli but are unable to interact or respond voluntarily or in any purposeful way to stimuli. PVS is a chronic condition and thus is typically not assigned unless a patient's state of altered consciousness persists for more than 30 days.
   - Patients in *MCS* exhibit deliberate or cognitively mediated behavior, may intermittently follow commands, or have intelligible but inconsistent verbal output. Patients may evolve to MCS from coma or PVS.
   - Patients with *locked-in syndrome* have intact cognition but complete paralysis of voluntary muscles in all parts of the body. They traditionally have been able to communicate through code systems by blinking or repeated up-and-down eye movements; however, recent breakthrough technology has allowed some patients to communicate via a human-machine computer interface that allows patients to initiate computer commands with only their thoughts through the use of a surgically embedded microchip in the cerebral cortex.

2. **Which are the major categories of disorders or injuries that cause coma?**
   - Coma can be caused by *structural brain injury* involving the relay nuclei and connecting fibers of the ascending reticular activation system (ARAS), which extends from upper brainstem through synaptic relays in the rostral intralaminar and thalamic nuclei to the cerebral cortex. The base of pons does not participate in arousal, and lesions such as central pontine myelinolysis do not usually profoundly impair consciousness. Instead, these lesions can interrupt all motor output except vertical eye movements and blinking that are initiated by nuclei in the mesencephalon (locked-in syndrome).
   - *Mesencephalic* and *thalamic injuries*, for example, as a result of occlusion of the tip of the basilar artery, or bilateral thalamic injuries, may result in somnolence, immobility, and decreased verbal output characteristic for MCS.
   - *Bihemispheric injuries* involving the cortex, white matter, or both may also result in impaired arousal.
   - Similarly, an acute *unilateral hemispheric* or *cerebellar mass* can lead to coma through destruction of the brain tissue and displacement of the falx and brainstem.
   - *Physiologic brain dysfunction* as a result of generalized tonic-clonic seizures, hypothermia, and poisoning or acute *metabolic and endocrine derangements* can also lead to coma. Typically, metabolic coma may spare the pupillary light reflex as it causes selected dysfunction of the cortex, whereas brainstem centers that control the pupils are spared. Hypoglycemia or nonketotic hyperosmolar coma, dysnatremia, thyroid storm, myxedema, fulminant hepatic failure, and acute hypopituitarism are examples in this category and should always be considered in a comatose patient. Asterixis, tremor, myoclonus, and foul breath may predominate the examination before these patients become unresponsive.

- Malignant catatonia and *psychogenic unresponsiveness* should also be considered in all unresponsive patients.
- *Acute muscle paralysis* (e.g., botulism or other toxins) should also be ruled out, because these patients may be awake and cognitively intact but unable to demonstrate responsiveness.

3. **Name common causes of structural brain injury in comatose patients.**
   Structural brain injuries may be caused by the following:
   - Bilateral cortical or subcortical infarcts (e.g., as a consequence of cardiac embolization or occlusion of major cerebral vessels)
   - Bleeding (e.g., hemorrhagic contusions, epidural or subdural hematoma, subarachnoid hemorrhage)
   - Infections (e.g., meningitis, cerebral abscess, subdural empyema, and herpes encephalitis)
   - Neoplasm (primary tumors and metastases)
   - Vasculitis and leukoencephalopathy, or lateral (acute midline shift of the brain of >1 cm) or downward herniation from mass effect or increased intracranial pressure (ICP) (e.g., massive brain edema, obstructive hydrocephalus)

4. **Describe the mechanisms of toxin-induced coma.**
   Depression of neuronal function can be caused by a reduction in the turnover of major neurotransmitters such as acetylcholine, dopamine, and serotonin through the γ-aminobutyric acid–benzodiazepine chloride iodophor receptor complex. Moreover, toxins can result in hypoxia (e.g., through respiratory depression or aspiration) or hypoglycemia (e.g., ethanol, β-blockers, and salicylates) leading to coma. Seizures can also be induced by toxins, as are acute cerebral bleedings, for example, caused by hypertension (cocaine, amphetamine) or coagulation abnormalities. Insulin is a common factor among patients with insulin-dependent diabetes.

5. **What are the initial steps in managing a patient with coma?**
   The immediate approach to the comatose patient includes measures to protect the brain by providing adequate cerebral blood flow and oxygenation, reversing metabolic derangements, and treating potential infections and anatomic or endocrine abnormalities.
   - The clinician must ensure that the patient has a patent and protected airway and adequate breathing. Supplemental oxygen should be administered and airway secured by intubating the trachea, if needed.
   - Vascular access should be obtained and hypotension corrected with vasopressor agents or fluid administration as required.
   - Blood samples should be obtained to rule out infection and metabolic or endocrine abnormalities.
   - Generalized seizures should be treated and metabolic abnormalities corrected as soon as possible.
   - If the cause of coma is uncertain and hypoglycemia cannot be excluded, 50% dextrose should be administered. Empirical therapy for Wernicke encephalopathy or narcotic or sedative overdose should be considered and thiamine, naloxone, or flumazenil administered if appropriate. Thiamine must be given before dextrose to prevent worsening of Wernicke encephalopathy.
   - If increased ICP with mass effect is suspected, the patient should have hyperventilation, mannitol, or hypertonic saline solution administered, and specific surgical measures to evacuate possible mass or hematoma should be initiated.
   - If meningitis is suspected, antibiotic treatment should be initiated, and then a computed tomography (CT) scan of the head performed to rule out mass effect or herniation, in combination with laboratory evaluation for coagulopathy or thrombocytopenia before lumbar puncture.

6. **Describe the diagnostic approach to the comatose patients.**

   The history may be obtained from relatives, friends, police, or paramedics and may suggest an obvious cause such as drug or alcohol overdose, sepsis, or abnormalities of glucose metabolism. Acute onset of coma in a previously healthy person suggests intracranial hemorrhage, generalized seizure, poisoning, or traumatic brain injury. Gradual worsening, on the other hand, can indicate metabolic derangement, inflammatory neurologic disorders, cortical venous sinus thrombosis, or a gradually expanding intracranial mass. Physical examination should aim at identifying localizing neurologic deficits and possible triggering mechanisms. Blood sample and, if feasible, cerebrospinal fluid should be obtained to rule out infection, hypoglycemia, and other metabolic and electrolyte abnormalities. The depth of coma should be documented and graded on arrival and periodically thereafter to assess any change. Imaging studies such as a CT of the brain are often required to assess for structural causes of coma. Electroencephalography (EEG) can be helpful in diagnosing seizures or to identify EEG patterns suggestive of toxic metabolic abnormalities.

7. **How can the respiratory pattern and brainstem reflexes help in the assessment of the comatose patient?**

   Respiratory pattern and rate are often helpful in identifying the cause of coma. Hyperventilation, as an example, may be a response to hypoxemia, metabolic acidosis, toxins, or dysfunction within the pons. Cheyne-Stokes breathing may indicate diencephalic lesions or bilateral cerebral hemisphere dysfunction, for example, increased ICP or metabolic abnormalities. Cluster breathing is associated with high medulla or lower pontine lesions. Brainstem reflexes should be examined and focal motor abnormalities, as well as reflex asymmetry, recorded. Equal and reactive pupils may indicate toxic or metabolic causes, whereas a unilateral fixed and dilated pupil usually indicates oculomotor palsy possibly as a result of uncal herniation. Bilateral pinpoint pupils with minute reaction suggest a pontine lesion, and bilateral fixed and dilated pupils may indicate medullary injury, global anoxia, or hypothermia. Ocular bobbing (a repetitive rapid vertical deviation downward and slow return to neutral position) indicates a pontine lesion often seen in basilar artery occlusion, whereas ping-pong or *windshield-wiper* eye movements usually indicate bilateral cerebral dysfunction. Eye movements can safely be elicited in the comatose patient without cervical spine injury by performing the oculocephalic maneuver (often called "doll's eyes"), that is, by rapidly rotating the head from side to side. If the paramedian pontine reticular formation and the vestibular system are intact, the eyes should move smoothly in the direction opposite to that in which the head is rotated.

   If cervical spine stability is in question, or no response to oculocephalic maneuvers occurs, the oculovestibular response (often called "cold calorics") can be tested instead. One tympanic membrane is irrigated with 30 mL of ice-cold water and the response observed. When the underlying brainstem structures are intact, both eyes will deviate laterally toward the side where the cold water is instilled. If cortical structures and parts of the frontal lobe are intact, there will be nystagmus with the fast phase toward the nonirrigated ear. In metabolic or toxic coma the clinician usually sees intact gaze deviation toward the irrigated ear but absent or abnormal nystagmus indicating cortical dysfunction. In many comatose patients with structural brainstem injury, the oculovestibular system is impaired, and deviation of the eyes is absent or abnormal.

8. **How do you manage a comatose patient after the initial work-up and stabilization?**

   After the initial assessment and treatment of the underlying cause of coma outlined in the answer to question 5, the comatose patient should be admitted to a specialized critical care unit for supportive care and to maximize the chance of recovery. Cardiorespiratory support should be maintained as appropriate with attention to maintenance of cerebral oxygenation. Care should be taken for prevention of ventilator-associated pneumonia. Electrolytes should be monitored closely and replaced as required. Early initiation of full enteral nutrition should be initiated whenever possible. Other essential steps in the care of the comatose patient include measures to reduce risk of infections, gastric ulcer prevention, thromboembolism prevention, physical therapy, splinting where appropriate, and skin care for pressure ulcer prevention. Early tracheostomy may be considered if prolonged mechanical ventilation is deemed necessary.

9. **What is diffuse axonal injury (DAI), and how is it diagnosed and graded?**
   DAI is a term that arose in the pre–magnetic resonance imaging (MRI) era and is commonly cited as the cause of coma in patients with traumatic brain injury (TBI) in the absence of space-occupying lesions or apparent structural injuries. It can, nevertheless, also be present with subdural or epidural hematomas. DAI is a primary lesion of rotational acceleration-deceleration head injury. In its severe form, hemorrhagic foci occur in the corpus callosum and dorsolateral and rostral brainstem with microscopic evidence of diffuse injury to axons (axonal retraction balls, microglial stars, and a generation of white matter fiber tracts). It can be clinically diagnosed after TBI when coma lasts >6 hours in the absence of intracranial mass, increased ICP, or cerebral ischemia. MRI is more sensitive than CT for detecting characteristics of DAI, and newer studies such as diffusion tensor imaging can demonstrate the degree of white matter fiber tract injury.
   - DAI is graded as *mild* when coma lasts up to 24 hours and is followed by mild to moderate memory impairment and disabilities.
   - Coma lasts >24 hours in *moderate* DAI and is followed by confusion and long-lasting amnesia, with memory, behavioral, and cognitive deficits.
   - In *severe* DAI, coma lasts for months, and the patient has flexor and extensor posturing, dysautonomia, cognitive impairment, and memory, speech, and sensory motor deficits.

10. **Describe the natural history and prognosis of coma, PVS, and MCS.**
    The prognosis of coma is dependent on the underlying cause and other comorbidities. Metabolic and toxic disturbances can often be fully reversed and have, therefore, generally a better prognosis. Coma after TBI has also a better outcome than after anoxic brain injury. Coma often evolves into PVS within a few weeks, but patients may remain in coma, PVS, or MCS permanently. The chance of meaningful recovery is minimal if PVS lasts >12 months after TBI, or >3 months in other cases. Typically, life expectancy is 2 to 5 years, but patients with MCS, particularly those who had TBI, have a better survival rate and an improved chance of functional recovery.
    EEG has not been validated as a prognostic tool, but recent advances in neuroimaging have improved the ability to predict outcome and may be helpful to guide decision making. As an example, injuries to the corpus callosum and dorsolateral brainstem on MRI are predictive of poor recovery. Of interest, functional MRI recently demonstrated that there are regions of preserved brain function and willful modulation of brain activity in a handful of patients with PVS and MCS. Thalamic deep brain stimulation is a promising approach to these patients and may improve responsiveness. Most patients undergo a trial of central nervous system stimulants to try to improve arousal.

11. **Describe the pattern of injury and prognosis in patients with hypoxic coma.**
    Hypoxemia (low arterial PO_2) and ischemia (e.g., after exsanguination or cardiac arrest) result in neuronal injury through a necrotic pathway or under certain circumstances through apoptosis or necrapoptotic cell death. Areas that are particularly vulnerable to this type of injury include cerebral gray matter, predominantly in the third cortical layer, hippocampus, and basal ganglia (selective vulnerability). Globus pallidus is often affected in hypoxemia, and caudate nucleus and putamen are usually affected after ischemia. Purkinje cells and dentate nuclei, as well as inferior olives, are also commonly affected. Patients with normal pupillary light reflex, Glasgow Coma Scale (GCS)–motor >1 and spontaneous extraocular movements within 6 hours of injury, or those with GCS-motor >3 and improved GCS-eye at 1 day have better chances of regaining independence. Absence of pupillary light reflexes, abnormal oculocephalic reflex, absent motor response to pain, and bilateral absence of early cortical somatosensory evoked potential are predictive of poor outcome. An EEG pattern of myoclonic status epilepticus after cerebral anoxia is also strongly predictive of poor outcome.

KEY POINTS: COMA

1. Coma can be caused by structural injury of the ARAS, metabolic and endocrine derangements, and psychogenic or physiologic brain dysfunction.

2. After adequate oxygenation and circulation are ensured, it is important to identify the cause of coma and employ measures to correct potentially reversible conditions.

3. If the cause of coma is unknown, dextrose and thiamine should be administered early, and reversal of opioids, benzodiazepines, and neurotoxins should be considered. Infections, metabolic derangements, and structural injuries should be ruled out.

BIBLIOGRAPHY

1. Adams JH, Graham DI, Murray LS, et al: Diffuse axonal injury due to nonmissile head injury in humans: an analysis of 45 cases. Ann Neurol 12:557-563, 1982.

2. Buettner UW, Zee DS: Vestibular testing in comatose patients. Arch Neurol 46:561-563, 1989.

3. Gennarelli TA, Thibault LE, Adams JH, et al: Diffuse axonal injury and traumatic coma in the primate. Ann Neurol 12:564-574, 1982.

4. Giacino JT, Ashwal S, Childs N, et al: The minimally conscious state: definition and diagnostic criteria. Neurology 58:349-353, 2002.

5. Giacino JT, Kalmar K: Diagnostic and prognostic guidelines for the vegetative and minimally conscious states. Neuropsychol Rehabil 15:166-174, 2005.

6. Giacino JT, Kalmar K: The vegetative and minimally conscious states: a comparison of clinical features and functional outcome. J Head Trauma Rehabil 12(4):36-51, 1997.

7. Levy DE, Caronna JJ, Singer BH, et al: Predicting outcome from hypoxic-ischemic coma. JAMA 253:1420-1426, 1985.

8. Liao YJ, So YT: An approach to critically ill patients in coma. West J Med 176:184-187, 2002.

9. Mercer WN, Childs NL: Coma, vegetative state, and the minimally conscious state: diagnosis and management. Neurologist 5:186-194, 1999.

10. Posner JB, Saper CB, Schiff N, et al: Plum and Posner's Diagnosis of Stupor and Coma. New York, Oxford University Press, 2007.

11. Ropper AH: Lateral displacement of the brain and level of consciousness in patients with an acute hemispheral mass. N Engl J Med 314:953-958, 1986.

12. Simeral JD, Kim SP, Black MJ, et al: Neural control of cursor trajectory and click by a human with tetraplegia 1000 days after implant of an intracortical microelectrode array. J Neural Eng 8(2):025027, 2011.

13. Wilson SL: Magnetic-resonance imaging and prediction of recovery from post-traumatic vegetative state. Lancet 352:485, 1998.

14. Zandbergen EG, deHaan RJ, Stoutenbeek CP, et al: Systematic review of early prediction of poor outcome in anoxic-ischaemic coma. Lancet 352:1808-1812, 1998.

CHAPTER 60

BRAIN DEATH

Corey R. Fehnel, MD, Ala Nozari, MD, PhD, and Lee H. Schwamm, MD, FAHA

1. **What is brain death?**
   Brain death is a universally accepted medical and legal standard for determining death.
   A determination of brain death is equivalent to cardiopulmonary death. Brain death is a complete and irreversible loss of brain and brainstem function when other body organ systems may persist. The advent of modern critical care intervention, primarily mechanical ventilation, necessitated a new definition of death because it was now possible to maintain vital functions for extended periods of time. The advent of organ transplantation in the 1950s brought into focus the need for a clear and precise definition of death of the brain in the face of preserved cardiopulmonary function to identify under what circumstances organ removal could occur.

2. **When should the diagnosis of brain death be considered?**
   Active debate continues regarding minimum time of observation before determining brain death. The diagnosis is rarely if ever considered before the first 6 to 24 hours after injury. A variety of toxic and metabolic derangements associated with the onset of critical illness make brain and brainstem function difficult to assess in the hyperacute setting. Patients being considered for brain death uniformly have endotracheal tubes in place and are receiving mechanical ventilation. Sedatives, narcotics, and paralytics used for intubation must be allowed several half-lives of elimination. Pharmacokinetics are often prolonged in patients with multiorgan dysfunction who make up many of these patients.

3. **What are the current guidelines for determination of brain death?**
   Mollaret and Goulon first reported 23 cases of irreversible coma in 1959. This was followed by early standards produced at Harvard Medical School in 1968. The Uniform Determination of Death Act (UDDA) has been adopted as law in most U.S. states. It defines as dead an individual who has sustained either:
   - Irreversible cessation of circulatory and respiratory functions, or
   - Irreversible cessation of all functions of the entire brain, including the brainstem.
     A determination of death must be made with accepted medical standards.
   The American Academy of Neurology (AAN) practice parameter for determining brain death in adults set forth "accepted medical standards" left open by the UDDA in 1995. In adults, there are no published reports of recovery of neurologic function after a diagnosis of brain death using the criteria presented in the 1995 AAN practice parameter. Brain death should be a diagnostic entity and never used as a prognostic statement about poor chances of recovery.

4. **Who can perform a brain death examination?**
   In most U.S. states, any physician is allowed to determine brain death. Neurologists, neurosurgeons, and intensive care specialists may have specialized expertise. Brain death statutes vary by states within the United States, and certain hospital guidelines may require examiners to have specific expertise. Given the complexity of the examination, the examiner should have extensive experience with the brain death examination and full understanding of accepted standards.

5. **What prerequisites must be met before performing a brain death examination?**
These are defined in Box 60-1.

BOX 60-1. PREREQUISITES TO BE MET BEFORE PERFORMING A BRAIN DEATH EXAMINATION

- Coma, irreversible and cause known. (Glasgow Coma Scale score must be 3)
- Neuroimaging explains coma
- CNS depressant drug effect absent (if indicated, perform toxicology screen; if barbiturates given, serum level should be <10 mcg/mL)
- No evidence of residual paralytics (verify by electrical nerve stimulation if paralytics used)
- Absence of severe acid–base, electrolyte, endocrine abnormality
- Normothermia or mild hypothermia (core temperature >36° C)
- Systolic blood pressure ≥100 mm Hg (pressor agents are okay to use)
- No spontaneous respirations

---

6. **What findings should be present on brain death examination?**
These are defined in Box 60-2.

BOX 60-2. FINDINGS THAT SHOULD BE PRESENT ON BRAIN DEATH EXAMINATION

- Pupils nonreactive to bright light, corneal reflex absent bilaterally
- Oculocephalic reflex absent (test only if C-spine *cleared*)
- Oculovestibular reflex absent (cold-water caloric testing)
- No facial movement to noxious stimuli at supraorbital ridge or temporomandibular joints
- Gag reflex absent
- Cough reflex absent to deep tracheal suctioning
- Absence of motor response to noxious stimuli in all four limbs (spinally mediated reflexes are permissible; see question 6)
- Apnea testing (see question 8)

---

7. **Can a patient make movements and still meet criteria for brain death?**
Yes. Spinally mediated reflexes and automatisms can be present in the setting of brain death. These movements are often misinterpreted by laypersons as signs of purposeful brain function. Careful neurologic examination can differentiate between reflexive movements and purposeful motor movements.

8. **What are the common spinally generated movements?**
These are **nonpurposeful** movements *released* by lack of descending inhibition of primitive spinal motor reflex pathways.
- *Deep-tendon reflexes:* For example, Achilles, patellar, and biceps are by definition monosynaptic spinally mediated reflexes and hence often preserved despite brain death.
- *Abdominal reflexes:* Deviation of the umbilicus toward a light stroking of the skin. Often preserved in brain-dead patients, it may be absent in normal or obese patients.
- *Triple flexion response or limb posturing:* Stereotyped, nonpurposeful flexion or extension and internal rotation in response to noxious stimulus. (A movement may be purposeful if the limb reliably moves away from, rather than toward, an applied noxious stimulus.)
- *Lazarus sign:* Considered a variant of opisthotonus. It consists of extensor posturing of the trunk, which may look like chest expansion, simulating a breath. It may be accompanied by raising and crossing of the arms in front of the chest or neck. This sign most often occurs in the setting of apnea testing or disconnection from the ventilator. Hence it may be upsetting for family members or health care providers to witness this reflex.

9. **What other movements may exist in brain-dead patients?**
   Rare reports exist of facial myokymia, transient bilateral finger tremor, repetitive leg movements, ocular microtremor, and cyclic constriction and dilatation in light-fixed pupils. Many patients may retain plantar reflexes, either flexion or transient stimulation-induced toe flexion.

10. **How do you perform apnea testing?**
    Brain-dead patients must demonstrate an absence of respiratory drive. This is defined by an increase in $PaCO_2$ and no discernible respiration. Prerequisites for apnea testing include the following:
    - Normal blood pressure (systolic blood pressure >100 mm Hg)
    - Normothermia
    - Euvolemia
    - Eucapnia ($PaCO_2$ 35-45 mm Hg)
    - Absence of hypoxia
    - No prior evidence of CO_2 retention (i.e., chronic obstructive pulmonary disease, severe obesity)
      See Box 60-3.

BOX 60-3. PROCEDURES FOR APNEA TESTING

- Preoxygenate for at least 10 minutes with 100% oxygen to a PaO_2 >200 mm Hg.
- Reduce ventilation frequency to 10 breaths per minute to eucapnia.
- Reduce positive end-expiratory pressure (PEEP) to 5 cm H_2O (oxygen desaturation with decreasing PEEP may suggest difficulty with apnea testing).
- If pulse oximetry oxygen saturation remains >95%, obtain a baseline blood gas level (PaO_2, $PaCO_2$, pH, bicarbonate, base excess).
- Disconnect the patient from the ventilator.
- Preserve oxygenation (e.g., place an insufflation catheter through the endotracheal tube and close to the level of the carina and deliver 100% O_2 at 6 L/min).
- Look closely for respiratory movements for 8 to 10 minutes. Respiration is defined as abdominal or chest excursions and may include a brief gasp.
- Abort if systolic blood pressure decreases to <90 mm Hg.
- Abort if oxygen saturation measured by pulse oximetry is <85% for >30 seconds.
- Retry procedure with T-piece, continuous positive airway pressure 10 cm H_2O, and 100% O_2 12 L/min.
- If no respiratory drive is observed, repeat blood gas analysis (PaO_2, $PaCO_2$, pH, bicarbonate, base excess) after approximately 8 minutes. If there is any reason to abort the test because of instability of the patient's condition, draw an arterial blood gas sample immediately before reconnecting the ventilator.
- If respiratory movements are absent and arterial $PaCO_2$ is $\geq$60 mm Hg (or 20 mm Hg increase in arterial PCO_2 over a baseline normal arterial PCO_2), the apnea test result is positive (i.e., supports the clinical diagnosis of brain death).
- If the test is inconclusive but the patient is hemodynamically stable during the procedure, it may be repeated for a longer period of time (10-15 minutes) after the patient is again adequately preoxygenated.

---

11. **Can brain-dead patients falsely trigger delivery of breaths on ventilators?**
    Yes. Numerous case reports exist of ventilator autocycling in patients who in fact have no respiratory drive. Pressure-triggered ventilation in pressure support modes can be seen with endotracheal tube cuff leak and bronchopleural fistula. Flow-triggered ventilators can be initiated by cardiogenic oscillations. These potential confounders may be accounted for by switching

between flow- and pressure-triggered ventilatory modes. In patients who meet all brain death clinical criteria yet continue to ventilate beyond the set ventilator rate, or breathe spontaneously, the patient should be closely observed off the ventilator circuit for evidence of spontaneous breathing. If no spontaneous breathing is present, then formal apnea testing may proceed as described above.

12. **Is there a single ancillary test that can confirm brain death?**
No. Brain death remains a clinical diagnosis, and no ancillary test can replace a clinical determination of brain death. However, situations occur where the full brain death examination is not possible (e.g., apnea testing due to hemodynamic instability, severe facial trauma, prolonged sedative exposure). In these situations, *one* additional test may help to confirm the diagnosis. Ordering multiple ancillary tests is not advisable. No data support superiority of one test over another. Multiple tests increase the odds of indeterminate or false-positive results due to artifact.

13. **What ancillary tests can help with diagnosing brain death?**
Testing can be divided into either cerebral arterial anatomic or flow studies versus studies of brain electrical activity.
- Flow studies
  - Cerebral scintigraphy (technetium Tc 99 m exametazime [HMPAO]):
  - A noninvasive and safe measure of cerebral blood flow. No patient transport required if a portable gamma camera is available. Sodium pertechnetate technetium 99 m (15–21 mCi per adult) is given by intravenous bolus. A gamma camera then obtains anterior images every 3 seconds for a total of 60 seconds. External carotid flow is either digitally subtracted or excluded by forehead tourniquet. The isotope should be injected within 30 minutes of its reconstitution. Anterior and lateral planar image counts of the head should be obtained immediately, at 30 to 60 minutes, and then at 2 hours. A positive scan reveals no radionuclide localization in the middle cerebral artery, anterior cerebral artery, or basilar artery territories of the cerebral hemispheres (hollow skull phenomenon). Because prior recent craniotomy may cause a false signal of extracranial blood flow to be suspected in the intracranial compartment, it is important to inform the nuclear medicine staff if this has occurred.
  - Conventional cerebral angiography:
  - Contrast medium is injected in the aortic arch under high pressure to reach both anterior and posterior circulations. A confirmatory test reveals absence of intracerebral filling beyond the carotid or vertebral arteries' entry to the skull. Patent external carotid (extracranial) circulation should be demonstrated.
  - Transcranial Doppler:
  - Useful only if a reliable waveform is found. Abnormalities should include either reverberating flow or small systolic peaks in early systole. Complete absence of flow may not be reliable if inadequate insonation windows exist. All traditional cranial windows should be evaluated for flow. The orbital window can be considered to obtain a reliable signal. Prior craniotomy can complicate the study.
- Measures of brain electrical activity
  - Electroencephalography (EEG):
  - A positive EEG for brain death reveals a lack of reactivity to intense somatosensory or audiovisual stimuli. Isoelectric EEG or the finding of electrocerebral silence may be mimicked by conditions such as hypothermia, systemic hypotension, barbiturates, or other central nervous system (CNS) depressants. Hence the patient should meet the same physiologic and hemodynamic standards during EEG as would be required during the brain death clinical examination.
  - Somatosensory evoked potential:

□ A peripheral stimulus is given, typically at the median nerve, and a response is measured at the contralateral primary sensory cortex. Absence of transmission measured 20 ms (N20 response) after stimulation suggests brainstem dysfunction.
□ Brainstem auditory evoked response:
□ May be useful in evaluating patients in whom coma of toxic etiology is suspected (i.e., barbiturate coma). Brainstem and auditory short-latency responses that are absent in brain death but preserved in toxic and metabolic disorders can make this a useful test.

14. **Are any blood tests helpful in establishing brain death?**
No. Neuron-specific enolase and the glial protein S100 are the most studied. Neither marker is used for brain death determination. Clinical examination remains paramount. In cases where brain death is not being considered, serum markers may aid in determining prognosis after hypoxic ischemic injury.

15. **What neuroimaging should be ordered to confirm brain death?**
There is no requirement for a particular neuroimaging modality to diagnose brain death. However, a structural cause by brain imaging must be established as prerequisite for brain death diagnosis. Hence computed tomography or magnetic resonance imaging of the head must be consistent with the diagnosis of brain death.

16. **How many examinations are required to pronounce a patient brain dead?**
Individual states have different guidelines and standards. Many states require only one full brain death examination. In states that require a second independent examination, organ donation rates may be adversely affected without any cases of incorrect brain death diagnoses being discovered.

KEY POINTS: BRAIN DEATH

1. Brain death is the irreversible loss of both brain and brainstem function from a known cause.

2. Brain death is rarely determined before 6 to 24 hours from neurologic injury.

3. The brain death examination should be performed by an experienced and knowledgeable physician.

4. It is not uncommon for brain-dead patients to make spinally mediated reflexive movements that are not indicative of preserved brain function. Families should be educated about this.

5. Brain death is a clinical diagnosis.

6. Ancillary tests may be helpful in confirming brain death but are not necessary or sufficient to make the diagnosis.

BIBLIOGRAPHY

1. American Encephalography Society : Guideline three: minimum technical standards for EEG recording in suspected cerebral death. J Clin Neurophysiol 11:10-13, 1994.

2. Greer DM, Varelas PN, Haque S, et al: Variability of brain death determination guidelines in leading US neurologic institutions. Neurology 70:284-289, 2008.

3. Imanaka H, Nishimura M, Takeuchi M, et al: Autotriggering caused by cardiogenic oscillation during flow triggered mechanical ventilation. Crit Care Med 28:402-407, 2000.

4. Lustbader D, O'Hara D, Wijdicks EFM, et al: Second brain death examination may negatively affect organ donation. Neurology 76:119-124, 2011.

5. McGee WT, Mailloux P: Ventilator autocycling and delayed recognition of brain death. Neurocrit Care 14:267-271, 2011.

6. Practice parameters for determining brain death in adults (summary statement): report of the Quality Standards Subcommittee of the American Academy of Neurology. Neurology 45:1012-1014, 1995.

7. Wijdicks EFM, Varelas P, Gronseth G, et al: Evidence based guideline update: determining brain death in adults. Neurology 74:1911-1918, 2010.

CHAPTER 61

STATUS EPILEPTICUS

Ala Nozari, MD, PhD, Corey R. Fehnel, MD, and Lee H. Schwamm, MD, FAHA

1. **What is the definition of status epilepticus (SE)?**
   SE has typically been defined as repetitive seizures lasting 30 minutes or longer, or seizures without full return of consciousness between episodes. This definition was recently challenged because it does not incorporate the practical considerations of patient management and because shorter periods of seizure activity can cause neuronal injury. Therefore others have recommended defining SE as seizures lasting ≥5 minutes or two or more seizures between which there is incomplete recovery of consciousness or function.

2. **Name important features of SE.**
   In patients with no prior seizure history, SE is usually a manifestation of cortical irritation or injury. Treatment of the underlying disorder is therefore critical. Relapse of seizure in patients with known seizure disorder, on the other hand, commonly reflects subtherapeutic levels of antiepileptic drugs (AED) and usually responds to a bolus of the maintenance drug. Most cases of convulsive SE in adults start as partial seizures that generalize.

3. **Describe the classification and clinical presentation of SE.**
   SE can be classified in several forms, including convulsive SE, focal SE, myoclonic SE, and nonconvulsive SE (NSE).
   - Generalized convulsive SE involves tonic flexion of the axial muscles, flexion in the arms and legs followed by extension, clenching of teeth, forced expiration, dilation of the pupils or sluggish pupillary light responses, and upward or lateral eye deviation. The uninterrupted jerking or shivering during the clonic phase may gradually resolve, but tonic spasm may occur again with a similar pattern of jerking and resolution. As the duration of the seizures increases, the movements and muscle contractions may become reduced despite continued generalized electrical activity in the brain.
   - Focal SE can be simple without loss of consciousness or complex with impaired consciousness. Jerking of one ipsilateral arm or leg or continuous clonic movements of one or two extremities can be observed. When confined to focal motor clonic seizures without Jacksonian march, it is often referred to as epilepsia partialis continua (EPC); the motor activity lasts for hours, days, weeks, or longer. Consciousness is not altered, but postictal weakness is frequent. In most cases, the ictal focus is cortical, and anticonvulsants help prevent generalization but are frequently ineffective at aborting the seizures. EPC is often caused by a structural lesion (e.g., tumor, chronic infarction) or a progressive neurodegenerative disease (particularly in children). Focal SE of all forms is often related to acute hemispheric lesions such as a hemorrhage or brain metastasis.
   - Myoclonic SE is seen in patients after cardiac arrest or asphyxiation and consists of synchronous brief jerking of the limbs, face, or diaphragm. It can also be seen after electrical injury, drug intoxication, or decompression sickness and often denotes severe cortical laminar necrosis in association with thalamic and spinal cord injuries.

4. **What defines NSE?**
   The same principles apply of prolonged duration (>5 minutes) or lack of return to baseline mental status in between seizures. However, NSE can be difficult to diagnose because of lack of

pronounced motor activity. NSE is commonly divided into complex partial status and absence status, which are often mistaken for behavioral abnormalities or a psychiatric disorder. Clinical presentation is diverse and can involve blank staring or eye movement abnormalities and subtle periorbital, facial, or limb myoclonus. Absence SE is characterized by a reduction in vigilance, lack of attention, and automatism. Given the challenge of clinical diagnosis of NSE, electroencephalography (EEG) is often required to establish the diagnosis. Careful examination of the fully undressed patient with attention to the eye movements *(versive saccades)* and hands and face can often reveal subtle rhythmic movements of the mouth or digits suggestive of subtle generalized motor status, especially in patients who have received anticonvulsants.

5. **Name common causes of convulsive SE.**
   The most common cause of SE in a patient with a known seizure disorder is subtherapeutic AED levels. However in young patients, febrile seizure is a common precipitator, and central nervous system (CNS) infection with common pathogens such as *Haemophilus influenzae* and *Streptococcus pneumoniae* should be ruled out by lumbar puncture. Metabolic and electrolyte disturbances, traumatic brain injury, tumor, and drug intoxication are among other common causes. Ischemic strokes rarely produce seizures in the acute period, but chronically areas of encephalomalacia can provide substrate for intractable seizures. Proconvulsant drugs include β-lactam antibiotics and quinolones, bronchodilators, certain antidepressants, and immunosuppressants. SE caused by low AED levels or alcohol abuse is associated with a relatively good prognosis, whereas outcome is generally poor after cerebrovascular disease or anoxic injury.

6. **Why is urgent treatment of SE a medical necessity?**
   SE can be life threatening with the development of pyrexia, deepening coma, and circulatory collapse. Aspiration is common and may result in respiratory failure with hypoxemia, systemic inflammatory response, and disseminated intravascular coagulation with multiple organ failure. Continuous seizures can result in rhabdomyolysis with risk for acute renal failure, lactic acidosis, and cardiac arrhythmias. Of importance, repetitive electric discharges can result in irreversible neuronal injury after as little as 5 to 20 minutes; cell death is common after 60 minutes. Neuronal injury can, understandably, also result from the acute insult that provoked the SE. A mortality rate of between 10% and 12% has been reported, of which the majority is related to the underlying process producing the SE. The highest mortality occurs in elderly patients and those with SE after a stroke or anoxia, whereas children, patients with SE related to subtherapeutic AED, or those who have unprovoked SE have usually a better outcome.

7. **Name general treatment measures for SE.**
   The immediate management of the patient should include measures to establish an airway, provide oxygenation, and stabilize circulation.
   - An oral airway can be used if feasible, although most patients with prolonged SE may benefit from early endotracheal intubation.
   - Supplemental oxygen should be provided, large-bore proximal intravenous (IV) access obtained, and liberal hydration with normal saline solution initiated.
   - Vital signs should be recorded regularly.
   - A blood sample should be collected as soon as possible to rule out hypoglycemia.
   - A complete blood cell count, anticonvulsant levels, serum electrolytes, serum osmolarity, blood urea nitrogen, creatinine, calcium, magnesium, phosphate, a drug screen, blood alcohol level, and arterial blood gas analysis should also be ordered.
   - If glucose testing reveals hypoglycemia, thiamine (100 mg IV) should be administered before the glucose bolus in patients with poor nutrition (e.g., patients with alcoholism).
   - Whenever appropriate, vasopressor agents should be used to support the circulation.
   - If CNS infection is suspected, empirical treatment followed by early lumbar puncture for cerebrospinal fluid analysis should be considered, especially in febrile children.

- EEG monitoring is particularly important in patients who have received neuromuscular blocking agents for intubation, as these agents may stop visible seizure manifestations despite electrical seizure activity in the brain.

8. **What are the first-line treatment options for generalized convulsive SE?**
There is no completely satisfactory approach to the treatment of SE, and the sequence of use of antiepileptic agents continues to evolve. Drugs should be given IV, but if IV access is not available, diazepam solution can be given rectally, intranasally, or via buccal mucosa. Lorazepam remains the first-line AED despite the risk for respiratory depression. A target total dose of 0.1 mg/kg can be given at a rate no faster than 2 mg/min and in 4-mg doses to a maximal adult dose of 10 mg.

9. **What are the second-line treatments for SE?**
Second-line drugs can be started simultaneously or, if seizure persists, 1 minute after the benzodiazepine dose. Phenytoin load with 18 to 20 mg/kg (if the patient is not already being given phenytoin) can be given only in normal saline solution to prevent precipitation and is usually administered at a maximum rate of <50 mg/minute. Blood pressure should be monitored for hypotension and electrocardiogram continuously recorded and monitored for arrhythmias. Sinus bradycardia is the most common cardiac arrhythmia, and the drug may also worsen any heart block. Asystole has been reported. If the patient is already receiving phenytoin but the phenytoin level is not known, 500 mg may be given at the preceding rate. Usually, 0.74 mg/kg to an adult raises the level by approximately 1 mcg/mL. Fosphenytoin is a water-soluble form of phenytoin and lacks the propylene glycol vehicle that has been implicated in the hypotension and cardiac arrhythmias that may be observed during traditional IV phenytoin loading. However, cardiac arrhythmias may still occur when fosphenytoin is infused at rates >150 mg phenytoin equivalent per minute. Phenytoin is albumin bound, and levels should be corrected for hypoalbuminemia.

10. **What are the third-line treatments for SE ?**
Only 7% of patients who have not responded to the above treatment will respond to a third-line drug, which is why many clinicians have proposed to skip the third-line drugs and proceed directly to continuous infusion therapy. Additional doses of 5 mg/kg phenytoin can be administered up to a total of 30 mg/kg. Traditionally, phenobarbital (15-20 mg/kg loading dose) has been recommended, given at a rate no faster than 50 to 100 mg/minute until the seizures stop. Maintenance therapy is then instituted at a dose of 1 to 4 mg/kg per day. Both phenobarbital and pentobarbital result in respiratory depression, which require close monitoring or sometimes intubation before initiation of treatment. Alternative treatments include sodium valproate at 15 to 30 mg/kg, followed by a maintenance dose of 500 mg three times a day, or levetiracetam 20 mg/kg IV bolus followed by a maintenance dose of 1500 mg twice a day.
 If the preceding treatment fails to stop the seizures within 30 minutes, many physicians now recommend inserting an endotracheal tube and beginning continuous infusion therapy with midazolam, pentobarbital, or propofol. Midazolam has a shorter half-life than lorazepam and produces sedation of shorter duration in SE. A loading dose of 0.2 mg/kg is followed by an hourly infusion of 0.75 to 10 mcg/kg per minute and should be continued for at least 12 hours before the dose is tapered. The absence of propylene glycol solution in midazolam reduces the risk of hypotension, bradycardia, and electrocardiogram changes, which are seen with diazepam or lorazepam infusions. Pentobarbital is administered as a loading dose of 3 mg/kg at a rate of 25 mg/minute, followed by a maintenance dose of 0.3 to 3 mg/kg per hour until the seizures stop clinically or burst suppression is reached on the EEG. Alternatively, propofol can be used in anesthetic doses (loading dose of 1-3 mg/kg followed by maintenance of 1-10 mg/kg per hour).
 These drugs are often associated with hemodynamic changes when administered in the doses mentioned and may require vasopressors to maintain adequate blood pressures. Prolonged infusion of high doses of propofol may also result in a rare complication known as the propofol

infusion syndrome, with refractory bradycardia, metabolic acidosis, rhabdomyolysis, renal failure, and cardiovascular collapse. Treatment includes discontinuation of the propofol infusion and supportive care. Additional drugs that may be tried, if seizures continue, include carbamazepine, oxcarbazepine, topiramate, lamotrigine, and gabapentin. See Table 61-1.

Other potential treatments include lidocaine infusion, inhalational anesthesia, electroconvulsive therapy, transcranial magnetic stimulation, and surgical intervention if a seizure focus is identified.

11. **How can you treat SE when you are unable to achieve IV access?**
If a peripheral IV access is difficult, initial management may include intramuscular or rectal administration of antiepileptic drugs. Benzodiazepines, such as rectal diazepam (0.2 mg/kg), or intramuscular midazolam (0.1 mg/kg), or lorazepam remain first-line agents. Intramuscular fosphenytoin at 20 mg/kg produces equal plasma concentrations of phenytoin as the oral dose within 1 to 2 hours of administration. An effective approach in patients with no IV access is the use of inhalational anesthetic agents, including isoflurane. In the past, placement of a central venous catheter or a brachial or saphenous vein cutdown was considered, but the advent of intraosseous cannulation makes this the access route of choice in emergency situations when traditional sites are unavailable.

12. **Describe the management of seizures in patients with preeclampsia.**
Magnesium sulfate remains the standard in prevention and treatment of preeclamptic seizures or SE. It is given at a dose of 4 to 5 g IV, followed by an IV infusion of 1 g/hour, with the aim to reach a therapeutic level of 3.5 to 7 mEq/L, which corresponds to 4.2 to 8.4 mg/dL. Recurrent seizures can be treated with a bolus of 2 to 4 g of magnesium sulfate. Additional antiepileptic agents are usually not needed and may cause respiratory depression in the newborn. Clinical signs for magnesium toxicity should be monitored, and reduced tendon reflexes (corresponding to a serum concentration of 8-12 mg/dL) or respiratory depression should prompt immediate discontinuation of the infusion. The most effective treatment of seizures relating to eclampsia remains delivery of the fetus if possible.

13. **Describe the pathogenesis and treatment of postanoxic myoclonic SE.**
Myoclonic SE is commonly seen in comatose patients who have survived asphyxia or cardiac arrest and indicates severe neurologic damage. It portends a very poor prognosis but must be distinguished from myoclonic jerks, which are often *asynchronous* and relate to muscle irritability rather than electrographic seizure activity. Myoclonic SE often consists of *synchronous* brief jerking in the limbs, face, or diaphragm and can be provoked by stimuli such as movement, touch, sound, or interventions such as intubation or placement of catheters. Myoclonic activity can be quite disconcerting to families and medical personnel.

Clonazepam has been advocated for treatment but is not consistently effective. Myoclonic status is also resistant to many other antiepileptic drugs such as phenobarbital, phenytoin, and benzodiazepines. Some anecdotal data suggest that valproate may be effective in treating this syndrome. Propofol infusion can be used when myoclonus causes marked contraction of diaphragm, hampering the ventilation of the lungs. Neuromuscular blocking agents may be considered to control the symptoms until the level of care has been discussed with the patient's family. It must be kept in mind that treatment of myoclonic status does not affect outcome though it may ease the distress of family and medical staff.

14. **What general measures should be considered after control of the seizures?**
It is important to establish the cause of the seizure once it is controlled and the patient's condition stabilized. Appropriate blood work and cultures should be completed. Lumbar puncture should be considered, if not already done, to rule out CNS infections and subarachnoid

TABLE 61-1. DRUGS THAT ARE TYPICALLY USED IN THE TREATMENT OF STATUS EPILEPTICUS

DRUG	LOADING DOSE	RATE OF ADMINISTRATION	MAINTENANCE DOSE	IMPORTANT ADVERSE EFFECTS
Diazepam	10-20 mg	Push	None	Hypotension, respiratory depression, sialorrhea
Lorazepam	4-8 mg	2 mg/min	None	Hypotension, respiratory depression, sialorrhea
Midazolam	0.2 mg/kg	0.4 mg/kg/hr	0.75-10 mcg/kg/min	Hypotension, respiratory depression, metabolic acidosis
Phenytoin	18-20 mg/kg	50 mg/min	Additional doses of 5 mg/kg up to 30 mg/kg	Cardiac depression, arrhythmias, hypotension, Stevens-Johnson syndrome
Fosphenytoin	18-20 mg/kg Phenytoin equivalent	150 mg/min	IV bolus one third of previous dose	Arrhythmias less frequent than with phenytoin
Phenobarbital	15-20 mg/kg	30-50 mg/min	1-4 mg/kg/day	Myocardial and respiratory depression, prolonged sedation
Pentobarbital	3 mg/kg	1-3 mg/kg/hr	0.3-3 mg/kg/hr	Myocardial and respiratory depression, prolonged sedation
Valproate	15-30 mg/kg	1.5-3 mg/kg/min	40 mg/kg/day in divided doses	Thrombocytopenia, hyperammonemia and hepatic toxicity, pancreatitis
Propofol	1-3 mg/kg	1-10 mg/kg/hr	1-3 mg/kg/hr	Hypotension, respiratory depression, hyperlipidemia, propofol infusion syndrome
Levetiracetam	20 mg/kg	Over 15 min	1500 mg twice daily	Psychosis and hallucination

hemorrhage, and imaging with computed tomography or magnetic resonance imaging should be obtained to rule out structural CNS causes. Empirical antibiotics should be started if an infectious cause is suspected, and maintenance doses of anticonvulsants should be administered and adjusted on the basis of serum levels.

KEY POINTS: STATUS EPILEPTICUS

1. SE is defined as seizures lasting ≥ 5 minutes or two or more seizures between which there is incomplete recovery of consciousness or function.

2. Morbidity and mortality are high in SE, and aggressive treatment strategies should be instituted immediately.

3. The most common cause of SE in a patient with known seizure disorder is low AED levels, whereas de novo SE is usually a manifestation of structural brain injuries or an illness that may require immediate diagnosis and treatment.

4. Treatment for SE is directed at stabilizing the patient's condition, controlling the seizure, and identifying the cause. The underlying disease should be treated promptly.

5. First-line treatment to control the seizures often includes a benzodiazepine, for example, IV lorazepam. Second-line antiepileptic drug (phenytoin or fosphenytoin) can be given simultaneously with the first-line drug, or 1 minute after its administration if seizure persists. If third-line antiepileptic drugs (phenobarbital, valproate, or levetiracetam) do not stop the seizures, proceed to continuous infusion therapy with midazolam, pentobarbital, or propofol.

BIBLIOGRAPHY

1. Bleck TP: Intensive care unit management of patients with status epilepticus. Epilepsia 48(Suppl 8):59-60, 2007.
2. Chen JW, Wasterlain CG: Status epilepticus: pathophysiology and management in adults. Lancet Neurol 5:246-256, 2006.
3. Costello DJ, Cole AJ: Treatment of acute seizures and status epilepticus. J Intensive Care Med 22:319-347, 2007.
4. DeLorenzo RJ, Pellock JM, Towne AR, et al: Epidemiology of status epilepticus. J Clin Neurophysiol 12:316-325, 1995.
5. Fountain NB, Lothman EW: Pathophysiology of status epilepticus. J Clin Neurophysiol 12:326-342, 1995.
6. Huff JS, Fountain NB: Pathophysiology and definitions of seizures and status epilepticus. Emerg Med Clin North Am 29:1-13, 2011.
7. Lowenstein DH, Bleck T, Macdonald RL: It's time to revise the definition of status epilepticus. Epilepsia 40:120-122, 1999.
8. Lucas MJ, Leveno KJ, Cunningham FG: A comparison of magnesium sulfate with phenytoin for the prevention of eclampsia. N Engl J Med 333:201-205, 1995.
9. Mayer SA, Claassen J, Lokine J, et al: Refractory status epilepticus: frequency, risk factors, and impact on outcome. Arch Neurol 59:205-210, 2002.
10. Mayhue FE: IM midazolam for status epilepticus in the emergency department. Ann Emerg Med 17:643-645, 1988.
11. Neligan A, Shorvon SD: Frequency and prognosis of convulsive status epilepticus of different causes: a systematic review. Arch Neurol 67:931-940, 2010.
12. Phillips SA, Shanahan RJ: Etiology and mortality of status epilepticus in children. A recent update. Arch Neurol 46:74-76, 1989.

13. Pritchard JA: The use of the magnesium ion in the management of eclamptogenic toxemia. Surg Gynecol Obstet 100:131-140, 1955.

14. Treiman DM, Meyers PD, Walton NY, et al: A comparison of four treatments for generalized convulsive status epilepticus. Veterans Affairs Status Epilepticus Cooperative Study Group. N Engl J Med 339:792-798, 1998.

15. Wijdicks EF, Parisi JE, Sharbrough FW: Prognostic value of myoclonus status in comatose survivors of cardiac arrest. Ann Neurol 35:239-243, 1994.

CHAPTER 62

STROKE

Corey R. Fehnel, MD, Ala Nozari, MD, PhD, and Lee H. Schwamm, MD, FAHA

1. **What is the definition of stroke?**

   Stroke is a sudden, focal neurologic syndrome due to cerebrovascular ischemia. Strokes are sudden, or apoplectic, by definition. A slow progression of neurologic symptoms should make the clinician consider alternative diagnoses. Strokes occur in two broad categories:
   - Ischemic stroke due to arterial occlusion
   - Hemorrhagic stroke due to vessel rupture

2. **Name two common conditions that mimic stroke symptoms.**

   Seizure and complicated migraine. Although at times difficult to distinguish, the clinician can often differentiate between these conditions on the basis of the temporal nature of symptom onset. Strokes generally produce a deficit that is sudden and maximal at onset. Seizures progress rapidly over a few seconds and may be associated with stereotyped motor movements and often impairment or loss of consciousness. Migraines can produce stereotypical visual, sensory, motor, or language symptoms in a predictable fashion because of the presumed mechanism of "cortical spreading depression" occurring over minutes. Spreading depression is an extracellular wave of neuronal depolarization thought to be related to rising levels of potassium concentration in the extracellular space that produces migratory symptoms as it spreads across the surface of the cortex.

3. **What are the most important aspects of evaluating an acute ischemic stroke?**

   The last time the patient was known to be at his or her baseline is key to all acute stroke interventions. The earlier a thrombolytic can be given, the greater the chance for saving neurons and reversing disability. Three- and 4.5-hour windows for intravenous (IV) thrombolysis relate primarily to the risk of hemorrhage, whereas patients receiving thrombolytic treatment within 90 minutes of symptom onset have the greatest benefit. Time is brain.

4. **Who should be administered IV recombinant tissue plasminogen activator (IVtPA)?**

   All patients seen within 3 hours of onset of acute neurologic deficit thought to result in significant disability (generally a National Institutes of Health Stroke Scale [NIHSS] score >3-4) and having intracerebral hemorrhage excluded by head computed tomography (CT) should be administered IVtPA.

5. **Who should *not* receive IVtPA?**

   See Box 62-1.

6. **Who are candidates for *extended-window* IVtPA?**

   Patients presenting between 3 and 4.5 hours after symptom onset may be candidates for extended-window IVtPA. There are *additional* exclusion criteria for extended-window tPA: age >80 years, NIHSS score >25, greater than one-third middle cerebral arteries (MCA) territory infarction by CT or magnetic resonance imaging (MRI), any oral anticoagulant use, prior stroke, or diabetes.

> **BOX 62-1. CONTRAINDICATIONS FOR IVtPA**
>
> **Absolute contraindications to IVtPA**
> - Presence of hemorrhage or large territory infarction on unenhanced head CT
> - Central nervous system lesion with high likelihood of hemorrhage (tumor, vascular malformation, aneurysm, abscess, contusion)
> - Known bacterial endocarditis
>
> **Relative contraindications to IVtPA (these are often interpreted widely and it may be reasonable to treat selected patients in the presence of one or more of these risk factors)**
> - Minor or rapidly improving symptoms
> - Seizure at stroke onset
> - Previous stroke or serious head trauma within 3 months
> - Major surgery within 14 days or minor surgery within 10 days
> - History of prior intracerebral hemorrhage
> - Blood pressure >185/110 mm Hg (may be corrected with antihypertensive)
> - Pregnant or less than 10 days post partum
> - Arterial puncture at noncompressible site within 7 days
> - International normalized ratio >1.7 (or prothrombin time >15/sec), partial thromboplastin time >40/sec, platelet count <100,000/μL
> - Glucose <50 mg/dL or >400 mg/dL
> - NIHSS score >22

7. **What are the benefits and risks of IVtPA?**
   IVtPA is supported by level I evidence and results in 30% reduction in disability at 3 months compared with placebo. Symptomatic hemorrhage rates vary depending on the study but range from 3% to 6%. An additional one in three patients given treatment with IVtPA will improve by one grade on the modified Rankin scale, and an additional one in eight will have complete reversal of deficits.

8. **When should you consider intraarterial thrombolysis or a catheter-based clot retrieval?**
   Intraarterial interventions remain an experimental therapy for acute ischemic stroke, although use of direct lytics via intraarterial catheter has a limited recommendation based on the Prolyse in Acute Cerebral Thromboembolism (PROACT) trial. Use of this intervention varies by institution. Intraarterial administration of thrombolytics is limited to 6 hours from last seen well time, whereas mechanical retrieval tends to be limited to 8 hours from symptom onset. Patients generally must have more severe neurologic deficits (NIHSS score >6) and a proximal arterial occlusion to be considered for intraarterial therapy. Full-dose IVtPA is not a contraindication to patients undergoing a catheter-based intervention.

9. **Describe the cerebral vasculature.**
   Four arteries supply the brain. Two common carotid arteries bifurcate into external and internal segments. The internal segment penetrates the base of the skull and travels within the cavernous sinus. The carotid emerges from the sinus to bifurcate into anterior cerebral arteries (ACA) and MCA. The carotid arteries terminating in ACA and MCA branches compose the *anterior circulation*. The *posterior circulation* is supplied by two vertebral arteries traveling within the lateral foramina of the sixth to second cervical vertebrae, which then penetrate the dura mater and join at the midline at the level of the pons to form the basilar artery. The basilar bifurcates to form the posterior cerebral arteries (PCA). Anterior and posterior circulations are joined by the posterior communicating arteries creating the circle of Willis.

10. **Describe a lacune and the common lacunar syndromes.**

A lacune literally means *pit*. Lacunar infarcts represent a series of small perforating vessel occlusions that result in clinical symptoms that differ from large artery infarctions. Lacunar strokes tend to be either motor or sensory and typically lack cortical findings such as alterations of consciousness or corticosensory modalities (i.e., graphesthesia, stereognosis). See Box 62-2.

BOX 62-2. LACUNAR SYNDROMES

Pure motor weakness: Face, arm and leg all involved equally. No cognitive, sensory, or visual field loss. Usually in contralateral pons or internal capsule.

Pure sensory syndrome: Numbness or paresthesias of face, arm, and leg without cognitive, motor, or visual field cut. Most commonly localized to the contralateral ventroposterolateral or medial thalamus.

Ataxic hemiparesis: Contralateral ataxia and weakness without cognitive, sensory, or visual field cut. Localizes to posterior limb of internal capsule or pons.

Dysarthria or clumsy hand: Contralateral hand clumsiness. Face or tongue weakness and slurred speech. Localizes to the pons.

---

11. **Describe the large artery infarction syndromes.**

See Box 62-3.

12. **What is a watershed syndrome?**

Infarction at border zones between major arterial territories typically occurs as the result of global brain hypoperfusion or hemispheric hypoperfusion (i.e., critical carotid stenosis). MCA-ACA is most common and results in a *person in a barrel* pattern of weakness affecting proximal greater than distal musculature.

13. **How do infarcts resulting from venous sinus thrombosis (VST) differ from arterial strokes?**

Visualized areas of infarction lie outside traditional arterial territories. Infarcts result from venous back pressure, have prominent vasogenic edema on imaging, and are often multifocal and associated with hemorrhage. VST is a less-common but significant cause of stroke in younger persons, particularly women. It is more common with venous thrombotic risk factors such as inherited hypercoagulable states (e.g., factor V Leiden mutation), and thrombophilia is encountered in approximately 80% of patients. Oral contraceptives in association with tobacco use, and late-term pregnancy or postpartum periods, present higher risk of VST. Despite the presence of hemorrhage, the risk of progression to devastating intracerebral hemorrhage appears to be lowered by anticoagulation with IV heparin. Treatment with heparin is not recommended for patients with isolated cortical vein thrombosis if the sinuses are patent.

14. **How should blood pressure be managed in acute ischemic stroke?**

A doctrine of permissive hypertension should be followed. Tissue bordering areas of infarction, or the penumbra, often has a loss of cerebral autoregulation and is at risk for hypoperfusion and hence further infarction in the setting of acutely lowered blood pressures (BP). The optimum BP goal for an individual patient depends on many factors, including baseline BP, pattern of cerebral collateral flow, and the degree of stenosis or occlusion of the intracerebral arteries. In the absence of evidence for other end-organ dysfunction (i.e., cardiac or renal), most clinicians tolerate BPs as high as 220/120 mm Hg. Pressures in excess of this are generally treated with labetalol or nicardipine as needed to gently lower the BP under careful observation for neurologic worsening. Aggressive treatment of hypertension in acute stroke often results in worsening of stroke symptoms and may result in greater disability. BP reduction occurs spontaneously outside the hyperacute period. Gradual pharmacologic reduction in BP can take

BOX 62-3. ARTERY INFARCTION SYNDROMES

Anterior Circulation Syndromes

Carotid artery occlusion: Often associated with transient monocular blindness (amaurosis fugax) due to ophthalmic artery involvement. Key symptoms are reflected by MCA involvement and include contralateral hemiparesis of the face and arm more than the leg, as well as loss of corticosensory modalities. If dominant hemisphere is involved, aphasia is present. Nondominant hemisphere results in neglect. If patient has poor collaterals, this occlusion may produce hemiplegia of face, arm, and leg with gaze deviation and decreased level of arousal.

MCA: Proximal occlusions result in contralateral hemiparesis of the face and arm more than the leg, as well as loss of corticosensory modalities. If complete proximal occlusion occurs, symptoms may resemble the carotid artery syndrome. If dominant hemisphere is involved, aphasia is present. Nondominant hemisphere results in neglect. The MCA has two major branches:

> **Superior division:** Results in anterior or Broca-type aphasia with more prominent motor symptoms of hemiparesis. Nondominant superior division occlusions spare language but result in anosognosia and aprosody of speech.

> **Inferior division:** Results in posterior or Wernicke-type aphasia with more prominent deficit of language comprehension, contralateral visual field loss. Nondominant hemisphere inferior division occlusions result in neglect, poor visual-spatial constructions, and sometimes agitation.

PCA: Most commonly results in contralateral hemianopia. Detailed review of other features, which depend on laterality of the brain, is outside the scope of this chapter. Readers are instead referred to the bibliography.

ACA: Weakness of foot and leg more than arm or face.

Posterior Circulation Syndromes

Basilar artery

Top of the basilar: These patients are somnolent with small, poorly reactive pupils and multiple gaze palsies. The condition is sometimes associated with involuntary movements of the extremities (basilar fits) that may resemble convulsions or hallucinations. Patients may have quadriparesis and become "locked in."

Pontine syndromes: Bilateral or crossed findings and gaze palsies (i.e., internuclear ophthalmoplegia) are key to localizing infarcts to the pons. These patients often have fluctuating symptoms in the early hours of the onset of symptoms.

Vertebral artery

Lateral medullary syndrome (Wallenberg): Vertigo, nystagmus, ipsilateral facial sensory loss, pharyngeal paresis, and Horner syndrome (autonomic dysfunction). Contralateral loss of pain and temperature to body and limbs.

Medial medullary syndrome: Ipsilateral tongue paresis (rarely seen), contralateral hemiparesis and posterior column dysfunction due to the medial lemniscus.

Cerebellar artery

Posterior inferior cerebellar artery: Vertigo, veering to ipsilateral side, ipsilateral limb ataxia, headache, and vomiting.

Superior cerebellar artery and anterior inferior cerebellar artery infarction rarely occur in isolation because of robust collaterals.

place over several days after an acute stroke. The one exception to this rule is among patients who are candidates for IVtPA where the BP should be <185/110 mm Hg to start treatment and be maintained at <180/105 mm Hg for the 24 hours after treatment.

15. **What is a transient ischemic attack (TIA)?**
The traditional definition of TIA was any ischemic stroke symptom that resolved within 24 hours. However, the definition has come under scrutiny because most deficits lasting greater than 1 hour are likely to cause infarction that is visible by MRI. For this reason, many centers manage patients with TIA with the same urgency as patients with acute ischemic stroke. A TIA should be considered an opportunity to rapidly intervene with appropriate medical or surgical therapies to prevent disability from an impending larger or more disabling stroke.

16. **What strokes require anticoagulation for secondary prevention?**
Anticoagulation is often used liberally in clinical settings, although the data do not support its use in unselected patients. The strongest indications for permanent anticoagulation for secondary prevention of ischemic stroke are atrial fibrillation, acute myocardial infarction complicated by left ventricular mural thrombus, mechanical prosthetic heart valves, and hypercoagulable disorders. Short-duration anticoagulation of up to 3 months followed by antiplatelet therapy is often used in the setting of arterial dissection or with severe cardiomyopathy, although specific studies addressing these populations are limited. Patients with noncardioembolic stroke due to other causes (large artery disease, small vessel disease, cryptogenic) are generally best treated with antiplatelet therapy. No evidence suggests that increasing the dose of aspirin in patients who have a stroke while taking aspirin will provide additional benefit.

17. **For what size infarctions should anticoagulation be withheld?**
This decision requires balancing the risk of recurrent infarction with the risk of hemorrhagic transformation of the index infarction. In general, if the area of infarction is large (i.e., more than one third of the MCA territory) or involves the deep lenticulostriate perforators, anticoagulation is often held for several weeks to reduce the risk of hemorrhagic transformation. However, anticoagulation may be initiated sooner in settings of high risk of recurrent stroke.

18. **Who should undergo hemicraniectomy for large hemispheric strokes?**
Very large territory strokes (so-called malignant MCA infarcts) with >50% of MCA territory involved on imaging or a measured estimated volume of >150 mL and major neurologic disability on presentation pose a risk of death of cerebral edema and subsequent herniation. Current data suggest both a functional and survival benefit from early decompressive surgery within 48 hours of stroke onset in persons under the age of 60 years. However, the decision should still be made on a case-by-case basis for the individual patient given the significant nature of remaining disability.

19. **What are the subtypes of primary hemorrhagic strokes?**
Primary intracerebral hemorrhage may be classified according to cause or location. Hypertensive hemorrhages more commonly involve deep brain structures because of the location of small arteries arising of large main trunk vessels that are most prone to hypertensive injury over time. Specific locations from most common to less common are the caudate, thalamus, pons, and cerebellum. Hemorrhages due to deposition of amyloid protein in the arterial wall, known as amyloid angiopathy, are lobar in location and spare the deep tissues. Although less common, ruptured aneurysms may present as intraparenchymal hemorrhages with minimal or no subarachnoid blood, and CT or traditional transfemoral angiography should be considered when the hematoma overlies the sylvian cistern.

20. **What BP goals should be met after acute intracerebral hemorrhage?**
This remains an active area of research. Optimum BP after a spontaneous intracerebral hemorrhage likely depends on the individual's normal BP range. Current guidelines suggest a

target systolic blood pressure (SBP) of less than 160 mm Hg, although ongoing trials suggest that an SBP of less than 140 mm Hg is probably also safe.

21. Describe the tools used for reversal of anticoagulation in warfarin-associated intracerebral hemorrhage.

Most centers currently use a combination vitamin K (safe, inexpensive, but slow reversal time) and fresh frozen plasma. A more rapid reversal is achieved with prothrombin complex concentrates and recombinant activated factor VII. Although these latter strategies rapidly correct measured laboratory abnormalities, it is unclear whether they provide long-term benefit over the traditional approaches. A randomized controlled trial of factor VII did not show clinical benefit despite promising phase II data and a reduction in hematoma growth. Practice varies significantly because of concerns over safety profile, cost, efficacy, and thrombotic complications.

22. When should an intracerebral hemorrhage be surgically evacuated?

Cerebellar hemorrhages require emergent surgical decompression, which has been shown to provide durable benefit. The role for surgical craniotomy and evacuation in spontaneous intracerebral hemorrhage in the supratentorial space is less clear, as a major randomized trial did not show benefit overall to early surgery, despite a trend toward benefit if the clot was located superficially.

23. Should patients with intracerebral hemorrhage receive empirical antiepileptic medications?

No data support the use of prophylactic antiepileptic drugs in spontaneous intracerebral hemorrhage. Some data suggest increased incidence of seizure within the first 7 days in the setting of traumatic intracerebral hemorrhage.

KEY POINTS: STROKE

1. Ischemic stroke is a medical emergency where treatment administered within accepted time frames (up to 4.5 hours for IVtPA) can dramatically improve functional outcome.

2. BP should not be treated in acute ischemic stroke unless it is greater than 220/110 mm Hg or SBP >185/110 mm Hg if IVtPA is to be administered.

3. Atrial fibrillation, acute myocardial infarction, mechanical heart valves, and hypercoagulable states are the proved indications for stroke prevention with therapeutic anticoagulation.

4. Intracerebral hemorrhage location suggests the likely cause with deep territory involvement suggesting hypertension and lobar location suggesting amyloid.

5. There is no role for surgical evacuation of spontaneous intracerebral hemorrhage in unselected patients. Cerebellar hemorrhage always warrants neurosurgical evaluation, and decompression should be undertaken in patients with declining examination results or large hemorrhages.

BIBLIOGRAPHY

1. Adams HP Jr, Del Zoppo GD, Alberts MJ, et al. Guidelines for the early management of adults with ischemic stroke. Circulation 115:e478-e534, 2007.

2. Broderick J, Connolly S, Feldmann E, et al: Guidelines for the management of spontaneous intracerebral hemorrhage in adults. Stroke 38:2001-2023, 2007.

3. Furie KL, Kasner SE, Adams RJ, et al: American Heart Association Stroke Council, Council on Cardiovascular Nursing, Council on Clinical Cardiology, and Interdisciplinary Council on Quality of Care and Outcomes Research. Guidelines for the prevention of stroke in patients with stroke or transient ischemic attack: a guideline for healthcare professionals from the American Heart Association/American Stroke Association. Stroke 42:227-276, 2011.

4. Furlan A, Higashida R, Wechsler L, et al: Intra-arterial prourokinase for acute ischemic stroke. The PROACT II study: a randomized controlled trial. Prolyse in Acute Cerebral Thromboembolism. JAMA 282:2003-2011, 1999.

5. Hacke W, Kaste M, Bluhmki E, et al: and for the European Cooperative Acute Stroke Study (ECASS) investigators: Alteplase compared with placebo within 3 to 4.5 hours for acute ischemic stroke. N Engl J Med 359:1317-1329, 2008.

6. Johnston SC, Albers GW, Gorelick PB, et al: National Stroke Association recommendations for systems of care for transient ischemic attack. Ann Neurol 69:872-877, 2011.

7. Levi M, Levy JH, Andersen HF, et al: Safety of recombinant activated factor VII in randomized clinical trials. N Engl J Med 363:1791-1800, 2010.

8. Marler JR, Tilley BC, Lu M, et al: Early stroke treatment associated with better outcome: the NINDS rt-PA stroke study. Neurology 55:1649-1655, 2000.

9. Mehdiratta M, Kumar S, Selim M, et al: Cerebral venous sinus thrombosis. In Caplan LR (ed): Uncommon Causes of Stroke, 2nd ed. New York, Cambridge University Press, 2008, pp 497-504.

10. Mendelow AD, Gregson BA, Fernandes HM, et al: Early surgery versus initial conservative treatment in patients with spontaneous supratentorial intracerebral haematomas in the International Surgical Trial in Intracerebral Haemorrhage (STICH): a randomised trial. Lancet 365:387-397, 2005.

11. The National Institute of Neurological Disorders and Stroke rt-PA Stroke Study Group : Tissue plasminogen activator for acute ischemic stroke. N Engl J Med 333:1581-1587, 1995.

12. Ropper AH, Samuels MA: Cerebrovascular diseases. In Adams and Victor's Principles of Neurology, 9th ed. New York, McGraw-Hill, 2009, pp 660-746.

13. Smith WS: Safety of mechanical thrombectomy and intravenous tissue plasminogen activator in acute ischemic stroke. Results of the multi Mechanical Embolus Removal in Cerebral Ischemia (MERCI) trial part I. AJNR Am J Neuroradiol 27:1177-1182, 2006.

14. Steiner T, Rosand J, Diringer M: Intracerebral hemorrhage associated with oral anticoagulant therapy: current practices and unresolved questions. Stroke 37:256-262, 2006.

15. Vahedi K, Hofmeijer J, Juettler E, et al: Early decompressive surgery in malignant infarction of the middle cerebral artery: a pooled analysis of three randomised controlled trials. Lancet Neurol 6:215-222, 2007.

CHAPTER 63

GUILLAIN-BARRÉ SYNDROME

Ala Nozari, MD, PhD, Corey R. Fehnel, MD, and Lee H. Schwamm, MD, FAHA

1. **What is Guillain-Barré syndrome (GBS)?**

   Also known as acute polyradiculoneuritis, GBS is an acute onset of peripheral neuropathy with progressive muscle weakness and areflexia that reaches maximum over 3 days to 3 weeks. It has a number of variants, including pure motor or motor-sensory variants, Miller Fisher variant, bulbar variant, and primary axonal GBS.

2. **Describe the pathophysiology of GBS.**

   GBS is a collection of syndromes with inflammatory demyelinating polyradiculoneuropathy. It is triggered by both humoral and cell-mediated autoimmune response to an immune sensitizing event such as an upper respiratory tract infection or cytomegalovirus, herpes simplex virus, *Campylobacter jejuni,* or mycoplasma infections. A clear antecedent infection is often difficult to identify. Antibodies to gangliosides and glycolipids trigger myelin disruption in the peripheral nervous system. Axonal antibodies occur in some cases, typically after campylobacter infection, and carry a worse prognosis for complete recovery. An increased incidence has been reported in patients with lymphoma or lupus. In the United States, it is a sporadic disease, but variants in Asia are often epidemic in the summer months, presumably because of increased human exposure to zoonotic infections from domesticated livestock.

3. **What is the typical clinical presentation of GBS?**

   GBS is an ascending paralysis that is typically characterized by symmetric weakness, sensory dysesthesias, and hyporeflexia. Mild cases may present with only mild weakness or as variants (e.g., ataxia, ophthalmoplegia, and hyporeflexia) without significant appendicular weakness. Fulminant cases may cause severe ascending weakness leading to complete tetraplegia and with paralysis of cranial nerves and respiratory muscles (involvement of the phrenic and intercostal nerves).

4. **Describe the diagnostic criteria for GBS.**

   Clinical features required for the diagnosis of GBS include areflexia and progressive motor weakness of more than one limb. Features strongly supportive of the diagnosis include progression of the motor weakness, relative symmetry, cranial nerve involvement, mild sensory symptoms, autonomic dysfunction, and recovery within 2 to 4 weeks after progression stops.

5. **What is the differential diagnosis of subacutely evolving, generalized motor weakness?**

   Disorders frequently mimicking GBS include acute intermittent porphyria, transverse myelitis, tick paralysis, myasthenia gravis, hypophosphatemia, and carcinomatous or lymphomatous meningitis. Severe peripheral neuropathies due to vasculitis or toxins such as lead, nitrofurantoin, dapsone, thallium, arsenic, and many others should also be considered.

6. **Describe laboratory and radiologic findings for GBS.**

   Cerebrospinal fluid (CSF) analysis shows elevated protein level without pleocytosis (albuminocytologic dissociation). Electromyogram and nerve conduction study results may be normal in the early acute period but after 1 to 2 weeks reveal characteristic segmental demyelination and reduction of conduction velocity. Dispersion or absence of F waves is an important early finding that is indicative of root demyelination. Although magnetic resonance imaging provides no characteristic findings, diffuse enhancement of cauda equina and nerve roots may occur as a result of disruption of the blood-nerve barrier caused by the inflammation. Conspicuous nerve root enhancement correlates with pain, disability grade, and duration of recovery.

7. **Describe the initial management of GBS in patients.**

Patients with GBS are often admitted to an intensive care unit for close observation, as some may have respiratory failure, autonomic instability, or hypotension during plasmapheresis. Patients with early cranial nerve dysfunction are more susceptible to aspiration and dysautonomia. Early tracheostomy should be considered in patients with severe weakness, particularly if it involves the bulbar musculature. Radicular thoracolumbar pain is often prominent and may benefit from treatment with neuropathic pain agents such as gabapentin. Aggressive skin care, physical therapy, and splinting are important to prevent skin breakdown and contractures. Low-molecular-weight heparin and graduated pressure stockings should be used to prevent deep vein thrombosis.

8. **When should patients with GBS have an endotracheal tube placed?**

Respiratory failure is often caused by a combination of respiratory muscle insufficiency and difficulty clearing secretions or inability to cough and protect the airway. This can be complicated by aspiration and respiratory tract infections. Bedside pulmonary function testing is helpful but may be difficult in patients with significant facial weakness because of the decreased ability to form a good seal. Clinical symptoms of neuromuscular respiratory failure include rapid and shallow breathing, restlessness, sweating, and increased accessory muscle use with the presence of paradoxical abdominal movements during inspiration.

Indications for intubation are not always clear, but the decision is supported by the presence of severe bulbar weakness with difficulty to handle secretions and protect airway, and rapidly evolving motor weakness. A vital capacity of less than 15 to 20 mL/kg and a maximum negative inspiratory pressure of less than −20 mm Hg can also indicate need for intubation. Because these patients often have facial weakness that prevents a tight seal around the lips, surrogate measures of vital capacity such as having the patient count out loud as high as he or she can in one breath may be useful (approximately 100 mL for each number counted slowly). Hypoxia by pulse oximetry or arterial blood gas measurements are only very late signs of respiratory muscle failure and if normal should not provide reassurance as to the stability of the condition of the patient with GBS. Hypercapnia and respiratory acidosis are also late signs of respiratory failure and should prompt rapid institution of ventilatory support.

9. **What considerations regarding anesthesia and neuromuscular blockade should be kept in mind when performing endotracheal intubation in a patient with GBS?**

Cranial and autonomic nervous dysfunction often predisposes these patients to an increased risk for aspiration. Aspiration precautions, including decompression of the stomach before the induction of anesthesia, should therefore be considered in all patients. A nondepolarizing neuromuscular blocking agent should be used whenever possible, as depolarizing neuromuscular blocking agents have been associated with an increased risk for hyperkalemia-induced cardiac arrest in immobilized or paralyzed patients.

10. **Describe autonomic dysfunction and its clinical implications in GBS.**

Dysautonomia consists of rapid fluctuations in blood pressure, heart rhythm disturbances including sinus bradycardia, or even sinus arrest. Gastric motility can also be affected. Dysautonomia results from excessive or insufficient sympathetic or parasympathetic activity. It is more commonly seen with the demyelinating form, as opposed to the axonal form of GBS and is usually present if the disease is severe enough to require mechanical ventilation. The hemodynamic instability is typically short-lived and self-limited, but small doses of short-acting and titratable vasoactive medications may be required.

11. **Do any specific therapies for GBS exist?**

Supportive therapy, mechanical ventilation, and measures to prevent aspiration are important. An arterial catheter may be placed to monitor blood pressure if hemodynamic instability is anticipated. Though debate remains, immunoglobulins are considered first-line treatment, particularly in the setting of dysautonomia or if a significant risk exists for catheter-related complications with plasmapheresis or exchange transfusion. Intravenous immunoglobulin (IVIG) is typically administered at a dose of 0.4 g/kg per day for 5 days. Side effects include anaphylaxis, aseptic meningitis, acute renal failure, and thromboembolic events. Patients who have immunoglobulin A (IgA) deficiency should receive IVIG that is also IgA deficient to reduce the risk of adverse reaction. Early plasma exchange may augment the recovery and can reduce the residual deficit. Typically it consists of five exchanges of 50 mL/kg over a 90- to 120-minute period, with 5% albumin repletion. Side effects include hypovolemia and hemodynamic instability, vasovagal reactions, anaphylaxis, hemolysis, thrombocytopenia, bleeding, and hypocalcemia. Relative contraindications to treatment include sepsis, recent myocardial infarction, marked dysautonomia, and active bleeding. Steroids are not helpful.

12. **Name other important components of the general care for patients with GBS.**

In case of facial dysplasia, the eyes should be protected from exposure keratitis. Aggressive skin care and measures to avoid pressure palsies of arms and legs are needed. Physical therapy and splinting are important to prevent contractures, and early enteral nutrition or total parenteral nutrition in patients with adynamic ileus should be considered. All patients require deep venous thrombosis prophylaxis with pneumatic compression devices and low-molecular-weight heparin, gastrointestinal prophylaxis, judicious use of analgesics and anxiolytics, and tremendous emotional support.

13. **Describe the outcome and appropriate timing for transfer out of the intensive care unit.**

Patients are usually admitted to the intensive care unit because of hemodynamic instability and acute consequences of respiratory muscle weakness, including hypercapnic respiratory failure, pneumonia, atelectasis, and difficulty to protect the airway. After the peak phase of the illness has resolved the patient must be prepared for discharge with use of a multidisciplinary approach incorporating potential caregivers. Recovery may not be complete for several months, and residual weakness and atrophy are present in up to 35% of patients. Most patients, however, have excellent recovery in muscle function, eventually returning to their baseline state with or without areflexia.

KEY POINTS: GUILLAIN-BARRÉ SYNDROME

1. GBS is an acute inflammatory demyelinating polyneuropathy with progressive muscle weakness and areflexia.

2. Cranial neuropathy is often present and may include facial diplegia, ophthalmoplegia, and bulbar symptoms.

3. Symptoms are often preceded by an infectious illness, immunization, or surgery.

4. Respiratory failure and autonomic dysfunction are major complications of GBS.

5. Diagnosis can be confirmed by clinical history, CSF findings showing albuminocytologic dissociation, and nerve conduction studies.

6. Specific therapies includes IVIG and plasmapheresis therapy.

BIBLIOGRAPHY

1. Asahina M, Kuwabara S, Suzuki A, et al: Autonomic function in demyelinating and axonal subtypes of Guillain-Barré syndrome. Acta Neurol Scand 105:44-50, 2002.

2. Asbury AK: Diagnostic considerations in Guillain-Barré syndrome. Ann Neurol 9 Suppl 1-5, 1981.

3. Gorson KC, Ropper AH, Muriello MA, et al: Prospective evaluation of MRI lumbosacral nerve root enhancement in acute Guillain-Barré syndrome. Neurology 47:813-817, 1996.

4. Guillain-Barre Syndrome Steroid Trial Group: Double-blind trial of intravenous methylprednisolone in Guillain-Barré syndrome. Lancet 341:586-590, 1993.

5. Hughes RA, Hadden RD, Gregson NA, et al: Pathogenesis of Guillain-Barré syndrome. J Neuroimmunol 100:74-97, 1999.

6. Hughes RA, Raphaël JC, Swan AV, et al: Intravenous immunoglobulin for Guillain-Barré syndrome. Cochrane Database Syst Rev 1:CD002063, 2006.

7. Hughes RA, Wijdicks EF, Benson E, et al: Supportive care for patients with Guillain-Barré syndrome. Arch Neurol 62:1194-1198, 2005.

8. Kehoe M: Guillain-Barré syndrome—a patient guide and nursing resource. Axone 22(4):16-24, 2001.

9. Lawn ND, Fletcher DD, Henderson RD, et al: Anticipating mechanical ventilation in Guillain-Barré syndrome. Arch Neurol 58:893-898, 2001.

10. Ropper AH: Further regional variants of acute immune polyneuropathy. Bifacial weakness or sixth nerve paresis with paresthesias, lumbar polyradiculopathy, and ataxia with pharyngeal-cervical-brachial weakness. Arch Neurol 51:671-675, 1994.

11. Ropper AH, Shahani BT: Pain in Guillain-Barré syndrome. Arch Neurol 41:511-514, 1984.

CHAPTER 64

MYASTHENIA GRAVIS

Corey R. Fehnel, MD, Ala Nozari, MD, PhD, and Lee H. Schwamm, MD, FAHA

1. **What is myasthenia gravis (MG)?**
   MG is an autoimmune disorder affecting the neuromuscular junction characterized by a T-cell–mediated response targeting the postsynaptic acetylcholine receptor or receptor-associated proteins. Patients typically have the classic pattern of *fatigable weakness*, where repetitive stimulation of a muscle results in progressive weakness.

2. **What are the classic patterns of weakness seen in patients with MG?**
   The disease is divided into ocular and generalized forms. Both forms can present similarly with extraocular, facial, and oropharyngeal muscles presenting early in the course of the disease. Weakness of these muscles is seen clinically as diplopia, ptosis, dysphagia, and hypophonia, respectively. The ocular form is restricted to these muscles, whereas the generalized form may present initially with, and/or progress to, weakness of flexors and extensors of the neck and proximal muscles of the trunk.

3. **List and describe the differential diagnosis of bulbar weakness.**
   - *Lambert-Eaton myasthenic syndrome (LEMS):* LEMS presents in the opposite fashion of MG. Patients present with weakness that improves on repetitive stimulation of the muscle. Autoantibodies are directed presynaptically and prevent Ca^{++}-mediated release of synaptic vesicles. LEMS is most often a paraneoplastic disorder.
   - *Miller Fisher variant Guillain-Barré syndrome (GBS):* Antibodies to GQ1b affect the bulbar musculature first resulting in the triad of ophthalmoplegia, ataxia, and areflexia. See Chapter 63 for description of classic GBS presentation.
   - *Thyrotoxicosis:* Presents with transient weakness and ocular findings. Hence thyroid function tests are part of the initial evaluation of any patient with suspected MG.
   - *Botulism:* Presents with blurred vision, midposition nonreactive pupils, dysphagia, and limb weakness.
   - *Amyotrophic lateral sclerosis (ALS):* Though early stage ALS can have protean manifestations, key differences are the presence of upper motor neuron signs such as spasticity and hyperreflexia not seen in MG.

4. **How is MG diagnosed?**
   The clinical syndrome of fatigable muscle weakness should raise clinical suspicion, often with better strength in the morning that progressively worsens throughout the day. Physical examination should include testing of sustained upgaze for >30 seconds with observation for eyelid twitch, ptosis, or diplopia. With ocular symptoms such as ptosis, an ice pack applied to the eyelid can speed synaptic transmission, which supports the diagnosis of MG; the reliability and specificity of this test are, nevertheless, questionable.

   Edrophonium (Tensilon) is no longer widely available. It is a very rapidly acting cholinesterase inhibitor and carries a small risk of heart block, warranting a small test dose and a monitored setting with access to external cardiac pacing pads when used. Reliable measurement of clinical symptoms is essential before considering the test, as improvement must be measured as objectively as possible.

Electromyography (EMG) is the current diagnostic test of choice in MG. The characteristic EMG pattern found in MG is progressively smaller action potentials with repetitive nerve stimulation (decrement). Single-fiber EMG can be a more sensitive method but requires great cooperation of the patient and hence rarely applies to the patient in the intensive care unit (ICU). Though often present, serum autoantibodies to the acetylcholine receptor are not required for the diagnosis of MG.

5. **Describe the pathophysiology of MG.**
Autoantibodies producing symptoms of MG are directed against the acetylcholine receptor (AChR) on the postsynaptic membrane. AChR antibodies are found in 80% to 90% of patients with generalized MG and 60% with ocular MG. Autoantibodies against the muscle-specific tyrosine kinase are found in 70% of patients with MG without AChR antibodies. A remaining small fraction of patients without identified autoantibodies have what is termed *seronegative MG*. The antibodies produce a functional deficit of acetylcholine receptors, as well as morphologic change in the neuromuscular junction visible by electron microscopy. Consequently, the effect of acetylcholine on the postsynaptic membrane is reduced, and the probability that a nerve impulse will cause a muscle action potential is reduced.

6. **What is myasthenic crisis?**
Myasthenic crisis is weakness from MG severe enough to necessitate intubation or to delay extubation after surgery. It can occur spontaneously or may be precipitated by surgery, infection, pregnancy, or a number of drugs including aminoglycosides, erythromycin, β-blockers, procainamide, quinidine, and magnesium. It should be distinguished from a cholinergic crisis in which weakness is due to inadvertent excess cholinergic medication.

7. **How should a patient in myasthenic crisis be evaluated?**
With increasing muscle weakness it is important to assess respiratory muscle strength and identify impending respiratory failure. Tachypnea is often the first sign of impending respiratory failure. Important respiratory parameters that should be monitored include vital capacity (VC) and maximum inspiratory force (MIF). Because neither measurement has been shown to be superior, the two are usually analyzed in combination. In a patient with progressive muscle weakness, a MIF <20 cm H_2O or VC <5 mL/kg indicates the need for elective intubation and mechanical ventilation. These measurements can often be difficult to obtain and are spurious in a patient with severe facial weakness, which can prevent a tight seal around the lips. Therefore surrogate measures of VC such as having the patient count out loud as high as he or she can in one breath may be useful (approximately 100 mL for each number counted slowly). Hypercarbia usually develops before hypoxia. Both are late signs of neuromuscular respiratory failure and should not be used as a decision for intubation in MG. After respiratory status has been stabilized, focus should be shifted to determining the underlying trigger for the exacerbation. Infections are a common trigger, often of pulmonary or urinary source, with further evaluation of other sources as clinical suspicion dictates. Great care should be taken to avoid medications that could worsen neuromuscular transmission. An extensive list of medications that aggravate MG can be found at http://www.myasthenia.org. The list should be reviewed for every patient with MG in your care. Key offenders are aminoglycosides and quinolones.

8. **How are intubation and airway management handled differently in patients with MG?**
Patients with MG are sensitive to nondepolarizing neuromuscular blocking agents but relatively resistant to depolarizing agents. As an example, the dose required to produce 95% depression of twitch height (ED95) for atracurium and vecuronium (nondepolarizing) is estimated to be 40% to 60% that of normal individuals. Preferably, short- or intermediate-acting

nondepolarizing neuromuscular blocking agents should be used. If muscle weakness is excessive, intubation of the trachea can also be performed without neuromuscular blocking agents (e.g., with remifentanil and propofol bolus only). If succinylcholine is used, a dose of 1.5 to 2.0 mg/kg should be adequate for rapid-sequence intubation in most patients with myasthenia, as the ED95 of succinylcholine is approximately 2.6 times that needed for patients without myasthenia (0.8 mg/kg vs. 0.3 mg/kg).

Patients with MG are more likely than normal patients to have a phase II block, and cholinesterase depletion with plasmapheresis or inhibition with pyridostigmine may prolong the blockade.

9. **What are the medical treatments for MG?**
   Acetylcholinesterase inhibitors represent the mainstay of symptomatic treatment. Pyridostigmine (Mestinon) is most commonly used as it has few muscarinic side effects. Onset of action is within 15 to 30 minutes (oral administration) and peak effect within 1 to 2 hours. Usual daily doses are between 30 to 120 mg, divided into three to six administrations per day. Corticosteroids cause a reduction in the number of antibodies to the acetylcholine receptors and are often used to initiate or maintain a remission. Care should be taken with sudden dose escalations of corticosteroids as there may be an initial period of worsening before improvement. Azathioprine and cyclosporine are popular steroid-sparing agents employed in refractory or steroid-dependent cases. Acute exacerbations require ICU care and are treated with intravenous immunoglobulin (IVIG) or plasmapheresis. Cholinesterase inhibitors are often held in the critical care setting to avoid toxicity, and restarting them can be tricky especially if the patient has reduced ability to handle oral secretions, which increase with use of these drugs. The oral dose of pyridostigmine is approximately 30 times the intravenous dose.

10. **Who should undergo thymectomy?**
    Hyperplasia of the thymus gland is seen in 65% of MG cases, whereas thymoma is seen in up to 15% of patients. Video-assisted thorascopic surgery–assisted thymectomy is often performed but is largely unproved. If a thymoma is present, then thymectomy appears to result in 35% remission rate if performed within 1 to 2 years of diagnosis. Thymectomy should be performed electively and not during a myasthenic crisis.

11. **Name the clinical signs of pyridostigmine toxicity.**
    Pyridostigmine toxicity (cholinergic crisis) can cause weakness and may be misdiagnosed as worsening of MG symptoms. Overstimulation of the nicotinic acetylcholine receptors results in involuntary twitching, fasciculations, and weakness (inability to coordinate muscle contraction and relaxation). Muscarinic side effects include excess salivation, lacrimation, urinary incontinence, diaphoresis, bronchorrhea, pulmonary edema, miosis, and blurred vision and are referred to as the "SLUDGE syndrome."

12. **What is the prognosis for patients with MG?**
    Prognosis for most patients is quite good. Most patients are able to return to their regular lifestyle. However, a wide spectrum of disease severity exists. Some patients respond well to minimal doses of pyridostigmine and do not require long-term immunosuppressive drugs. Others require long-term corticosteroids and powerful immunomodulatory agents and may still have frequent exacerbations. Time of diagnosis from symptom onset and age at onset are predictors of clinical remission. History of intubation from respiratory failure is a negative prognostic sign. Pregnancy has variable effects on the course of MG and can lead to exacerbation, remission, or no change in disease. The first trimester and immediate postpartum period are times of highest risk for exacerbation.

KEY POINTS: MYASTHENIA GRAVIS

1. MG is an autoimmune disorder with antibodies directed against the postsynaptic acetylcholine receptors.

2. In a majority of cases MG preferentially affects ocular and bulbar musculature followed later by muscles of the trunk and limbs.

3. Myasthenic crisis is weakness resulting in respiratory failure best measured by respiratory rate and serial measurement of MIF and VC. Hypoxia and hypercarbia develop very late in myasthenic crisis and should not be used as intubation criteria.

4. Plasmapheresis and IVIG are the mainstays of treatment of severe myasthenic exacerbations. A careful evaluation for infection and review of all potentially harmful medications (an extensive list) should occur for every patient with exacerbation of MG.

BIBLIOGRAPHY

1. Drachman DB: Myasthenia gravis. N Engl J Med 330:1797-1810, 1994.

2. Gomez AM, Van Den Broeck J, Vrolix K, et al: Antibody effector mechanisms in myasthenia gravis-pathogenesis at the neuromuscular junction. Autoimmunity 43:353-370, 2010.

3. Jani-Acsadi A, Lisak RP: Myasthenic crisis: guidelines for prevention and treatment. J Neurol Sci 261:127-133, 2007.

4. Mao ZF, Mo XA, Qin C, et al: Course and prognosis of myasthenia gravis: a systematic review. Eur J Neurol 17:913-921, 2010.

5. Scherer K, Bedlack R, Simel D: Does this patient have myasthenia gravis? JAMA 293:1906-1914, 2005.

CHAPTER 65

ALCOHOL WITHDRAWAL

Bruce A. Crookes, MD, FACS, and William Peery, MD

1. **What are alcohol use disorders (AUDs)?**
   AUDs are a spectrum of disorders that range from excessive use, to abuse, to dependence, to addiction.
   - *Abuse* is defined as being when an individual has adverse socioeconomic or health consequences related to the use of a substance.
   - *Dependence* is manifested when a patient has withdrawal symptoms when the substance is discontinued or when larger amounts are required to obtain the same effect.
   - *Addiction* is present when the individual has a compulsive craving for the substance. It is important to realize that, at any one time, an individual may be experiencing a combination of abuse, dependence, and/or addiction.

2. **How much alcohol is too much? How big a problem is it in the intensive care unit (ICU)?**
   The National Institutes of Health has published guidelines that serve to quantify and define excessive alcohol use. Men aged $\leq$65 years are thought to have excessive alcohol consumption if they consume more than four drinks per day or more than 14 drinks in a week. For men >65 years and for women, these volumes are halved. It is thought that patients who consume excessive amounts of alcohol are at increased risk for health problems. It has been estimated that AUDs are seen in as many of 15% to 20% of primary care and hospitalized patients, in 10% to 33% of ICU admissions, and in approximately 50% of trauma patients.

3. **Are AUDs associated with any alterations in patient outcomes?**
   The outcomes of patients with AUDs appear to vary by the reason for admission. Trauma patients with AUDs seem to have no difference in mortality or length of stay as compared with controls, although trauma patients with a history of chronic alcohol abuse have a higher incidence of pneumonia and cardiac complications. Burn patients with AUDs have higher mortality and poorer shorter and long-term outcomes. Surgical patients are at greater risk for pneumonia, wound infections, sepsis, poor wound healing, and cardiac complications. In the medical ICU, AUDs increase the need for mechanical ventilation and are independent risk factors for sepsis.

4. **How is immune function altered by alcohol ingestion?**
   Neutrophil and macrophage response is altered by the ingestion of alcohol, and leukopenia may result from depressed levels of granulocyte colony-stimulating factor. In surgical and trauma patients, aberrant cytokine concentrations have been noted, including decreased levels of interleukin (IL)-1, IL-6, IL-12, tumor necrosis factor-α, and interferon-β. Overall, in surgical and trauma patients, an imbalance appears to exist between proinflammatory cytokines and antiinflammatory cytokines.

5. **What are the criteria for alcohol withdrawal, and when does it typically occur?**
   First, the patient must have cessation of (or reduction in) alcohol use that has been heavy and prolonged. In addition, the patient must have two or more of the following, developing several hours to a few days after cessation: autonomic hyperactivity (i.e., sweating or heart rate >100 beats/minute); increased hand tremor; insomnia; nausea or vomiting; transient visual,

tactile, or auditory hallucinations or illusions; psychomotor agitation; anxiety; and grand mal seizures, typically tonic-clonic in nature. Alcohol withdrawal typically manifests itself 48 to 96 hours after abstinence from alcohol.

6. **What is delirium tremens (DTs)? What is the mortality associated with DTs in the ICU?**

According to the American Psychiatric Association *Diagnostic and Statistical Manual of Mental Disorders,* fourth edition, DTs is alcohol withdrawal and associated with either a:
- Disturbance of consciousness (i.e., reduced clarity of awareness in the environment) with reduced ability to focus, sustain, or shift attention; delirium; confusion; and frank psychosis
- *or*
- Change in cognition (such as memory deficit, disorientation, language disturbance)
- *or*
- Development of a perceptual disturbance that is not better accounted for by a preexisting, established, or evolving dementia

ICU patients in whom DTs develop have a mortality rate of 5% to 15%.

7. **What are the four clinical states of alcohol withdrawal?**

Alcohol withdrawal has four clinical states: autonomic hyperactivity, hallucinations, neuronal excitation, and DTs. Note that these states occur along a timeline relative to time at which alcohol intake was reduced, but patients do not progress linearly from one stage to the next, often skipping one or more of the stages.

8. **Is there a methodology to predict the severity of alcohol withdrawal?**

The severity of alcohol withdrawal may be predicted by the severity of previous detoxifications or the presence of a history of detoxification-related seizures. The Clinical Institute Withdrawal Assessment for Alcohol revised 10-item scale is a validated, 10-item assessment tool that can be used to monitor and medicate patients, while functioning as a predictor of severe withdrawal symptoms. It examines several symptoms, including nausea or vomiting, tremors, agitation, anxiety, paroxysmal sweats, orientation, tactile and auditory disturbances, visual disturbances, and headache.

9. **What is the pathophysiology of alcohol use?**

Acutely, alcohol ingestion inhibits excitatory N-methyl-D-aspartate (NMDA) receptors, which leads to a reduction in the release of the neurotransmitter glutamate. Activation of the inhibitory γ-aminobutyric acid A (GABA-A)–type receptor during alcohol exposure leads to anxiolytic and sedative, as well as impairment of motor coordination. As alcohol ingestion becomes chronic, GABA-A receptor function is decreased, and the NMDA receptors are up-regulated, leading to tolerance.

10. **What is the pathophysiology of alcohol withdrawal?**

When alcohol is abruptly discontinued, NMDA receptor function is increased, and the tonic inhibition provided by GABA-A receptors is reduced. This phenomenon of increased excitation and loss of suppression results in the clinical manifestations of autonomic excitability and psychomotor agitation.

11. **What class of medications are primarily used to treat alcohol withdrawal?**

Benzodiazepines enhance GABA transmission, thereby balancing the surge of glutamate that is responsible for the effects of alcohol withdrawal. Current recommendations in the United States and Europe favor the use of benzodiazepines for the treatment of severe to moderate alcohol withdrawal symptoms, including seizures and DTs. In a recent Cochrane review, it was thought that benzodiazepines showed a protective benefit against alcohol withdrawal symptoms, in particular seizures.

12. **What are the advantages and disadvantages of *symptom-triggered* benzodiazepine therapy?**
Short-acting benzodiazepines (i.e., lorazepam, oxazepam) are typically used in a *symptom-triggered* capacity, in response to the severity of withdrawal. The downside of this approach is that it requires frequent patient assessment, and many of the symptoms of alcohol withdrawal (i.e., agitation) are not uncommon in the typical ICU population. The advantage to this approach is that patients generally receive a lower total dose of benzodiazepines over the course of their ICU stay and generally have fewer days using the ventilator.

13. **What are the advantages and disadvantages of *fixed-dose* benzodiazepine therapy?**
Longer-acting benzodiazepines (i.e., diazepam, chlordiazepoxide) are usually used in a "fixed-dose" strategy and may afford a smoother withdrawal. Unfortunately, this strategy may result in patients receiving too much or too little of the benzodiazepine, resulting in uncontrolled symptoms or oversedation. Generally, in the ICU, lorazepam (Ativan) is preferred because of a lack of active metabolites, because it can be administered intravenously, and because it does not need to be adjusted in renal failure. No specific benzodiazepine has been shown to be superior to another when used in the ICU setting.

14. **Are there any risks to lorazepam use?**
Lorazepam is suspended in propylene glycol, and continuous infusions of lorazepam could result in elevated levels of propylene glycol. Accumulation of propylene glycol is associated with hyperosmolar metabolic acidosis, lactic acidosis, acute tubular necrosis, intravascular hemolysis, central nervous system depression, seizures, cardiac arrhythmias, and hypotension.

15. **Is intravenous alcohol safe in the treatment of alcohol withdrawal?**
Intravenous alcohol has been used to treat withdrawal and was shown in one trial to be as effective as diazepam for the management of withdrawal. Unfortunately, in the group that received the alcohol infusion, the majority of patients did not have detectable levels of alcohol in their blood, and the patients had wide fluctuations in their level of sedation. This would suggest that dosing is difficult, at best. Most authors recommend that intravenous alcohol not be used to treat withdrawal in the ICU, because of the risks of intoxication, delirium, and gastritis.

16. **Can I use carbamazepine or oxcarbazepine to treat alcohol withdrawal?**
Carbamazepine and oxcarbazepine are nonbenzodiazepine anticonvulsants that possess GABA-nergic activity and have been used to treat alcohol withdrawal in Europe for more than 30 years. Both of these drugs are nonaddictive, have no sedating effects, and seem to promote a reduction in withdrawal symptoms. Although carbamazepine has demonstrated efficacy, safety, and tolerability in the treatment of moderate to severe alcohol symptoms, the literature is inconclusive in its ability to prevent DTs or seizures relative to benzodiazepines.

17. **Are any other new therapies available for the treatment of alcohol withdrawal?**
Pregabalin, a newer anticonvulsant drug, has been examined in two small studies and was found to be safe and efficacious in alcohol withdrawal. Unfortunately, not enough evidence exists to develop a recommendation for its use over benzodiazepines. The prototype GABA B receptor antagonist baclofen may also represent an effective alternative in the treatment of alcohol withdrawal, but evidence recommending it in the treatment of alcohol withdrawal is insufficient at this time.

KEY POINTS: ALCOHOL WITHDRAWAL

1. AUD in trauma patients is associated with higher morbidity but not a higher mortality in the ICU.

2. DTs is associated with a 5% to 15% mortality.

3. Alcohol withdrawal manifests *48 to 96 hours after cessation*.

4. Benzodiazepines are the *drug of choice* for treating alcohol withdrawal.

BIBLIOGRAPHY

1. Amato L, Davoli M, Vecchi S, et al: Cochrane systematic reviews in the field of addiction: what's there and what should be. Drug Alcohol Depend 113:96-103, 2011.

2. American Psychiatric Association: Diagnostic and statistical manual of mental disorders. 4th ed. Text revision. Washington, D.C, American Psychiatric Association, 2000.

3. Baldwin WA, Rosenfeld BA, Breslow MJ, et al: Substance abuse-related admissions to adult intensive care. Chest 103:21-25, 1993.

4. Delgado-Rodriguez M, Gomez-Ortega A, Mariscal-Ortiz M, et al: Alcohol drinking as a predictor of intensive care and hospital mortality in general surgery: a prospective study. Addiction 98:611-616, 2003.

5. de Wit M, Jones DG, Sessler CN, et al: Alcohol-use disorders in the critically ill patient. Chest 138:994-1003, 2010.

6. Jurkovich GJ, Rivara FP, Gurney JG, et al: The effect of acute alcohol intoxication and chronic alcohol abuse on outcome from trauma. JAMA 270:51-56, 1993.

7. Mariani JJ, Levin FR: Pharmacotherapy for alcohol-related disorders: what clinicians should know. Harv Rev Psychiatry 12:351-366, 2004.

8. Moss M, Burnham EL: Chronic alcohol abuse, acute respiratory distress syndrome, and multiple organ dysfunction. Crit Care Med 31:S207-S212, 2003.

9. National Institute on Alcohol Abuse and Alcoholism: Helping patients who drink too much: a clinician's guide. Rockville, Md., Department of Health and Human Services, National Institutes of Health, updated 2005 ed. (rev. Jan. 2007).

10. Sarff M, Gold JA: Alcohol withdrawal syndromes in the intensive care unit. Crit Care Med 38:S494-S501, 2010.

11. Spies C, Tonnesen H, Andreasson S, et al: Perioperative morbidity and mortality in chronic alcoholic patients. Alcohol Clin Exp Res 25:164S-170S, 2001.

12. Turner RC, Lichstein PR, Peden JG Jr, et al: Alcohol withdrawal syndromes: a review of pathophysiology, clinical presentation, and treatment. J Gen Intern Med 4:432-444, 1989.

13. Weinberg JA, Magnotti LJ, Fischer PE, et al: Comparison of intravenous ethanol versus diazepam for alcohol withdrawal prophylaxis in the trauma ICU: results of a randomized trial. J Trauma 64:99-104, 2008.

BURNS AND FROSTBITE

Shawn P. Fagan, MD, and Jeremy Goverman, MD, FACS

CHAPTER 66

1. **What determines the degree of tissue destruction after a thermal injury?**
   The degree of tissue injury is directly related to the temperature and duration of contact with the heat source. Children are particularly susceptible to thermal injury because of the thinner dermal layer. At 156° F (68.9° C), it requires less than 1 second to have a full-thickness thermal injury. As temperature of the heat source decreases, the time necessary for a clinical significant thermal injury is prolonged. This is evident by the 10 seconds required to produce a full-thickness thermal injury at 130° F (54.4° C). For this reason, the American Burn Association recommends setting the thermostat of a household water heater to 120° F (48.9° C) to prevent clinically significant thermal injuries in the household.

2. **What determines the physiologic impact of a thermal injury on the human body?**
   The physiologic impact of the thermal injury is directly related to the extent of second- and third-degree thermal injury. This is why most burn fluid resuscitative formulas are based on the extent of second- and third-degree thermal injury. Of interest, the depth of thermal injury does not affect the physiologic consequences but may affect the wound management techniques required for effective wound healing. Most second-degree thermal injuries can be managed until healing with topical antimicrobials, whereas third-degree thermal injuries, dependent on size, generally require excision of nonviable tissue and closure with skin grafts.

3. **How are thermal injuries classified?**
   Thermal injuries are classified by the depth of injury to the underlying skin's structure. The skin is composed of an outer epidermis and inner dermis. The regenerative capacity of the skin, the stem cells, reside in the dermis and hair follicles. Thus the ability to heal a thermal injury is directly related to the degree of damage of the dermis and the presence of hair follicles at the site of thermal injury. Burn wounds are classified from first through fourth degree:
   - **First degree:** Thermal injury only affects the epidermis—sunburn.
   - **Second degree:** Thermal injury affects the epidermis and superficial dermis. The injury results in blistering and mild to moderate edema to the affected area. The wound is painful because of damaged nerves but should heal with simple topical antimicrobials in approximately 14 to 21 days.
   - **Third degree:** The thermal injury affects both the epidermis and dermis. A true third-degree thermal injury should be without pain because of the complete destruction of the sensory nerves. However, few thermal injuries are composed of only one class of injury. The majority of deep thermal injuries are a mixture of depths, thus making lack of sensation a poor marker to classify depth of injury. A more specific marker of a third-degree thermal injury is the white and leathery appearance. Healing of a third-degree thermal injury will require excision and grafting.
   - **Fourth degree:** Thermal injuries that affect structure deep to the skin–fat, fascia, muscle, and/or bone. Treatment and presentation are similar to those of third-degree thermal injuries.

4. **What are the initial steps in the management of an individual who had a thermal injury?**
   The management of a thermally injured patient should proceed in a similar manner as the clinician would evaluate any trauma patient with the understanding of a few burn-specific nuances. The first step is to stop the burning process. This may be as simple as removing

smoldering clothing or copious irrigation of chemical or radiation injuries. As the burning process is being addressed, the patient should undergo a primary survey consisting of airway, breathing, circulation, disability, and exposure.

Airways can be challenging in a burn patient. Therefore clinicians must be aware of potential inhalation injuries that may affect the supraglottic airway (airway obstruction) and/or infraglottic airway (chemical pneumonitis). Children are particularly susceptible to supraglottic obstruction because of progressive edema and relatively narrow upper airways. Individuals demonstrating airway compromise or having large thermal injuries should have an endotracheal tube placed to avoid airway issues. The important point to remember is that maximal edema occurs approximately 24 hours after thermal injury.

Appropriate and rapid resuscitation is critically important to avoid future morbidity and mortality after a thermal injury. Studies have demonstrated that the timing of initial resuscitation is directly related to mortality. Delay in resuscitation must be avoided, but the rate of fluids administered must be appropriate. Recently, studies have demonstrated increased morbidity and mortality associated with overresuscitation. Thus calculating the estimated fluid requirement for a thermally injured patient should be performed early in the evaluation process and titrated on the basis of urine output and normalization of resuscitative laboratory results.

It is critically important not to be distracted by the extent or depth of thermal injury during the initial evaluation. All thermally injured patients should have a comprehensive trauma evaluation to avoid missed injuries. It is not uncommon for thermal injuries to be associated with significant trauma.

5. **What is burn shock?**
   Classically, burn shock was simply defined by a state of hypovolemia. However, it is now realized that burn shock is a complex process not only affecting preload but also influencing cardiac output and systemic vascular resistance. During the first 8 hours after thermal injury a substantial increase in capillary permeability occurs resulting in a state of intravascular volume depletion. This relative intravascular volume depletion is coupled with a decrease in cardiac output and increased systemic vascular resistance. The degree of impaired cardiac output and increased vascular tone cannot be completely attributed to the state of post–burn injury hypovolemia. Therefore a goal-directed approach to the resuscitation of a thermally injured patient is warranted. The specific impairment (preload, cardiac output, systemic vascular resistance) should be identified and appropriate therapeutic measures initiated to improve the specific problem. Simply stated, burn shock is not simply a state of hypovolemia.

6. **How do you determine the initial fluid requirements of a thermally injured patient?**
   Although burn shock can influence preload, cardiac output, and systemic vascular resistance, burn patients do differ from other intensive care unit populations with the substantial intravascular fluid depletion that occurs over the first 24 hours. This is directly related to increased capillary permeability. Therefore thermally injured patients require a considerable amount of volume administration in the first 24 hours.

   The Parkland Burn Center published the most widely used burn resuscitation formula. The formula states that the total amount of lactated Ringer's solution necessary during the first 24 hours is directly related to the size of thermal injury (second and third degree) and the preburn weight (kilograms) of the patient. The Parkland formula is 2 to 4 mL/kg body weight/Total body surface area (TBSA) thermal injury. Half of the volume is administered during the first 8 hours from time of injury with the remaining amount administered over the following 16 hours. The formula is an *estimate* of the fluids necessary during the initial 24 hours; therefore the rate of fluid administration must be adjusted on the basis of the monitoring of resuscitative parameters with the primary goal of avoiding overresuscitation.

   Some centers modify the resuscitative formula for children because of the larger surface area per kilogram body weight compared with an adult. The Galveston resuscitation formula is based on TBSA affected by thermal injury but also includes a maintenance infusion rate. The Galveston formula is 5000 mL lactated Ringer's/TBSA thermal injury +1200 mL/TBSA. In addition, infants and young children should have a continuous source of glucose administered via the maintenance fluids. Similar to that for adults, the resuscitative formula is an estimate of the fluids necessary during the first 24 hours; adjustment must be made on the basis of response to the initial resuscitation.

7. **Should a primary survey be repeated during the first 24 hours after thermal injury?**
The primary survey must be repeated frequently during the first 24 hours to avoid complications associated with progressive edema after thermal injury. Airway and breathing may be initially stabilized with early endotracheal intubation but can progressively deteriorate during the first 24 hours because of edema. This is particularly true for individuals who have circumferential thermal injuries to the chest. Progressive edema of the underlying soft tissues with restriction of chest expansion by eschar can limit tidal volumes and thus influence minute ventilation. Constant monitoring of airway pressures and tidal volumes are necessary to identify and treat this potential airway emergency. Should constriction of the chest cavity become physiologically significant, bilateral anterior axillary line escharotomies coupled with an escharotomy across the costal margin to join the axillary line escharotomies should be performed. The goal is to allow expansion of the chest cavity and to separate the chest cavity from the abdominal cavity.

   Similar to the chest, extremities must also be monitored for compromise due to progressive edema limited by circumferential eschar. Initially, all thermally injured extremities should be elevated to 45 degrees and monitored on an hourly basis. All constricting jewelry should be removed immediately. If possible, patients should be encouraged to move the affected extremities. Should vascular compromise be identified, by increasing pain on passive movement or diminished pulses, lateral escharotomies should be performed with documentation of return of perfusion. If perfusion is not reestablished with a lateral escharotomy, medial escharotomies should be performed initially followed by fasciotomies if necessary to establish effective perfusion.

8. **How do you determine the fluid needs of a thermally injured patient after the first 24 hours?**
Although everyone is exposed to the Parkland Burn Resuscitation Formula at sometime during his or her career, the fluid needs after the initial 24 hours are not as well known or published. The exact fluid requirement is individualized on the basis of the TBSA affected by thermal injury, the body's physiologic response to the thermal injury, and ambient environment surrounding the patient.

   The goal is always to administer the appropriate amount of fluid and to avoid a hypervolemic state and/or a generalized edematous state. Proper fluid administration can be achieved by adjusting the infusion rate frequently on the basis of the urine output. If the urine output is greater than 0.5 mL/kg per hour, the infusion rate can be decreased by one third and resuscitative laboratories and urine output monitored. After 3 hours of monitoring, fluid rates should again be adjusted on the basis of the urine output and trends of resuscitative parameters. To aid in estimating this fluid requirement, the Galveston burn group developed a formula to calculate this fluid requirement. The formula is 3750 mL/TBSA affected by thermal injury +1200 mL/TBSA.

9. **Who should be referred to a verified burn center?**
The American Burn Association recommends that individuals with the following conditions be referred to a verified burn center for evaluation and treatment:
   - Partial thickness burns greater than 10% TBSA
   - Burns involving the face, hands, feet, genitalia, perineum, or major joints
   - Third-degree burns in any age group
   - Electrical burns, including lightning injury

- Chemical burns
- Inhalation injury
- Burn injury in patients with preexisting medical disorders that could complicate management, prolong recovery, or affect mortality
- Any patient with burns and concomitant trauma in which the burn injury poses the greatest risk of morbidity or mortality
- Burned children in hospitals without qualified personnel or equipment for the care of children
- Burn injury in patients who will require special social, emotional, or long-term rehabilitative intervention

10. **How should potential ocular involvement be evaluated after thermal injury?**
Potential ocular involvement requires immediate attention during the first 24 hours after thermal injury. Appropriate referral to an ophthalmologist is critical not only for initial assessment of direct ocular injury but to monitor ocular pressures during the time of resuscitation. Most direct ocular injuries can be treated conservatively with ocular ointments or the application of amniotic membranes. Increases in ocular pressures due directly to the thermal injury or resulting from a generalized edematous state require aggressive monitoring and treatment. Initially, conservative therapy should be initiated with head-of-bed elevation to 30 degrees. However, high initial or progressively increasing ocular pressures should be aggressively treated with a lateral canthotomy. The goal is to prevent ocular compartment syndrome.

11. **What is burn-induced hypermetabolism?**
After a major thermal injury (TBSA >30%), several metabolic derangements have been identified and include the following:
- A relative decrease in insulin secretory capacity
- Peripheral insulin resistance
- Exaggerated protein catabolism
- A significantly elevated resting energy expenditure
   The catecholamine surge after thermal injury results in a reset of the hypothalamus thermostat by $2°$ C and alterations in the neuroendocrine axis. Combined, this results in an elevated resting energy expenditure that can be approximately 60% to 80% greater than the normal basal metabolic rate. Therefore appropriate nutrition must be instituted immediately supplying approximately 30 to 35 kcal/kg body weights with 20% to 25% of the total caloric requirement being composed of protein. In addition, several techniques are routinely used to reduce the impact of the postburn generalized hypermetabolic state:
- Maintenance of appropriate ambient temperature surrounding the burn patient
- Early excision and grafting of all third-degree thermal injuries
- Administration of anabolic agents, isolated or in combination (oxandrolone, propranolol, insulin)
- Early range of motion and exercise

12. **What are the four main advances in burn care that have dramatically reduced mortality over the last 50 years?**
- **Appropriate resuscitation:** Restoration of end-organ perfusion while avoiding overresuscitation.
- **Control of infection:** Application of topical antimicrobial agents to prevent wound infections and using systemic antimicrobials only after documentation of invasive wound infection (cellulitis), not colonization, and presence of systemic infection (bacteremia).
- **Modulation of hypermetabolism:** Early and appropriate nutrition, anabolic agents, early occupational and physical therapy.
- **Early excision and grafting:** Protein catabolism progressively worsens with the presence of third-degree thermal injury. The goal is to remove all nonviable tissue within 96 hours to lessen the degree of catabolism.

13. **What is the treatment of hydrofluoric acid exposure?**

The treatment begins the same for any potential chemical burn. First stop the burning process, remove all saturated items, irrigate the wound bed, and arrange for burn center transfer. Next determine the exact agent involved, concentration of agent, duration of contact, and mechanism of action of the specific agent. Never attempt to neutralize any chemical injury.

For hydrofluoric acid exposure it is critically important to determine the concentration of the agent. Hydrofluoric acid is a weak acid, but the fluoride can prove to be very toxic. Fluoride has a high affinity for free calcium and can potentially create a life-threatening hypocalcemia. Dilute hydrofluoric acid exposure (<10%) can be managed conservatively. The patient typically has a delayed presentation of severe pain to the affected region. It can be safely treated with topical calcium gluconate gel. Unknown or high-concentration exposure to hydrofluoric acid requires aggressive and specialized wound management coupled with serial serum calcium measurements to avoid severe hypocalcemia. Burn center transfer should not be delayed.

14. **How are electrical injuries treated?**

Electrical injuries can range from a minor "shock" without any consequences to significant morbidity due to complete conduction of the electrical current. The key concept to remember when evaluating an electrical injury is that the superficial cutaneous injuries may underestimate the total extent of injury specifically to the deeper tissues. The tissue damage caused by an electrical source is directly dependent on the strength of the current and duration of contact. This is summarized by the Joule effect, which states that the heat generated (tissue damage) is directly dependent on the current (I) squared times the resistance (tissue type) (R) times the duration of contact (T) ($J = I^2 \times R \times T$). Surprisingly, the epidermis has one of the highest resistances in the human body and thus, when overcome, the affected body part acts as a volume conductor. When this occurs, the current can pass along the very dense and highly resistant skeletal bone resulting in significant muscular damage.

All electrical burn patients should undergo a standard trauma and burn primary and secondary evaluation with particular attention to a few specific items:

- First, all patients must be evaluated for potential cardiac dysrhythmias; however, if absent, the most recent data would suggest no clinical need for continued cardiac monitoring.
- Second, all patients should be suspected of having deep tissue damage, particularly when voltages are greater than 600 V.
- Finally, all patients should have a baseline eye examination to rule out cataracts because of the potential for cataract formation after any significant electrical injury.

15. **How are frostbite injuries treated?**

Until recently, frostbite injuries were treated with rapid, moist rewarming followed by conservative management. This included allowing damaged digits and extremities to autoamputate to preserve as much length as possible after the cold injury.

Within the last few years, the concept of frostbite injuries has significantly changed from one of local tissue damage to one of local tissue damage combined with vascular occlusion. Several groups have demonstrated significant reduction in the need for amputation when rapid tissue rewarming is coupled with urgent angiography and catheter-directed fibrinolysis. Currently, all patients presenting within 24 hours from time of injury with second- and third-degree frostbite injuries should have the affected body part rapidly rewarmed and, if an extremity, urgent angiography for evaluation of potential fibrinolytic therapy.

16. **What are the known and common complications of topical antimicrobials?**

Topical antimicrobial therapy is the mainstay of the treatment for small and large thermal injuries. Although most antimicrobials have a broad range of activity against gram-positive and gram-negative organisms (silver sulfadiazine [Silvadene], silver nitrate, mafenide [Sulfamylon]), some have a narrow spectrum of activity but work well on minor thermal injuries (bacitracin, mupirocin [Bactroban]). As with any pharmacologic agent, a physician must know the indications and potential complications of the agent being prescribed. Although most topical antimicrobials are well tolerated, several have known complications associated with them. See Table 66-1.

TABLE 66-1. TOPICAL ANTIMICROBIAL THERAPY				
TOPICAL ANTIMICROBIAL	**SPECTRUM OF ACTIVITY**			**COMPLICATION**
	GRAM +	**GRAM −**	**FUNGAL**	
Bacitracin	×			Allergic rash—often delayed in presentation
Silver sulfadiazine	×	×	×	Leukopenia—self-resolving with continued treatment
Silver nitrate	×	×	×	Hyponatremia—degree directly related to surface area treated
Mafenide	×	×	×	Carbonic anhydrate inhibitor—metabolic acidosis

KEY POINTS: BURNS AND FROSTBITE

1. Thermal injuries are classified by the extent of damage to the skin's underlying structure; the physiologic impact is dependent on the extent of second- and third-degree injury.

2. All patients who have a thermal injury should have a complete primary and secondary survey performed with particular attention to airway (potential obstruction) and circulation (potential compartment syndrome).

3. Burn shock is not simply a state of hypovolemia; appropriate resuscitation is mandatory to avoid morbidity and mortality.

4. Burn-induced hypermetabolism is a significant metabolic disturbance following a major thermal injury. Proper nutrition coupled with early excision, grafting, and exercise is the best treatment.

5. Hypocalcemia can develop after exposure to concentrated hydrofluoric acid.

6. Frostbite injuries should be treated with rapid rewarming and potential catheter-directed thrombolysis.

BIBLIOGRAPHY

1. American Burn Association: Advanced burn life support providers manual. Chicago, American Burn Association, 2005.

2. Barrow RE, Jeschke MG, Herndon DN: Early fluid resuscitation improves outcomes in severely burned children. Resuscitation 45:91-96, 2000.

3. Bruen KJ, Ballard JR, Morris SE, et al: Reduction of the incidence of amputation in frostbite injury with thrombolytic therapy. Arch Surg 142:546-551, 2007.

4. Greenhalgh DG: Topical antimicrobial agents for burn wounds. Clin Plast Surg 36:597-606, 2009.

5. Hart DW, Wolf SE, Chinkes DL, et al: Effects of early excision and aggressive enteral feeding on hypermetabolism, catabolism, and sepsis after severe burn. J Trauma 54:755-761, 2003.

6. Herndon DN, Tompkins RG: Support of the metabolic response to injury. Lancet 363:1895-1902, 2004.

7. Jeschke MG, Chinkes DL, Finnery CC, et al: Pathophysiologic response to severe burn injury. Ann Surg 248:387-401, 2008.

8. Kirkpatrick JJ, Enion DS, Burd DA: Hydrofluoric acid burns: a review. Burns 21:483-493, 1995.

9. Klein MB, Hayden D, Elson C: The association between fluid administration and outcome following major burn: a multicenter study. Ann Surg 245:622-628, 2007.

10. Krammer GC, Lund T, Beckum OL: Pathophysiology of burn shock and burn edema. In Herndon DN (ed): Total Burn Care, 3rd ed. Philadelphia, Saunders, 2007, pp 93-106.

11. Pham TN, Gibran NS, Heimbach DM: Evaluation of the burn wound: management decisions. In Herndon DN (ed): Total Burn Care, 3rd ed. Philadelphia, Saunders, 2007, pp 119-126.

12. Rosen CL, Adler JN, Rabban JT, et al: Early predictors of myoglobinuria and acute renal failure following electrical injury. J Emerg Med 17:783-789, 1999.

13. Sheridan RL: Comprehensive treatment of burns. Curr Probl Surg 38:657-756, 2001.

14. Sheridan RL, Ryan CM, Quinby WC Jr, et al: Emergency management of major hydrofluoric acid exposures. Burns 21:62-64, 1995.

15. Sullivan SR, Ahmadi AJ, Singh CN, et al: Elevated orbital pressure: another untoward effect of massive resuscitation after burn injury. J Trauma 60:72-76, 2006.

CHAPTER 67

PNEUMOTHORAX

Madison Macht, MD, and Michael E. Hanley, MD

1. **What are the major etiologic classifications of pneumothoraces?**
   Pneumothoraces are classified as spontaneous or traumatic:
   - **Spontaneous:** Spontaneous pneumothoraces occur without antecedent trauma or other obvious cause. A primary spontaneous pneumothorax occurs in a person without underlying lung disease. Secondary spontaneous pneumothoraces occur as a complication of underlying lung disease.
   - **Traumatic:** Traumatic pneumothoraces result from direct or indirect trauma to the chest and are further classified as iatrogenic or noniatrogenic.

2. **What are the common causes of pneumothorax in critically ill patients?**
   Secondary spontaneous pneumothoraces occasionally require admission to the intensive care unit because of acute respiratory failure resulting from the combination of the pneumothorax and underlying lung disease. In addition, secondary spontaneous pneumothoraces may develop in patients with lung disease who are already in the intensive care unit. This occurs more commonly in patients with chronic obstructive lung disease, asthma, interstitial lung disease, necrotizing lung infections, and *Pneumocystis jiroveci* pneumonia. However, most pneumothoraces that develop in the intensive care unit are due to either antecedent noniatrogenic chest trauma or iatrogenic causes. Box 67-1 lists the common causes of iatrogenic pneumothorax.

BOX 67-1. COMMON CAUSES OF IATROGENIC PNEUMOTHORAX

- Positive pressure ventilation
- Central venous catheter placement
- Thoracentesis
- Tracheostomy
- Nasogastric tube placement*
- Bronchoscopy†
- Pericardiocentesis
- Transthoracic needle aspiration
- Cardiopulmonary resuscitation

*Because of inadvertent insertion of the nasogastric tube into the tracheobronchial tree.
†Especially if transbronchial biopsy is performed.

---

3. **What measures reduce the risk of iatrogenic pneumothorax in patients receiving positive pressure ventilation?**
   End-inspiratory plateau pressure should be kept < 35 cm H_2O, and both positive end-expiratory pressure (PEEP) and auto-PEEP levels should be minimized. Approaches that may help achieve these goals include using the following:
   - Smaller tidal volumes in patients with underlying lung disease
   - Permissive hypercapnia when high minute ventilation is required
   - High inspiratory flow rates

In addition, thoracentesis and subclavian or internal jugular venous line insertion should be performed with utmost care (including under ultrasound guidance) in high-risk patients.

4. **Describe the clinical manifestations of pneumothoraces.**
Dyspnea and unilateral chest pain are the most common manifestations of primary spontaneous pneumothorax. Physical examination findings include tachycardia, ipsilateral chest expansion, hyperresonance to percussion, decreased tactile fremitus, and decreased breath sounds on the affected side. The trachea may also be deviated toward the contralateral side. On rare occasions patients with primary pneumothoraces may have no symptoms.

In contrast, most patients in whom secondary spontaneous pneumothoraces develop have preexisting lung pathologic conditions and resultant decreased pulmonary reserve. Therefore their symptoms are often more severe than in those with primary pneumothoraces. Dyspnea occurs in virtually all patients with secondary pneumothoraces and is commonly out of proportion to the size of the pneumothorax. Cyanosis and hypotension are common. Side-to-side differences in the examination of the chest may not be so apparent because many of the physical signs associated with the underlying lung disease are similar to those associated with pneumothoraces.

5. **What subtle signs or symptoms should prompt consideration of pneumothorax in patients receiving mechanical ventilation?**
The sudden onset of any of the following should raise the possibility of a pneumothorax in patients receiving mechanical ventilation:
- Decline in oxygen saturation
- Agitation
- Respiratory distress
- Patient-ventilator dyssynchrony
- Sudden increase in peak inspiratory and/or static airway pressure
- Hypotension
- Cardiovascular collapse
- Pulseless electrical activity

6. **How is the diagnosis of pneumothorax established in critically ill patients?**
Chest radiography is the most common tool used to confirm the presence of a pneumothorax. A thin pleural line and the absence of lung parenchymal markings between the pleural line and chest wall adequately support the diagnosis. Upright radiographs are most helpful, as the supine position commonly allows free pleural air to collect anteriorly and avoid detection. Evidence of an increase in the size of the ipsilateral hemithorax, including contralateral shift of the mediastinum and heart, as well as depression of the ipsilateral hemidiaphragm, may be the only radiographic clues to the presence of a pneumothorax in such cases. A wide, deep radiolucency along the costophrenic angle is referred to as the deep sulcus sign and may be the only clue to the presence of a pneumothorax on supine chest radiography. Chest roentgenograms obtained at expiration are often requested, although some data suggest that inspiratory and expiratory films are equally sensitive for the diagnosis. Radiographs taken with the patient in the lateral decubitus position or from the cross-table lateral view may be useful in confirming the diagnosis in select cases. If chest radiographs are nondiagnostic and the patient's condition is sufficiently stable for transport, computed tomography of the chest may be required to prove the diagnosis.

7. **What is the role of ultrasonography in the diagnosis of pneumothorax in critically ill patients?**
Ultrasonography has several important advantages in the diagnosis of pneumothoraces in critically ill patients. Pneumothoraces can be detected by ultrasound with certainty at the bedside, without the need for conventional radiography, thus potentially saving time and sparing patients radiation exposure. Other advantages include portability and real-time imaging. These features are especially important when a diagnosis must be made emergently. Large

dressings, agitation, significant subcutaneous emphysema, and posterior or mediastinal air collections may decrease the sensitivity of ultrasonography. Several studies have shown that the sensitivity and specificity of ultrasonography for the detection of pneumothorax is greater than 90% in the initial management of trauma patients.

8. **What findings on ultrasound suggest the presence of a pneumothorax?**
Sonographic findings suggestive of a pneumothorax include absence of *lung sliding* and *comet tail* artifacts. Lung sliding refers to the normal horizontal back-and-forth movement of the visceral pleura as it slides over the parietal pleura during the respiratory cycle. Comet tail artifacts, also called "B-lines," are echogenic raylike shadows that radiate from the visceral-parietal pleural interface and extend to the bottom of the ultrasound screen. False-positive results have been reported in patients with bullous emphysema and pleural adhesions.

   The presence of these findings excludes a pneumothorax. For this reason, ultrasound may be especially valuable as a quick, safe, and reliable method of excluding this diagnosis in emergent situations (such as when a tension pneumothorax may be the cause of a clinically unstable patient) or after invasive procedures that may be complicated by a pneumothorax (such as thoracentesis or central venous catheter placement).

9. **Describe the treatment of a pneumothorax in critically ill patients.**
Tube thoracostomy should be performed in almost all secondary spontaneous or noniatrogenic, traumatic pneumothoraces, especially if mechanical ventilation is required. Proper positioning of the thoracostomy tube is important in obtaining complete evacuation of pleural air. The tube should be directed to an anterior-apical position. For isolated pneumothoraces a 20 F to 24 F thoracostomy tube is frequently adequate. However, if an associated pleural effusion or hemothorax is present, 32 F to 36 F tubes are usually preferred. Tube thoracostomy should also be performed for all iatrogenic pneumothoraces because of positive pressure ventilation. Other forms of iatrogenic pneumothorax require tube thoracostomy only if the pneumothorax:
   - Is large (>40%)
   - Is associated with significant symptoms or arterial blood gas abnormalities
   - Progressively enlarges
   - Does not respond to simple aspiration
   - Occurs in a patient requiring positive pressure ventilation

   Pleural air resorbs at a rate of approximately 1.5% per day. Because nitrogen is the largest component of the atmosphere and is not metabolized, the usual partial pressure gradient between pleural air and the pulmonary capillary blood is small. Decreasing the nitrogen content by increasing inhaled oxygen content may therefore hasten pleural air resorption. For this reason patients who are treated conservatively with observation alone should at minimum be given high levels of supplemental oxygen.

10. **Does the development of a pneumothorax portend a worse prognosis for patients with acute respiratory distress syndrome (ARDS)?**
Not necessarily. The association of pneumothorax and other air leaks (i.e., extrusion of any air outside the tracheobronchial tree) with mortality was studied in 725 patients with ARDS in the late 1990s. The 30-day mortality rate for patients in whom a pneumothorax developed was 46% compared with 40% in patients without pneumothorax ($P = 0.35$). Similarly, the 30-day mortality rate for patients with any type of air leak was 45.5% compared with 39.0% for patients without air leaks ($P = 0.28$).

   However, it should be pointed out that both groups of patients received ventilation with higher tidal volumes than are currently recommended for ARDS (mean 11.4 ± 3 mL/kg in those without pneumothorax and 11.7 ± 3.3 mL/kg in those without). It is not known whether the same results would be observed in the era of lower tidal volumes and lung-protective ventilator strategies.

11. **What are the potential physiologic consequences of a bronchopleural fistula (BPF) in patients receiving mechanical ventilation?**
The potential consequences of a BPF are highlighted in Box 67-2. It should be emphasized, however, that BPFs are extremely well tolerated by most patients.

BOX 67-2. PHYSIOLOGIC CONSEQUENCES OF A BRONCHOPLEURAL FISTULA IN PATIENTS RECEIVING MECHANICAL VENTILATION

- Inability to maintain adequate alveolar ventilation through loss of effective tidal volume
- Inappropriate cycling of the ventilator
- Incomplete lung reexpansion
- Inability to apply PEEP

---

12. **Describe the initial management of a BPF.**
BPFs are managed by minimizing the flow of air through the fistula while maintaining complete evacuation of the pleural space. This is primarily accomplished in spontaneously breathing patients (negative-pressure ventilation) by altering the level of suction applied to the pleural space. The optimal amount of suction must be determined on an individual basis.
   Gas flow across a BPF in patients with mechanical ventilation is also influenced by peak inspiratory and mean airway pressures. Management in this setting includes measures that minimize alveolar distention and minute ventilation. This is accomplished by minimizing PEEP, tidal volume, inspiratory time, and the number of mechanically delivered breaths per minute. Permissive hypercapnia should be considered if not contraindicated. Mechanical ventilation should be discontinued as soon as possible.

13. **How is a persistent BPF managed?**
Most BPFs close spontaneously once the underlying lung injury improves and positive pressure ventilation is discontinued. However, if a BPF in a patient no longer receiving positive pressure ventilation does not close after 5 to 7 days of chest tube drainage, or if adequate ventilation cannot be maintained because of the size of the air leak, suturing or resection of the fistula with scarification of the pleura by either thoracoscopy or open thoracotomy should be considered. The decision to perform this procedure should include a consideration of the operative risk to the patient. Prolonged chest tube drainage, intrabronchial bronchoscopic instillation of materials (e.g., Gelfoam or tissue adhesives such as cyanoacrylate-based or fibrin glues) designed to occlude the fistula, differential lung ventilation, or synchronized chest tube occlusion should be considered in patients whose operative risk is increased by significant underlying lung disease or other medical problems.

14. **What is reexpansion pulmonary edema?**
Reexpansion pulmonary edema involves the development of unilateral pulmonary edema after reexpansion of a collapsed lung. The risk and severity of reexpansion pulmonary edema appear to be related to the duration of the pneumothorax, as well as the magnitude of negative pressure applied to the pleural space to reexpand the lung. The exact incidence of reexpansion pulmonary edema after treatment of pneumothoraces in humans is unknown, but it is rare. The mortality of reexpansion pulmonary edema can be as high as 10% to 20%.

15. **How can the risk of reexpansion pulmonary edema be minimized?**
The risk can be minimized by withholding pleural suction during the immediate treatment of pneumothoraces of either unknown duration or duration greater than 3 days. If the pneumothorax is not completely evacuated after 24 to 48 hours of water seal, or if significant respiratory compromise requires more rapid evacuation, low levels of negative pressure (<20 cm H_2O) should be applied to the pleural space. Nonetheless, reexpansion pulmonary edema has been reported even under these conditions.

16. **What is a tension pneumothorax?**
A tension pneumothorax occurs when the pressure within a pneumothorax is greater than atmospheric pressure throughout expiration and often during inspiration. Tension pneumothoraces generally result from a one-way valve phenomenon and most frequently occur in patients receiving positive pressure ventilation. They are a medical emergency that may rapidly lead to death if not recognized and treated expeditiously.

17. **Describe the treatment for a tension pneumothorax.**
Time should not be wasted pursuing radiographic confirmation if a clinician suspects the diagnosis of tension pneumothorax in a hemodynamically unstable patient. The patient should be immediately given 100% oxygen and the pneumothorax evacuated. This is best accomplished by emergent placement of a tube thoracostomy. If the diagnosis is in question, or if a tube thoracostomy is not readily available, an alternative approach includes insertion into the pleural space of a large-bore needle attached by a three-way stopcock to a 50-mL syringe partially filled with sterile saline solution. The needle is inserted under sterile conditions through the second anterior intercostal space in the midclavicular line while the patient is supine. After the needle has been inserted, the plunger is withdrawn from the syringe. The presence of a pneumothorax is confirmed if air bubbles up through the saline solution. If a pneumothorax is present, the needle should be left in place until air ceases to bubble through the saline solution, and a tube thoracostomy is performed. If air does not bubble up into the syringe, a pneumothorax is not present and the needle may be removed.

CONTROVERSY

18. **Should a tube thoracostomy be removed immediately in patients receiving positive pressure ventilation once the air leak has resolved and the lung is completely reexpanded?**
Pro:
- The tube thoracostomy is no longer required to evacuate air after the BPF has closed and all air has been evacuated. At this point, the chest tube is only a potential source of infection, both at its insertion site and in the pleural space.
- Patients can be closely monitored and chest tubes reinserted if a pneumothorax recurs.
- Routine insertion of a prophylactic tube thoracostomy is not indicated in patients receiving mechanical ventilation.

Con:
- Risk of a recurrent pneumothorax remains high in patients receiving mechanical ventilation, especially if they have ARDS or a necrotic lung process.
- Many pneumothoraces in patients receiving mechanical ventilation present under tension. Tension pneumothoraces are associated with a higher mortality, especially if delay occurs in diagnosis or treatment.

KEY POINTS: CLINICAL MANIFESTATIONS OF TENSION PNEUMOTHORAX

1. Sudden deterioration often occurs in patients with tension pneumothorax.

2. Respiratory distress is another manifestation.

3. Cyanosis may occur.

4. Diaphoresis is often present.

5. Cardiovascular instability, including tachycardia and hypotension, sometimes occurs.

6. Another manifestation of tension pneumothorax is ipsilateral hyperresonance.

7. Ipsilateral diminished breath sounds also occur.

8. Tension pneumothorax is sometimes accompanied by an increase in the size of the ipsilateral hemithorax.

9. Contralateral shift of the trachea may be present.

BIBLIOGRAPHY

1. Anzueto A, Frutos-Vivar F, Esteban A, et al: Incidence, risk factors and outcome of barotraumas in mechanically ventilated patients. Intensive Care Med 30:612-619, 2004.

2. Baumann MH: What size chest tube? What drainage system is ideal? And other chest tube management questions. Curr Opin Pulm Med 9:276-281, 2003.

3. Boussarsar M, Thierry G, Jaber S, et al: Relationship between ventilatory settings and barotrauma in the acute respiratory distress syndrome. Intensive Care Med 28:406-413, 2002.

4. Chen KY, Jerng JS, Liao WY, et al: Pneumothorax in the ICU: patient outcomes and prognostic factors. Chest 122:678-683, 2002.

5. de Lassence A, Timsit JF, Tafflet M, et al: Pneumothorax in the intensive care unit: incidence, risk factors, and outcome. Anesthesiology 104:5-13, 2006.

6. Heffner JE, McDonald J, Barbieri C: Recurrent pneumothoraces in ventilated patients despite ipsilateral chest tubes. Chest 108:1053-1058, 1995.

7. Kempainen RR, Pierson DJ: Persistent air leaks in patients receiving mechanical ventilation. Semin Respir Crit Care Med 22:675-684, 2001.

8. Leigh-Smith S, Harris T: Tension pneumothorax—time for a re-think? Emerg Med J 22:8-16, 2005.

9. Lichtenstein DA: Ultrasound in the management of thoracic disease. Crit Care Med 35(5 Suppl):S250-S261, 2007.

10. Lichtenstein DA, Meziere G, Lascols N, et al: Ultrasound diagnosis of occult pneumothorax. Crit Care Med 33:1231-1238, 2005.

11. Lois M, Noppen M: Bronchopleural fistulas: an overview of the problem with special focus on endoscopic management. Chest 128:3955-3965, 2005.

12. O'Connor A, Morgan WE: Radiological review of pneumothorax. BMJ 330:1493-1497, 2005.

13. Powner DJ, Cline CD, Rodman GH: Effect of chest tube suction on gas flow through a bronchopleural fistula. Crit Care Med 13:99-101, 1985.

14. Reissig A, Copetti R, Kroegel C: Current role of emergency ultrasound of the chest. Crit Care Med 39:839-845, 2011.

15. Seow A, Kazerooni EA, Pernicano PG, et al: Comparison of upright inspiratory and expiratory chest radiographs for detecting pneumothoraces. AJR Am J Roentgenol 166:313-316, 1996.

16. Sherman SC: Reexpansion pulmonary edema: a case report and review of the current literature. J Emerg Med 24:23-27, 2003.

17. Theodoro D, Bausano B, Lewis L, et al: A descriptive comparison of ultrasound-guided central venous cannulation of the internal jugular vein to landmark-based subclavian vein cannulation. Acad Emerg Med 17:416-422, 2010.

18. Vezzani A, Brusasco C, Palermo S, et al: Ultrasound localization of central vein catheter and detection of postprocedural pneumothorax: an alternative to chest radiography. Crit Care Med 38:533-538, 2010.

19. Weg J, Anzueto S, Balk RA, et al: The relation of pneumothorax and other air leaks to mortality in the acute respiratory distress syndrome. N Engl J Med 338:341-346, 1998.

20. Wilkerson RG, Stone MB: Sensitivity of bedside ultrasound and supine anteroposterior chest radiographs for the identification of pneumothorax after blunt trauma. Acad Emerg Med 17:11-17, 2010.

21. Xirouchaki N, Magkanas E, Vaporidi K, et al: Lung ultrasound in critically ill patients: comparison with bedside chest radiography. Intensive Care Med 37:1488-1493, 2011.

CHAPTER 68

FLAIL CHEST AND PULMONARY CONTUSION

Susan R. Wilcox, MD, and Edward A. Bittner, MD, PhD

1. **What are the most common injuries in patients sustaining blunt chest trauma?**
   Rib fractures are the most common injury after chest trauma, and multiple rib fractures leading to flail chest occur in 15% to 25% of patients. Pulmonary contusion is the most common intrathoracic injury, occurring in 40% to 60% of patients with blunt chest trauma. Although isolated pulmonary contusion may occur after an explosion injury, most trauma patients have concurrent injury to the chest wall.

2. **What are the risk factors for adverse outcomes after blunt thoracic injury?**
   Thoracic injury and its complications are responsible for up to 25% of blunt trauma mortality. Increasing age and a larger number of rib fractures are most closely linked with increased complications. The greatest risk factors for mortality in patients with blunt chest trauma are age of 65 years or more, sustaining three or more rib fractures, and the presence of medical comorbidities, especially cardiopulmonary disease. Rib fractures cause intense pain and can lead to *splinting* of the chest with a rapid, shallow breathing pattern, as well as poor secretion clearance, increasing the risk for development of pneumonia. After injury, the development of pneumonia is a significant risk factor for mortality.

3. **What is the sensitivity of chest radiograph for diagnosis of rib fractures?**
   Compared with a computed tomography (CT) scan, chest radiography misses approximately 50% of rib fractures. For stable patients with mild injury, the diagnosis of rib fracture is often clinical, with findings of significant pain and tenderness on examination. However, for patients with more severe injuries, any rib fracture or pulmonary contusion visible on the initial chest radiograph significantly increases the incidence of pulmonary morbidity or mortality.

4. **What is a flail chest, and how is it diagnosed?**
   Flail chest is defined as fractures of three or more consecutive ribs or costal cartilages fractured in two or more places (Fig. 68-1). These fractured segments give rise to a free-floating portion of the thorax, which moves paradoxically throughout the respiratory cycle, with inward motion with inspiration and outward motion with exhalation. Although rib fractures may be diagnosed radiographically, flail chest is a clinical diagnosis. Patients often present with chest wall pain, tenderness, bruising, and palpable step-offs of the ribs, but flail chest is distinguished from other chest trauma by noting the paradoxical movement of the chest wall during spontaneous respiration. Patients receiving positive pressure ventilation usually do not demonstrate the classic paradoxical movements. Respiratory dysfunction usually does not arise from the paradoxical chest motion but rather is due to underlying contusions and splinting from pain.

5. **What is a pulmonary contusion?**
   Pulmonary contusion is a bruise of the lung, with alveolar and interstitial hemorrhage and destruction of the pulmonary parenchyma. The subsequent inflammation leads to asymmetric edema, atelectasis, and poor mucous clearance from the airways. These factors lead to progressive ventilation-perfusion mismatch and loss of pulmonary compliance, which may be

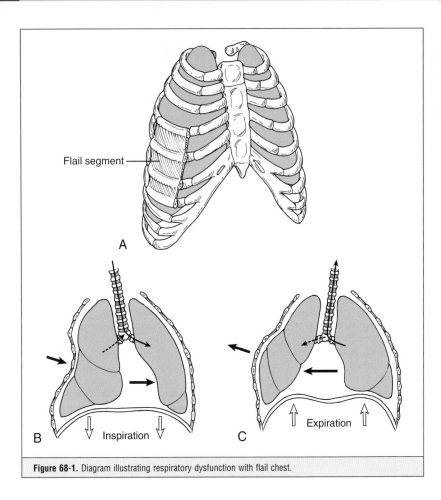

Figure 68-1. Diagram illustrating respiratory dysfunction with flail chest.

manifested clinically as progressive respiratory failure develops over the first 6 to 24 hours after the injury. Contusions tend to worsen over the 24 to 48 hours after injury and then slowly resolve within 7 days.

6. **What is the role of radiographs in the diagnosis of pulmonary contusion?**
   Pulmonary contusions are diagnosed radiographically. Although initial chest radiographs may be unremarkable, a nonsegmental infiltrate typically develops over a 6-hour period. If the contusions are visible on the initial chest radiograph, the injury is likely to be more severe, and enlargement of the contused area on the radiograph over the next 24 hours is a poor prognostic sign. Classic radiograph patterns include irregular consolidations or a diffuse patchy pattern (Fig. 68-2). Even after development of chest radiograph findings, plain radiographs may underestimate the severity of the contusions. CT scan is more sensitive for diagnosis of pulmonary contusions and can quantify the volume of lung involved.

7. **What is the relationship among rib fractures, flail chest, and pulmonary contusions?**
   Pulmonary contusions often occur without flail chest and may even be present in the setting of minimal to no rib fractures. Flail chest, however, indicates that the chest wall sustained a large

force, and therefore more than 90% of patients with flail chest have associated intrathoracic injuries, often pulmonary contusions. These patients also frequently have a hemothorax, a pneumothorax, or both. Patients with flail chest are likely to have additional traumatic injuries, including head injury and intraabdominal injuries. The pattern of rib fractures on imaging has been shown to be suggestive of other injuries in a recent series of trauma patients. Lower rib fractures were highly predictive of solid organ injury when compared with upper and midzone rib fractures, and scapular and sternal fractures were more common with upper zone fractures.

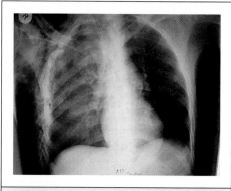

Figure 68-2. Radiograph of a patient with a pulmonary contusion.

8. **What is the relationship between pulmonary contusions and acute respiratory distress syndrome (ARDS)?**
Patients with a pulmonary contusion are at higher risk than other patients for development of pneumonia and ARDS. The volume of lung parenchyma involved as determined by CT scan has been shown to be a risk factor for the development of ARDS, with patients having contusion volumes of greater than 20% being at the highest risk. Of these patients, ARDS has been shown to develop in approximately 80%.

9. **What is the mortality rate and cause of death for patients with flail chest and pulmonary contusions?**
The overall mortality rate of patients with blunt chest trauma is 16% with either a pulmonary contusion or flail chest to 42% when patients had both. Although these patients have severe thoracic injury, the most common cause of death in patients with flail chest and pulmonary contusions is brain injury.

10. **What are the basic treatment strategies for flail chest or pulmonary contusions?**
All trauma patients should be assessed with use of the principles of advanced trauma life support, directed at diagnosing and intervening in life-threatening injuries immediately. Using a primary survey, verifying the ABCs (airway, breathing, and circulation) is paramount. Prompt endotracheal intubation, tube thoracostomy for suspected hemopneumothorax, and mechanical ventilation are warranted in the unstable patient with chest trauma. For the stable patient with chest trauma, management centers around close monitoring of the respiratory status, pain control, aggressive lung physiotherapy, early mobilization, and adequate nutrition.

11. **What are the pitfalls in pain management of patients with blunt chest trauma without an endotracheal tube in place?**
Pain control is fundamental to the management of rib fractures to decrease chest wall splinting and alveolar collapse. Patients with pain due to rib fractures seek to minimize their chest wall motion by reducing their tidal volume and coughing effort. Delayed and inadequate pain control are common pitfalls in management of these patients. Effective pain control is a vital adjunct that permits patient mobilization, deep breathing, and secretion clearance, thereby decreasing the risk for pneumonia. Traditionally, intravenous narcotics were used in an attempt to control pain. Narcotic medications can be effective in relieving pain but can result in

oversedation with resulting hypoventilation and can depress respiratory efforts and the cough reflex and increase the risk for aspiration. These drawbacks have prompted investigations into alternative therapies for pain control including intrapleural blocks, intercostal blocks, and paravertebral blocks. Several studies suggest that epidural analgesia provides optimal pain relief and may improve outcome in patients with blunt chest trauma. Unfortunately many trauma patients have spinal fractures or coagulopathy that precludes the use of epidural catheters.

12. **Does the type of pain control influence the rate of pneumonia in patients with multiple rib fractures?**

Pain is recognized as a contributing factor in the morbidity associated with rib fractures and pulmonary contusion. Multiple analgesia modalities have been used to manage pain in patients with rib fractures including oral analgesia, intermittent parenteral opioids, patient-controlled opioid analgesia, interpleural blocks, intercostal blocks, paravertebral blocks, and epidural analgesia. Retrospective studies of trauma patients with rib fractures have shown inconsistent benefits of epidural analgesia compared with other analgesic modalities. In one small (46 patients) prospective randomized trial, Bulger et al. found that the incidence of nosocomial pneumonia was reduced (18% vs. 38%) by epidural analgesia compared with parenteral opioids. However, a recent meta-analysis of epidural analgesia in patients with traumatic rib fractures failed to find a benefit in mortality, intensive care unit (ICU) length of stay, hospital length of stay, or duration of mechanical ventilation. Additional controlled studies comparing analgesic modalities are clearly needed.

13. **What is the optimal fluid management strategy in patients with blunt chest trauma?**

Judicious fluid resuscitation is required during the initial resuscitation of the patient with blunt chest trauma as the injured lung is prone to fluid overload while at the same time significant secondary injury can result from undertransfusion of fluids. Increased permeability of pulmonary capillaries that occurs early after a pulmonary contusion predisposes the patient to the development of tissue edema and worsening gas exchange. The use of colloid solutions for patients with pulmonary contusion has been advocated by some with the aim of maintaining plasma oncotic pressure and possibly withdrawing water from the contused lung, although no randomized trials exist that demonstrate a clear benefit from colloid administration in this setting. Current opinion on fluid replacement is in favor of ensuring adequate resuscitation to ensure end-organ perfusion followed by avoidance of further unnecessary fluid administration. This may be best achieved with early use of invasive monitoring or echocardiography to guide fluid replacement.

14. **Which respiratory therapy procedure(s) should be used for patients with significant blunt chest trauma?**

For patients with blunt chest trauma without an endotracheal tube in place, lung expansion therapy using incentive spirometry (IS), deep breathing, and coughing are critical to reduce secretions, prevent atelectasis, and avoid the need for intubation. All patients should have pain assessed and received maximal lung expansion therapy on an hourly basis. Underlying reactive lung disease should be optimized as well. In patients not meeting predicted goals with IS, either intermittent or continuous positive airway pressure (CPAP) therapy should be initiated. These modalities are often limited by the requirement of an awake, cooperative patient. Chest physical therapy consists of postural drainage, enhanced coughing maneuvers, chest vibration, and percussion. Prospective studies are lacking for efficacy, and chest percussion is obviously not well tolerated in patients with thoracic trauma. Nasotracheal suctioning is reserved for patients not able to effectively mobilize their secretions. Vigorous ambulation, when possible, remains the best method of restoring normal respiratory physiology.

15. **Do all patients with flail chest require mechanical ventilation?**

    Recent studies have shown that a significant number of patients with flail chest and/or pulmonary contusion can be safely and effectively managed with aggressive pulmonary care including face mask oxygen, CPAP, and chest physiotherapy. CPAP restores functional residual capacity, improves compliance, and stabilizes the flail segment until the underlying pulmonary contusion resolves. CPAP, compared with intermittent positive pressure ventilation, has also been shown to lower mortality and nosocomial infections in patients who required mechanical ventilation. Noninvasive ventilation is particularly attractive for the patient who initially does not require emergent intubation and may decrease the need for subsequent intubation. Patients with frank shock or head injury do not make good candidates for noninvasive ventilation and are at high risk for aspiration. If noninvasive ventilation is attempted then close follow-up is essential as patients may fail and require endotracheal intubation. Early intubation and mechanical ventilation are essential in patients with refractory respiratory failure, shock, or other serious traumatic injuries.

16. **What is the optimal mode of ventilation for patients with flail chest or pulmonary contusion?**

    The optimal mode of ventilation for patients with flail chest or pulmonary contusion continues to be debated. When required, mechanical ventilation strategies should be tailored to optimize oxygenation while minimizing the potential for secondary lung injury. In patients with ARDS, lung protective ventilation strategies using a volume- and pressure-limited approach have resulted in reductions in mortality. This strategy, although not clearly proved in the setting of pulmonary contusion, is aimed at reducing further ventilator trauma. Many of the newer modes of ventilation are consistent with a lung protective strategy and have shown promising results, but data are lacking showing superiority.

17. **What is the role of positive end-expiratory pressure (PEEP) in the management of blunt chest trauma?**

    Providing a constant pressure throughout the respiratory cycle (PEEP) may recruit atelectatic lung regions and prevent the cyclic opening and closing of the airways, thereby reducing additional lung injury. Identifying optimal PEEP is complex, but in general the goal is to select a PEEP level that prevents derecruitment and allows for FiO_2 reduction. PEEP can have significant physiologic effects relevant to the trauma patient. Most notably, PEEP can significantly reduce venous return in the patient with hypovolemia. This can worsen hemodynamics in the setting of hemorrhagic shock. PEEP may also exacerbate ventilation-perfusion mismatch in patients with asymmetric pulmonary injury.

18. **What are the indications for surgical stabilization of flail chest injuries?**

    Surgical stabilization of rib fractures and flail chest remains a controversial issue. Rib fixation can theoretically aid in a patient's recovery by allowing the patient to mobilize and ventilate comfortably. Studies comparing surgical stabilization and conservative management are few and difficult to conduct because of the heterogeneity of thoracic trauma and other associated injuries.

    The proponents of surgical stabilization claim a reduction in ventilator days, pulmonary complications, pain, and chest wall deformity. Proposed indications for rib fracture repair include flail chest; painful, movable rib fractures refractory to conventional pain management; chest wall deformity or defect; rib fracture nonunion; and during thoracotomy for other traumatic indication. A variety of fixation methods have been proposed, including pins, plates, wires, and struts. A prospective study by Tanaka et al. randomly assigned patients to either surgical fixation within 7 days of injury or mechanical ventilation alone. They demonstrated a reduction in pneumonia and ventilator and ICU days in those patients undergoing surgery. These results have not been duplicated in larger trials. Despite these reported benefits, stabilizations are seldom performed.

19. **What is the long-term morbidity in flail chest injuries?**

Few long-term follow-up studies regarding disability after flail chest injury are available. Outcome in patients with flail chest injuries with or without pulmonary contusion is difficult to delineate without accounting for the presence of other injuries. Flail chest appears to be associated with a worse outcome when compared with multiple rib fractures despite similar rates of lung contusion and extrathoracic injuries. A significant increase in mortality is related to increasing age in patients with a flail chest injury.

Patients with flail chest express fairly consistent symptoms in the few studies completed. Most complaints are subjective, such as chest tightness, pain, and decreased activity level. In a prospective study in 28 patients surviving severe chest injury, Livingston and Richardson found severe pulmonary dysfunction with pulmonary function tests (PFTs) at 40% to 50% of predicted within 2 weeks of hospital discharge but a trend of marked improvement that continued out to at least 18 months after discharge, with PFTs 65% to 90% of predicted. Only 5% of patients met criteria for pulmonary disability. In another study, Kishikawa et al. prospectively followed 18 patients with severe blunt chest trauma. They found that pulmonary function recovered within 6 months in patients without pulmonary contusion, even in the presence of severe residual chest wall deformity. However, patients with pulmonary contusion had decreased functional residual capacity and decreased supine PaO_2 for years afterward. Additional studies are clearly needed.

20. **Are prophylactic antibiotics indicated in patients requiring a tube thoracostomy after chest trauma?**

Use of antibiotics in patients with isolated chest trauma is controversial. Available studies offer conflicting results because of methodological limitations including small sample sizes, suboptimal antibiotic regimens, prolonged dosing, or variation in the patient populations involved. A recent meta-analysis suggests that prophylactic antibiotics in patients requiring tube thoracostomy can reduce the incidence of empyema and pneumonia. A level III recommendation by the Eastern Association for the Surgery of Trauma guidelines supports administration of a first-generation cephalosporin before tube thoracostomy placement and continued no longer than 24 hours. Although the question of prophylactic antibiotics is not settled, it appears that adequate drainage of a hemothorax and the use of appropriate sterile techniques are the key factors in reducing the risk for infection.

KEY POINTS: FLAIL CHEST AND PULMONARY CONTUSION

1. Increasing age places patients with multiple rib fractures at high risk for pulmonary complications.

2. Pulmonary contusions place patients at increased risk for pneumonia and ARDS.

3. Management of flail chest or pulmonary contusion includes immediate assessment of airway, breathing, and circulation and, for stable patients, monitoring the respiratory status, pain control, lung physiotherapy, early mobilization, and adequate nutrition.

4. Fluid replacement for patients with pulmonary contusion should focus on ensuring adequate resuscitation to ensure end-organ perfusion followed by avoidance of further unnecessary fluid administration.

5. Lung protective strategies should be used when patients with a flail chest or pulmonary contusion require mechanical ventilation because of ARDS.

BIBLIOGRAPHY

1. Al-Hassani A, Abdulrahman H, Afifi I, et al: Rib fracture patterns predict thoracic chest wall and abdominal solid organ injury. Am Surg 76:888-891, 2010.

2. Bastos R, Calhoon JH, Baisden CE: Flail chest and pulmonary contusion. Semin Thorac Cardiovasc Surg 20:39-45, 2008.

3. Battle CE, Hutchings H, Evans PA: Risk factors that predict mortality in patients with blunt chest wall trauma: a systematic review and meta-analysis. Injury 43:8-17, 2012.

4. Bulger EM, Edwards T, Klotz P, et al: Epidural analgesia improves outcome after multiple rib fractures. Surgery 136:426-430, 2004.

5. Carrier FM, Turgeon AF, Nicole PC, et al: Effect of epidural analgesia in patients with traumatic rib fractures: a systematic review and meta-analysis of randomized controlled trials. Can J Anesth 56:230-242, 2009.

6. Cohn SM, DuBose JJ: Pulmonary contusion: an update on recent advances in clinical management. World J Surg 34:1959-1970, 2010.

7. Hernandez G, Fernandez R, Lopez-Reina P, et al: Noninvasive ventilation reduces intubation in chest trauma-related hypoxemia: a randomized clinical trial. Chest 137:74-80, 2010.

8. Kiraly L, Schreiber M: Management of the crushed chest. Crit Care Med 38(9 Suppl):S469-S477, 2010.

9. Kishikawa M, Yoshioka T, Shimazu T, et al: Pulmonary contusion causes long-term respiratory dysfunction with decreased functional residual capacity. J Trauma 31:1203-1208, 1991.

10. Livingston DH, Richardson JD: Pulmonary disability after severe blunt chest trauma. J Trauma 30:562-566, 1990.

11. Livingston DH, Shogan B, John P, et al: CT diagnosis of rib fractures and the prediction of acute respiratory failure. J Trauma 64:905-911, 2008.

12. Nirula R, Mayberry JC: Rib fracture fixation: controversies and technical challenges. Am Surg 76:793-802, 2010.

13. Sanabria A, Valdivieso E, Gomez G, et al: Prophylactic antibiotics in chest trauma: a meta-analysis of high-quality studies. World J Surg 30:1843-1847, 2006.

14. Simon B, Ebert J, Bokhari F, et al: Practice management guideline for "pulmonary contusion—flail chest" June 2006. Eastern Association for the Surgery of Trauma www.east.org Accessed April 15, 2011.

15. Tanaka H, Yukioka T, Yamaguti Y, et al: Surgical stabilization of internal pneumatic stabilization? A prospective randomized study of management of severe flail chest patients. J Trauma 52:727-732, 2002.

CHAPTER 69

CARDIAC TRAUMA

Ali Y. Mejaddam, MD, and Marc A. DeMoya, MD

1. Describe the causes of blunt cardiac injury (BCI).

BCIs occur most often after motor vehicle collisions, and falls or crush injuries constitute a smaller proportion of the causes. Rapid deceleration is the mechanism of injury in these cases. Abrupt pressure fluctuations in the chest, shearing forces, and compression of the heart between the spine and sternum traumatize the heart. A rare cause of BCI occurs when a projectile strikes the chest during sports (e.g., baseball), which may cause cardiac arrest if the strike happens during a period of electrical susceptibility (commotio cordis). BCIs are commonly described in terms of anatomic injuries (e.g., valvular or septal rupture) or myocardial contusion (e.g., arrhythmia, decreased contractility).

2. What is a myocardial contusion?

The definition of myocardial contusion is established on pathologic examination as myocardial cell necrosis and interstitial hemorrhage. Histologically, contusion differs from ischemic infarction in that the transition zone is sharper and necrosis occurs in a patchy pattern. This can be established on autopsy, which means that other, less reliable, diagnostic tools are needed in the clinical setting (e.g., electrocardiography [ECG], echocardiography, laboratory markers). The incidence of BCI, including myocardial contusion, ranges from 20% to 78% of all blunt thoracic trauma, depending on the criteria and diagnostic modality used.

3. What is the pattern of injury in BCI?

The right side of the heart has the most anterior surface area and therefore is the most commonly injured chamber. Injuries may include rupture of the interventricular septum, a valve, or the ventricle (Fig. 69-1). Patients with a ruptured chamber will rarely reach the hospital alive. Less commonly, injury to coronary arteries occurs that may lead to myocardial infarction. Arrhythmias and decreased contractility may follow myocardial contusion or the previously mentioned injuries.

4. Are there associated chest injuries that make BCI more likely after blunt trauma?

BCI often presents with concomitant chest injuries, but it is important to note that cardiac injury may occur without apparent signs of chest trauma. Fractures of the sternum or clavicle, flail chest, and great vessel injury may suggest associated cardiac injury. Any patient with a heavy trauma burden should raise the level of suspicion for cardiac injury.

5. Describe clinical features that could suggest BCI.

Few signs and symptoms are specific for BCI. Although chest pain is frequently reported by patients with suspected cardiac injury, often concurrent chest injury (e.g., musculoskeletal) of confounding nature exists. Specific signs such as cardiac arrhythmias, murmurs, or precordial thrills warrant further testing to rule out heart injury. In severe cases, patients may present with distended jugular veins and hypotension as signs of cardiogenic shock. On the other hand, myocardial contusion is commonly clinically silent, and the diagnosis may be missed unless the clinician conducts further testing.

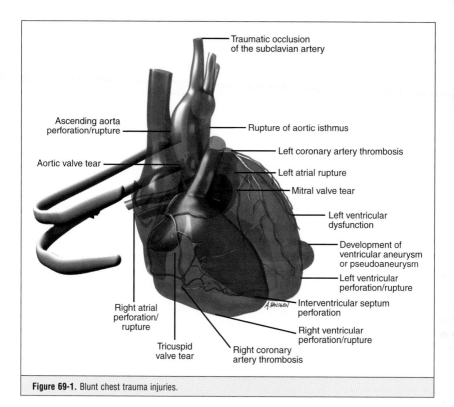

Figure 69-1. Blunt chest trauma injuries.

6. **What is the role of ECG in the diagnosis of myocardial contusion?**

The ECG is the most frequently used screening test for patients with suspected BCI. Suggestive findings on the ECG include ventricular or atrial arrhythmias, bundle-branch block, and ST-wave abnormalities. The prevalence of abnormal ECGs in patients with myocardial contusion ranges from 40% to 83% in the literature. An abnormal ECG may also be related to noncardiac causes such as hypovolemia, electrolyte abnormalities, head injury, and illicit drug use. The ECG will not conclusively rule in or rule out BCI, but recent guidelines propose that hemodynamically stable patients with no history of cardiac disease do not need further work-up for BCI if the ECG is normal.

7. **What is the role of cardiac enzyme determination in the diagnosis of myocardial contusion?**

Cardiac enzymes may be measured to evaluate possible cell necrosis in myocardial contusion. Historically, creatine kinase, myocardial bound (CKMB) has been used for this purpose, but its sensitivity and specificity for myocardial contusion are poor. A meta-analysis in patients with BCI reported a positive correlation between abnormal CKMB and cardiac complications requiring treatment, but further studies have failed to corroborate these results. Currently, CKMB is not recommended as a routine screening test for BCI.

Cardiac troponins are more specific for myocardial cellular injury than CKMB but remain an inaccurate tool for diagnosing myocardial contusion. In the setting of an abnormal ECG, troponin levels are unlikely to affect clinical management, and such patients will require admission with further evaluation. However, in those patients with a nonspecific sinus tachycardia otherwise unexpected, measuring cardiac troponins in 6 hours from the time of injury can effectively rule out a significant cardiac contusion.

8. **How is echocardiography used in the diagnosis of BCI?**

   Transthoracic echocardiography (TTE) provides rapid visualization of the heart and is a useful diagnostic tool for BCI. It can be used to identify anatomic abnormalities (e.g., valvular injury, pericardial effusion), ventricular dyskinesia, shunting of blood, and intracardiac thrombi. It provides necessary information in patients who manifest hemodynamic instability or abnormal screening tests (ECG, cardiac enzymes) but has lower sensitivity in the patient whose condition is stable.

   Transesophageal echocardiography (TEE) provides better visualization of wall motion abnormalities and valvular injuries than TTE, albeit in a more invasive fashion. It has superior sensitivity to TTE for injuries that require therapeutic intervention and can be performed with relative ease in the bedside or concurrent with other surgical procedures.

   Either form of echocardiography is indicated only if the patient is hemodynamically unstable.

9. **What is the optimal approach to the diagnosis of myocardial contusion?**

   Patients should initially be evaluated according to the principles of advanced trauma life support. On arrival, a clinician should identify any life-threatening conditions of BCI through physical examination, ECG, and bedside ultrasound (i.e., focused abdominal sonography for trauma [FAST]). An ECG is routinely performed in trauma patients with complaints of chest pain, history of heart disease, or other symptoms and signs suggestive of active cardiac pathologic condition. If the FAST is negative or equivocal for hemopericardium in patients with significant arrhythmias or unexplained hemodynamic instability, a formal TTE should be performed. In cases of continued diagnostic uncertainty, patients may undergo TEE. Routine examination of cardiac biomarkers (troponin, CKMB) is not recommended because of their poor sensitivity and specificity for BCI and myocardial contusion. However, serial laboratory examinations are warranted in cases of symptoms or ECG signs of cardiac ischemia.

10. **Describe the standard management of BCI.**

    The management of patients with no symptoms and with minimal or no associated injuries is debated, but discharge from the hospital after a short observation period (6 to 8 hours) with negative or minimal ECG findings and negative troponin levels at 6 hours is supported. Patients who are elderly, have a history of cardiac disease, or are hemodynamically unstable require close continuous cardiac monitoring. The use of antiarrhythmic agents in patients with myocardial contusion is controversial and should occur in close concert with cardiologists. Also, consultation of cardiothoracic surgeons should occur in suspected cases of surgically amenable injuries.

11. **Is follow-up needed in patients with BCI?**

    Long-term prognosis of patients with myocardial contusion is good, and functional recovery of the heart should be expected. As such, follow-up is not routinely required in patients with an uneventful cardiac course in the hospital. For those patients with a complicated course, a follow-up echocardiography is warranted to exclude formation of an aneurysm, cardiac thrombus, or valve anomaly.

12. **When should penetrating cardiac injury (PCI) be suspected?**

    The presentation of PCI is variable and depends on the location of the wound and cardiorespiratory compensation. Any gunshot wound or stab wound to the *cardiac box*, defined as the region medial to the midclavicular lines, inferior to the clavicles, and superior to the costal margin, is highly concerning for cardiac injury (Fig. 69-2). Of note, an injury outside of the *box* does not exclude PCI; mortality has been reported as higher for cardiac injuries through wounds outside of the *box*, possibly because of delayed diagnosis.

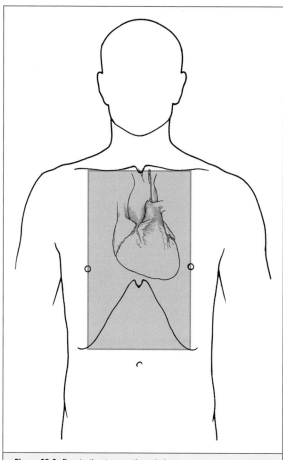

Figure 69-2. Penetrating trauma thoracic box.

13. **Describe the clinical presentation of patients with PCI.**
    Clinical presentation varies widely from hemodynamic stability to cardiac arrest. PCI can cause exsanguinating hemorrhage or cardiac tamponade. The classical findings of cardiac tamponade are described as Beck triad (distended neck veins, hypotension, and muffled heart sounds) but are present only infrequently and should not create a false sense of security if absent. Other signs of shock, such as tachycardia, hypotension, and agitation, are more useful indicators of severity and should be assessed. Less commonly, patients may present with myocardial infarction after coronary artery transection due to PCI.

14. **What is the optimal method of diagnosis of PCI?**
    An initial focused physical examination along with a rapid FAST examination of the pericardium offers the optimal method of preoperative diagnosis of PCI. FAST has an excellent sensitivity (90%-100%), specificity (96%-97%), and accuracy (96%-100%) in prospective studies with trained operators. A pericardial window was previously considered the gold standard for diagnosing hemopericardium but has been largely replaced with echocardiography today.

Pericardiocentesis has low specificity and sensitivity as well as a limited therapeutic role, and, in light of better alternatives, it is generally not recommended in trauma.

15. How should PCI be treated?

It has classically been mentioned for PCIs that "perhaps in no other injury is rapid transport of such paramount importance" as traditional means of resuscitation provide limited improvement in pathophysiology. Expeditious surgical repair is necessary, and access to the heart can be gained through a median sternotomy (preferred approach) or an anterolateral thoracotomy. Digital control of cardiac wounds is an effective method to control bleeding ahead of definitive repair. If possible, intubation should occur after the patient is prepared and draped in the operating room because of potential cardiovascular collapse after anesthetic induction. In cases of cardiac collapse before arrival in the operating room, an emergency department thoracotomy can be performed; its benefit is highest in patients with previously witnessed signs of life.

16. Describe factors associated with survival in PCI.

Mortality remains high, 41% to 84%, and, despite many surgical advances, survival has not improved significantly over several decades. This could possibly be due to an increasing proportion of gunshot wounds and faster prehospital transport of patients in extremis who previously would have been declared dead in the field. Predictors of survival include initial hemodynamic stability, stab wounds, and cardiac tamponade. Gunshot wounds often cause devastating cardiac injury and have a reported mortality of 77% to 86%. Unlike wounds causing exsanguinating hemorrhage, injuries associated with cardiac tamponade may have a protective effect by limiting bleeding, which can prolong survival until therapeutic intervention.

KEY POINTS: CARDIAC TRAUMA

1. A sternal fracture should raise the suspicion of cardiac injury, but its absence does not exclude injury.

2. Echocardiography, transthoracic or transesophageal, is a useful diagnostic tool in hemodynamically unstable patients with suspected blunt cardiac injury.

3. Patients with no symptoms and with negative ECG findings during a short observation period may be safely discharged home.

4. Any penetrating injury to the thorax or upper abdomen should raise the suspicion of cardiac injury.

5. FAST examination is the method of choice for diagnosing hemopericardium.

BIBLIOGRAPHY

1. Bansal MK, Maraj S, Chewaproug D, et al: Myocardial contusion injury: redefining the diagnostic algorithm. Emerg Med J 22:465-469, 2005.

2. Chirillo F, Totis O, Cavarzerani A, et al: Usefulness of transthoracic and transoesophageal echocardiography in recognition and management of cardiovascular injuries after blunt chest trauma. Heart 75:301-306, 1996.

3. Degiannis E, Loogna P, Doll D, et al: Penetrating cardiac injuries: recent experience in South Africa. World J Surg 30:1258-1264, 2006.

4. Kang N, Hsee L, Rizoli S, et al: Penetrating cardiac injury: overcoming the limits set by Nature. Injury 40:919-927, 2009.

5. O'Connor J, Ditillo M, Scalea T: Penetrating cardiac injury. J R Army Med Corps 155:185-190, 2009.

6. Prêtre R, Chilcott M: Blunt trauma to the heart and great vessels. N Engl J Med 336:626-632, 1997.

7. Schultz JM, Trunkey DD: Blunt cardiac injury. Crit Care Clin 20:57-70, 2004.

8. Türk EE, Tsokos M: Blunt cardiac trauma caused by fatal falls from height: an autopsy-based assessment of the injury pattern. J Trauma 57:301-304, 2004.

9. Velmahos GC, Karaiskakis M, Salim A, et al: Normal electrocardiography and serum troponin I levels preclude the presence of clinically significant blunt cardiac injury. J Trauma 54:45-51, 2003.

LIVER AND HEART TRANSPLANTATION

Claus U. Niemann, MD, and Abbas Ardehali, MD, FACS

CHAPTER 70

LIVER TRANSPLANTATION

1. **How many liver transplantations are performed in the United States annually?**
   Approximately 6000 to 6500 liver transplantations are performed annually in the United States. This includes a small number (3%-5%) from living liver donors. An estimated 17,000 to 18,000 patients are on the waiting list for liver transplantation. Approximately 1600 to 1800 patients die annually while awaiting liver transplantation. One-year, 3-year, and 5-year patient survival after primary transplantation is approximately 88%, 80%, and 74%, respectively.

2. **What are the reasons for liver transplantation?**
   The list of diseases treatable by liver transplantation has expanded steadily over the last decade. Most commonly, the disease process leading to liver transplantation is chronic. Less frequent is acute-on-chronic disease and acute liver failure. Chronic viral hepatitis B or C and alcoholic liver remain the most common reasons for transplantation. Increasingly, nonalcoholic fatty liver disease is an indication for liver transplantation.
   Overall, the etiology of chronic liver disease can be classified as follows:

   - **Noncholestatic cirrhosis:** Alcohol; hepatitis A, B, C, D; cryptogenic; autoimmune.
   - **Cholestatic cirrhosis:** Primary biliary cirrhosis, secondary biliary cirrhosis, primary sclerosing cholangitis.
   - **Metabolic disease:** Wilson disease, hemochromatosis, primary oxalosis, glycogen storage disease, α_1-antitrypsin deficiency, tyrosinemia, homozygous hyperlipidemia.
   - **Malignant neoplasm:** The single most common neoplasm presenting for liver transplantation is hepatocellular carcinoma. Eligibility for transplantation is most commonly based on tumor burden as defined by the Milan or University of California, San Francisco (UCSF) criteria. Cholangiocarcinoma, hepatoblastoma, and hemangiosarcoma are all very rare indications for transplantation.
   - **Miscellaneous:** Biliary atresia (in children most common indication), cystic fibrosis, polycystic liver disease, Budd-Chiari syndrome, neonatal hepatitis.
   - **Acute hepatic necrosis:** Etiology unknown, drug induced, acute hepatitis, environmental exposure (i.e., *Amanita phalloides* mushrooms).

   The severity of liver disease is calculated on a numeric scale that ranges from 6 (less ill) to 40 (gravely ill). The scoring system, *model for end-stage liver disease* (MELD), was introduced almost a decade ago and is also used for allocation of organs. The MELD risk score is a mathematical formula that includes creatinine, bilirubin, and international normalized ratio. It does not include the cause of liver disease. Exception points can be earned with hepatocellular carcinoma and comorbidities such as hepatopulmonary syndrome.
   Priority exception to MELD is category *status 1,* which defines acute severe onset of liver failure (fulminant hepatic failure).

3. **Why is a patient rejected for liver transplantation?**
   Reasons to deny transplantation may be due to medical conditions and psychosocial reasons and may vary from center to center. Liver transplantation is considered a medium- to high-risk procedure. Significant coronary artery disease, compromised cardiac function (reduced ejection

fraction), and uncontrolled pulmonary hypertension are considered contraindications for liver transplantation. Nevertheless, patients may be eligible once cardiopulmonary disease is adequately treated (i.e., percutaneous transluminal coronary angioplasty). Significant vasopressor support and intubation (other than airway protection) immediately before transplantation may exclude eligibility for transplantation. Uncontrolled infection or sepsis is also considered a contraindication. A positive HIV test, without evidence of AIDS, is *not* a contraindication, and reasonable survival has been reported. Advanced hepatocellular carcinoma (outside Milan or UCSF criteria) or metastatic disease is generally considered to be a contraindication because of high risk of recurrence and poor 5-year survival. In fulminant hepatic failure, uncontrolled and markedly elevated intracerebral pressure (ICP) is the most common reason for exclusion.

Psychosocial factors such as active drug or alcohol abuse or the lack of a good social support system may lead to the exclusion of the patient from transplantation. Thorough preoperative evaluation and periodic review of the patient's medical and psychosocial condition are crucial for successful transplantation and long-term survival.

Older age per se is not a reason to deny liver transplantation. Increasingly, patients older than 65 years of age receive liver transplants.

4. **What is the patient pathophysiology before liver transplantation?**
   Every organ system can be affected by end-stage liver disease. Frequently, patients with end-stage liver disease have considerable comorbidities:
   - **Central nervous system:** Hepatic encephalopathy (grade I-IV in chronic and acute-on-chronic disease) and elevated ICP in acute hepatic failure.
   - **Cardiac system:** Hyperdynamic circulation with high cardiac output and low systemic vascular resistance. This may be blunted in patients receiving nonselective β-blockade for secondary prevention of upper gastrointestinal bleeding; cirrhotic cardiomyopathy.
   - **Respiratory system:**
     - Pleural effusions (right > left).
     - Hepatic hydrothorax, atelectasis, hepatopulmonary syndrome (orthodeoxia, $PaO_2 < 70$ mm Hg on room air, or $A - aO_2$ gradient > 20 mm Hg, intrapulmonary vascular dilatation).
     - Portopulmonary hypertension (presence of portal hypertension, precapillary or arteriolar pulmonary hypertension, mean pulmonary artery pressure > 25 mm Hg, pulmonary vascular resistance [PVR] > 240 dyne/second/cm^{-5}). Pulmonary capillary wedge pressure < 15 mm Hg (all at rest and primary pulmonary hypertension ruled out). Estimation of systolic pulmonary pressure on transthoracic echocardiography can be used as a valuable screening tool. Increasingly, the transpulmonary pressure gradient is also used for evaluation.
   - **Gastrointestinal system:** Portal hypertension with possible upper gastrointestinal bleeding, (refractory) ascites.
   - **Hematologic system:** Anemia, thrombocytopenia (mainly sequestration into the spleen), prolonged prothrombin time–partial thromboplastin time, and decreased fibrinogen. Hypercoagulability (especially in patients with malignant disease).
   - **Renal system:** Hepatorenal syndrome type I or II, acute kidney injury.
   - **Miscellaneous:** Significant electrolyte disturbances (sodium, potassium, glucose), immunosuppression with increased risk for infection, malnutrition.

5. **What are common complications of patients undergoing liver transplantation?**
   Perioperative complications depend largely on the medical condition and surgical history of the recipient (see question 4). Poor organ quality can also lead to a complicated perioperative course. The organ quality depends on multiple factors including donor age, organ ischemia time, and mechanism of death. Frequently the donor risk index is used to assess donor organ quality. Slow graft function may result in significantly increased resource utilization. Primary

nonfunction of the implanted organ, often still manifesting during surgery, requires immediate relisting and retransplantation of the patient.

Overall, hemodynamic instability requiring multiple vasopressors, significant blood loss, severe coagulopathy, electrolyte or glucose abnormalities, renal dysfunction, and respiratory compromise are not uncommon during liver transplantation.

6. **What are indicators of good graft function in the immediate perioperative period?**
Bile production (during surgery), correction of negative base excess, normalization of prothrombin time, reduction of diffuse bleeding, decreasing fresh frozen plasma (FFP) requirements, and hemodynamic stability after implantation of the liver.

7. **Does every patient receiving a liver transplant need to continue to have an endotracheal tube in place and be admitted to the intensive care unit (ICU) after surgery?**
Postoperative intubation is not required per se, as long as commonly accepted extubation criteria are followed and good organ function is established. Blood loss alone should not be considered as an indication for postoperative intubation. Patients can have the endotracheal tube removed either in the operating room or shortly after arrival in the ICU.

Most centers still will admit patients to the ICU for monitoring purposes. However, some centers established fast-track protocols admitting patients with uncomplicated cases to the postanesthesia care unit and subsequently discharge them to the ward (step-down unit).

8. **How do you manage the liver transplant patient in the immediate postoperative period?**
As for the intraoperative course, the immediate postoperative course is primarily dictated by the medical condition of the recipient and donor organ function. In most cases, therapy is supportive and follows guidelines established for all intensive care patients. However, certain aspects require special attention:
- **Hypocoagulable or hypercoagulable states:** Overall, treatment should be dictated by clinical evidence of bleeding (i.e., drain output, drop in hematocrit). Occasionally, patients require postoperative FFP therapy to offset an initially slow graft function. Platelets may be needed with persistent low platelet counts and evidence of diffuse bleeding. With the exception of a confirmed rapidly dropping hematocrit requiring red blood cell transfusion, transfusion of FFP, platelets, and cryoprecipitate should not be based on laboratory values alone. The threshold for reexploration should be low in the setting of persistent hematocrit drops. Leakage from vascular anastomosis sites and small arterial or venous bleeding should always be considered.
- **Renal function:** Renal dysfunction is frequently present before surgery, and acute kidney injury can develop during the immediate postoperative period. This can be due to temporary renal outflow obstruction during surgery when the inferior vena cava is entirely clamped for insertion of the donor liver. Significant hemodynamic instability requiring large doses of vasopressors and blood loss can contribute to postoperative acute kidney injury. Intraoperative venovenous bypass may ameliorate the outflow obstruction but is not used at most centers. More commonly a piggyback technique is used with preservation of the inferior vena cava. Postoperative supportive therapy of renal function follows ICU standard protocols. In some cases, continuous renal replacement therapy (continuous venovenous hemofiltration) through the immediate postoperative period will help with recovery of renal function.
- **Glucose and electrolytes:** With adequate postoperative liver function and steroid administration, patients tend to have hyperglycemia, which may warrant a continuous insulin infusion. In most cases, the infusion can be tapered off within the first 24 to 48 hours. Depending on the renal function and diuretic or insulin therapy, potassium can be either high or low. If necessary, sodium levels should be corrected cautiously and

according to implemented protocols. Calcium homeostasis is not significantly altered in the postoperative period.

- **Immunosuppression:** Allograft rejection can occur at any given point after surgery and is classified as hyperacute, acute, and chronic. Immunosuppressive therapy is usually started immediately after surgery. Commonly used drugs, often in combination, are cyclosporine, tacrolimus, sirolimus, mycophenolate mofetil, and steroids. These agents can cause a variety of side effects, including undesired drug interactions, hypertension, hyperlipidemia, and osteoporosis.
- **Infection:** After transplantation, recipients are at a significant risk for bacterial, fungal, and viral infections. Infections in this patient population have increased morbidity and mortality and unique infectious risks compared with immunocompetent ICU patients.

HEART TRANSPLANTATION

9. **How many heart transplantations are performed in the United States annually?**
   In the year 2010, 2333 heart transplantations were performed in the United States. As of May 2011, 3138 patients were on the waiting list for heart transplantation. Approximately 402 patients die annually while awaiting heart transplantation. Nationwide, the 1-year and 3-year patient survival after transplantation is approximately 89% and 81%, respectively.

10. **What are the reasons for heart transplantation?**
    Cardiac transplantation has become an accepted treatment for selected patients with end-stage heart failure. As with liver transplantation, the number of candidates and the waiting time have increased over the last years. The most common causes of end-stage heart disease leading to heart transplantation are cardiomyopathy and coronary artery disease. The etiology of end-stage heart disease can be classified as follows:
    - **Dilated cardiomyopathy:** viral, idiopathic, post partum, familial, doxorubicin (Adriamycin), myocarditis, ischemic
    - **Restricted cardiomyopathy:** sarcoidosis, amyloidosis, endocardial fibrosis, idiopathic, secondary radiation, chemotherapy
    - **Retransplantation or graft failure:** primary failure, hyperacute, acute, chronic rejection, nonspecific, restrictive-constrictive, accelerated allograft coronary artery disease
    - **Other:** congenital disease, valvular disease, hypertrophic cardiomyopathy

    It is important to keep in mind that medical treatment of patients with end-stage heart disease continuously improves, selected patients can be managed medically, and survival outcomes have become similar to those of heart transplantation. Hence heart transplantation should be offered to patients who have severe disability due to their cardiac disease despite optimal medical treatment and also have no major contraindications for heart transplantation. More recently the ventricular assist device has emerged as another option for patients with end-stage heart disease that is refractory to medical therapy.

11. **Why is a patient rejected for heart transplantation?**
    Contraindications may vary slightly from center to center. Common contraindications include significant or irreversible pulmonary hypertension; renal, hepatic, cerebrovascular disease; uncontrolled infection or sepsis; and cancer of uncertain status. Patients with systematic diseases that affect multiple organs, such as amyloidosis, may not be suitable candidates for heart transplantation. In addition, noncompliance, psychological instability, lack of social support, and active drug use may exclude a patient from heart transplantation. Old age per se is not a reason to deny heart transplantation. Indeed, increasingly, patients older than 65 years of age are transplant recipients.

12. **What is the physiology after heart transplantation?**

Although baseline cardiac function is generally preserved, the cardiac response to demand is significantly altered. Cardiac denervation is nearly always permanent after transplantation. Because of the lack of sympathetic innervation, heart rate can only increase slowly via increased circulating catecholamine levels. Maintaining an adequate stroke volume therefore becomes paramount to sustain cardiac output in these patients. Hence, patients after heart transplantation are very preload dependent. Denervation also affects the pharmacologic therapy in these patients. Drugs that act indirectly on the heart, through either the sympathetic or parasympathetic nervous system, are ineffective. Drugs acting directly on the heart are the agents of choice to modify cardiac physiology. In addition, denervation of the heart usually prevents the recipient from experiencing chest pain when myocardial ischemia is present.

13. **What are common complications seen in patients undergoing heart transplantation?**

Long-term survival has significantly improved for patients undergoing heart transplantation. However, a number of complications may occur after transplantation. The complications include right or left ventricular failure, pulmonary hypertension, systemic hypertension, heart block, bradyarrhythmias, tachyarrhythmias, early graft failure, allograft rejection, accelerated allograft coronary artery disease, renal dysfunction, infection, and malignancy.

The postoperative stability of the patient is also affected by donor characteristics and by the operative technique chosen. The use of the bicaval techniques over the biatrial technique has resulted in less atrioventricular valve dysfunction and arrhythmia. Use of these newer techniques has also shown improvements in hemodynamics, exercise capacity, and overall patient survival.

14. **How do you manage the heart transplant patient in the immediate postoperative period?**

Similar to other post–cardiac surgical patients, post–heart transplantation patients require close monitoring via electrocardiography, arterial blood pressure, central venous pressure, pulmonary artery pressure, cardiac output, arterial blood gas measurements, and chest tube output. Most patients will require chronotropic and inotropic support in the form of pacing and/or β-adrenergic agonist infusion (isoproterenol, epinephrine, dobutamine, dopamine). If cardiac function is still depressed despite pacing and pharmacologic support, mechanical support in the form of intraaortic balloon pumps, ventricular assist devices, or extracorporeal membrane oxygenators (ECMO) may be instituted. Once the hemodynamic state and postoperative bleeding have stabilized, patients may undergo extubation. Certain aspects warrant special attention:

- **Preload dependence:** As mentioned, patients are very preload dependent because of cardiac denervation. This renders them sensitive to positive pressure ventilation, bleeding or tamponade, and pneumothorax.
- **Increased PVR or right ventricular failure:** Although fixed pulmonary hypertension will have been excluded before surgery, postoperative increased PVR may still develop. If severe and untreated, it can lead to right ventricular failure in the newly grafted heart. Management of increased PVR includes inhaled vasodilators such as prostacyclin and nitric oxide. Intravenous vasodilators such as nitroglycerin and nitroprusside are also options. Unfortunately, intravenous vasodilators are associated with systemic hypotension, and their use may require an additional α-agonist infusion. Right ventricular dysfunction can also be treated with atrial pacing, β-adrenergic agonists, and phosphodiesterase inhibitors. If these measures are ineffective, right ventricular assist devices or ECMO may be required.
- **Cardiac arrhythmias:** In addition to bradycardia and heart block, atrial and ventricular tachyarrhythmias are also quite common after heart transplantation. Atrial arrhythmias may be associated with allograft rejection.
- **Rejection or graft failure:** Allograft rejection can occur at any given point after surgery and is classified as hyperacute, acute, and chronic. Diagnosis of cellular rejection of the transplanted

TABLE 70-1.	DRUGS USED FOR IMMUNOSUPPRESSIVE THERAPY
AZATHIOPRINE	**MYELOSUPPRESSION**
Cyclosporine	Hypertension, ↓renal function, ↑K^+, ↓Mg^{++}, ↓seizure threshold
Mycophenolate mofetil	Myelosuppression, gastrointestinal bleeding
Prednisone	Hypertension, ↑Glu, adrenal suppression
Tacrolimus	↓Renal function, ↓seizure threshold, ↑Glu, ↑K^+, ↓Mg^{++}

Glu, Glucose.

heart relies mainly on endomyocardial biopsy particularly in view of vague clinical symptoms and no reliable serologic markers. Serial biopsies are performed after surgery to detect any sign of rejection. Antibody-mediated rejection is difficult to diagnose; it is usually detected by the rising titer of donor-specific antibodies, when other causes have been excluded.

- **Immunosuppression:** Patients usually start immunosuppressive therapy immediately after surgery. Common drugs, often used in combination, are calcineurin inhibitors (such as cyclosporine, tacrolimus), cell cycle inhibitors (such as mycophenolate mofetil, azathioprine), and steroids. These agents can cause a variety of side effects, as well as drug interactions (see Table 70-1).

15. **How will the denervated heart respond to medications after transplantation?**
    - **Indirect cardiac agents:** Drugs, such as ephedrine and atropine, are mediated via the sympathetic and parasympathetic nervous system. These drugs will have minimal effects. Digitalis will also have no effect on atrioventricular nodal conduction but retains its direct inotropic effect.
    - **Direct cardiac agents:** β-Adrenergic agents (isoproterenol, epinephrine, dobutamine, dopamine, norepinephrine) are unaffected and will improve both chronotropy and inotropy. Phosphodiesterase inhibitors (amrinone, milrinone) are also unaffected and improve cardiac output, as well as cause vasodilation.
    - **Vasodilators:** Nitrates are unaffected and cause both venous and arterial vasodilation. However, because of the denervation, reflex tachycardia is severely depressed.
    - **Vasoconstrictors:** Phenylephrine, norepinephrine, and vasopressin are still effective, but less reflex bradycardia is seen.
    - **β-Blockers and calcium channel blockers:** These agents retain the ability to decrease heart rate and blood pressure.

KEY POINTS: TRANSPLANTATION

Postoperative complications of liver transplantation:
1. Donor risk index and poor organ function

2. Significant metabolic disturbances (e.g., hyperglycemia)

Denervated hearts:
1. Are preload dependent

2. Are responsive only to direct-acting cardiac medications

3. Do not display reflex bradycardia or tachycardia

BIBLIOGRAPHY

1. Ardehali A, Hughes K, Sadeghi A, et al: Inhaled nitric oxide for pulmonary hypertension after heart transplantation. Transplantation 72:638-641, 2001.

2. Ashary N, Kaye AD, Hegazi AR, et al: Anesthetic considerations in the patient with a heart transplant. Heart Dis 4:191-198, 2002.

3. Augoustides JG, Riha H: Recent progress in heart failure treatment and heart transplantation. J Cardiothorac Vasc Anesth 23:738-748, 2009.

4. Findlay JY, Fix OK, Paugam-Burtz C, et al: Critical care of the end-stage liver disease patient awaiting liver transplantation. Liver Transpl 17:496-510, 2011.

5. Hlava N, Niemann CU, Gropper MA, et al: Postoperative infectious complications of abdominal solid organ transplantation. J Intensive Care Med 24:3-17, 2009.

6. Kamath PS, Kim WR: Advanced Liver Disease Study Group. The model for end-stage liver disease (MELD). Hepatology 45:797-805, 2007.

7. Khush KK, Valantine HA: New developments in immunosuppressive therapy for heart transplantation. Expert Opin Emerg Drugs 14:1-21, 2009.

8. Luckraz H, Goddard M, Charman SC, et al: Early mortality after cardiac transplantation: should we do better? J Heart Lung Transplant 24:401-405, 2005.

9. Mehra MR, Kobashigawa J, Starling R, et al: Listing criteria for heart transplantation: International Society for Heart and Lung Transplantation guidelines for the care of cardiac transplant candidates. J Heart Lung Transplant 25:1024-1042, 2006.

10. Miniati DN, Robbins RC: Heart transplantation: a thirty-year perspective. Annu Rev Med 53:189-205, 2002.

11. Morgan JA, Edwards NM: Orthotopic cardiac transplantation: comparison of outcome using biatrial, bicaval, and total techniques. J Card Surg 20:102-106, 2005.

12. Razonable RR, Findlay JY, O'Riordan A, et al: Critical care issues in patients after liver transplantation. Liver Transpl 17:511-527, 2011.

13. Stehlik J, Edwards LB, Kucheryavaya AY, et al: The Registry of the International Society for Heart and Lung Transplantation: twenty-seventh official adult heart transplant report—2010. J Heart Lung Transplant 29:1089-1103, 2010.

14. Stobierska-Dzierzek B, Awad H, Michler RE: The evolving management of acute right-sided heart failure in cardiac transplant recipients. J Am Coll Cardiol 38:923-931, 2001.

15. Weiss ES, Nwakanma LU, Patel ND, et al: Outcomes in patients older than 60 years of age undergoing orthotopic heart transplantation: an analysis of the UNOS database. J Heart Lung Transplant 27:184-191, 2008.

16. Yost SC, Niemann CU: Organ transplantation. In Miller RD (ed): Miller's Anesthesia, 7th ed. New York, Churchill Livingstone, 2009, pp 2155-2184.

USE OF PARALYTIC AGENTS IN THE INTENSIVE CARE UNIT

David W. Miller, MD, and Jean-François Pittet, MD

CHAPTER 71

1. **What are neuromuscular blocking agents (NMBs)?**
   NMBs (also called muscle relaxants or paralytics) are agents that act primarily on acetylcholine (ACh) receptors located on the postsynaptic motor end plate of the neuromuscular junction to cause skeletal muscle paralysis. They do not have any effect on cardiac or smooth muscle. Muscle relaxants do not have any sedating properties; therefore appropriate sedatives and analgesics are needed to avoid awareness (being alert without the ability to move).

2. **How are NMBs classified?**
   NMBs are broadly separated into depolarizing and nondepolarizing agents. The only clinically significant depolarizing agent is succinylcholine (SCh). Nondepolarizing agents are divided into the benzylisoquiniliniums, which include agents such as cisatracurium, and the aminosteroids, of which vecuronium and rocuronium are examples.

3. **Why are NMBs used in the intensive care unit (ICU)?**
   The most common reason for using muscle relaxants in the ICU is for facilitation of endotracheal intubation and mechanical ventilation. Examples include securing the airway for hypoxemic respiratory failure, severe patient-ventilator dyssynchrony, and increasing effectiveness of inverse ratio ventilation. Management of increased intracerebral pressure (ICP) is another indication. There are case reports of using muscle relaxants for control of muscle spasms whether from tetanus, drug overdoses, or seizures. Many protocols for controlled hypothermia after cardiac arrest advocate the use of muscle relaxants to prevent shivering. Continuous electroencephalogram monitoring should be used if muscle relaxants are used in conjunction with a hypothermia protocol or to prevent lactic acidosis in seizures. Muscle relaxants are advocated for decreasing oxygen consumption, although no study has definitively shown that they reduce oxygen consumption. NMBs will improve pulmonary compliance, however. Muscle relaxants may also be used to facilitate the transport of critically ill patients, aid in radiologic imaging, or improve conditions for bedside surgical procedures, such as bronchoscopies and tracheostomies, in the ICU. Sedation alone should always be used if feasible.

4. **How does the neuromuscular junction work?**
   The neuromuscular junction contains the prejunctional motor nerve ending and the postsynaptic membrane on the skeletal muscle cell. Action potentials cause the release of ACh from synaptic vesicles stored in the motor nerve ending. ACh diffuses across the synaptic cleft to the postsynaptic membrane (approximately 20 nm). When two ACh molecules bind to one nicotinic cholinergic receptor within this motor end plate, depolarization occurs with the subsequent influx of calcium from the sarcoplasmic reticulum of the skeletal muscle cell. This results in contraction of the cell. ACh is rapidly hydrolyzed by acetylcholinesterase at the motor end plate, which terminates depolarization. ACh also diffuses away from the synaptic cleft or undergoes reuptake into the motor nerve ending.

5. **Explain the mechanism of action of SCh.**
   SCh is the only clinically significant depolarizing muscle relaxant in use. Its chemical structure is similar to that of ACh, and it acts as an *agonist* at nicotinic cholinergic receptors on the

postsynaptic membrane of the neuromuscular junction. While succinylcholine is bound to the receptor further transmission is blocked. Calcium is not being shuttled back into the sarcoplasmic reticulum of the skeletal muscle cell while SCh remains bound to the receptor, which results clinically in muscle relaxation. SCh is hydrolyzed by plasma cholinesterase, which is not located at the neuromuscular junction; therefore the rate of blockade is dependent on the rate at which SCh diffuses away from the neuromuscular junction. The depolarization caused by SCh is prolonged compared with that caused by ACh, and relaxation persists as long as SCh is present.

6. **What type of patients should not receive SCh?**
   Because of its ability to raise serum potassium concentration even in healthy patients, succinylcholine should be avoided in patients with hyperkalemia. The hyperkalemic response is pronounced in patients with extrajunctional ACh receptors. These extrajunctional receptors are more common in patients with burns or severe crush injuries and in neuromuscular disease (i.e., Duchenne muscular dystrophy, Guillain-Barré syndrome, and previous stroke). SCh should also not be used in patients with sepsis, in patients with significant immobility (>3-5 days), or in pediatric patients (concern for undiagnosed neuromuscular disease). If a patient has a personal or known family history of pseudocholinesterase deficiency, the duration of action of SCh may be prolonged unpredictably. It may also cause sinus bradycardia via its stimulation of cardiac muscarinic receptors; therefore SCh should be used with caution in patients with bradycardia. SCh is a known trigger of malignant hyperthermia; therefore it should be avoided if personal or family history suggests a possibility of malignant hyperthermia. Evidence supports that SCh will elevate intraocular pressure (IOP) and ICP. The use of SCh to avoid aspiration in a rapid-sequence intubation should consequently be weighed against any possible harm from raising IOP or ICP in patients with open globe injuries or severe brain pathologic conditions. The rise in ICP can be avoided by pretreatment with a small dose of a nondepolarizing agent. SCh can also increase gastric pressure, but this response is inconsistent and of concern only if there is an impaired lower esophageal sphincter (i.e., hiatal hernia, esophagectomies).

7. **When should SCh be used in the ICU?**
   Rapid-sequence intubations to avoid aspiration in patients without contraindications to its use would be the main reason. Circumstances also exist in which the brief duration of action of SCh may be desired, such as after a patient's motor or neurologic examination after emergent intubation. In one meta-analysis, SCh was shown to give better intubating conditions than with a nondepolarizing agent.

8. **What are the enzymes that metabolize SCh and ACh?**
   Butyrylcholinesterase (pseudocholinesterase or plasma cholinesterase), located in the plasma and liver, metabolizes SCh into succinylmonocholine, an active metabolite, and choline. It also metabolizes mivacurium, ester-type local anesthetics, and trimethaphan. Acetylcholinesterase (true cholinesterase) is present at the neuromuscular junction and metabolizes ACh. Unspecific esterases are located in plasma and certain tissue that degrade atracurium and remifentanil.

9. **What is a phase II blockade?**
   After prolonged administration of SCh, fade will appear on train-of-four (TOF) and tetanic stimulation. This block can be reversed by anticholinesterases. The onset of this block coincides with tachyphylaxis to SCh.

10. **What is the mechanism of action for nondepolarizing muscle relaxants?**
    Nondepolarizing NMBs are competitive antagonists of nicotinic cholinergic receptors. A single molecule is able to bind to the receptor in its resting closed state to cause blockade. This compares with SCh, which enacts its effects through a prolonged depolarization of the motor end plate, which results in no further action potentials being propagated.

11. **How do nondepolarizing agents differ in their dosing and duration of action?**
A summary of the pharmacology of the commonly used NMBs is given in Table 71-1.

TABLE 71-1.	NEUROMUSCULAR BLOCKING AGENTS USED IN THE INTENSIVE CARE UNIT					
	ED95 (MG/ KG)	INTUBATING DOSE (MG/ KG)	ONSET (MIN)	DURATION OF ACTION (MIN)	CONTINUOUS INFUSION DOSE (MCG/KG/MIN)	PRIMARY ELIMINATION
Depolarizing NMBs						
SCh	0.3	1-1.5	0.5-1	Under 10	NA	Ester hydrolysis
Benzylisoquinolinium agents						
Atracurium	0.25	0.5	1.5-3	25-35	4-12	Hofmann, ester hydrolysis
Cisatracurium	0.05	0.15	2-4	45-60	2.5-3.0	Hofmann, ester hydrolysis
Aminosteroidal agents						
Rocuronium	0.3	0.6-1	1-2	30	10-12	Hepatic
Vecuronium	0.05	0.1	3-4	35-45	1-2	Hepatic
Pancuronium	0.07	0.1	2-3	90-100	1-2	Renal, hepatic

ED95, Dose required to produce 95% reduction in twitch height; *NA*, not applicable.

12. **How do the aminosteroid and benzylisoquinolinium differ in side effects?**
Aminosteroids such as rocuronium and pancuronium can to some degree block cardiac muscarinic receptors resulting in tachycardia. The benzylisoquinoliniums cause some degree of histamine release, especially older drugs such as mivacurium, which may result in hypotension and bronchoconstriction. Atracurium has only slight histamine release, and cisatracurium has none. The aminosteroid rocuronium has been associated with cases of anaphylaxis.

13. **What is Hofmann elimination?**
This is the method by which atracurium and cisatracurium are primarily metabolized. It is an organ-independent process that makes these drugs useful in patients with liver and renal failure. The process is decreased by hypothermia and acidosis, which should prompt closer monitoring and dose adjustments.

14. **What nondepolarizing agent is the best alternative to SCh when it is contraindicated?**
Rocuronium has the shortest onset of action with an intubating dose of 0.6 to 1.0 mg/kg resulting in adequate relaxation within 2 minutes. The drug should be used for rapid-sequence intubations if SCh cannot be used.

15. **What are some unique features of pancuronium?**
Pancuronium has a vagolytic effect that can cause a modest increase in heart rate, cardiac output, and blood pressure. Because it is metabolized by the liver and eliminated in the bile and urine, doses should be modified in hepatic and renal failure.

16. **Explain how the depth of neuromuscular blockade is monitored in the ICU. What equipment is used?**

A peripheral nerve stimulator is used to monitor the degree of neuromuscular blockade. Generally contraction of the adductor pollicis muscle in response to ulnar nerve stimulation is measured. The peroneal nerve or facial nerve may be substituted.

Electrode pads or needles are placed on or in the skin over the nerve of interest and a supramaximal, monophasic current with a square wave is passed through the electrodes with the motor response being monitored by feeling or watching the muscle contract. The TOF and double-burst stimulation (DBS) are the most commonly used methods of delivering current. The TOF current is four stimuli being applied over a 2-second period. The result can be reported as the number of twitches felt out of four. A TOF ratio can be calculated as well by dividing the amplitude of the fourth twitch by the amplitude of the first twitch. DBS is performed by the stimulator giving two 50-Hz tetanic bursts 750 milliseconds apart. Each burst lasts 0.2 second and contains three impulses. DBS may improve tactile detection of residual blockade. More accurate measurements of TOF ratios may be obtained by using mechanomyography, electromyography, or acceleromyography, which quantitates the degree of movement or contraction. Of note, only nondepolarizing muscle relaxants will demonstrate fade. The TOF ratio with SCh is always 1.0; only amplitude of the twitches changes, unless a phase II blockade has occurred.

17. **How does TOF count correlate with degree of neuromuscular blockade?**

During a partial nondepolarizing blockade, when one twitch is detectable, the degree of neuromuscular blockade is 90% to 95%. The second twitch is detected when 80% to 90% blockade is present. The third represents 70% to 80% blockade. When the fourth twitch becomes detectable, there is still 65% to 75% of blockade remaining. In the operating room, most surgical procedures only need one to two twitches. Note that if no twitches are present, it is difficult to assess degree of blockade.

18. **What depth of paralysis is necessary in most circumstances in the ICU?**

It is first always encouraged to use sedation if possible instead of neuromuscular blockade. If neuromuscular blockade is needed as an infusion the lowest dose possible to obtain the clinical response should be used. If this is unclear, then it is recommended to keep the TOF count to one to two twitches. Frequent (daily) drug holidays are also useful to make sure that no accumulation of active metabolites occurs and that no other neurologic process (i.e., cerebrovascular accident or neuropathy) has occurred.

19. **Name the potential adverse outcomes from the use of nondepolarizing muscle relaxants in the ICU.**

The main risks include awareness from inadequate sedation, generalized deconditioning and muscle atrophy, skin breakdown, corneal abrasions, ICU-acquired weakness, peripheral nerve injury from improper positioning, myositis ossificans (ossification of connective tissue), central nervous system toxicity, and the inability to clear secretions from cough suppression.

20. **What is ICU-acquired weakness, and what are its risk factors?**

ICU-acquired weakness is the main clinical sign of critical illness neuromyopathy (CINM), which results in either structural or functional changes in skeletal muscle. This disease prolongs ventilator time, makes ventilator weaning more difficult, and increases ICU length of stay.

Five main risk factors are multiple organ failure, muscle immobilization, hyperglycemia, use of corticosteroids, and neuromuscular blockade. A decrease in muscle action potential with spontaneous electrical activity during electrophysiologic testing diagnoses the disease. NMBs either have a direct toxic effect or increase the toxic effect of corticosteroids on muscles.

21. **What are some ways ICU-acquired weakness can be treated?**
    Multiple studies now show that early mobilization of patients with acute respiratory failure when coupled with an aggressive sedation weaning protocol and daily physical and occupational therapy will shorten total ventilator time and ICU days. Reports also exist that daily electrical muscle stimulation will shorten ventilator time and prevent onset of CINM.

22. **How do muscle relaxants interact with other commonly used drugs in the ICU?**
    A variety of drugs either augments or inhibits the actions of nondepolarizing muscle relaxants. A summary is given in Table 71-2.

TABLE 71-2. DRUG–DRUG INTERACTION OF NEUROMUSCULAR BLOCKING AGENTS	
DRUGS THAT POTENTIATE THE ACTION OF NONDEPOLARIZING NMBS	**DRUGS THAT ANTAGONIZE THE ACTIONS OF NONDEPOLARIZING NMBS**
Local anesthetics	Phenytoin
Lidocaine	Carbamazepine
Antimicrobials (aminoglycosides, polymyxin B, clindamycin, tetracycline)	Sodium valproate
Antiarrhythmics (procainamide, quinidine)	Ranitidine
Magnesium	Steroids
Calcium channel blockers	Azathioprine
β-Adrenergic blockers	
Immunosuppressive agents (cyclophosphamide, cyclosporine)	
Dantrolene	
Diuretics	
Lithium carbonate	
Inhaled anesthetics	
Tamoxifen	

23. **Describe how serum electrolyte, acid–base status, and temperature alter the action of neuromuscular blockade.**
    The duration of action of nondepolarizing muscle relaxants is prolonged by hypothermia, especially if core temperatures drop below 36° C. This is due to altered renal and hepatic clearance and by altered enzyme function. Hypermagnesemia potentiates neuromuscular blockade by nondepolarizing muscle relaxants. This is probably due to inhibition of calcium channels at the presynaptic membrane, which trigger the release of ACh. Magnesium also makes the postjunctional membrane less excitable. Hypercalcemia, on the other hand, shortens the time course for neuromuscular blockade recovery. Both metabolic and respiratory acidosis augments nondepolarizing muscle relaxant blockade, but only respiratory acidosis limits adequate reversal with neostigmine. Hypophosphatemia and hypokalemia also potentiate the effects of muscle relaxants. Patients with elevated liver function tests or creatinine may have accumulation of NMBs and their metabolites.

24. **What are the active metabolites of muscle relaxants, and what effects do they cause?**
    3-Deacetylvecuronium is a potent (approximately 80%) metabolite of vecuronium and has a longer duration of action with slower plasma clearance. Vecuronium should not be used in

patients with hepatic and renal dysfunction, especially as a continuous infusion, because a prolonged blockade may occur. Laudanosine is an active metabolite of atracurium. It is dependent on the liver and kidney for elimination. It theoretically has central nervous system stimulatory (seizures) and cardiovascular (hypotension) effects, but these require high levels to be of concern. Cisatracurium is a more potent isomer of atracurium; therefore approximately five times less laudanosine is produced, which is not thought to be clinically significant.

25. **What steps can be taken to prevent long-term muscle relaxant use?**
Every effort should be given to avoid muscle relaxants and to use infrequent boluses compared with long-term infusions if possible. If infusions are needed, close monitoring both clinically and with a peripheral nerve stimulator should be undertaken. The depth of paralysis should be adjusted until one or two twitches are obtained. Deepening of sedation can usually prevent the need for neuromuscular blockade.

26. **How can the effects of nondepolarizing muscle relaxants be reversed?**
The easiest and most effective way for the effect of muscle relaxants to terminate is to wait for the drug to be metabolized and eliminated from the body. The effects of nondepolarizing muscle relaxants may be actively reversed in two ways, however. The first involves increasing the amount of ACh in the neuromuscular junction to overcome the muscle relaxant competing for the receptor. Drugs called cholinesterase inhibitors (anticholinesterases) inhibit the enzyme that hydrolyzes ACh, thus effectively overwhelming the muscle relaxant so that it cannot work. A list of these agents is in Table 71-3. Of note, physostigmine is another cholinesterase inhibitor that crosses the blood–brain barrier and is not used for the reversal of neuromuscular blockade. Pyridostigmine is primarily used for the treatment of myasthenia gravis and not for reversal of neuromuscular blockade. The second way muscle relaxants may be actively reversed involves the use of a novel drug that binds aminosteroid muscle relaxants. See question 28.

TABLE 71-3.	REVERSAL AGENTS OF NEUROMUSCULAR BLOCKADE		
DRUG	**DOSE (MG/KG)**	**ONSET (MIN)**	**DURATION (MIN)**
Edrophonium	0.5-1	2	45-60
Neostigmine	0.035-0.07	7	60-90
Pyridostigmine	0.15-0.25	11	60-120

27. **What are the side effects of anticholinesterases, and how are they attenuated?**
The most significant side effects are due to these drugs increasing ACh at muscarinic cholinergic receptors (parasympathetic stimulation) in addition to the neuromuscular junction. This may result in bradycardia or asystole, increased motility of the gastrointestinal tract, pulmonary bronchospasm, increased bladder tone, and pupillary constriction (miosis). Anticholinergics with similar onset of action are given to avoid these side effects.

28. **What is sugammadex?**
Sugammadex is a cyclodextrin compound and is the first selective muscle relaxant–binding agent. Its three-dimensional structure forms a hydrophobic central cavity that can accommodate steroidal NMBs. These agents bind in a 1:1 fashion (rocuronium>vecuronium>>pancuronium). This drug causes a rapid drop in the serum muscle relaxant concentration with the resulting gradient leading to more agent leaving the neuromuscular junction. This terminates the action of the muscle relaxant and eliminates the need for anticholinesterases. It is currently available in Europe but not the United States.

29. **Are any good effects associated with neuromuscular blockade use in the ICU?**
Neuromuscular blockade with cisatracurium when compared with placebo has been shown to improve mortality in early acute respiratory distress syndrome (ARDS). Some evidence also supports a decrease in the proinflammatory state in ARDS when cisatracurium is used.

KEY POINTS: ADVERSE EFFECTS OF PROLONGED NEUROMUSCULAR BLOCKADE

1. Corneal abrasions and peripheral nerve injury

2. Skin breakdown and decubitus ulcers

3. Muscle atrophy, deconditioning, connective tissue ossification

4. Deep venous thrombosis and embolus

5. Pooling of pulmonary secretions, pneumonia

6. ICU-acquired weakness, myopathy, neuropathy

BIBLIOGRAPHY

1. Akha AS, Rosa J, Jahr JS, et al: Sugammadex: cyclodextrins, development of selective binding agents, pharmacology, clinical development, and future directions. Anesthesiology 28:691-708, 2010.

2. De Jonghe B, Lacherade JC, Sharshar T, et al: Intensive care unit-acquired weakness: risk factors and prevention. Crit Care Med 37(Suppl):S309-S315, 2009.

3. Forel J, Roch A, Marin V, et al: Neuromuscular blocking agents decrease inflammatory response in patients presenting with acute respiratory distress syndrome. Crit Care Med 34:2749-2757, 2006.

4. Griffiths RD, Hall JB: Intensive care unit–acquired weakness. Crit Care Med 38:779-787, 2010.

5. Murray MJ, Cowen J, DeBlock H, et al: Clinical practice guidelines for sustained neuromuscular blockade in the adult critically ill patient. Crit Care Med 30:142-156, 2002.

6. Naguib M, Lien CA: Pharmacology of muscle relaxants and their antagonists. In Miller RD (ed): Miller's Anesthesia, 7th ed. New York, Churchill Livingstone, 2009, pp 859-911.

7. Papazian L, Forel J, Gacouin A, et al: Neuromuscular blocking agents in early acute respiratory distress syndrome. N Engl J Med 363:1107-1116, 2010.

8. Perry JJ, Lee JS, Sillberg VA, et al: Rocuronium versus succinylcholine for rapid sequence induction intubation. Cochrane Database Syst Rev 2: CD002788, 2008.

9. Routsi C, Gerovasili V, Vasileiadis I, et al: Electrical muscle stimulation prevents critical illness polyneuromyopathy: a randomized parallel intervention trial. Crit Care 14:R74, 2010.

CHAPTER 72

PAIN MANAGEMENT IN THE INTENSIVE CARE UNIT

Philip McArdle, MB, BCh, BAO, FFARCSI, and Jean-François Pittet, MD

1. **Do critically ill patients require analgesia?**

   Intensive care unit (ICU) patients experience pain from underlying medical disease, immobility, surgery, and trauma. Insertion and maintenance of monitoring and therapeutic devices (venous and arterial catheters, chest tubes, drains, and endotracheal tubes) and routine bedside care (dressing changes, mobilization, physical therapy, and airway suctioning) may also cause pain and discomfort in ICU patients.

2. **Is pain relief generally adequate in ICU patients?**

   The degree of analgesia in critically ill patients is often inadequate. Level of pain is harder to assess in ICU patients because patients are often confused, unable to communicate, or even paralyzed. Inadequate use of analgesic agents, together with routine use of sedatives, may result in oversedation and even delirium, and impaired ability of the patient to cooperate with pain assessment and management.

3. **How can pain be assessed in critically ill patients?**

   Pain should be assessed and documented at regular intervals. Pain is a subjective experience and is most reliably measured by using a subjective scale such as the numeric rating scale (Fig. 72-1), which can be employed in patients as young as 5 years. Younger patients' pain is assessed by using the faces scale (Fig. 72-1), which is a modified visual analog scale. In patients unable to communicate, reliance on objective measures (physiologic or behavioral) becomes necessary. Whereas use of physiologic measures (blood pressure, heart rate, tearing, diaphoresis, mydriasis) can cause underreporting and overreporting of pain, use of behavioral measures such as observation of facial expression has been demonstrated to correlate with subjective reporting.

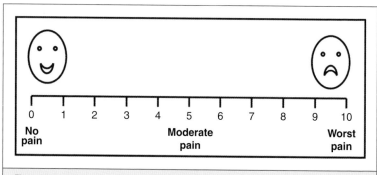

Figure 72-1. Visual analog and numeric rating scales.

4. **Is pain harmful?**
   Through activation of the stress response, pain exacerbates the negative effects of the sympathoadrenal response to critical illness at a multisystem level. Pain can contribute to the development of delirium, which is increasingly recognized as a contributor to poor outcomes and even long-term cognitive dysfunction. Myocardial ischemia is exacerbated through both increased myocardial oxygen demand and decreased supply. Pain after thoracic or upper abdominal surgery induces an acute restrictive respiratory defect (reflex muscle rigidity, splinting, loss of functional residual capacity) exacerbated by a reflex reduction in phrenic nerve activity with decrease in diaphragmatic contractility. The result is impaired cough, atelectasis, and pneumonia. Sympathoadrenal activation prolongs the adynamic ileus that follows abdominal surgery and that is recognized as a contributor to prolongation of hospital stay. Neuroendocrine components of the stress response interact with the cytokine system to cause a catabolic state with muscle wasting and impaired immunity and to promote a hypercoagulable state with the attendant risks of myocardial infarction and venous thrombosis.

5. **What are the treatment options for a critically ill patient in pain?**
   - *Nonpharmacologic treatment* of pain includes proper positioning of patients, stabilization of fractures, elimination of irritating physical stimulation, and environmental modification to promote comfort. Because sleep deprivation as well as anxiety and delirium may diminish the pain threshold, it is important to minimize stimuli that can disturb the normal diurnal sleep pattern (noise, artificial light) and treat anxiety and delirium promptly.
   - *Pharmacologic treatment* of pain works by inhibition of the release of local mediators in damaged tissue (nonsteroidal antiinflammatory drugs [NSAIDS], acetaminophen), blocking nerve conduction (regional anesthesia), or altering pain neurotransmission in the central nervous system (opioids, acetaminophen, ketamine, dexmedetomidine).

6. **What is the role of opioids in the ICU, and how do they act?**
   Opioids are the mainstay of analgesic therapy in the ICU. Long-standing familiarity has fostered relative safety in their use. They are mainly effective against visceral pain of a static nature but relatively ineffective against somatic and dynamic pain; analgesic efficacy tends to dissipate once movement including out-of-bed mobilization and respiratory therapy maneuvers are instituted.
   The term *opioid* refers to any agent with activity at an opioid receptor. There are at least four discrete opioid receptors in the central and peripheral nervous system; the analgesic effects of opioids are mediated mostly via mu (μ) or kappa (κ) receptors. These are G protein–coupled receptors that mediate inhibition of adenyl cyclase.

7. **Which opioids are recommended for routine administration in ICU patients?**
   Morphine, fentanyl, hydromorphone, and sufentanil are the analgesic agents most commonly used and recommended in the ICU (Table 72-1).

8. **How do you decide which opioid to use?**
   Before an opioid is ordered, the goal of analgesia is determined and a therapeutic plan developed. The patient's cardiovascular status and subsystem organ function are assessed.
   - **Morphine** is a naturally occurring, relatively hydrophilic opioid with a long clinical history and therefore familiarity with its use. The onset of action is slow (effect site equilibration time 15-30 minutes), and duration of action is 2 to 4 hours. However, it has relatively rapid hepatic clearance and tends not to accumulate because of its water solubility, which limits the volume of distribution, although glucuronide metabolites with sedative-analgesic properties may accumulate in the setting of renal insufficiency.
   - **Fentanyl** is a synthetic, potent, and highly lipid-soluble opioid. The lipid solubility is responsible for the rapid onset of action (effect site equilibration time 1-3 minutes). This makes it a preferable analgesic in the acutely distressed patient. Fentanyl has a short duration of action

TABLE 72-1. PHARMACOLOGY OF OPIOID ANALGESICS IN THE ADULT INTENSIVE CARE UNIT

	RELATIVE POTENCY	BOLUS DOSE* (IV)	HALF-LIFE (HR)	CONTINUOUS DOSE* (MG/HR; IV)	COMMENT
Morphine	1	2-5 mg	3-7	2-10	Histamine release Accumulation of active metabolite (morphine-6-glucuronide), especially in renal insufficiency
Fentanyl	80-100	25-100 mcg	1.5-6	0.025-0.2	Marked accumulation of parent drug after prolonged infusion
Hydromorphone	5-10	0.25-0.75 mg	2-3	0.5-2	
Sufentanil	500-1000	5-20 mcg	2-4	0.005-0.04	
Meperidine[†]	0.1	12.5-50 mg	3-4	NA	Efficient to treat shivering Histamine release Accumulation of active, neuroexcitatory metabolite (normeperidine), especially in renal insufficiency or high doses Interaction with antidepressants

NA, Not applicable.
*Doses are approximate for a 70-kg adult patient; bolus dose may be repeated every 5 to 15 minutes.
[†]Not recommended for routine use in ICU patients.

(30-45 minutes after one bolus); however, repeated dosing may cause accumulation and prolonged action (long context-sensitive half-life). Cardiovascular side effects are minimal.

- **Hydromorphone** is a semisynthetic opioid that is approximately 10 times more potent than morphine and has lipid solubility between those of morphine and fentanyl. Compared with morphine, its onset and duration of action are slightly shorter (effect site equilibration time 10-20 minutes, duration of action 1-3 hours). There is less histamine release and greater hemodynamic stability, and there is no clinically significant active metabolite.

- **Sufentanil** is a synthetic, highly lipid-soluble opioid with high selectivity for the μ-receptor. It has been shown to cause less respiratory depression compared with other opioids; thus it may be preferred in patients with spontaneous ventilation. Sufentanil accumulates less compared with fentanyl (shorter context-sensitive half-life).

9. **What is the place of meperidine in the ICU?**
   Meperidine is useful in the treatment of *postoperative shivering* and has been demonstrated to be superior to morphine and fentanyl for this indication. A small intravenous (IV) dose of 10 to 25 mg is usually sufficient. Postoperative shivering can increase oxygen consumption and may be detrimental if it occurs in patients with ischemic heart disease. However, meperidine is not recommended for repetitive use in ICU patients because of its active metabolite (normeperidine), which may cause central nervous system excitation and its interactions with antidepressants (contraindicated with monoamine oxidase inhibitors, best avoided with selective serotonin reuptake inhibitors).

10. **Which other opioids should be avoided in the ICU for routine analgesia?**
    - **Mixed agonist-antagonists** (e.g., nalbuphine) may reverse other opioids and may precipitate a withdrawal syndrome in patients in whom tolerance or dependence has developed.
    - **Methadone** prolongs the QT interval and can induce *torsades de pointes* ventricular arrhythmia. It is metabolized by the hepatic cytochrome P-450 system, and a risk exists for drug interactions and accumulation after repeated dosing.
    - **Codeine** is not useful for most patients because it lacks analgesic efficacy.

11. **How should opioids be administered for acute pain management in the ICU?**
    The IV route is considered superior because regional hypoperfusion due to shock or edema may render the absorption of opioids less reliable via the subcutaneous and intramuscular routes. IV opioids can be delivered in three different modes:
    - **IV bolus injections** are often used for moderate pain. The doses are titrated to analgesic requirements avoiding respiratory depression and hemodynamic instability.
    - In clinical situations with moderate to severe pain, which is only poorly controlled with repeated boluses, a **continuous IV infusion** may be considered.
    - Alternatively, a **patient-controlled analgesia (PCA)** regimen may be preferable in conscious patients.

12. **Explain the concept of PCA.**
    PCA is managed with microprocessor-based pumps that allow the patient to self-administer analgesics according to a predetermined limit set by the physician. The goal of PCA is to produce a relatively stable and effective level of analgesia by allowing the patient to receive multiple small boluses after an initial loading dose. Patients prefer this pain relief technique because they control analgesia administration themselves. The following basic parameters can be set on a PCA pump: *bolus* (dose administered when the patient pushes the button), *lockout interval* (minimal length of time between two doses), *maximal dose* to be given, *background infusion* (continuous infusion in addition to the boluses). Morphine is commonly prescribed because of its relatively rapid clearance; typical adult doses are 1 to 2 mg bolus, 10-minute lockout interval, and 24 to 30 mg 4-hour limit. Background infusion is probably better avoided in opioid-naïve patients because of the risk of respiratory depression.

13. **Why should you avoid routinely prescribing background infusions by PCA?**
    PCA continuous infusions (background infusion) bypass the intrinsic safety feature of standard, bolus-only PCA by allowing opioids to be continuously delivered even if sedation is excessive. Studies have demonstrated that patients after surgery treated with PCA plus continuous infusion have no improvement in analgesia but have a significantly greater number of side effects compared with patients after surgery receiving standard PCA.

14. **What are the side effects of opioids? (See Table 72-2.)**
    Although seldom a problem in the euvolemic patient, opioids can cause *hypotension* through reduction in sympathetic tone or histamine release. The latter is more frequent with the traditional phenanthrene derivatives (morphine), and the newer semisynthetic phenylpiperidines (fentanyl, sufentanil) offer greater hemodynamic stability.

    Opioids are *respiratory depressants*. Classically described as central respiratory depressants that blunt the ventilatory response to elevated arterial carbon dioxide tension, these analgesics also appear to produce an obstructive sleep apnea state. Weakened and delayed phasic inspiratory contraction of pharyngeal dilator muscles may be a major cause of opioid-induced hypoxemia, particularly in patients with an underlying diagnosis of obstructive sleep apnea. Opioids are relatively ineffective at reversing the dynamic pain associated with deep breathing and coughing maneuvers after thoracic and upper abdominal surgery that are responsible for much of the associated postoperative atelectasis, impaired gas exchange, and pneumonia.

    Pain-induced *delayed gastrointestinal transit* time is exacerbated by opioids, which cause sphincter contraction and increased gastrointestinal resting tone through μ-receptor stimulation. Resumption of oral intake is further exacerbated by these agents' tendency to cause nausea. Judicious use of prokinetic and antiemetic agents is recommended.

TABLE 72-2. SIDE EFFECTS OF OPIOID ANALGESICS	
CENTRAL NERVOUS SYSTEM	**MIOSIS** **EUPHORIA, DYSPHORIA, SEDATION** **ADDICTION**
Pulmonary	Respiratory depression Muscle rigidity (especially highly lipid-soluble opioids)
Cardiovascular	Bradycardia, hypotension
Gastrointestinal	Nausea, emesis Constipation, ileus
Urogenital	Urinary retention Antidiuretic hormone release (water retention)
Other	Histamine release: flushing, tachycardia, hypotension, bronchospasm Pruritus

15. **What is the role of nonopioid analgesics in the ICU, and what are their characteristics?**
    Acetaminophen and NSAIDs have been shown to decrease the need for opioids and are particularly effective in reducing muscular and skeletal pain. They are often more effective than opioids in reducing pain from pleural or pericardial rubs, a pain that responds poorly to opioids. Basic pharmacology is summarized in Table 72-3.

16. **What are the side effects of nonopioid analgesics?**
    ■ **Acetaminophen** may be potentially hepatotoxic, especially in patients with depleted glutathione stores. Therefore acetaminophen should be avoided in acute liver failure, and the drug should be maintained at less than 2 g/day in patients with a significant history of alcohol intake or poor nutritional status.
    ■ **NSAIDs** may cause bleeding as a result of platelet function inhibition, gastrointestinal side effects such as ulcers and bleeding, and the development of acute renal failure. Risk factors for the development of acute renal failure are patient age, preexisting renal impairment,

TABLE 72-3.   PHARMACOLOGY OF SELECTED NONOPIOID ANALGESICS IN THE ADULT INTENSIVE CARE UNIT

	DOSE RECOMMENDATIONS	HALF-LIFE (HR)	COMMENT
Acetaminophen	PO: 325-650 mg every 4-6 hr IV: 500-1000 mg every 6-8 hr (avoid >2 days use)	2-3	Maximal dose ≤4 g daily
Diclofenac	PO: 50 mg every 6-12 hr IV: 75 mg (maximum 150 mg/day, avoid >2 days use)	1-2	
Ibuprofen	PO: 400 mg every 4-6 hr	1.5-2.5	Reduce dose if: age >65 yr, weight <50 kg, or renal impairment
Ketorolac	IV: 15-30 mg every 6 hr (avoid >5 days use)	2.5-8.5	

PO, Oral.

hypovolemia, and shock. The prolonged use of NSAIDs should be avoided. For example, it has been shown that ketorolac applied for ≥5 days has been associated with a twofold increased risk of acute renal failure. Furthermore, NSAIDs should be avoided in patients with asthma and aspirin allergy. The role of the newer NSAIDs in the ICU, the selective cyclooxygenase (COX)-2 inhibitors, remains unknown. Although initially believed to offer protection from the renal and gastrointestinal side effects of traditional nonselective NSAIDs, this does not appear to be the case as both the gut and kidney depend on constitutive activity of the COX-2 enzyme to regulate organ perfusion.

17. **What is dexmedetomidine?**
Dexmedetomidine is a highly selective α_2-agonist with both sedative and analgesic properties but without respiratory depression. It appears useful in discontinuing mechanical ventilation in patients after surgery. Its opioid-sparing effect may be useful in patients with obstructive sleep apnea and pulmonary disease. Recent research demonstrates a reduction in ventilator days and delirium with its use. The maintenance infusion dose of dexmedetomidine is 0.2 to 0.7 mcg/kg/hour. Although an initial loading dose can be prescribed, caution is advised given its tendency to produce bradycardia.

18. **Does ketamine have a role as an analgesic agent in the ICU?**
Ketamine is a phencyclidine derivative with unique properties. Originally used in 1964, it has had long-standing use for its intensely analgesic effect, hemodynamic stability, and relative lack of respiratory depression. IV boluses of ketamine (0.5-2 mg/kg) have been used in ICU patients to enhance tolerance of limited but painful procedures, such as dressing changes for burns. More recently, its value as an infusion (0.1 mg/kg/hour) has been recognized because of its bronchodilator and anticonvulsant properties. Although traditionally used with caution in acute brain injury owing to a cerebral vasodilator effect, it appears safe if hypercarbia is avoided,

and the *N*-methyl-ᴅ-aspartate antagonist properties of ketamine may be neuroprotective. Furthermore, small doses of ketamine may be a valuable adjunct to routine analgesia to decrease opioid requirements.

19. **Does epidural analgesia have a role in ICU patients?**
Epidural analgesia with use of a local anesthetic agent offers several theoretic advantages in patients admitted to the ICU after surgery including reduction in pneumonia, myocardial infarction, and venous thrombosis. Improved outcomes should particularly result from the use of thoracic epidural technique after thoracic or upper abdominal surgery in patients with underlying cardiac or pulmonary disease. However, studies demonstrate varying results. There does appear to be improved analgesia, particularly from pain on mobilization, and earlier return of gut function. The latter factors may allow earlier rehabilitation and hospital discharge as part of a well-coordinated recovery program. Other potential advantages of epidural analgesia may result from reduction in opioid administration. As a general practice, physicians insert epidural catheters most commonly at mid- or low-thoracic level for patients undergoing thoracic or upper abdominal surgery, respectively. The physicians use a solution of bupivacaine 0.1% with hydromorphone 10 mcg/mL, which is run at 4 to 6 mL/hour.

20. **Is epidural analgesia safe in the setting of deep vein thromboprophylaxis?**
Regional anesthesia may be performed in this setting, although practitioners are advised to follow the guidelines of the American Society of Regional Anesthesia and Pain Medicine (www.asra.com) and be vigilant for the development of epidural hematoma. If low-dose unfractionated heparin is being used, needle placement and/or catheter removal should be done ≥ 2 hours after discontinuing heparin, and reheparinization may be started ≥ 1 hour after an uncomplicated epidural insertion. If fractionated low-molecular-weight heparin (LMWH) is being used in prophylactic doses, a waiting period of ≥ 12 hours for any neuraxial technique should be applied after the last dose of LMWH, and the next LMWH dose should be given ≥ 2 hours after an uncomplicated procedure.

KEY POINTS: ADEQUATE ANALGESIA IN THE CRITICALLY ILL PATIENT

Adequate analgesia in the critically ill patient is necessary because of the following:
1. Patient comfort, ethical aspects

2. Attenuation of potentially deleterious physiologic responses to pain
   a. Sympathetic activation

   b. Increased myocardial oxygen consumption

   c. Persistent catabolism

   d. Hypercoagulability

   e. Immunosuppression

BIBLIOGRAPHY

1. Bonnet F, Marret E: Influence of anaesthetic and analgesic techniques on outcome after surgery. Br J Anaesth 95:52-58, 2005.
2. Domino E: Taming the ketamine tiger. Anesthesiology 113:678-684, 2010.

3. Jacobi J, Fraser GL, Coursin DB, et al: Clinical practice guidelines for the sustained use of sedatives and analgesics in the critically ill adult. Crit Care Med 30:119-141, 2002.

4. Mehta S, McCullagh I, Burry L: Current sedation practices: lessons learned from international surveys. Crit Care Clin 25:471-488, 2009.

5. Riker RR, Shehabi Y, Bokesch PM, et al: Dexmedetomidine vs midazolam for sedation of critically ill patients: a randomized trial. JAMA 301:489-499, 2009.

CHAPTER 73

SEDATION AND DELIRIUM

Pratik Pandharipande, MBBS, MSCI, and Arna Banerjee, MD

1. **What is delirium?**

   Delirium is defined by the *Diagnostic and Statistical Manual of Mental Disorders* (DSM-IV) as:
   - Disturbance of consciousness (i.e., reduced clarity of awareness of the environment) with reduced ability to focus, sustain, or shift attention.
   - A change in cognition (such as memory deficit, disorientation, language disturbance) or the development of a perceptual disturbance that is not better accounted for by a preexisting, established, or evolving dementia.
   - The disturbance develops over a short period of time (usually hours to days) and tends to fluctuate during the course of the day.

2. **Why is it important to diagnose delirium?**

   The true prevalence and magnitude of delirium have been poorly documented because a myriad of terms, such as acute confusional state, intensive care unit (ICU) psychosis, acute brain dysfunction, and encephalopathy have been used historically to describe this condition. Although the overall prevalence of delirium in the community is only 1% to 2%, the prevalence increases with age, rising to 14% among those more than 85 years old. It may range from 14% to 24% with incidence rates up to 60% among general hospital populations, especially in older patients and those in nursing homes or post–acute care settings. In critically ill patients in the ICU (medical, surgical, trauma, and burn units) the reported prevalence of delirium is 20% to 80%, depending on the severity of illness, and may be closer to 80% in those who are receiving mechanical ventilation. In spite of this, the condition is often unrecognized by clinicians or the symptoms are incorrectly attributed to dementia or depression or considered an expected, inconsequential complication of critical illness. Numerous national and international surveys have shown a disconnect between the perceived importance of delirium, the accuracy of diagnosis, and the implementation of management and treatment techniques. Given that delirium is the most common organ dysfunction seen in critically ill patients and is associated with worse acute and long-term outcomes, it is important to diagnose and manage the disease by implementation of validated screening protocols.

3. **What morbidity and mortality are associated with delirium?**

   Delirium is a strong predictor of a longer hospital stay, longer times receiving mechanical ventilation, higher costs, and increased risk for death. Additionally, each additional day with delirium increases the risk for dying by 10%. Patients with longer periods of delirium are also associated with more cognitive decline, when evaluated after 1 year, attesting to the importance of detecting and managing delirium early in the course of illness.

4. **Describe the clinical features of delirium.**

   The most important feature of delirium is a disturbance of consciousness accompanied by inattention and a change in cognition that cannot be explained by preexisting or evolving dementia. The condition develops over a short period of time, usually hours to days, and tends to fluctuate during the course of the day.

   Delirium may be manifested by a reduced clarity of awareness of the environment and ability to focus, sustain, or shift attention. This may be accompanied by memory impairment, disorientation, or language disturbance. Speech or language disturbances may be evident as dysarthria, dysnomia, dysgraphia, or even aphasia. In some cases, speech is rambling and irrelevant, in others pressured and incoherent, with unpredictable switching from subject to subject. Perceptual disturbances may include misinterpretations, illusions, or hallucinations. Delusion is often associated with a disturbance in the sleep-wake cycle. Patients may also exhibit anxiety, fear, depression, irritability, anger, euphoria, and apathy.

5. **What are the subtypes of delirium?**
   Delirium can be classified by psychomotor behavior into the following:
   - **Hypoactive** delirium is characterized by decreased physical and mental activity and inattention. Patients may be sluggish and lethargic, approaching stupor, and may be associated with a worse prognosis.
   - **Hyperactive** delirium is characterized by combativeness and agitation. Manifestations may include groping or picking at the bedclothes or attempting to get out of bed when it is unsafe or untimely. This puts both patients and caregivers at risk for serious injuries. Fortunately, this form of delirium occurs in the minority of critically ill patients.
   Patients with both features have mixed delirium.

6. **Describe risk factors for delirium.**
   Many risk factors for delirium exist, and these can be divided by host, acute illness, and iatrogenic and environmental factors (Table 73-1). Many of these factors are modifiable. Fortunately, several mnemonics can aid clinicians in recalling the list; two common ones are IWATCHDEATH and DELIRIUM (Table 73-2).

TABLE 73-1. RISK FACTORS FOR DELIRIUM		
HOST FACTORS	**ACUTE ILLNESS**	**IATROGENIC OR ENVIRONMENTAL**
Age	Sepsis	Metabolic disturbances*
Baseline comorbidities	Hypoxemia*	Anticholinergic medications*
Baseline cognitive impairment	Global severity of illness score	Sedative and analgesic medications*
Genetic predisposition (?)	Metabolic disturbances	Sleep disturbances*

*Modifiable risk factors.

7. **How is delirium diagnosed?**
   The diagnosis of delirium is primarily clinical and is based on careful bedside observation of key features. It is a two-step process. Level of arousal is first measured, and, if the patient is arousable, delirium evaluation can be performed by instruments such as the Confusion Assessment Method or the Delirium Rating Scale–Revised 98 (DRS-R 98) in hospitalized patients. The DRS-R 98 provides a measure of severity of delirium in addition to the ability to diagnose delirium. In the ICU, delirium can be diagnosed by using a sedation scale to assess arousal followed by either the Confusion Assessment Method for the ICU (CAM-ICU) or the Intensive Care Delirium Screening Checklist (ICDSC); both these instruments are reliable and have been validated in critically ill patients.

TABLE 73-2. MNEMONICS FOR RISK FACTORS FOR DELIRIUM	
IWATCHDEATH	**DELIRIUM**
Infection	Drugs
Withdrawal	Electrolyte and physiologic abnormalities
Acute metabolic	Lack of drugs (withdrawal)
Trauma/pain	Infection
Central nervous system pathology	Reduced sensory input (blindness, deafness)
Hypoxia	Intracranial problems (CVA, meningitis, seizure)
Deficiencies (vitamin B_{12}, thiamine)	Urinary retention and fecal impaction
Endocrinopathies (thyroid, adrenal)	Myocardial problems (MI, arrhythmia, CHF)
Acute vascular (hypertension, shock)	
Toxins/drugs	
Heavy metals	

CHF, Congestive heart failure; *CVA,* cerebrovascular accident; *MI,* myocardial infarction.

8. **How can detection of delirium be improved?**
The Society of Critical Care Medicine (SCCM) has published guidelines for the use of sedatives and analgesics in the ICU. They recommend routine monitoring of pain, anxiety, and delirium with use of validated tools and documentation of responses to therapy for these conditions. A number of tools have been developed recently and validated for use, in both patients with endotracheal tubes in place and those without endotracheal tubes, and measured against a *gold standard*, the DSM criteria. These are the following:
- CAM-ICU
- ICDSC
- Nursing Delirium Screening Scale (Nu-DESC)
- Delirium Detection Score
- Neelon and Champagne (NEECHAM) Confusion Scale

Of these, the CAM-ICU and the ICDSC are the most frequently used instruments that have been translated into a number of languages.

These screening instruments differ in the components of delirium they evaluate, the threshold for diagnosing delirium, and their ability to be used in patients with impaired vision and hearing and in those who have endotracheal tubes and are receiving mechanical ventilation. Hence, it is important to consider the patient population when choosing the instrument.

9. **What causes delirium?**
The pathophysiology of delirium is poorly understood, although a number of hypotheses exist.
- **Neurotransmitter imbalance.** Multiple neurotransmitters have been implicated, including dopamine (excess), acetylcholine (relative depletion), γ-aminobutyric acid, serotonin, endorphins, norepinephrine, and glutamate.
- **Inflammatory mediators.** Tumor necrosis factor-α, interleukin-1, and other cytokines and chemokines have been implicated in the pathogenesis of endothelial damage, thrombin formation, and microvascular dysfunction in the central nervous system (CNS), contributing to delirium.
- **Impaired oxidative metabolism.** Delirium may be a result of cerebral insufficiency caused by a global failure of oxidative metabolism.

- **Large neutral amino acids.** Increased cerebral uptake of tryptophan and tyrosine (amino acid precursors) can lead to elevated levels of serotonin, dopamine, and norepinephrine in the CNS, leading to an increased risk for development of delirium.

10. Which drugs are most likely to be associated with delirium?
Many drugs are considered to be risk factors for the development of delirium.

Marcantonio found that delirium was significantly associated with postoperative exposure to meperidine and benzodiazepines, although not to other commonly prescribed opiates. Long-acting benzodiazepines had a trend toward stronger association with delirium than the short-acting agents, and high-dose exposures had a trend toward stronger association than low-dose exposures. Although targeted pain control has been shown to be associated with improved rates of delirium, overzealous administration of opiates has been associated with worse outcomes. Similarly in the ICU, studies have shown that opioids and benzodiazepines are risk factors for delirium in medical and surgical ICU patients, though trauma and burn patients who have pain appear to be protected from development of delirium with intravenous opiates. The class of benzodiazepines does not seem to change the risk profile, with both lorazepam and midazolam being significant risk factors for delirium.

11. What psychiatric diagnoses may be confused with delirium?
Dementia can be difficult to distinguish from delirium, particularly when information about baseline cognitive functioning is unavailable, and is the most common differential diagnosis. Memory impairment is common to both delirium and dementia, but the person with dementia alone is alert and does not have the disturbance in consciousness that is characteristic of delirium. In delirium, the onset of symptoms is much more rapid and fluctuates during a 24-hour period. Delirium that is characterized by vivid hallucinations, delusions, language disturbances, and agitation must be distinguished from psychotic disorder, schizophrenia, schizophreniform disorder, and mood disorder with psychotic features. Finally, delirium associated with fear, anxiety, and dissociative symptoms such as depersonalization must be distinguished from acute stress disorder. Delirium must also be distinguished from malingering and factitious disorder.

12. How should the work-up of delirium be pursued?
The SCCM recommends routine monitoring of delirium with use of validated tools. A rapid assessment should be performed, including assessment of vital signs and physical examination to rule out life-threatening problems (e.g., hypoxia, self-extubation, pneumothorax, hypotension) or other acutely reversible physiologic causes (e.g., hypoglycemia, metabolic acidosis, stroke, seizure, pain). The IWATCHDEATH and DELIRIUM mnemonics can be particularly helpful for guiding this initial evaluation. See Table 73-2.

13. What studies should be considered in the work-up of delirium?
Routine laboratory tests are important but not the mainstay of diagnosis. These include a complete blood cell count, electrolytes, blood urea nitrogen, creatinine, glucose, calcium, pulse oximetry or arterial blood gas, urinalysis, urine drug screens, liver function tests with serum albumin, cultures, chest radiograph, and electrocardiogram. Cerebrospinal fluid examination should also be considered for cases in which meningitis or encephalitis is suspected. Other tests that need to be considered are VDRL, for the human immunodeficiency virus, B_{12} and folate, heavy metal screen, antinuclear antibody, ammonia level, thyroid-stimulating hormone, measurement of serum medication levels (e.g., digoxin), and urinary porphyrins. Electroencephalogram changes have been seen in patients with delirium. Other tests that are still experimental include brain imaging and measures of serum anticholinergic activity.

14. How is delirium treated?

Once delirium is noted, an underlying cause should be ruled out before attempting pharmacologic intervention. Once life-threatening causes are ruled out, focus should be on the following:

- Reorienting patients
- Improvement of sleep hygiene
- Visual and hearing aids if previously used
- Removing medications that can provoke delirium
- Discontinuing invasive devices not required (e.g., bladder catheters, restraints)

To improve patient outcome, an evidence-based organizational approach referred to as the ABCDE bundle (*A*wakening and *B*reathing trials, *C*hoice of appropriate sedation, *D*elirium monitoring, and *E*arly mobility and exercise) is presented.

- ***Awaken the patient daily:*** Studies have shown that protocolized target-based sedation and daily spontaneous awakening trials reduce the number of days of mechanical ventilation. This strategy also exposes the patient to smaller cumulative doses of sedatives.
- ***Spontaneous breathing trials:*** This involves daily interruption of mechanical ventilation. Spontaneous breathing trials were shown to be superior to other varied approaches to ventilator weaning. Thus incorporation of spontaneous breathing trials into practice reduced the total time of mechanical ventilation.
  - ○ Coordination of daily awakening and daily breathing: The awakening and breathing controlled trial combined the spontaneous awakening trial with the spontaneous breathing trial, which showed shorter duration of mechanical ventilation, a 4-day reduction in hospital length of stay, a remarkable 15% decrease in 1-year mortality, and no long-term neuropsychological consequences of waking patients during critical illness.
- ***Choosing the right sedative regimen in critically ill patients:*** Numerous studies have identified that benzodiazepines are associated with worse clinical outcomes. The Maximizing Efficacy of Targeted Sedation and Reducing Neurological Dysfunction (MENDS) study showed more days alive without delirium or coma (7.0 vs. 3.0 days; $P = 0.01$), with a lower risk for delirium developing on subsequent days if the patient is taking dexmedetomidine compared with lorazepam. The Safety and Efficacy of Dexmedetomidine Compared with Midazolam (SEDCOM) study also showed a decrease in delirium prevalence in the dexmedetomidine group (54% vs. 76.6% [95% confidence interval, 14% to 33%]; $P < 0.001$) compared with midazolam, with those with shorter times receiving mechanical ventilation.
- ***Delirium management:*** The SCCM has published guidelines recommending routine monitoring for delirium in all ICU patients. Pharmacologic therapy for delirium should be attempted only after correcting any contributing factors or underlying physiologic abnormalities.
- ***Exercise and early mobility:*** Morris et al. showed that initiating physical therapy early during the patient's ICU stay was associated with decreased length of stay both in the ICU and in the hospital. Schweickert et al. found that patients who underwent early mobilization had a significant improvement in functional status at hospital discharge. These patients also had a significant decrease in the duration of delirium (50%) in the ICU, as well as during the hospital stay.

15. Describe the pharmacologic management of delirium.

Patients who manifest delirium should be treated with a traditional antipsychotic medication (haloperidol) per the SCCM guidelines. Newer *atypical* antipsychotic agents (e.g., risperidone, ziprasidone, quetiapine, or olanzapine) also may prove helpful for the treatment of delirium. Although the Modifying the Incidence of Delirium (MIND) study showed no difference in the duration of delirium between haloperidol, ziprasidone, or placebo when used for prophylaxis and treatment, a smaller study done by Devlin et al. showed that quetiapine was more effective than placebo in resolution of delirium when supplementing ongoing haloperidol therapy. Data from the MENDS study and the SEDCOM trial support the view that dexmedetomidine can decrease the duration and prevalence of delirium when compared with lorazepam or midazolam. Benzodiazepines remain the drugs of choice for the treatment of delirium tremens (and other withdrawal syndromes) and seizures (Table 73-3).

TABLE 73-3. PHARMACOLOGIC TREATMENT OF DELIRIUM IN HOSPITALIZED PATIENTS	
CLASS AND DRUG	**DOSE**
Antipsychotic	
Haloperidol	0.5-1 mg PO twice daily*, with additional doses every 4 hr as needed up to a maximum of 20 mg daily
	0.5-1 mg IM; observe after 30-60 min and repeat if needed
Atypical antipsychotics	
Risperidone	0.25-1 mg/day up to a maximum of 6 mg/day
Olanzapine	2.5-10 mg once or twice daily
Quetiapine	25-50 mg PO once or twice daily
Ziprasidone	20-40 mg PO once or twice daily
Benzodiazepine	
Lorazepam	0.5-1 mg PO, with additional doses every 4 hr as needed; reserve for use in alcohol withdrawal, Parkinson disease, and neuroleptic malignant syndrome
Antidepressant	
Trazodone	25-150 mg PO at bedtime

IM, Intramuscular; *PO*, orally.
*Note: See text for more rapid effects with IV/IM dosing.

16. **Describe the use of haloperidol in delirium.**
   The SCCM guidelines recommend haloperidol as the drug of choice. It is a butyrophenone *typical* antipsychotic. It does not suppress the respiratory drive and works as a dopamine receptor antagonist by blocking the D_2 receptor, treating the positive symptoms (hallucinations and unstructured thought patterns).
   Adverse effects include hypotension, acute dystonias, extrapyramidal effects, laryngeal spasm, malignant hyperthermia, glucose and lipid dysregulation, and anticholinergic effects. Perhaps the most immediately life-threatening adverse effect of antipsychotics is torsades de pointes, and these agents should not be given to patients with prolonged QT intervals unless thought to be absolutely necessary.

17. **How is haloperidol dosed in delirium?**
   A recommended starting dose is 2 to 5 mg (IV or IM) every 6 to 12 hours; the maximum effective doses are usually around 20 mg/day.

18. **How are second-generation antipsychotic agents used in delirium?**
   Newer *atypical* antipsychotic agents (e.g., risperidone, ziprasidone, quetiapine, and olanzapine) may also prove helpful for delirium. The advantage over haloperidol is theoretic and may be

related to its effect not only on dopamine but also on other neurotransmitters such as serotonin, acetylcholine, and norepinephrine. Studies need to be repeated with larger patient populations before any concrete recommendations can be made regarding the efficacy of typical or atypical antipsychotics in delirium.

KEY POINTS: DELIRIUM

1. Delirium is a disturbance of consciousness with inattention, accompanied by a change in cognition or perceptual disturbances that develop over a short period of time and fluctuate over days.

2. Delirium is associated with significant morbidity and mortality.

3. Diagnosis of delirium is a two-step process. Level of arousal is first measured, and, if the patient is arousable, delirium evaluation is performed with use of validated instruments.

4. Pharmacologic treatment should be used only after giving adequate attention to correction of modifiable contributing factors.

5. Pharmacologic treatments:
   - Haloperidol is considered to be the first-line drug and should be started at a low dose.

   - Atypical antipsychotics have also been used when risk for adverse events such as QTc prolongation or extrapyramidal side effects is estimated to be high. These drugs include olanzapine, risperidone, quetiapine, and ziprasidone.

   - Benzodiazepines should be reserved for use only in delirium associated with alcohol withdrawal.

WEBSITES

ICU Delirium and Cognitive Impairment Study Group: www.icudelirium.org
American Psychiatric Association guidelines (including treatment of delirium): www.psych.org/psych_pract/treatg/pg/prac_guide.cfm

BIBLIOGRAPHY

1. American Psychiatric Association : Diagnostic and statistical manual of mental disorders, 4th ed. Washington, D.C, American Psychiatric Association, 2000.

2. Banerjee A, Pandharipande P: Delirium. In Bope ET, Rakel RE, Kellerman RD: Conn's Current Therapy 2010, Philadelphia, Saunders, 2010, pp 1117.

3. Devlin JW, Roberts RJ, Fong JJ, et al: Efficacy and safety of quetiapine in critically ill patients with delirium: a prospective, multicenter, randomized, double-blind, placebo-controlled pilot study. Crit Care Med 38:419-427, 2010.

4. Ely E, Shintani A, Truman B, et al: Delirium as a predictor of mortality in mechanically ventilated patients in the intensive care unit. JAMA 291:1753-1762, 2004.

5. Ely EW, Inouwe SK, Bernard GR, et al: Delirium in mechanically ventilated patients: validity and reliability of the confusion assessment method for the intensive care unit (CAM-ICU). JAMA 286:2703-2710, 2001.

6. Girard TD, Jackson JC, Pandharipande P, et al: Delirium as a predictor of long-term cognitive impairment in survivors of critical illness. Crit Care Med 38:1513-1520, 2010.

7. Girard TD, Kress JP, Fuchs BD, et al: Efficacy and safety of a paired sedation and ventilator weaning protocol for mechanically ventilated patients in intensive care (Awakening and Breathing Controlled trial): a randomised controlled trial. Lancet 371:126-134, 2008.

8. Girard TD, Pandharipande P, Ely E: Delirium in the intensive care unit. Crit Care 12(Suppl 3):S3, 2008.

9. Gunther M, Morandi A, Ely E: Pathophysiology of delirium in the intensive care unit. Crit Care Clin 24:45-65, 2008.

10. Marcantonio ER, Juarez G, Goldman L, et al: The relationship of postoperative delirium with psychoactive medications. JAMA 272:1518-1522, 1994.

11. Morris PE, Goad A, Thompson C, et al: Early intensive care unit mobility therapy in the treatment of acute respiratory failure. Crit Care Med 36:2238-2243, 2008.

12. Pandharipande P, Cotton BA, Shintani A, et al: Motoric subtypes of delirium in mechanically ventilated surgical and trauma intensive care unit patients. Intensive Care Med 33:1726-1731, 2007.

13. Pandharipande P, Cotton BA, Shintani A, et al: Prevalence and risk factors for development of delirium in surgical and trauma intensive care unit patients. J Trauma 65:34-41, 2008.

14. Pandharipande P, Morandi A, Adams JR, et al: Plasma tryptophan and tyrosine levels are independent risk factors for delirium in critically ill patients. Intensive Care Med 35:1886-1892, 2009.

15. Pandharipande P, Pun BT, Herr DL, et al: Effect of sedation with dexmedetomidine vs lorazepam on acute brain dysfunction in mechanically ventilated patients: the MENDS randomized controlled trial. JAMA 298:2644-2653, 2007.

16. Pandharipande P, Sanders RD, Girard TD, et al: Effect of dexmedetomidine versus lorazepam on outcome in patients with sepsis: an a priori–designed analysis of the MENDS randomized controlled trial. Crit Care 14:R38, 2010.

17. Pandharipande P, Shintani A, Peterson J, et al: Lorazepam is an independent risk factor for transitioning to delirium in intensive care unit patients. Anesthesiology 104:21-26, 2006.

18. Riker R, Shehabi Y, Bokesch PM, et al: Dexmedetomidine vs midazolam for sedation of critically ill patients: a randomized trial. JAMA 301:489-499, 2009.

19. Schweickert W, Pohlman MC, Pohlman AS, et al: Early physical and occupational therapy in mechanically ventilated, critically ill patients: a randomised controlled trial. Lancet 373:1874-1882, 2009.

DISASTER MEDICINE: IMPACT ON CRITICAL CARE OPERATIONS

CHAPTER 74

John R. Benjamin, MD, MSc, and Edward E. George, MD, PhD

Disaster medicine encompasses extraordinarily wide and disparate scenarios. Despite the heterogeneity of scope and nature, many components are common to virtually all situations. The impact on health care resources at all levels of care most often requires adjusting the routine manner(s) of delivering care in response to these challenges. Better appreciation of the generic components of disaster medicine may help individuals involved in critical care medicine prepare and optimize response to these challenging situations.

1. **What are the two general categories of disasters?**
   Natural and manmade

2. **What are the most commonly encountered disasters?**
   Hurricanes, earthquakes, industrial accidents, acts of terror

3. **How does the public health sector plan for disaster medicine–related events?**
   The Department of Homeland Security (DHS) in conjunction with the Department of Health and Human Services (HHS) bears a prominent role in the National Response Plans of the federal government. In the National Preparedness Guidelines issued by the DHS are listed 15 National Planning Scenarios (Box 74-1).

   In reviewing the various situations listed by government agencies exercising oversight for the public welfare, it is apparent that many of the envisioned scenarios could or would result in victims requiring medical care in facilities ranging in echelon from community hospitals to tertiary-level academic institutions.

   For a comprehensive discussion of disaster planning from the level of the federal government please refer to the National Preparedness Guidelines website: www.dhs.gov/xlibrary/assets/National_Preparedness_Guidelines.pdf.

BOX 74-1. UNITED STATES NATIONAL PLANNING SCENARIOS

Improvised nuclear device	Major earthquake
Aerosol anthrax	Major hurricane
Pandemic influenza	Radiological dispersal device
Plague	Improvised explosive device
Blister agent	Food contamination
Toxic industrial chemicals	Foreign animal disease
Nerve agent	Cyber attack
Chlorine tank explosion	

From Department of Homeland Security: National Preparedness Guidelines September 2007: www.dhs.gov/xlibrary/assets/National_Preparedness_Guidelines.pdf.

---

4. What mechanisms are commonly employed in acts of terror?
Explosives, chemical agents, biologic agents

5. What are common categories of injuries encountered in the disaster victim?
- Burns
- Crush
- Fractures
- Cardiopulmonary: Commonly seen with inhalation agents such as mustard or blistering agents causing both a direct insult to pulmonary tissue(s) and indirect as a result of marked pulmonary edema with potential compromise of cardiac function.
- Systemic (biologics or chemicals): Infectious agents, such as anthrax and smallpox, present obvious systemic effects, with an appreciable delay between exposure and manifestation of systems, thereby presenting a further challenge in timely therapy. Chemical agents (e.g., cyanide) with direct effects on cellular respiration and nerve gases (e.g., sarin) by inhibition of acetylcholinesterase exhibit systemic effects ranging from respiratory collapse to paralysis.

6. What are the four phases of disaster response?
See Table 74-1.

Personnel responding to disasters vary in training and experience, in part as a function of the phase of response. After the chaotic component, initial response is almost exclusively local personnel. Specifically police, fire, and emergency medical assets (emergency medical technicians and paramedics) will be the first trained personnel arriving at the scene. As on-scene assessments are conducted and contingency plans engaged, the process of bringing additional specially trained personnel and equipment into the area and establishing a coordinated process of command and control for triage and evacuation relies more heavily on teams trained in

TABLE 74-1. FOUR PHASES OF DISASTER RESPONSE

1. CHAOS	2. INITIAL RESPONSE/ REORGANIZATION (CRISIS MANAGEMENT)	3. SITE CLEARING	4. LATE/RECOVERY
	Establish command post	Search and rescue/ recovery	Rebuilding infrastructure
	Needs assessment	Casualty distribution from CCAs to hospital	Definitive hospital medical care/ secondary casualty distribution
	Security and safety procedures	Clearing debris	Provider and casualty mental health follow-up
	Casualty evacuation to CCAs	Initial hospital medical care	Postevent critique and analysis of disaster response Community recovery

CCA, Casualty collection area.

the management of disaster scenes, as well as coordination with evacuation centers. Training and exercise for such contingencies are ongoing at the municipal, state, and federal level with guidance and oversight provided by numerous federal agencies to include the Federal Emergency Management Agency, as well as the DHS and HHS. With training directed and coordinated at the national level, personnel from every tier of the response system benefit from understanding the overall approach to a specific disaster, as well as expectations and capabilities of support at and from all levels.

7. **What are the four categories of blast injury?**
   - **Primary:** Injuries resulting from the overpressurization wave that affects gas-filled structures such as the lungs, gastrointestinal tract, and middle ear
   - **Secondary:** Injuries resulting from flying debris affecting any body part
   - **Tertiary:** Resultant injuries from personnel being thrown by the blast wind
   - **Quaternary:** Exacerbations from existing conditions (i.e., chronic obstructive pulmonary disease exacerbations, myocardial infarctions) or complications from blast injuries (i.e., burns, crush injuries, closed head injuries)

8. **Describe *blast lung*.**
   - Lung injury is a result of a blast wave passing through lung tissue, causing tissue disruption at the capillary-alveolar interface. Effectively a pulmonary contusion caused by the traversing of a shock wave (associated with a blast) through the various structures of the lung, the process can be *magnified* as a result of the blast occurring in a confined structure thereby magnifying the effect with the pressure wave rebounding from the walls, floor, and ceiling. This type of injury may be mimicked by a shotgun blast to the thorax; however, injuries associated with high-velocity projectiles and knives do not present a similar pattern of injury.
   - Blast lung is clinically diagnosed by the presence of respiratory distress, hypoxia, and *butterfly* or batwing infiltrates (perihilar infiltrates caused by the reflection of the blast wave of mediastinal structures).
   - If patients require mechanical ventilation, the Acute Respiratory Distress Syndrome Network (ARDSNet) protocol is appropriate.

TRIAGE

9. **Describe the history of triage.**
   Triage is a concept originating with the French (*trier*, to sort) during the Napoleonic Wars, although the principles have been applied for centuries. Napoleon's surgeon, Baron Dominique-Jean Larrey, also credited with establishing the ambulance corps, popularized a system for sorting wounded soldiers in the field and prioritizing which casualties to evacuate first. Military and disaster triage differs from standard civilian emergency medical service (EMS) systems because often the most critically ill patients are evacuated last to ensure that injured casualties who have a greater chance of survival receive expedited medical treatment.

10. **What are the secondary triage categories?**
    - **Priority I:** immediate, life-threatening injuries requiring simple urgent intervention
    - **Priority II:** delayed, not life-threatening but urgent injuries that can tolerate a delay before further medical care is needed
    - **Priority III:** minimal, not life-threatening and not urgent injuries; also known as the *walking wounded*
    - **Priority IV:** expectant, unsalvageable injuries due to either severity or limits to resources
    - **Priority V:** dead

11. **What is *overtriage*?**

    Sending low-priority patients to major trauma centers because they are incorrectly assigned as priority I or II. This triage error leads to increased mortality in mass casualty incidents.

12. **How can overtriage be reduced or prevented?**
    - Secondary and tertiary triage sites set up away from the disaster scene allow for a more methodical process to prioritize casualties.
    - Although primarily designed to reduce overtriage, reevaluating patients may also identify deteriorating casualties. This process is also known as dynamic triage.
    - A vital component to the triage process is the means and manner of patient evacuation, from the perspective of both personnel involved in the process and the assets used for transport. Initial casualty staging areas are commonly evacuated by ground ambulance or helicopter, with the bulk of personnel associated in this process drawn from local assets (police, fire, EMS, local Red Cross). However, given the magnitude of the disaster and the requirements for more extensive evacuation, additional assets are provided by state and federal institutions to assist in both local transport and secondary evacuations to more specialized (and often more distant) treatment facilities. In that a local disaster can easily overwhelm the resources of care facilities proximal to the scene of the disaster, contingency plans exist at the municipal, state, and federal levels to *redistribute* the burden of casualties to more remote and/or more specialized treatment facilities. Given the special care requirements of critically injured victims, a coordinated process with close collaboration between public health and military assets may be employed to use civilian personnel, with specialized training in the evacuation by air transport of critically ill patients, in conjunction with the Department of Defense to provide aircraft, facilities, and additional personnel.

13. **What is the *second-hit* phenomenon of disaster scenes?**
    - This describes the additional events that occur after the initial disaster and may result in significant loss of life and equipment.
    - A well-known example of this is the collapse of the World Trade Center towers on September 11, 2001.
    - This also applies to a common terrorist strategy where a second attack is planned to target first responders. For example, a vehicular bomb may be detonated in a marketplace, with additional explosive devices strategically placed around the initial explosion site, either set with delayed timers or remotely detonated by an observer to injure responding rescue personnel.

PLANNING AND RESPONSE

14. **Does the Joint Commission require hospitals to engage in disaster drills?**

    Hospitals are required to conduct disaster drills twice a year and annually test the integration with the local community.

15. **How has Walmart affected hospital disaster preparedness?**

    Walmart's pioneering supply system, known as just-in-time inventory, has revolutionized the way businesses resupply inventory. As a result, many hospitals no longer have significant stores of supplies. A hospital near a disaster zone and receiving a large number of casualties may quickly experience a material crisis if the supply chain is interrupted. This *leaner* philosophy of resupply operation reinforces the need to examine institutional contingency plans with a distinct focus on the impact of logistics.

16. **What is the Incident Command System (ICS)?**
    - The ICS was first introduced in the 1970s in an effort to more effectively coordinate the response to large-scale wildfires in the West.

- The ICS is a modular system that provides a command structure to disaster scenes. It assembles the key components of a response (i.e., fire, EMS, law enforcement) to an individual event at a location in close proximity to the scene.
- Although the size and scope of an ICS vary, five functional requirements are inherent to the organization. They are command, operations, planning, logistics, and finance and administration.
- Although the ICS is commonly a prehospital concept, many medical centers have a hospital emergency ICS (HEICS) set up in the event of a disaster or mass casualty situation.

17. **What are critical supply issues during Emergency Mass Critical Care (EMCC) events?**
   Institutions faced with responding to an EMCC will certainly experience shortages of supplies, equipment, space, and personnel. Although institutional resources may be capable of absorbing the initial requirements for support, the challenges associated with large-scale disaster will rapidly exhaust any reserve in place. Planning with local or municipal authorities in advance of any real event will facilitate any response to shortfalls. Systems such as HEICS will not only optimize the use of any institutional assets but also coordinate identified and anticipated needs with extramural resources commonly coordinated by state and federal agencies. Assets such as the Strategic National Stockpile for medications can be used, via regionalized distribution sites, to provide vital agents in a timely manner.
   - **Ventilators:** Most institutions have few ventilators not in use at any given time. Vendors supplying inventory on hand or shipments from hospitals not affected by a surge in patients may provide extra capacity. The United States has a strategic reserve of ventilators that may be shipped to hospitals. Adapting anesthesia machines as ventilators may be a possibility if the disaster has a low surgical patient population.
   - **Oxygen:** Many hospitals rely on liquid oxygen stores that must be replenished periodically. The limited number of producers of medical oxygen and the specialized transportation requirement hamper hospital resupply.
   - **Medications:** The United States has experienced numerous shortages of medications routinely used in the intensive care unit (ICU) including vasopressors, sedatives, and diuretics, to name a few. Such inherent shortages would be exacerbated during a sudden surge in critically ill patients. Contingency plans within the institution to utilize substitute medications (and equipment) in time of shortage can help attenuate the logistical challenges associated with shortages across the spectrum of operations.
   - **Staff:** Although major events and crises are often accompanied by a surge of volunteers and altruistic staff willing to work extended hours, high absenteeism commonly follows. It is vital to have established emergency staffing plans in place to ensure that all institutions maintain a longitudinal response and staffing capability. Although extended hours and physical demands are characteristic of disaster and emergency operations, it is critical that all personnel appreciate the potential compromise of care resulting from overstressed or exhausted personnel.
   - **Beds:** Critical care requires specialized equipment, medical gas access, suction, and electrical resources not available throughout most areas of the hospital. This requirement also limits the ability of an ICU standing up in a public space (i.e., gymnasiums) or a temporary shelter, such as a tent.

18. **In what manner are hospital surge operations defined?**
   Surge operations are variable depending on not only the nature of the causative factor(s) but also the individual institution's resources. Surge operations are characterized by the ability to rapidly expand the capacity of an institution to respond to an increased patient volume that would otherwise challenge or exceed routine capacity of the facility. These challenges may occur as the result of events ranging from day-to-day acute demands to the demands of an emergent event encountered in disaster medicine.

19. **What is the estimated patient surge during a mass critical care illness?**
Hospitals should prepare for triple their usual ICU capacity and not to expect significant resupply for 10 days.

20. **How can a hospital, with an average census of 90%, expect to handle a significant patient influx?**
Data indicate that up to 20% of hospital inpatients can be discharged home within a few hours. Another 40% could be quickly transported to other hospitals with community resources (buses, taxis, vans). What should not be overlooked with these data is that a hospital's priority is to take care of its current patient load first.

KEY POINTS: DISASTER MEDICINE

1. Disasters come in many shapes and sizes; however, an appreciation of commonalities of response can serve as the basis of an executable disaster plan.

2. Realistic on-scene training is vital to an efficient and effective disaster plan.

3. Caregivers may also be impacted (friends and family) by disasters, and contingency plans must be prepared and understood to ensure an adequate and sustainable response plan.

4. Although disasters by nature are chaotic and information may be limited and/or conflicting, reliance on training will always provide the best likelihood of a successful response effort.

BIBLIOGRAPHY

1. Department of Homeland Security: National Preparedness Guidelines September 2007: www.dhs.gov/xlibrary/assets/National_Preparedness_Guidelines.pdf.

2. Ritenour AE, Baskin TW: Primary blast injury: update on diagnosis and treatment. Crit Care Med 36:S311-S317, 2008.

3. Rubinson L, Hick JL, Hanfling DG, et al: Definitive care for the critically ill during a disaster: a framework for optimizing critical care surge capacity. Chest 133:18S-31S, 2008.

4. Stein M, Hirshberg A: Medical consequences of terrorism: the conventional weapons threat. Surg Clin North Am 79:1537-1552, 1999.

5. Wise RA: The creation of emergency health care standards for catastrophic events. Acad Emerg Med 13:1150-1152, 2006.

6. Zoraster RM, Amara R, Fruhwirth K: Transportation resource requirements for hospital evacuation. Am J Disaster Med 6:173-178, 2011.

CHAPTER 75

ALLERGY AND ANAPHYLAXIS

Susan A. Vassallo, MD

1. **When was anaphylaxis first described?**

   In 2641 BC, a wasp from the Hymenoptera order (wasps, bees, ants, sawflies) stung Pharaoh Menes. The events were described in hieroglyphics, and this is believed to be the first recorded death of anaphylaxis. Another important event occurred during a cruise on the yacht of Prince Albert of Monaco when the prince asked Professor Charles Richet to apply his immunology skills in the study of the Portuguese man-of-war (*Physalia* or jelly). These invertebrates live in the Mediterranean Sea and are highly poisonous. In the early 1900s Richet worked at the Musée Océanographique de Monaco. Along with Paul Portier, he extracted the *Physalia* poison with glycerol, injected dogs with this mixture, and was able to reproduce the symptoms of *Physalia* poisoning (1902). He expected a second injection would be harmless, but instead his dogs "showed serious symptoms: vomiting, blood diarrhea, syncope, unconsciousness, asphyxia and death" (Nobel Lecture, 1913). Richet created the word *anaphylaxis* to describe this phenomenon. *Phylaxis* is protection in Greek, and the prefix *ana* implies away from protection. Anaphylaxis therefore means "that state of an organism in which it is rendered hypersensitive, instead of being protected." Richet was awarded the Nobel Prize in Physiology and Medicine in 1913 for his discovery of anaphylaxis.

2. **How often does anaphylaxis occur?**

   The incidence of anaphylaxis ranges from one to three people per 10,000. This includes allergic reactions to food, drugs, latex, and Hymenoptera. Lethal anaphylaxis probably occurs in 0.65% to 2.0% of recorded allergic events or in one to three per million people.

3. **What are the immune mechanisms that lead to anaphylaxis?**

   The final common pathway for anaphylaxis is mast cell activation and subsequent release of vasoactive mediators—both preformed and newly generated substances. Preformed mediators include histamine and tryptase stored in cell granules. Newly generated mediators are synthesized at the time of antigen exposure and include leukotrienes (LTC_4, LTD_4, LTE_4), prostaglandins (PGD_2), platelet-aggregating factor (PAF), and cytokines. In the past, the leukotrienes were not well defined and were simply called "slow-reacting substances of anaphylaxis," or SRS-A. It is now known that leukotrienes, prostaglandins, and PAF are much more potent bronchoconstrictors than histamine.

4. **How are immunologic reactions in anaphylaxis classified?**

   The Gell and Coombs classification (1963) described four types of immunologic reactions (see Table 75-1). A fifth type of reaction, termed *idiopathic*, was added to the classification system several years later.

5. **What substances activate mast cells?**

   - Immunoglobulin (Ig) E (IgE) antibodies. IgE antibodies fixed to mast cell surfaces are cross-linked on exposure to an antigen. This initiates cell degranulation and release of mediators.

TABLE 75–1. GELL AND COOMBS CLASSIFICATION OF IMMUNOLOGIC REACTIONS

TYPE	DESCRIPTION	MEDIATOR
I	Immediate hypersensitivity	IgE usually
II	Cytotoxic or cytolytic	IgG, IgM
III	Immune complex disease	Antigen-antibody
IV	Delayed hypersensitivity	T cells
V	Idiopathic	Unknown

- IgG and IgM antibodies. Immunologists have created *knockout mice* that lack the gene for synthesis of IgE antibody. These mice can still develop anaphylaxis via IgG antibodies and complement.
- Complement-mediated reactions. Complement is the term given to plasma and cell membrane proteins that activate the release of inflammatory mediators. Complement activation occurs as a cascade of reactions. IgG or IgM antibody-antigen binding, heparin-protamine complexes, and radiocontrast dye activate the classic pathway. Endotoxins, certain drugs, and radiocontrast dyes can activate the alternate pathway.
- Activated T cells can stimulate mast cell degranulation in a delayed hypersensitivity reaction.
- Direct mast activation. Direct mast cell activation can occur in the absence of antibody or complement. Drugs such as morphine, vancomycin, and d-tubocurarine can cause histamine release, especially if administered quickly.
- Bradykinin is thought to be involved in the systemic inflammatory response system and in angioedema associated with angiotensin-converting enzyme inhibitors. Kinins can mediate a nonhistamine anaphylactoid reaction. Certain polygeline plasma expanders (e.g., Haemaccel) have been implicated in anaphylactoid reaction during anesthesia.

6. **How frequently do neuromuscular blocking drugs (NMBDs) cause anaphylaxis, and what is the mechanism?**
   NMBDs have long been considered the most common cause of intraoperative anaphylaxis in adults. This is true in all published studies from Australia, New Zealand, the United Kingdom, France, Norway, Belgium, and Spain. These drugs have accounted for 54% to 69% of reactions, depending on the study. Within this drug class, succinylcholine and rocuronium are the most common causes. Succinylcholine is a quaternary ammonium ion and is a flexible molecule that can cross-link two IgE molecules more easily than nondepolarizing muscle relaxants with a rigid backbone (e.g., pancuronium or vecuronium).

   There are five important points to remember when considering allergy, anaphylaxis, and NMBDs:
   - Quaternary and tertiary ammonium ions are present in many drugs, cosmetics, and food products. Sensitization can occur outside of the operating room, and a serious reaction can occur with first exposure to a NMBD.
   - Cross-sensitivity between NMBDs can occur in up to 60% of people.
   - NMBDs can cause adverse reactions without IgE antibody mediation. This mechanism of action is via direct mast cell degranulation and release of histamine and other inflammatory mediators. Isoquinolinium compounds such as d-tubocurarine, metocurine, atracurium, and mivacurium are more likely to cause mast cell degranulation.
   - Anaphylaxis to NMBDs is rare in the United States but is reported more frequently in Europe, especially France. An important recent paper has challenged the results of previous French skin test studies. This investigation found that undiluted rocuronium and vecuronium extracts produced a positive wheal and flare response in 50% and 40% of nonatopic anesthesia-naïve

volunteers, respectively. However, a dilution of 1:1000 did not yield any skin response at 15 minutes. Although their study was small (30 healthy adults), the authors questioned the reliability of skin prick testing with undiluted solutions of rocuronium and vecuronium when making the diagnosis of allergy. An accompanying editorial supported the recommendations for using dilute test extracts and suggested that the incidence of NMBD allergy may be overestimated.
- No demonstrated evidence exists for improved outcomes with preoperative screening of sensitivity to NMBDs.

7. How common are latex allergies?
Although its incidence is decreasing, it is still the second most common cause of intraoperative anaphylaxis in adults. Latex is harvested from the *Hevea brasiliensis* tree and is used in hundreds of medical products. Latex remains the most common cause of intraoperative anaphylaxis in children. Certain subsets of patients have a higher risk of latex allergy:
- Children with myelodysplasia or bladder exstrophy or children who have had multiple surgeries
- Health care workers exposed to latex
- Atopic individuals who have asthma, allergic rhinitis, and certain food allergies (e.g., bananas, kiwi, avocado)
- Workers in the rubber industry

Latex allergy can present as a type I immediate hypersensitivity reaction mediated by IgE antibodies with the prototypical features of anaphylaxis: hypotension, tachycardia, bronchoconstriction, or cardiovascular collapse. Latex allergy also can present as a type IV T cell–mediated delayed hypersensitivity reaction that is due to chemicals added as accelerators in the manufacture of latex gloves.

8. How often are antibiotics involved in anaphylaxis?
Penicillin is still the most common cause of anaphylaxis among the general population of the United States and the leading cause of death from anaphylaxis; it accounts for a few hundred deaths each year. Most reactions occur in patients with history of prior exposure to penicillin.

Penicillin is a low-molecular-weight drug. Penicillin can produce four types of the reactions described in the Gell and Coombs classification. It is immunogenic only after binding to tissues and forming a protein hapten complex. The β-lactam ring of penicillin opens to form a penicilloyl group, which is termed the *major determinant*. Derivatives of penicillin are formed in small amounts and are termed *minor determinants*. IgE antibodies specific for these derivatives also can mediate anaphylaxis to penicillin.

9. How do you treat the patient who reports a reaction to penicillin? Is it safe to administer a cephalosporin?
- Patients with an allergy to penicillin have three times the risk for having anaphylaxis to any other drugs.
- A patient with a history of penicillin allergy should not receive antibiotics with a similar structure (e.g., imipenem).
- A patient with a positive skin test to penicillin should not receive cephalosporins.
- Most patients who report an allergy to penicillin had never been skin tested.
- Some authors suggest that it appears to be safe to administer cephalosporins to patients who claim to be allergic to penicillin. However, no conclusion can be made concerning patients who report severe or anaphylactic reactions to penicillin, because these patients were excluded from studies.

10. How frequent is anaphylaxis to propofol?
The original preparations of propofol contained Cremophor EL and caused hypersensitivity reactions on injection. Today, both the brand and generic formulations contain propofol, soybean

oil, glycerol, and sodium hydroxide. The trade brand (Zeneca) contains egg lecithin and the preservative disodium edetate. The generic brand (Baxter) contains egg yolk phospholipid and sodium metabisulfite as a preservative.

Most studies report an incidence of propofol anaphylaxis of 1 in 60,000. One group in France has reported an incidence of 1%. Propofol can cause adverse reactions via IgE antibodies. Occasionally it is associated with nonspecific local histamine release, rash, pruritus, or flushing.

A frequent question regarding propofol is the potential for cross-sensitivity in a patient who is allergic to eggs. The egg lecithin in propofol is purified egg yolk, and most people with egg allergy are sensitive to ovalbumin, the primary protein in egg white. Theoretically, there should be no risk of cross-sensitivity. During phase I trials, propofol was inadvertently given to people with egg allergies without obvious complications. However, the manufacturers of propofol warn that it should not be given to people with egg allergies or soybean allergies. Propofol should not be given to anyone with a history of soybean allergy.

11. How frequent is anaphylaxis to heparin?

Heparin is a large-molecular-weight acidic mucopolysaccharide, and it is derived from bovine or porcine lung. Type 1 IgE immediate hypersensitivity reactions have occurred in humans, although they are rare. More commonly, heparin can induce a thrombocytopenia (HIT), which is mediated by IgG and IgM antibodies directed against platelet factor 4 antigen. This is a delayed adverse reaction usually seen after a few days of heparin therapy. HIT is very rare when low-molecular-weight heparin is used.

12. Are there cases of anaphylaxis to skin and oral disinfectants?

Chlorhexidine is used commonly as a disinfectant before surgery or invasive procedures, including central line placement. Allergy to chlorhexidine is usually mild and limited to cutaneous reactions. In the past few years, reports of intraoperative anaphylaxis to this compound have increased. Typically, hypotension, tachycardia, and cardiovascular collapse occur 24 minutes after application. Because chlorhexidine is also used in toothpastes, mouthwashes, contact lens solutions, and topical antiseptic ointments, significant potential exists for exposure and sensitization to this chemical in the general population.

13. What happens to the patient when anaphylaxis occurs?

Histamine, a preformed mediator, causes vasodilatation, resulting hypotension, and reflex tachycardia. Increased vascular permeability causes edema and urticaria. Cytokines (e.g., tumor necrosis factor), PGD_2, the leukotrienes, and PAF are also potent vasodilators.

Bronchoconstriction, increased mucus secretions, and airway edema can occur in varying stages. A patient might complain of rhinitis, dyspnea, wheezing, or agitation. An anesthetized patient might have decreased airway compliance and increased inspiratory pressure.

Vasodilatation causes erythema, and increased vascular permeability can lead to a wheal and flare, which is an area of local edema and redness. In more severe episodes, angioedema can occur. An awake patient might complain of itching, nausea, abdominal pain, or cramping.

14. How should anaphylaxis be treated?

See Box 75-1.

15. What tests can confirm or negate the diagnosis of anaphylaxis in a patient?

In vitro tests:
- **Histamine.** Histamine has a very short half-life, on the order of minutes. Histamine levels are not usually performed because it is easy to miss the peak, especially if the team is resuscitating the patient.

BOX 75-1. MANAGEMENT OF ANAPHYLAXIS

1. Remove antigen if detected.
2. Administer 100% oxygen.
3. Administer intravenous fluids.
4. Discontinue antibiotic infusion; discontinue blood, fresh frozen plasma, platelet transfusion, if in progress.
5. Adjust epinephrine dose for the clinical scenario:

   For bronchospasm: Start at low doses 0.1 to 0.5 mcg/kg IV (or 5-10 mcg), and increase as needed.

   For hypotension: Start at 1 to 5 mcg/kg IV, and increase as needed.

   For an infusion: Start at 0.05 to 0.1 mcg/kg/min IV (or 0.5-5 mcg/min), and increase as needed.

   For cardiac arrest:

   Pediatric: 10 mcg/kg (0.1 mL/kg of a 1:10,000 solution)

   Adult: 0.5 to 1 mg; titrate to response, as higher doses may be needed
6. Vasopressin can be used when anaphylaxis is refractory to epinephrine therapy. Start with low doses: 5 to 10 units IV, and increase to 40 units if necessary. Infusion: 0.4 units per minute.
7. Secondary therapy: antihistamine

   H_1: diphenhydramine: 0.5 to 1 mg/kg IV

   Optional: H_2: ranitidine: 1 mg/kg IV
8. Secondary therapy: steroids (dose for anaphylaxis)

   Hydrocortisone: 1 to 1.5 mg/kg IV

   Methylprednisolone: 1 mg/kg IV

IV, Intravenous.

- **Tryptase.** Serum tryptase is a protease, and it is a marker only for mast cell degranulation. Its half-life is 2 hours, and the level may remain elevated for a few hours after an acute event. However, occasionally tryptase can be released by mast cells without evidence of IgE, IgG, or IgM antibody mediation. Tryptase levels do not always increase during vancomycin administration or with peanut food allergy.
- **IgE, IgG, IgM levels.** Total antibody levels are not routinely measured unless there is a concern of immunologic disease (such as multiple myeloma) or absence of certain antibody classes (e.g., congenital IgA deficiency).
- **Radioallergosorbent test (RAST).** A radioactive marker is used to identify IgE antibodies to a specific antigen. The key point is to isolate and test for the active antigen; otherwise a false-negative result might occur. A substance can have several antigenic components. For example, at least 11 natural rubber latex antigens exist. In the allergy world in general, RAST is considered less reliable (lower sensitivity and lower specificity) than skin testing, although these rates have improved since the introduction of the Pharmacia CAP RAST method.
- **Enzyme-linked immunosorbent assay (ELISA).** This test uses enzyme activity rather than radioactivity to measure IgE levels for a specific antigen. Both RAST and ELISA have false-positive and false-negative rates, specific for each test and antigen. The availability of a test and its clinical utility can be very different things.
- **Antigens**
  - RAST for measurement of IgE antibodies is available for some NMBDs, propofol, morphine, meperidine, penicillin, barbiturates, aprotinin, protamine, and latex.
  - ELISA looking for IgE antibodies and IgG antibodies is available for most of these drugs. Both RAST and ELISA have turnaround times of 4 to 7 days because they must be sent out to regional immunology laboratories.

In vivo tests:

- In vivo tests include skin tests (subcutaneous and intradermal); provocation and challenge tests are performed in an allergist's office. The tests must be done at least 4 to 6 weeks after a suspected allergic reaction because recent mast cell degranulation may have depleted mediator stores. If skin tests are performed shortly after a reaction, there is the possibility of a false-negative result. Antihistamines must be discontinued 5 days before skin testing. Skin testing can demonstrate whether hypersensitivity is mediated by antibodies; skin tests do not evaluate whether a nonantibody-mediated sensitivity reaction has occured (e.g., nonspecific mast cell degranulation, which is a side effect of some medications).
- Skin tests are available for NMBDs, propofol, fentanyl, latex, chlorhexidine, and local anesthetics. Skin testing before local anesthetics are needed is helpful, especially if the diagnosis is unclear. Although skin testing is the best available method for identification of sensitivity to NMBDs, it is not infallible. Anaphylaxis to cisatracurium after negative skin testing has occurred. The sensitivity and specificity of skin tests to NMBDs are greater than 95%. No skin tests exist for cefazolin, hydromorphone, or midazolam.
- Penicilloyl polylysine (Pre-Pen) is a commercially available skin test reagent to look for IgE antibodies associated with penicillin. It is positive in up to 85% of patients with β-lactam allergy. The remaining 15% of allergic patients react to minor determinants. These antigens are not commercially available and are prepared in a few specialty centers only for in-house use. Curiously, the anaphylactic reactions are seen more commonly in patients who react to the minor determinants of penicillin.

16. **Is there any role for anti-IgE therapy in acute anaphylaxis?**
Omalizumab (Xolair; Genentech) is a monoclonal IgG antibody that binds to the $C\varepsilon3$ domain of IgE. It is a second-line drug in patients with moderate to severe asthma.

   TNX-901 is a humanized IgG1 monoclonal antibody against IgE; it inhibits the binding of IgE to mast cells and basophils. This drug has been studied in people with peanut allergy and was associated with an increase in the threshold of sensitivity to oral peanut challenge.

KEY POINTS: ALLERGY AND ANAPHYLAXIS

1. Five possible immunologic reactions are involved in anaphylaxis, including immediate hypersensitivity, cytotoxicity, immune complex disease, delayed hypersensitivity, and idiopathic.

2. Several things can activate mast cells and cause anaphylaxis including antibodies (IgE, IgG, IgM), drugs directly activating mast cells, complement-mediated reactions, bradykinin, and activated T cells.

3. Penicillin is still the most common cause of anaphylaxis in the general population.

4. Patients who have anaphylaxis have vasodilation and increased endothelial permeability that leads to hypotension, tachycardia, edema, erythema, and urticaria. Bronchoconstriction leads to hypoxia and tachypnea.

BIBLIOGRAPHY

1. Baumgart KW, Baldo BA: Cephalosporin allergy. N Engl J Med 346:380-381, 2002.
2. Brozovic G, Kvolik S: Anaphylactic reaction after rocuronium. Eur J Anaesthesiol 22:72-73, 2005.
3. Cohen SG: The Pharaoh and the wasp. Allergy Proc 10:149-151, 1989.

4. de Leon-Casasola O, Weiss A, Lema MJ: Anaphylaxis due to propofol. Anesthesiology 77:384-386, 1992.

5. Djonneur G, Combes X, Chassard D, et al: Skin sensitivity to rocuronium and vecuronium: a randomized controlled prick-test study in healthy volunteers. Anesth Analg 98:986-989, 2004.

6. Goodman EJ, Morgan MJ, Johnson PA, et al: Cephalosporins can be given to penicillin-allergic patients who do not exhibit an anaphylactic response. J Clin Anesth 13:561-564, 2001.

7. Kay AB: Advances in immunology: allergy and allergic diseases. First of two parts. N Engl J Med 344:30-37, 2001.

8. Kay AB: Advances in immunology: allergy and allergic diseases. Second of two parts. N Engl J Med 344:109-113, 2001.

9. Laxenaire MC: Epidemiology of anesthetic anaphylactoid reactions. Fourth multicenter survey (July 1994-December 1996). Ann Fr Anesth Reanim 18:796-809, 1999.

10. Laxenaire MC: Substances responsible for perianesthetic anaphylactic shock. A third French multicenter study (1992–1994). Ann Fr Anesth Reanim 15:1211-1218, 1996.

11. Leung DYM, Sampson HA, Yunginger JW, et al: Effect of anti-IgE therapy in patients with peanut allergy. N Engl J Med 348:986-993, 2003.

12. Levy JH: Anaphylactic reactions to neuromuscular blocking drugs: are we making the correct diagnosis? Anesth Analg 98:881-882, 2004.

13. Mertes PM, Laxenaire MC: Adverse reactions to neuromuscular blocking agents. Curr Allergy Asthma Rep 4:7-16, 2004.

14. Moneret-Vautrin DA, Morisset M, Flabbee J, et al: Epidemiology of life-threatening and lethal anaphylaxis: a review. Allergy 60:443-451, 2005.

15. Oettgen HC, Martin TR, Wynshaw-Boris A, et al: Active anaphylaxis in IgE-deficient mice. Nature 370:367-370, 1994.

16. O'Sullivan S, McElwain JP, Hogan TS: Kinin-mediated anaphylactoid reaction implicated in acute intra-operative pulseless electrical activity. Anaesthesia 56:771-772, 2001 (comment).

17. Richet C: Nobel Prize presentation speech, 1913. Nobel Lectures, Physiology or Medicine, 1901–1921, Amsterdam, Elsevier, 1967.

18. Vetter RS: Wasp or hippopotamus? J Allergy Clin Immunol 106:196, 2000 (letter).

CHAPTER 76

HYPOTHERMIA

Peter J. Fagenholz, MD, and Edward A. Bittner, MD, PhD

1. **How is hypothermia defined?**

   Hypothermia is defined as a core temperature < 35° C (95° F) and is further classified as follows: mild 35° C to 32° C, moderate 32° C to 28° C, severe 28° C to 20° C, and profound < 20° C. In suspected hypothermia, the temperature is best measured via the rectum or esophagus. A rectal probe should be inserted 10 to 15 cm and not placed into cold feces. Care should be taken to use a thermometer without a minimum temperature; many commonly used thermometers have a minimum temperature of 35° C.

2. **What are the five modes of heat loss?**

   Heat is lost through the following:
   - Radiation
   - Conduction
   - Convection
   - Respiration
   - Evaporation

   Radiation normally accounts for approximately 60% of heat loss and is dependent on the ambient temperature and the amount of body surface exposed. Conduction normally accounts for a small percentage of heat loss, but in patients lying uninsulated on the ground, wearing wet clothing, or, in the most extreme example, immersed in cold water it may account for the majority of heat loss. Convection normally accounts for 10% to 15% of heat loss, though this increases in minimally clothed people and in windy conditions. Inspiration of cold air can account for 2% to 9% of heat loss. Evaporation from the skin and respiratory tract accounts for approximately 25%.

   Accidental hypothermia usually results from increases in heat loss through one of the mechanisms listed previously. It may also be caused by decreased heat production (as can occur in hypothyroidism or adrenal insufficiency) or impaired thermoregulation (as sometimes occurs with central nervous system injury or certain toxic ingestions).

3. **What is the significance of shivering?**

   Shivering is an intrinsic mechanism for augmenting heat production in response to hypothermia. It occurs at core temperatures between 32° C and 37° C. Shivering can result in a fivefold increase in basal metabolic rate but cannot continue when muscles fatigue, their glycogen stores are depleted, or body temperature falls below 32° C. The cessation of shivering in a patient still exposed to the cold should be considered an ominous sign of progressive hypothermia.

4. **What is the J wave?**

   Also known as the Osborn wave, or hypothermic hump, the J wave is a hypothermia-related elevation of the J point at the junction of the QRS complex and ST segment (Fig. 76-1). J waves appear at temperatures at or below 32° C and are usually first seen in leads II and V_6. As the temperature decreases further, they increase in size and may appear in the precordial leads. The J wave is neither specific, nor sensitive, nor prognostic in hypothermia. Automated electrocardiographic interpretation software may misinterpret the J wave as ischemic injury (ST elevation), and it is important not to fall into this trap.

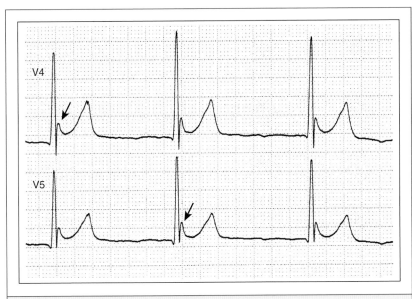

Figure 76-1. J waves in lateral leads during moderate hypothermia.

5. **What is core temperature afterdrop?**
   Core temperature afterdrop is the phenomenon of continued decrease in core temperature when a patient with hypothermia is removed from the cold. It likely results from a combination of thermal equilibration between the relatively warmer core and colder extremities and an increase in convective heat loss due to peripheral vasodilation. It can be avoided by confining active external rewarming to the torso and stabilizing core temperature before thawing frozen extremities. Limiting activity, which stimulates peripheral blood flow, may also be helpful.

6. **Which patients with hypothermia should receive cardiopulmonary resuscitation (CPR)?**
   CPR should be instituted in the patient with hypothermia with no signs of life and no verifiable spontaneous circulation. Tissue destruction, dependent lividity, rigor mortis, and fixed dilated pupils are not reliable indicators of death in hypothermia.
   Even extremely limited perfusion and circulation, which can be difficult to detect, may be sufficient to meet the reduced metabolic needs in hypothermia. Because mechanical agitation is a possible source of arrhythmias in hypothermia, unnecessary CPR (as can occur if a hypothermic bradyarrhythmia is not appreciated) may be especially detrimental to the patient with hypothermia. A Doppler device to detect blood flow or an ultrasound machine to identify cardiac activity may be useful to identify otherwise difficult-to-detect perfusion. At least 1 minute should be spent seeking evidence of a pulse in the patient with hypothermia before instituting CPR.
   Once CPR is initiated, it should be continued until the patient has return of spontaneous circulation, cardiopulmonary bypass (CPB) is initiated, or the patient remains unresuscitated despite reaching a core temperature >35° C. Many cases of prolonged CPR resuscitating patients with hypothermia have been documented. Guidance is provided by the aphorism that "you're not dead until you're warm and dead."

7. **You said mechanical agitation can cause arrhythmias. Is it acceptable to endotracheally intubate? What about central venous or pulmonary artery catheterization?**

    Endotracheal intubation is safe in the patient with hypothermia, and the indications are the same as in normothermia. It will often be necessary to secure the airway because patients with severe hypothermia are obtunded and have depressed airway reflexes, bronchorrhea, and ileus.

    The hypothermic heart is extremely prone to arrhythmia. Even central venous line placement may induce arrhythmias if the guidewire or tip of the catheter enters the atrium. It is best to avoid internal jugular or subclavian placement or to be extremely cautious about the depth to which the guidewire and catheter are advanced. If central access is indicated, it is safest to establish via the femoral vein. Pulmonary artery catheters should be avoided because of the potential for induced arrhythmias, as well as a possible increased risk for pulmonary artery rupture.

8. **How should arrhythmias be treated in the patient with hypothermia?**

    Atrial fibrillation and other supraventricular arrhythmias are common and almost universally benign. They will nearly always resolve with rewarming and should not be treated pharmacologically. Asystole in the patient with severe hypothermia is not as ominous a rhythm as in normothermia and may resolve with rewarming.

    For ventricular fibrillation (VF), experts have traditionally recommended avoiding pharmacotherapy or repeated attempts at defibrillation until rewarming has been achieved. Although durable cardioversion of VF has been reported at a temperature as low as 20° C, this was thought to be the exception rather than the rule, meriting perhaps a single attempt at cardioversion, with further attempts avoided until rewarming to a temperature >30° C. Pharmacotherapy has traditionally been avoided on the basis of concerns that slowed metabolism of antiarrhythmics and increases in serum levels during rewarming could result in toxic levels. Although convincing human trials do not exist to support one strategy or another, on the basis of animal data and isolated clinical reports, the American Heart Association endorses the use of standard advanced cardiac life support (ACLS) protocols concurrent with rewarming, including cardioversion and administration of amiodarone for VF.

9. **Aside from the life support measures described, what other initial management should be undertaken?**

    Volume resuscitation is necessary in most patients with severe hypothermia. Throughout the onset of hypothermia, patients are typically unable to maintain plasma volume both because of impairment of the normal thirst mechanism and because they may not be able to access water. Hypothermia also induces a cold diuresis, with loss of copious dilute urine even in the setting of dehydration. As rewarming reverses peripheral vasoconstriction, hypovolemia may become apparent. In neonates with hypothermia, adequate fluid resuscitation significantly reduces mortality. Such definitive mortality data are lacking in adults, though volume resuscitation does improve hemodynamics. Intravenous administration of 500 to 1000 mL of 5% dextrose in 0.9% sodium chloride is a reasonable starting point for adults, with ongoing resuscitation dictated by clinical response. The hypothermic liver may not be able to metabolize lactate, and therefore lactated Ringer solution is generally avoided.

10. **What are the methods for rewarming patients?**

    Because no controlled studies of various rewarming methods have been rigorously carried out, no rigid protocol can be justifiably instituted. Clinicians should be aware of their own institutional capacities. A recommended algorithm for rewarming is presented in Figure 76-2.

    The first decision for the clinician is whether to choose active or passive rewarming. Passive external rewarming (PER) is the treatment of choice for patients with mild hypothermia (temperature ≥32° C). PER involves covering the patient with insulating material in a warm environment (ambient temperature >21° C). This minimizes the normal processes of heat loss

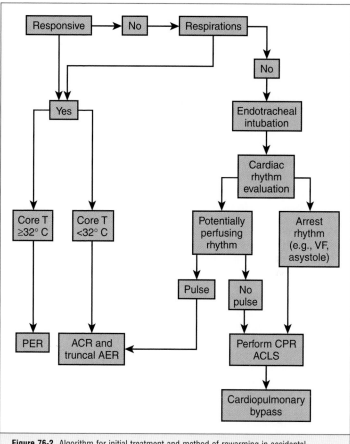

Figure 76-2. Algorithm for initial treatment and method of rewarming in accidental hypothermia. *T*, Temperature.

while relying on the patient's own metabolism to generate the heat necessary for rewarming. PER has the advantages of being simple and noninvasive and is usually effective in mild hypothermia. However, patients with primary defects that prevent adequate endogenous heat production such as glycogen depletion, endocrine deficiencies, untreated sepsis, central nervous system lesions, or hypovolemia need to have their primary abnormalities addressed and may require active rewarming.

Active rewarming can be divided into active external rewarming (AER) and active core rewarming (ACR).

- AER involves applying heat directly to the skin. There are a variety of methods for doing this, including forced air external rewarming, warm water immersion, heating pads, and radiant sources. AER is probably safe, though usually unnecessary in mild hypothermia. It has been associated with poor outcomes in moderate to severe hypothermia. Most of these problems have been attributed to peripheral vasodilation and resulting core temperature afterdrop with decreased overall rewarming rate. These effects may be mitigated by limiting AER to patients with brief hypothermic exposures (e.g., witnessed immersion), by restricting rewarming to the trunk, and by combining AER with ACR techniques listed next.

- ACR includes airway rewarming by the administration of heated, humidified inhalant; administration of warmed intravenous fluids; and lavage of various body cavities (gastrointestinal tract, bladder, peritoneum, pleural cavities, mediastinum) with warm fluids. Airway rewarming and heated intravenous fluid administration are safe and simple. Temperatures from 40° to 45° C are appropriate for both. Irrigation techniques are less effective and invasive and have potentially serious technical complications. They should be avoided at centers where extracorporeal rewarming (ECR) techniques are available. Endovascular rewarming using systems designed for therapeutic hypothermia (see later) have recently been described for rewarming of accidental hypothermia victims. Diathermy is an ACR technique that can transmit heat to deep tissues via ultrasonic or microwave radiation, but clinical experience is limited.

    ECR involves removing blood from the patient's circulation, warming it, and reinfusing it. The available techniques include hemodialysis, venovenous rewarming, continuous arteriovenous rewarming, and CPB. Except for CPB, all these modalities require the patient to have spontaneous circulation. Hemodialysis is widely available and portable and requires only cannulation of a single blood vessel. It has the added advantages of correcting electrolyte abnormalities and allowing clearance in cases of intoxication with a dialyzable substance. In patients with severe hypothermia and circulatory arrest, CPB is the ideal modality. It offers the fastest rewarming and simultaneously provides circulatory support while rewarming is underway. It is usually performed via a femoral-femoral circuit. The principal disadvantages are its limited availability, the time required to initiate bypass, and the need for anticoagulation.

11. **Which patients with hypothermia should undergo CPB?**

    Any patient with severe hypothermia who is hemodynamically unstable should be considered for CPB. CPB is probably the best hope for patients with severe hypothermia without spontaneous circulation. Patients must have no contraindication to anticoagulation, or a CPB circuit that does not require heparinization must be available. Various centers have established different exclusion criteria aimed at identifying those in whom attempted resuscitation is fruitless including pH <6.5, serum potassium level >10 mmol/L, and temperature $<12°$ C, though none of these are extensively validated. One physician with a core temperature of 13.7° C survived after CPB and was able to return to work.

12. **What are the therapeutic uses of hypothermia?**

    Therapeutic hypothermia is most widely accepted as a neuroprotective therapy for adults in cardiac arrest who remain comatose after return of spontaneous circulation. It is also routinely used during cardiovascular surgery requiring circulatory arrest. It is under investigation and used in some centers, for treatment after ischemic cerebral vascular accidents, traumatic brain injury, spinal cord injury, trauma resuscitation, and neonatal asphyxia. The appropriate indications for the use of therapeutic hypothermia in these various disease states are still being defined. Relative contraindications include severe coagulopathy and active bleeding.

13. **What is the usual target temperature in therapeutic hypothermia?**

    Few studies directly compare different cooling mechanisms and protocols. Standard cooling regimens (as for cardiac arrest) target a core temperature of 30° to 34° C with cooling rates of 2° to 4° C per hour. This temperature range has demonstrated neuroprotective effects, with a low incidence of arrhythmias and other complications of more severe hypothermia.

14. **How are patients cooled to the target temperature?**

    Cooling frequently must be initiated in an environment (such as the emergency department) where complex, self-regulating cooling equipment is not available. The cooling process can be begun by placing ice packs around the groin, axillae, head, and neck; administering refrigerated (4° C) intravenous fluids; and covering the patient in a mist of water or alcohol and applying a fan. Intravascular and surface cooling methods have recently been shown to be equivalent in a retrospective review. Intravascular cooling devices circulate cold water through a specially designed intravascular catheter. Surface cooling similarly circulates cold water through pads applied to the patient's skin. In both systems the cooling device is attached to a patient thermometer that provides feedback control. Unless central blood temperature is measured directly, a lag time will exist between measured temperature (via the esophagus, rectum, tympanic membrane) and true core temperature. This can result in an overshoot below the desired core temperature during induction of hypothermia. The faster the cooling rate, the greater the potential to overshoot.

15. **What should be done if a patient shivers during therapeutic hypothermia?**
Shivering must be suppressed for effective cooling. Some centers use routine paralysis to prevent shivering, though suppression of shivering can be achieved without paralytics in most patients through the appropriate use of medications such as propofol, narcotics, and magnesium. Avoiding paralysis has some advantages. It:
- Decreases the incidence of critical illness polyneuropathy
- Allows simple monitoring for seizure, which is a real concern in patients with anoxic or traumatic brain injury and would otherwise require continuous electroencephalographic monitoring
- Allows for simple monitoring of the adequacy of sedation

16. **How long are patients kept in hypothermia?**
Hypothermia is usually discontinued after a specified period of time (24–48 hours) based on protocol. For certain disease processes, such as traumatic brain injury, alternative end points such as the normalization of intracranial pressure have been investigated. The cooling systems (intravascular or surface) described above can be used to regulate rewarming. A typical rate of rewarming is 0.2° to 0.5° C per hour.

17. **What are the important side effects of therapeutic hypothermia?**
Hypothermia affects nearly every organ system and so has myriad side effects of variable clinical significance. Electrolyte abnormalities and infectious complications are most likely to concern the clinician. Electrolyte abnormalities commonly require management and must be actively monitored. During cooling, hypomagnesemia and hyperglycemia are common, whereas, during rewarming, hypoglycemia and hyperkalemia are dangers. Most centers check electrolyte panels every 30 to 60 minutes during cooling and every 4 to 6 hours during the maintenance of hypothermia. Hypothermia may be immunosuppressive via a number of mechanisms and masks the normal febrile response to infection. Many centers draw routine daily blood cultures during induced hypothermia to monitor for infection. An aggressive stance toward investigation and empiric treatment of other potential infectious sources is appropriate, though routine antibiotic prophylaxis is not justified.

KEY POINTS: HYPOTHERMIA

1. Rigor mortis, dependent lividity, and fixed pupils do not reliably indicate death in severe hypothermia.
2. Endotracheal intubation is safe and has the same indications as in normothermia.
3. VF should be treated with standard ACLS in conjunction with rewarming, but multiple rounds of cardioversion and amiodarone should be avoided when the temperature is < 30° C.
4. CPR should be performed in patients with hypothermia without spontaneous circulation.
5. CPB should be initiated in patients with severe hypothermia without return of spontaneous circulation.
6. Therapeutic hypothermia (temperature = 30° C-34° C) is recommended for comatose survivors of cardiac arrest and is likely to be used for more conditions in the future.

BIBLIOGRAPHY

1. Bernard SA, Gray TW, Buist MD, et al: Treatment of comatose survivors of out-of-hospital cardiac arrest with induced hypothermia. N Engl J Med 346:557-563, 2002.
2. Cohen JA, Blackshear RH, Gravenstein N, et al: Increased pulmonary artery perforating potential of pulmonary artery catheters during hypothermia. J Cardiothorac Vasc Anesth 5:234-236, 1991.
3. Crawshaw LI, Wallace HL, Dasgupta S: Thermoregulation. In Auerbach PS, Wilderness Medicine, 5th ed. Philadelphia, Mosby, 2007, pp 110-124.
4. Danzl DF: Accidental hypothermia. In Auerbach PS: Wilderness Medicine, 5th ed. Philadelphia, Mosby, 2007, pp 125-160.
5. Danzl DF, Pozos RS, Auerbach PS, et al: Multicenter hypothermia survey. Ann Emerg Med 16:1042-1055, 1987.
6. Epstein E, Anna K: Accidental hypothermia. BMJ 332:706-709, 2006.
7. Gilbert M, Busund R, Skagseth A, et al: Resuscitation from accidental hypothermia of 13.7 degrees C with circulatory arrest. Lancet 355:375-376, 2000.
8. Goheen MSL, Ducharme MB, Kenny GP, et al: Efficacy of forced-air and inhalation rewarming using a human model for severe hypothermia. J Appl Physiol 83:1635-1640, 1997.
9. Graham CA, McNaughton GW, Wyatt JP: The electrocardiogram in hypothermia. Wilderness Environ Med 12:232-235, 2001.
10. Gregory JS, Bergstein JM, Aprahamian C, et al: Comparison of three methods of rewarming from hypothermia: advantages of extracorporeal blood warming. J Trauma 31:1247-1251, 1991.
11. Grissom CK, Harmston CH, McAlpine JC, et al: Spontaneous endogenous core temperature rewarming after cooling due to snow burial. Wilderness Environ Med 21:229-235, 2010.
12. Holzer M: Targeted temperature management for comatose survivors of cardiac arrest. N Engl J Med 363:1256-1264, 2010.
13. Hypothermia After Cardiac Arrest Study Group: Mild therapeutic hypothermia to improve the neurologic outcome after cardiac arrest. N Engl J Med 346:549-556, 2002.
14. Laniewicz M, Lyn-Kew K, Silbergleit R: Rapid endovascular warming for profound hypothermia. Ann Emerg Med 51:160-163, 2008.
15. Mattu A, Brady WA, Perron AD: Electrocardiographic manifestations of hypothermia. Am J Emerg Med 20:314-326, 2002.
16. Nunnally ME, Jaeschke R, Bellingan GJ, et al: Targeted temperature management in critical care: a report and recommendations from five professional societies. Crit Care Med 39:1113-1125, 2011.
17. Pitoni S, Sinclair HL, Andrews PJ: Aspects of thermoregulation physiology. Curr Opin Crit Care 17:115-121, 2011.
18. Polderman KH: Mechanisms of action, physiological effects, and complications of hypothermia. Crit Care Med 37 (7 Suppl):S186-S202, 2009.
19. Polderman KH, Herold I: Therapeutic hypothermia and controlled normothermia in the intensive care unit: practical considerations, side effects, and cooling methods. Crit Care Med 37:1101-1120, 2009.
20. Tømte Ø, Drægni T, Mangschau A, et al: A comparison of intravascular and surface cooling techniques in comatose cardiac arrest survivors. Crit Care Med 39:443-449, 2011.
21. Vanden Hoek TL, Morrison LJ, Shuster M, et al: Part 12: Cardiac arrest in special situations: 2010 American Heart Association Guidelines for Cardiopulmonary Resuscitation and Emergency Cardiovascular Care. Circulation 122:S829-S861, 2010.
22. Walpoth BH, Walpoth-Aslan BN, Mattle HP, et al: Outcome of survivors of accidental deep hypothermia and circulatory arrest treated with extracorporeal blood warming. N Engl J Med 337:1500-1505, 1997.

CHAPTER 77

HEAT STROKE

William J. Benedetto, MD

1. **What is heat stroke?**

   Heat stroke is a life-threatening illness characterized by a core body temperature above 40° C and central nervous system (CNS) dysfunction. The CNS abnormalities may include delirium, lethargy, convulsions, or coma. Anhidrosis (lack of sweating) may or may not be present, depending on the type and presentation of the illness.

2. **What is the pathophysiology of heat stroke?**

   The body gains heat from metabolism and from the environment, and this heat must be dissipated to maintain a normal temperature of 37° C. This process (thermoregulation) relies primarily on cutaneous vasodilatation and evaporation of sweat. When these processes are overwhelmed, core temperature will rise. When the core temperature exceeds 40° C, an acute phase response is elicited from heat-stressed cells including cytokines and heat shock proteins.

3. **What are the two types of heat stroke? How do they present?**
   - Classic heat stroke is associated with high environmental heat and humidity with inadequate cooling. There is generally no history of significant exercise or exertion. Classic heat stroke typically has a slow onset, often developing over days. It generally afflicts the elderly and the chronically ill, who may present with anorexia, nausea, vomiting, headache, dizziness, confusion, and hypotension. Anhidrosis is a common finding. Up to 25% of patients present with hypotension.
   - Exertional heat stroke usually affects young people in good health who are exercising in a hot, humid environment, often with clothing or equipment that restricts cooling. It is rapid in onset, and nausea, dizziness, and confusion are common. Fatigue, ataxia, coma, and nuchal rigidity or posturing may also occur. Profuse sweating is a typical finding on examination.

4. **Which populations are at greater risk for heat stroke?**
   - Extremes of age—because of relatively poor temperature regulation in the young and old, especially during heat waves
   - Chronically ill—especially those taking drugs that predispose to heat illness
   - Military recruits—especially Northerners not acclimated to the weather in the Southern region of the United States
   - Athletes—most commonly football players and runners
   - Laborers—especially if water losses have not been replaced
   - Obese individuals—because heat dissipation is compromised

5. **Which medications predispose a person to heat stroke?**
   - Drugs increasing heat production through increased motor activity: cocaine, amphetamines, ephedrine, phencyclidine, lysergic acid diethylamide, alcohol withdrawal
   - Drugs decreasing thirst: for example, haloperidol
   - Drugs decreasing sweating: antihistamines, anticholinergics, phenothiazines, β-blockers

6. **What is the mortality rate of heat stroke?**

When treatment is prompt and effectively lowers core temperature, mortality in young, healthy patients is minimal. In the setting of delayed effective treatment and significant comorbidities, mortality can be as high as 70%.

7. **What are the common sequelae and complications of heat stroke?**

Heat stroke can lead to multiorgan dysfunction syndrome including the following:
- Encephalopathy
- Renal failure or rhabdomyolysis (most commonly in exertional heat stroke)
- Acute respiratory distress syndrome
- Myocardial injury and circulatory collapse
- Hepatocellular injury
- Intestinal ischemia and infarction
- Pancreatic injury
- Hemorrhagic complications and disseminated intravascular coagulation, which are common complications and important mechanisms in heat stroke morbidity and mortality

8. **Which other diagnoses should be considered in a patient presenting with hyperthermia?**
- Other hyperthermic syndromes
  - □ Malignant hyperthermia
  - □ Neuroleptic malignant syndrome
  - □ Drug-induced hyperthermia
- Infections
  - □ Especially meningitis, encephalitis, and sepsis
- Endocrinopathies
  - □ Such as thyroid storm and pheochromocytoma
- CNS lesions
  - □ Hypothalamic bleeding, acute hydrocephalus

9. **How can heat stroke be prevented?**

Heat stroke is currently more preventable than treatable. Efforts to prevent heat stroke should focus on acclimatization (gradual exposure to higher temperature environments and increasing work loads), rescheduling activities to cooler times of day, increasing consumption of nonalcoholic fluids, and removing vulnerable populations from high-heat areas.

10. **What is the most important aspect in the treatment of heat stroke?**

Rapid cooling is the main therapeutic goal for treatment of heat stroke. Mortality increases dramatically with even relatively short delays in cooling. Delay in cooling is a better predictor of poor patient outcome than the degree of hyperthermia.

11. **What treatment modalities are effective for rapid cooling?**

Immersion in ice water is effective though can be difficult to do and is often poorly tolerated. This modality may not be appropriate in the comatose or combative patient. Aggressive evaporative cooling, consisting of treatment with tepid water spray (40° C [104° F]) and a forced air stream from a fan, has proved successful and is an easy therapy to apply. Ice packs and massage may be used. Techniques such as iced gastric lavage and peritoneal lavage have also been reported. Though a cooling target has not been clearly established, a core temperature of 39° C or less is considered safe.

12. **In addition to cooling, what other treatment is appropriate?**

Heat stroke can lead to multiorgan dysfunction, and supportive therapy is indicated, as appropriate:
- Airway protection and mechanical ventilation
- Seizure control with benzodiazepines

- Monitoring of circulatory status and fluid therapy or pressors as needed
- Volume expansion and renal monitoring in the setting of rhabdomyolysis
- Correction of electrolyte abnormalities

13. **Which laboratory abnormalities are seen in heat stroke?**
    - Acid/base disturbance.
        □ Classic heat stroke commonly presents with a respiratory alkalosis.
        □ Exertional heat stroke presents with a respiratory alkalosis and lactic acidosis.
    - Hypophosphatemia is common in classic heat stroke, though heat stroke associated with exertion may present with hyperphosphatemia from rhabdomyolysis.
    - Hypokalemia is common except in the setting of rhabdomyolysis.
    - Serum proteins and hypercalcemia increase because of volume contraction.

14. **What prognostic signs predict outcome?**
    Longer duration of hyperthermia is associated with poorer outcome. Coma, hypotension, hyperkalemia, and an aspartate aminotransferase level > 1000 units are associated with a poor prognosis.

15. **What steps can be taken to prevent heat stroke?**
    - Maintain adequate fluid intake during periods of high temperature, high humidity, or increased activity levels.
    - Decrease levels of activity during time of high heat and humidity.
    - Control ambient temperature and humidity if possible.
    - Dress appropriately for the weather.
    - Use prudence during acclimation to a hotter environment.
    - Adjust dosages of predisposing drugs, if possible, during hot weather.
    - Be aware of symptoms of impending heat stroke.

16. **What other medications have been considered for treatment of heat stroke?**
    - Activated protein C has been shown to be useful treatment for heat stroke in a rodent model and has generated some interest in the critical care community, though currently no human trials have been published.
    - Dantrolene has been investigated for treatment of heat stroke, and a nonrandomized trial demonstrated some efficacy. However, a randomized and blinded trial did not confirm this result, and dantrolene is *not* indicated for the treatment of heat stroke.

KEY POINTS: DIAGNOSTIC CRITERIA FOR HEAT STROKE

1. Exposure to increased heat stress: exercise and/or increased temperature and humidity.

2. Altered mental status.

3. Core (rectal) temperature greater than 40° C.

4. Sweating may or may not be present.

BIBLIOGRAPHY

1. Bouchama A, Dehbi M, Chaves-Carballo E: Cooling and hemodynamic management in heatstroke: practical recommendations. Crit Care 11:R54, 2007.
2. Bouchama A, De Vol EB: Acid–base alterations in heat stroke. Intensive Care Med 27:680-685, 2002.

3. Bouchama A, Knochel J: Heat stroke. N Engl J Med 346:1978-1988, 2002.

4. Curley FJ, Irwin RS: Disorders of temperature control part II: hyperthermia. In Irwin RS, Rippe JM (eds): Intensive Care Medicine, 5th ed. Philadelphia, Lippincott Williams & Wilkins, 2003, pp 762-777.

5. Leon L, Helwig B: Heat stroke: role of the systemic inflammatory response. J Appl Physiol 109:1980-1988, 2010.

6. Marini JJ, Wheeler AP: *Thermal disorders*. Critical Care Medicine, The Essentials, Philadelphia, Lippincott Williams & Wilkins, 2006, pp 466–476.

7. O'Connor F, Casa D, Bergeron M, et al: American College of Sports Medicine Roundtable on Exertional Heat Stroke—Return to Duty/Return to Play: Conference Proceedings. Curr Sports Med Rep 9:314-321, 2010.

8. Xiao-Jing L, Yi-Lei L, Gui-Ping M, et al: Activated protein C can be used as a prophylactic as well as a therapeutic agent for heat stroke in rodents. Shock 32:524-529, 2009.

XVI. TOXICOLOGY

GENERAL TOXICOLOGY AND TOXIDROMES

Aaron B. Skolnik, MD, and Susan R. Wilcox, MD

CHAPTER 78

1. What are the most common causes of death by poisoning?

In order from most to least commonly reported, the following categories of drugs are the 10 associated with toxin-related fatalities:

- Miscellaneous sedatives
- Miscellaneous hypnotics
- Miscellaneous antipsychotics
- Miscellaneous cardiovascular drugs
- Opioids
- Acetaminophen combinations
- Acetaminophen alone
- Miscellaneous antidepressants
- Miscellaneous stimulants and street drugs
- Miscellaneous muscle relaxants and cyclic antidepressants

2. What are the common toxidromes?

Toxidromes are syndromes associated with particular classes of toxins. They may be useful in making the diagnosis of poisoning and initiating treatment as patients are often too ill to wait for the results of laboratory or other testing (Table 78-1).

3. What laboratory testing is indicated in the poisoned patient?

Laboratory testing in critically ill poisoned patients should be dictated by the suspected toxin(s) and the findings of the history and physical examination. Laboratory testing should include serum electrolytes and calculation of the anion gap. If the anion gap is elevated, serum osmolarity and calculation of the osmolar gap are often useful. Further laboratory testing might include transaminase and prothrombin time (PT) for a patient who has ingested acetaminophen. Arterial blood gas testing is useful in a critically ill patient poisoned by salicylates as is a carboxyhemoglobin level in a patient with carbon monoxide exposure. Urinalysis may show oxalate crystals suggesting ethylene glycol poisoning or may even fluoresce under a Wood lamp if a patient has ingested a commercial antifreeze preparation.

4. What is the value of serum and urine toxicology screens in the poisoned patient?

In many hospitals, a *basic* serum toxicology screen includes levels of acetaminophen, salicylate, and volatile alcohols. This is a good starting point when ingestants are unknown as it includes treatable toxins for which serum levels guide therapy. Quantitative levels of tricyclic antidepressants are of *no* value in determining treatment, and many hospitals use a qualitative screen. Urine drug screens are often used to test for metabolites of drugs of abuse and are often not valuable in making a toxicologic diagnosis. Some hospitals have comprehensive blood or urine toxicology testing that can isolate many obscure compounds. However, the results of these tests often become available long after the window for appropriate treatment has closed for patients. It is important to know the availability of toxicologic testing at your hospital and to be aware of the limitations of testing. Cross-reactivity with particular assays may also lead to

TABLE 78-1. TOXIDROMES

TOXIDROME	CLINICAL FINDINGS	EXAMPLE AGENTS
Cholinergic	Diarrhea, fecal incontinence, enuresis, miosis, tachycardia followed by bradycardia, lacrimation, sialorrhea, sweating, muscle fasciculations followed by weakness and/or paralysis, altered mental status	Organophosphate and carbamate insecticides *Amanita muscaria* Nicotine
Anticholinergic	Agitated delirium, flushing, decreased sweating, tachycardia, mydriasis, urinary retention, decreased peristalsis, hyperthermia	Atropine Benztropine Scopolamine Diphenhydramine
Sympathomimetic	Mydriasis, hyperthermia, seizures, hyperactivity, hypertension, tachycardia, diaphoresis, delusions, piloerection	Cocaine Methamphetamine MDMA
Sympatholytic	Miosis, hypotension, bradycardia or reflex tachycardia, CNS depression	Clonidine Methyldopa Oxymetazoline
Opioid	Miosis, CNS depression, respiratory depression or apnea, may have hypotension	Heroin Morphine Fentanyl Oxycodone
Serotonin syndrome	Mental status changes, autonomic hyperactivity, neuromuscular abnormalities, akathisia, tremor, clonus, muscle hypertonicity, hyperthermia	Sertraline Fluoxetine Citalopram Linezolid Trazodone Meperidine Tramadol
Neuroleptic malignant syndrome	Fever, "lead pipe" muscular rigidity, altered mental status, autonomic dysfunction (in setting of recent treatment with neuroleptics)	Haloperidol Chlorpromazine Promethazine Prochlorperazine Ziprasidone Quetiapine

CNS, Central nervous system; *MDMA*, methylenedioxymethamphetamine.

false positives. Treating patients on the basis of their clinical status rather than their test results is often the safest plan.

5. **What other diagnostic testing is useful in the poisoned patient?**
Electrocardiography is a noninvasive test that rapidly supplies a great deal of information about a number of potential toxins and has prognostic value in cyclic antidepressant and sodium channel blocker poisoning. It is sound practice to obtain at least one electrocardiogram in all poisoned patients. Chest radiography should be obtained if a patient has significant pulmonary symptoms or findings or requires airway management.

6. **What is the role of gastric lavage in the management of the poisoned ICU patient?**
Usually, there is no role for gastric lavage (*stomach pumping*) in the critically poisoned patient. Gastric lavage involves the passage of a large-bore orogastric tube and the repeated instillation and aspiration of fluid to remove potentially toxic stomach contents. In animal and volunteer studies, the recovery of drugs is highly variable and declines quickly as the time from ingestion increases. Clinical studies have not confirmed a benefit of gastric lavage alone even when performed rapidly (<60 minutes) after ingestion. Given that significant time typically elapses before arrival of a poisoned patient in the intensive care unit (ICU), gastric lavage in the ICU is likely to be of no benefit. In addition, orogastric lavage has been associated with complications including aspiration, hypoxia, hypercapnia, electrolyte disturbances, and mechanical injuries to the pharynx, esophagus, and stomach.

7. **What is the role of activated charcoal in the treatment of poisoned patients?**
A single dose of activated charcoal may be useful in the management of some patients. Activated charcoal reduces the bioavailability of some substances, with the magnitude of reduction declining with increasing time from the ingestion. Evidence is insufficient from clinical studies that single-dose activated charcoal improves outcomes in poisoned patients. Most of the time, the decision to give activated charcoal is made in the emergency department because of the proximity to the time of ingestion. Consider ICU administration of activated charcoal on a case-by-case basis if the risk of the ingested poison outweighs the aspiration risk of charcoal administration, if the patient has a patent or protected airway, and if the ingested toxin is well adsorbed to activated charcoal (Box 78-1).

BOX 78	XINS POORL
▪ Acids	▪ Inorganic salts
▪ Alcohols including ethanol	▪ Iron
▪ Alkali	▪ Lithium
▪ Ethylene glycol	▪ Pesticides
▪ Heavy metals	▪ Potassium

8. **Does multiple-dose activated charcoal (MDAC) reduce the absorption of poisons from the gastrointestinal tract?**
MDAC is repeated administration of enteral activated charcoal in an effort to increase drug elimination via diffusion along concentration gradients into the gut and preventing the reabsorption of drugs with significant enterohepatic circulation. The process has been referred to

as "gastrointestinal dialysis," and drugs amenable to MDAC share some characteristics with dialyzable drugs, including a low (<1 L/kg) volume of distribution and low protein binding. MDAC has demonstrated enhanced elimination of carbamazepine, dapsone, theophylline, quinine, and phenobarbital. It has been proposed as treatment for a number of other agents, including salicylate and digoxin, and may also be considered for poisoning by sustained-release preparations of drugs.

9. **Is there a role for syrup of ipecac in treating poisoning?**
   Syrup of ipecac no longer has a role in acute poisoning treatment. Ipecac syrup induces vomiting, but its recovery of drugs in experimental models is erratic and unreliable. In the pediatric population, administration of ipecac in the home did not improve outcomes or reduce emergency department utilization. In addition, the induction of persistent vomiting poses a risk for aspiration and inability to cooperate with further therapies. The American Academy of Clinical Toxicology and the American Academy of Pediatrics recommend against the routine administration of ipecac to poisoned patients in the emergency department and in the home.

10. **What is whole-bowel irrigation (WBI), and does its use benefit poisoned patients?**
    WBI is the administration of large volumes of polyethylene glycol solution, with the intent of flushing drugs or toxins out of the gastrointestinal tract via liquid stools. Data on the efficacy of WBI for removing drugs from the body are mixed, and clinical evidence is insufficient to recommend its routine use. In addition, the administration of WBI is likely to cause significant discomfort to patients. WBI is an option for possibly expediting the gastrointestinal luminal clearance of sustained-release preparations, toxic heavy metals, or packets of illicit drugs smuggled within the body ("body packers").

11. **What is the role of dialysis in the care of the poisoned patient?**
    Drugs amenable to removal via hemodialysis share a number of important characteristics. They must:
    - Be small enough and lack charge such that they will cross a dialysis membrane
    - Be highly water soluble and have a small volume of distribution (<1 L/kg is a good rule of thumb) so that they are concentrated in the blood (rather than the tissues) in sufficient quantity for removal
    - Have low protein binding in general, although dialysis can occasionally be used to remove free drug when protein binding is fully saturated in a massive overdose

12. **Which drugs can be removed from the body via hemodialysis?**
    Lithium and salicylate are two drugs commonly removed via hemodialysis in overdose. When considering hemodialysis in a poisoned patient, the risks of the procedure including venous and/or arterial access, discomfort, transient anticoagulation, and hemodynamic shifts must be weighed carefully against the severity of the poisoning. Acetaminophen can easily be removed by hemodialysis, but this is rarely done, because antidotal treatment with *N*-acetylcysteine usually works well, is noninvasive, and carries less risk to the patient.

13. **What antidotes are commonly useful in the ICU?**
    See Table 78-2.

TABLE 78-2. ANTIDOTES COMMONLY USED IN THE INTENSIVE CARE UNIT

ANTIDOTE	PHARMACOLOGIC EFFECTS	TYPICAL USES
Benzodiazepines	Potentiator of GABA inhibitory neurotransmission in the CNS	• Alcohol or sedative/hypnotic withdrawal • Antiepileptic • Anxiolysis, sedation • Relaxation of muscle rigidity • Treatment of agitation associated with sympathomimetic or anticholinergic syndromes
Sodium bicarbonate	Can produce alkalemia in the serum and in urine, provides sodium ion load	Treatment of sodium channel blockade due to: • Tricyclic antidepressants • Class Ia and Ic antiarrhythmics • Cocaine, diphenhydramine Serum and urinary alkalinization to prevent tissue distribution and improve renal clearance of: • Salicylates
Flumazenil	CNS benzodiazepine receptor antagonist	• Reversal of CNS and respiratory depression due to benzodiazepines (in patients *without* history of long-term benzodiazepine use)
Glucose	Cellular energy source	• Hypoglycemia • Empiric treatment for altered mental status or seizure without clear cause • With high-dose insulin infusion for calcium channel blocker poisoning
Naloxone	Opioid mu, kappa, and delta receptor antagonist	• Reversal of respiratory and/or CNS depression suspected to be caused by opiates, opioids
Octreotide	Long-acting somatostatin analog, inhibits pancreatic insulin release	Suppression of drug-induced insulin secretion caused by: • Sulfonylureas, quinine
Hydroxocobalamin	Binds cyanide ions to form cyanocobalamin, which is excreted in the urine	• Treatment of cyanide toxicity

(Continued)

TABLE 78-2. ANTIDOTES COMMONLY USED IN THE INTENSIVE CARE UNIT—*cont'd*		
ANTIDOTE	**PHARMACOLOGIC EFFECTS**	**TYPICAL USES**
Physostigmine	CNS and peripheral acetylcholinesterase inhibitor, increasing stimulation of nicotinic and muscarinic ACh receptors	• Transient reversal of severe antimuscarinic syndromes *not* caused by cyclic antidepressants
Deferoxamine	Binds free iron in the blood, enhances urinary elimination	• Treatment of iron toxicity

ACh, Acetylcholine; *CNS,* central nervous system; *GABA,* γ-aminobutyric acid.

KEY POINTS: TOXICOLOGY

1. The diagnostic evaluation for the poisoned critically ill patient should be determined by the history and physical examination.

2. Urine and serum toxicology screens vary among hospitals and may not be of significant clinical utility.

3. Gastric lavage no longer has a role in the management of the poisoned patient.

4. Hemodialysis is beneficial in the management of several common poisonings.

5. Poisonings with antidotes must be recognized and treatment initiated promptly.

BIBLIOGRAPHY

1. Alapat PM, Zimmerman JL: Toxicology in the critical care unit. Chest 133:1006-1013, 2008.

2. Anonymous: Position paper: ipecac syrup. J Toxicol Clin Toxicol 42:133-143, 2004.

3. Boyle JS, Bechtel LK, Holstege CP: Management of the critically poisoned patient. Scand J Trauma Resusc Emerg Med 17:29, 2009.

4. Chyka PA, Seger D, Krenzelok EP, et al: Position paper: single-dose activated charcoal. Clin Toxicol 43:61-87, 2005.

5. Erickson TB, Thompson TM, Lu JJ: The approach to the patient with an unknown overdose. Emerg Med Clin North Am 25:249-281, 2007.

6. Higgins RM, Connolly JO, Hendry BM: Alkalinization and hemodialysis in severe salicylate poisoning: comparison of elimination techniques in the same patient. Clin Nephrol 50:178-183, 1998.

7. Holstege CP, Dobmeier SG, Bechtel LK: Critical care toxicology. Emerg Med Clin North Am 26:715-739, viii-ix, 2008.

8. Kolecki PF, Curry SC: Poisoning by sodium channel blocking agents. Crit Care Clin 13:829-848, 1997.

9. Mokhlesi B, Leiken JB, Murray P, et al: Adult toxicology in critical care: part I: general approach to the intoxicated patient. Chest 123:577-592, 2003.

10. O'Malley GF: Emergency department management of the salicylate-poisoned patient. Emerg Med Clin North Am 25:333-346, 2007.

11. Vale JA, Kulig K: American Academy of Clinical Toxicology, European Association of Poisons Centres and Clinical Toxicologists: Position paper: gastric lavage. J Toxicol Clin Toxicol 42:933-943, 2004.

12. Wells K, Williamson M, Holstege CP, et al: The association of cardiovascular toxins and electrocardiographic abnormality in poisoned patients. Am J Emerg Med 26:957-959, 2008.

13. Wu AH, McKay C, Broussard LA: National Academy of Clinical Biochemistry laboratory medicine practice guidelines: recommendations for the use of laboratory tests to support poisoned patients who present to the emergency department. Clin Chem 49:357-379, 2003.

CHAPTER 79

ANALGESICS AND ANTIDEPRESSANTS

Aaron B. Skolnik, MD, and Susan R. Wilcox, MD

1. **What are the signs and symptoms of salicylate poisoning?**
   Supratherapeutic levels of salicylate produce characteristic tinnitus. Salicylate poisoning induces a central nervous system (CNS)–mediated respiratory alkalosis, while producing a metabolic acidosis. Aspirin in particular is highly irritating to the gastrointestinal tract, and patients may present with nausea, vomiting, abdominal pain, or hematemesis. Severe poisoning can induce hypoglycemia and hyperthermia due to uncoupling of oxidative phosphorylation and may also cause acute respiratory distress syndrome. Aspirin significantly inhibits platelet function, and any salicylate-containing product can inhibit vitamin K–dependent clotting factors when taken in overdose. The most serious poisonings involve the CNS and may present with confusion, agitation, delirium, hallucinosis, seizures, coma, or death.

2. **When patients die of salicylate poisoning, of what do they usually die?**
   Usually, they die of cerebral edema or refractory shock with terminal arrhythmias. Their shock, in turn, is often related to severe and refractory acidemia.

3. **What constitutes a toxic dose of aspirin?**
   Acute ingestion of greater than 150 mg/kg of aspirin or equivalent is sufficient to produce toxicity that may include gastrointestinal symptoms, metabolic disturbances, tinnitus, and tachypnea and/or hyperpnea. Acute ingestion of greater than 300 mg/kg of aspirin may be lethal. Be aware that chronic salicylate toxicity may also develop in elderly patients, dehydrated patients, or those taking carbonic anhydrase inhibitors. This can happen even at stable *therapeutic* dosing depending on the patient's underlying health status and salicylate clearance.

4. **What are the initial steps in treating salicylate poisoning?**
   - First, delay and prevent absorption of salicylate. Early initial management of an acute ingestion should include administration of activated charcoal, when possible. Multiple dose activated charcoal may also be considered.
   - Patients should also be resuscitated.
   - Patients with moderate or severe poisoning are typically volume depleted, and intravenous fluids should be administered via bolus.
   - It is important to remember that salicylate-poisoned patients have a very high minute ventilation, both from primary respiratory alkalosis and to compensate for metabolic acidosis. Physicians must be especially cautious in administering sedation or initiating mechanical ventilation so as not to worsen acidosis.

5. **What is the role of bicarbonate in the treatment of salicylate poisoning?**
   Alkalinization of serum is important in limiting the distribution of salicylate into tissues, especially the CNS. The ensuing urinary alkalinization traps salicylate in its ionized form in the urine and enhances renal clearance. Sodium bicarbonate solutions (typically dextrose 5% with 150 mEq/L sodium bicarbonate) should be infused to a goal serum pH of 7.5 to 7.55.

Administration of intravenous bicarbonate will also help to alkalinize the urine, with a goal urinary pH of 8. To maintain alkaluria, potassium must also be replaced. Often, 40-50 mEq/L of potassium chloride is added to sodium bicarbonate infusions to maintain normokalemia.

6. **What laboratory values are important in salicylate toxicity?**
   To guide therapy, arterial pH, serum electrolytes, and urinary pH must be measured frequently and high urine output maintained. As salicylate's absorption from the gastrointestinal tract can be erratic, salicylate levels must also be checked serially, as often as every 1 to 2 hours in the most severely poisoned patients.

7. **What are the indications for hemodialysis in salicylate poisoning?**
   Patients with renal failure, hemodynamic instability, any sign of CNS toxicity, or rising serum salicylate levels despite maximal medical therapy should undergo hemodialysis. Most patients with any salicylate level more than 100 mg/dL will require hemodialysis at some point in their treatment. Hemodialysis should be also considered for those with salicylate levels greater than 80 mg/dL on the basis of their clinical status. Failure to initiate hemodialysis promptly for neurotoxic patients is a common error in management, and salicylate-poisoned patients can very rapidly decompensate.

8. **What are the signs and symptoms of acetaminophen poisoning?**
   The challenge of recognizing and treating acetaminophen toxicity is that patients are often asymptomatic after acute acetaminophen ingestion. Nausea, vomiting, anorexia, and/or lethargy may occur within hours of ingestion. Very rarely, massive overdose can cause altered mental status and metabolic acidosis within 6 hours of an overdose. Twenty-four to 48 hours after overdose, hepatic injury with transaminitis may develop or even acute or hyperacute liver failure with accompanying hyperbilirubinemia, jaundice, coagulopathy, and encephalopathy. Acute renal failure, which is probably multifactorial in origin, may also occur. Acetaminophen toxicity should be considered in any patient with unexplained liver failure.

9. **What is the mechanism of acetaminophen-induced hepatotoxicity?**
   Acetaminophen's hepatotoxicity is due to a reactive metabolite called N-acetyl-p-benzoquinone imine (NAPQI). Under therapeutic dosing conditions, most acetaminophen is metabolized in the liver by glucuronidation and sulfation. A tiny amount is excreted unchanged in the urine, and about 4% is metabolized by the cytochrome system (mostly cytochrome P 2E1) into NAPQI. NAPQI is then safely detoxified by the antioxidant effects of hepatic glutathione. However, under overdose conditions, hepatic glutathione stores become depleted, allowing NAPQI to bind to and cause death of hepatocytes.

10. **How is the Rumack-Matthew acetaminophen treatment nomogram used?**
    The Rumack-Matthew treatment nomogram is used to identify patients who have taken a single, acute acetaminophen overdose and who are at risk for hepatotoxicity and require treatment. To use the nomogram, the time of ingestion must be known and a serum acetaminophen level must be drawn at a known time at least 4 hours after ingestion. The time after ingestion is plotted on the x-axis and the acetaminophen level on the y-axis. If the intersection point of these two values falls above the treatment line, the patient is treated with N-acetylcysteine (NAC). In the United States, this treatment line is labeled "possible hepatic toxicity" and corresponds with a 4-hour postingestion acetaminophen level of 150 mcg/mL (Fig. 79-1).

11. **How does NAC work?**
    NAC works by replenishing hepatic glutathione stores and acting as a glutathione substitute, allowing the detoxification of NAPQI. This prevents the resulting NAPQI-induced hepatocyte damage and death. It also increases sulfation of acetaminophen, thereby reducing NAPQI formation.

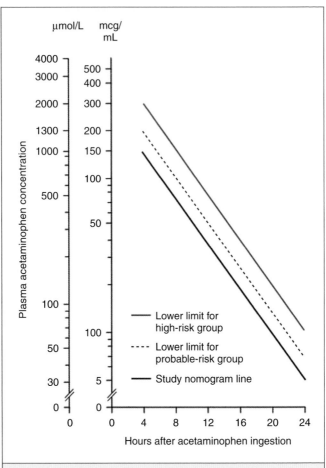

Figure 79-1. The Rumack-Matthew nomogram identifies patients with a single ingestion of acetaminophen at risk for hepatotoxicity. (From Heard KJ: Acetylcysteine for acetaminophen poisoning. N Engl J Med 359:285–292, 2008.)

12. **Which is better: intravenous or oral NAC?**

Two common regimens exist for treatment and prevention of acetaminophen-induced hepatotoxicity, a 72-hour regimen of oral NAC and a 20-hour regimen of intravenous NAC. On the basis of the literature at the time of this writing, both regimens seem to have good safety profiles for patients, though more anaphylactoid reactions occur when NAC is administered intravenously and more gastrointestinal intolerance when administered orally (NAC smells like rotten eggs). No good, prospective data at this time suggest that either IV or oral NAC is superior in preventing clinically significant hepatotoxicity (i.e., that resulting in liver failure or need for transplantation). Intravenous NAC has the advantage of parenteral administration in patients unable to take or tolerate oral NAC and necessitates a shorter hospital stay. Many toxicologists favor a patient-tailored approach, wherein one of the above protocols is initiated and the final duration of NAC therapy is based on the patient's laboratory values and clinical course.

13. **What are the receptor effects and clinical effects of tricyclic antidepressant (TCA) poisoning?**

    TCAs have seven pharmacologic effects. Understanding these effects is helpful in remembering the associated clinical syndrome of TCA toxicity (Table 79-1).

TABLE 79-1. PHARMACOLOGIC EFFECTS OF TRICYCLIC ANTIDEPRESSANTS

MECHANISM	EFFECT
Presynaptic biogenic amine reuptake inhibition (norepinephrine and serotonin)	Therapeutic antidepressant effect
	Early sympathomimesis
	Myoclonus
	Hyperreflexia
Fast sodium channel influx blockade	QRS duration prolonged
	PR interval prolonged
	Right axis deviation
	Bundle branch blockade
	Ventricular dysrhythmias
	Negative inotropy
Potassium channel efflux blockade	QTc prolongation
Muscarinic acetylcholine receptor blockade	Tachycardia
	Mydriasis
	Decreased sweating
	Hyperthermia
	Flushing
	Ileus
	Urinary retention
Histaminic receptor blockade	Sedation
Alpha receptor blockade	Sedation
	Orthostatic hypotension
	Miosis
	Reflex tachycardia
GABA-A receptor blockade	Seizures
	Status epilepticus

GABA-A, γ-Aminobutyric acid-A.

14. **What value is the electrocardiogram in patients with TCA poisoning?**

    The electrocardiogram is the best early screen for TCA toxicity. Electrocardiographic findings usually manifest within the first few hours of poisoning and allow this potentially fatal diagnosis to be made early. The combination of the following classic electrocardiographic findings in a patient with an unknown ingestion strongly suggests TCA poisoning. These findings include the following:
    - Sinus tachycardia
    - PR prolongation
    - Widened QRS complex (greater than 100 milliseconds)
    - QTc prolongation
    - Terminal R complex in aV_R greater than 3 mm in height

In addition, electrocardiographic features are predictive of the clinical course and guide treatment in severe toxicity. The risk of seizures increases if the QRS duration is greater than 100 milliseconds, and a terminal R wave greater than 3 mm in aV_R predicts an increased risk of both seizures and ventricular dysrhythmias. The presence of either of these findings warrants immediate treatment.

15. **How is cardiovascular toxicity of TCAs treated?**
Cardiovascular toxicity of TCAs is treated first with sodium bicarbonate therapy, titrating initial bolus therapy to resolution of QRS prolongation and following this with continuous infusion of bicarbonate solution to alkalinize the serum and provide a loading dose of sodium ions. If the patient continues to have QRS prolongation or significant right axis deviation, despite alkalemia to pH of 7.55, hypertonic saline solution can also be administered. Lidocaine is the historical second-line agent in treating dysrhythmias, but the physician must be aware that lidocaine is also a sodium channel blocker and administration could potentiate seizures. Synchronous cardioversion should be used in patients with TCA overdose on the basis of current advanced cardiac life support guidelines when indicated. Torsades de pointes can be treated with magnesium sulfate infusion. Despite the QTc prolongation associated with TCA use, the tachycardia due to the antimuscarinic effects of TCAs often limits the likelihood of "R-on-T" phenomena. Finally, in recent years, lipid emulsion rescue has emerged as an antidotal treatment in life-threatening poisoning by lipophilic drugs. All TCAs are highly lipophilic, given their therapeutic targets in the CNS, and animal and human data suggest that TCAs and related compounds respond well to lipid rescue. Patients with known or suspected TCA cardiotoxicity and hemodynamic instability or malignant dysrhythmias are candidates for lipid emulsion therapy, discussed in more detail in Chapter 81 on cardiovascular drug toxicity.

KEY POINTS: ANALGESICS AND ANTIDEPRESSANTS

1. Patients with salicylate toxicity should start alkalinization therapy and have serum salicylate levels checked every 1 to 2 hours.

2. Hemodialysis should be initiated promptly in any patient with salicylate levels over 100 mg/dL or those with levels greater than 80 mg/dL with significant clinical deterioration or neurotoxicity.

3. Acetaminophen levels may be plotted on the Rumack-Matthew nomogram only if the patient has had a single, acute ingestion of acetaminophen at a known time at least 4 hours before presentation.

4. Any suspected or confirmed acetaminophen-toxic patient should immediately start receiving NAC, by either the oral or IV route.

5. Sodium bicarbonate is the treatment of choice to prevent seizures and arrhythmias in TCA overdose and should be administered as boluses until the QRS is <100 milliseconds.

BIBLIOGRAPHY

1. Bailey B, Buckley NA, Amre DK: A meta-analysis of prognostic indicators to predict seizures, arrhythmias or death after tricyclic antidepressant overdose. J Toxicol Clin Toxicol 42:877-888, 2004.

2. Bradberry SM, Thanacoody HK, Watt BE, et al: Management of the cardiovascular complications of tricyclic antidepressant poisoning: role of sodium bicarbonate. Toxicol Rev 24:195-204, 2005.

3. Body R, Bartram T, Azam F, et al: Guidelines in Emergency Medicine Network (GEMNet): guideline for the management of tricyclic antidepressant overdose. Emerg Med J 28:347-368, 2011.

4. Engels PT, Davidow JS: Intravenous fat emulsion to reverse haemodynamic instability from intentional amitriptyline overdose. Resuscitation 81:1037-1039, 2010.

5. Heard KJ: Acetylcysteine for acetaminophen poisoning. N Engl J Med 359:285-292, 2008.

6. Higgins RM, Connolly JO, Hendry BM: Alkalinization and hemodialysis in severe salicylate poisoning: comparison of elimination techniques in the same patient. Clin Nephrol 50:178-183, 1998.

7. Johnson MT, McCammon CA, Mullins ME, et al: Evaluation of a simplified N-acetylcysteine dosing regimen for the treatment of acetaminophen toxicity. Ann Pharmacother 45:713-720, 2011.

8. Khandelwal N, James LP, Sanders C, et al: the Acute Liver Failure Study Group. Unrecognized acetaminophen toxicity as a cause of indeterminate acute liver failure. Hepatology 53:567-576, 2011.

9. Kolecki PF, Curry SC: Poisoning by sodium channel blocking agents. Crit Care Clin 13:829-848, 1997.

10. O'Malley GF: Emergency department management of the salicylate-poisoned patient. Emerg Med Clin North Am 25:333-346, 2007.

11. Pentel PR, Benowitz NL: Tricyclic antidepressant poisoning. Management of arrhythmias. Med Toxicol 1:101-121, 1986.

12. Pierog JE, Kane KE, Kane BG, et al: Tricyclic antidepressant toxicity treated with massive sodium bicarbonate. Am J Emerg Med 27:1168.e3-e7, 2009.

13. Wells K, Williamson M, Holstege CP, et al: The association of cardiovascular toxins and electrocardiographic abnormality in poisoned patients. Am J Emerg Med 26:957-959, 2008.

CHAPTER 80

TOXIC ALCOHOL POISONING

Aaron B. Skolnik, MD, and Susan R. Wilcox, MD

1. **What are the compounds commonly referred to as the *toxic alcohols*?**
   Typically, the term *toxic alcohols* includes isopropanol, methanol, and ethylene glycol. Ethanol, of course, may also be toxic.

2. **What household or commercial products commonly contain toxic alcohols?**
   - Isopropanol (or isopropyl alcohol) is most commonly sold as *rubbing alcohol*, in a 70% solution. It can also be found in antifreezes, glass cleaners, jewelry cleaner, stain removers, deicers, household disinfectants, and hand sanitizers.
   - Methanol can be found in windshield washer fluid, antifreeze, copy machine fluid, canned fuel (Sterno), and some solvents. Perhaps most famously, methanol is a frequent contaminant in illicitly distilled alcoholic beverages—hence the term *moonshine blindness*, originating from methanol retinal toxicity.
   - Ethylene glycol is often the main ingredient in automobile antifreeze and is sometimes used as a solvent.

3. **What are potentially lethal doses of isopropanol, methanol, and ethylene glycol?**
   - Isopropanol ingestion of 150 to 250 mL can be lethal because of central nervous system (CNS) and myocardial depression.
   - The reported lethal dose of methanol is 1.2 mL/kg; however, as little as 30 mL (6 teaspoons) may cause permanent vision impairment.
   - The lethal dose of ethylene glycol in untreated patients varies, but 100 mL is a common conservative approximation.

4. **What are the mechanisms of toxicity for isopropanol?**
   Isopropanol is estimated to be twice as intoxicating by volume as ethanol. It is a CNS depressant and may cause peripheral vasodilation, myocardial depression, and subsequent shock at high doses. It is metabolized by alcohol dehydrogenase (ADH) to acetone, which appears to contribute to further CNS depression. Isopropanol is extremely irritating to the gastric mucosa and classically causes severe gastritis, which may be hemorrhagic.

5. **What are the mechanisms of toxicity for methanol?**
   Methanol is first metabolized by ADH to formaldehyde, which is then rapidly converted to formic acid by aldehyde dehydrogenase. Formic acid inhibits mitochondrial electron transport, leading to acidemia and production of reactive species. It also depletes glutathione, which is an endogenous antioxidant. The combination of these effects leaves cells that are under significant oxidative stress such as those in the retina and putamen, exposed to oxidant cytotoxicity.

6. **What are the mechanisms of toxicity for ethylene glycol?**
   Ethylene glycol is metabolized to toxic glycolic acid, glyoxylic acid, oxalic acid, and several other minor metabolites. Oxalic acid precipitates with calcium into calcium oxalate crystals. In addition to causing hypocalcemia, deposition of oxalate in the renal tubules and other tissues causes cell death. The resulting metabolic acidosis, renal failure, pulmonary edema, and cerebral injury contribute to mortality in these patients.

7. **What are the signs and symptoms of toxic alcohol poisoning?**

CNS depression is the common element in toxic alcohol poisoning, ranging from typically mild in the case of methanol to profound intoxication in the case of isopropanol or ethylene glycol poisoning. Patients who ingest any of these substances may ultimately have coma, shock, and death. Each of the toxic alcohols has key clinical features that distinguish one from the other. Isopropanol-intoxicated patients typically have prominent gastrointestinal symptoms and may present with severe abdominal pain, vomiting, or hematemesis. Because acetone is the metabolite of this alcohol, ketosis without acidosis develops, and patients have fruity breath odor.

Retinal toxicity is the hallmark of methanol poisoning and may develop many hours after ingestion. Visual complaints may vary, with complete vision loss, afferent pupillary defects, and optic disc hyperemia on funduscopic examination being late findings.

Ethylene glycol toxicity usually begins with CNS depression. Hypocalcemia may cause tetany or myoclonus. Untreated, patients may progress to seizure, pulmonary edema, and ultimately renal failure, cerebral edema, and death.

8. **What is the osmolal gap, and how is it used in diagnosing toxic alcohol poisoning?**

The osmolal gap (OG) is the difference between the calculated serum osmolality (oc) and the measured serum osmolality (om). This value approximates the quantity of unmeasured osmoles in the serum. To calculate the serum osmolality:

$$oc = (2 \times \text{Serum sodium}) + (\text{Blood urea nitrogen}/3) + (\text{Glucose}/18) + (\text{Ethanol}/4.6)$$

The osmolal gap:

$$OG = om - oc$$

An osmolal gap greater than 20 mOsm/L should always raise suspicion for ingestion of exogenous osmoles. All of the toxic alcohols discussed in this chapter increase the serum osmolality, and serum levels of these compounds may be approximated by calculating the osmolal gap and using conversion factors based on their molecular weight. As the parent compounds are metabolized, the osmolal gap closes. In the case of methanol and ethylene glycol poisoning, the acid products of metabolism accumulate, which causes the anion gap to rise as the osmolal gap decreases. In isopropanol poisoning, the osmolal gap simply closes, as acetone is not a strong acid.

9. **What is the value of obtaining serum levels for the toxic alcohols?**

Generally, the value of serum levels is in confirming the diagnosis of toxic alcohol poisoning. However, serum levels are not readily available at most hospitals and often result hours to days after the patient's initial evaluation. There are also no absolute values that determine when to start or end therapy for toxic alcohol–poisoned patients. When in doubt, basing treatment decisions on the clinical status of the patient is the right way to proceed, as in most of toxicology.

10. **How does fomepizole work, and when should it be given?**

Fomepizole (4-methylpyrazole) is a competitive ADH inhibitor. It is used to block metabolism of ethylene glycol and methanol to their toxic metabolites. It should be given when a known or suspected toxic ethylene glycol or methanol ingestion has occurred and the patient has metabolic acidosis and elevated osmolar gap. Because the drug is given every 12 hours, empiric treatment with a single dose allows sufficient time to evaluate the patient, perhaps obtain access and begin hemodialysis, and/or obtain serum levels of the toxins. Many sources recommend giving fomepizole on the basis of a serum ethylene glycol or methanol concentration greater than 20 mg/dL. The loading dose of fomepizole is 15 mg/kg infused intravenously over 30 minutes. If dialysis is initiated, fomepizole will also be dialyzed from the serum, and the dosing interval is decreased to every 4 hours.

11. **Can ethanol be used as an antidote to toxic alcohols?**
Ethanol can be used, much like fomepizole, as a competitive substrate for ADH to allow time for clearance or extracorporeal removal of methanol or ethylene glycol. Ethanol was widely used in this fashion until the introduction of fomepizole. However, because ethanol retains its intoxicating properties when used in this fashion, the risk of CNS depression and adverse events is higher than with fomepizole use. Fomepizole has been recommended as the first-line ADH-inhibiting agent in toxic alcohol poisoning, and ethanol use should be reserved for when fomepizole is unavailable or the patient is severely allergic.

12. **When is hemodialysis indicated for toxic alcohol poisoning?**
Patients poisoned with toxic alcohols may meet conventional indications for hemodialysis, such as severe metabolic acidosis or uremia, and this treatment should not be withheld. Those poisoned with isopropanol rarely require dialysis, though it has been suggested in patients who have hypotension or extremely high serum levels.
    For patients who have ingested methanol, any vision disturbance is an indication for dialysis. Other methanol-poisoned patients with severe metabolic acidosis unresponsive to medical therapy or methanol levels greater than 50 mg/dL should also undergo dialysis.
    Ethylene glycol–poisoned patients should undergo dialysis on the basis of the severity of their metabolic acidosis and their renal function. If oliguric or anuric renal failure develops, hemodialysis must be initiated as ethylene glycol elimination in the presence of fomepizole depends exclusively on renal clearance.

13. **What are some common errors in the management of patients poisoned by toxic alcohols?**
The most common error is delay to diagnosis. This disease remains relatively uncommon and may not be considered until late in the clinical course. Also, as the ingestant is being metabolized, the osmolal gap will be closing, while the anion gap is opening. Therefore poisoned patients may be evaluated at a time when osmolal and anion gaps are normal or near normal. To avoid this mistake, patients with suspected toxic alcohol poisoning should undergo serial laboratory testing before dismissing the diagnosis from the differential. Delay to inhibiting ADH is another common mistake. When methanol or ethylene glycol ingestion is being considered, giving one empiric dose of fomepizole may prevent further harm to the patient for hours while the diagnosis is being formally made. Clinicians must also remember that both ethanol and fomepizole are removed via hemodialysis, and these should be replaced to maintain ADH inhibition. Finally, patients poisoned with methanol should undergo formal ophthalmologic evaluation initially and after treatment.

KEY POINTS: TOXIC ALCOHOL POISONING

1. Toxic alcohols are commonly found in numerous household products, with methanol commonly being a component of windshield washer fluid and ethylene glycol being a main ingredient in antifreeze.

2. Ingestion of toxic alcohols frequently starts with CNS depression, often associated with myocardial depression. Isopropanol may lead to hemorrhagic gastritis, methanol to visual disturbances, and ethylene glycol to renal failure, as well as eventual coma and death.

3. Toxic alcohol ingestions present with an elevated osmolal gap that closes with metabolism but develops an increasing anion gap in the case of methanol and ethylene glycol poisoning.

4. Fomepizole, a competitive ADH inhibitor, should be administered when toxic alcohol poisoning is suspected.

5. Patients with toxic alcohol poisonings and any vision disturbance, severe metabolic acidosis, or renal failure should undergo urgent hemodialysis.

BIBLIOGRAPHY

1. Brent J: Fomepizole for the treatment of pediatric ethylene and diethylene glycol, butoxyethanol, and methanol poisonings. Clin Toxicol (Phila) 48:401-406, 2010.

2. Brent J, McMartin K, Phillips S, et al: Methylpyrazole for Toxic Alcohols Study Group. Fomepizole for the treatment of ethylene glycol poisoning. N Engl J Med 340:832-838, 1999.

3. Glaser DS: Utility of the serum osmol gap in the diagnosis of methanol or ethylene glycol ingestion. Ann Emerg Med 27:343-346, 1996.

4. Jammalamadaka D, Raissi S: Ethylene glycol, methanol and isopropyl alcohol intoxication. Am J Med Sci 339:276-281, 2010.

5. Kraut JA, Kurtz I: Toxic alcohol ingestions: clinical features, diagnosis, and management. Clin J Am Soc Nephrol 3:208-225, 2008.

6. Mégarbane B, Borron SW, Baud FJ: Current recommendations for treatment of severe toxic alcohol poisonings. Intensive Care Med 31:189-195, 2005.

CHAPTER 81

POISONING BY CARDIOVASCULAR DRUGS

Aaron B. Skolnik, MD, and Susan R. Wilcox, MD

1. **What are the clinical effects of digoxin toxicity?**

   Although all nodal agents such as digoxin, β-blockers, and calcium channel blockers delay conduction through the atrioventricular node, each has distinct properties that can help distinguish one from the other in a poisoning or overdose. Because digoxin stimulates automaticity in addition to delaying nodal conduction, frequent junctional or ventricular ectopy may be seen. The appearance of *regularized* atrial fibrillation, actually an accelerated junctional rhythm, is classic for digoxin poisoning. Bidirectional ventricular tachycardia, though rare, is pathognomonic for digoxin toxicity. Patients poisoned with digoxin may also have characteristic noncardiac symptoms, including scotomata, color aberrancy, confusion, hallucinosis, vomiting, and diarrhea.

2. **What is the role of potassium in digoxin overdose?**

   Digoxin exerts its effects in part by binding to the sodium-potassium–adenosine triphosphatase (Na^+, K^+–ATPase) pump on cardiac cell membranes, competing with potassium for binding sites. When a patient taking digoxin has hypokalemia, the low serum potassium level decreases the competition for binding, leading to increased effects of digoxin and potentiating toxicity.

   Conversely, once a patient is digoxin toxic, the Na^+, K^+–ATPase pumps are thoroughly bound and inhibited. This leads to decreased uptake of potassium into the cells, with resultant increases in the serum potassium concentration. Therefore hypokalemia can potentiate toxic effects of digoxin, and hyperkalemia is a marker for digoxin toxicity.

3. **Should you avoid giving calcium to digoxin-poisoned patients?**

   Historically, the administration of calcium to treat hyperkalemia in patients with digoxin toxicity was contraindicated. The concern, based on case reports and animal models, was that resulting high levels of myocardial calcium could produce a *stone heart* by impairing diastolic relaxation and precipitate ventricular dysrhythmias. In recent years, a retrospective study suggests that patients who (possibly inadvertently) received intravenous calcium while digoxin toxic had no increase in mortality or any life-threatening dysrhythmias within 1 hour of administration, a finding supported by more recent animal models. Currently, avoiding calcium in suspected digoxin overdose is still recommended, although this may change in the future as data continue to emerge.

4. **What is digoxin immune Fab, and how is it used as an antidote?**

   Digoxin immune Fab is a preparation of antibody fragments with specificity for digoxin. It is produced by preparing monoclonal antibodies to digoxin and then chemically cleaving off the immunogenic Fc portion. Digoxin immune Fab binds to digoxin, as well as a number of naturally occurring cardiac glycosides, and neutralizes their effects on the myocardium and other end-organs. Dosing of Fab fragments is based on the amount required to neutralize the total body burden of digoxin, which can be estimated on the basis of the amount ingested or on the serum digoxin level, if available. In patients who have chronic toxicity, a smaller dose is sometimes administered initially to avoid fully reversing the therapeutic effects of digoxin while treating toxicity.

5. **How can the clinician distinguish between β-blocker and calcium channel blocker poisoning?**

β-Blockers and calcium channel blockers may be difficult to distinguish clinically from one another in poisoning. Both classes have similar negative effects on cardiac conduction, inotropy, and blood pressure. Also, many patients with cardiovascular disease are taking medications of both types. However, serum blood glucose determination can help tell the two drug classes apart. β-Blockers may cause and/or mask hypoglycemia by blocking stimulation of hepatic glycogenolysis and the release of pancreatic glucagon in response to falling serum glucose levels. Calcium channel blockers may prevent the release of insulin from the pancreas, a process normally mediated by influx of calcium through voltage-gated calcium channels. The ensuing hypoinsulinemia can lead to impressive hyperglycemia in patients without diabetes.

6. **What vasopressor(s) should be used in patients with hypotension poisoned by β-blockers or calcium channel blockers?**

No good prospective comparisons of the various vasopressors in these patients exist, but, in general, direct-acting mixed sympathetic agonists such as norepinephrine and epinephrine are preferred over dopamine. Part of dopamine's effect on blood pressure is exerted via the presynaptic release of norepinephrine and epinephrine, a calcium-mediated process that may be impaired in the setting of calcium channel antagonism. Furthermore, patients with either β-blocker or calcium channel blocker poisoning may be depleted of endogenous catecholamines by the time that treatment is initiated, and this may lead to a lack of response or tachyphylaxis to dopamine's indirect vasopressor effects.

7. **Is glucagon useful in poisoning with cardiovascular drugs?**

Glucagon is a first-line therapy in treatment of β-blocker toxicity. Glucagon works by stimulating increases in intracellular cyclic adenosine monophosphate, independent of the β-receptors. This, in turn, leads to activation of phosphokinase A (PKA), which phosphorylates a number of intracellular targets important to increase cardiac inotropy and chronotropy. Evidence also exists to support glucagon's use in cases of calcium channel blocker poisoning, as PKA activation also leads to increases in influx of calcium into poisoned myocytes. One dosing regimen consists of a 2- to 10-mg bolus, followed by continuous infusion at 1 to 5 mg/hour, intravenously.

8. **What is hyperinsulinemia-euglycemia therapy?**

Hyperinsulinemia-euglycemia therapy involves administration of high doses of insulin while maintaining a normal serum glucose level. It has become a widely used therapy in calcium channel blocker poisoning. Insulin is a positive inotrope but is obviously not used as such under normal circumstances given the high risk for hypoglycemia. In addition, stunned heart seems to develop some acute insulin resistance and prefers carbohydrate to its normal free fatty acid fuel. By offering large amounts of insulin with accompanying appropriate amounts of dextrose, it is thought that carbohydrate is directed to the energy-starved cardiac myocytes. Furthermore, insulin or glucose administration leads to shifts of potassium into the cells. The resulting relative hypokalemia prolongs phase II of the cardiac action potential, during which calcium influx occurs. This may also be beneficial in raising intracellular calcium levels and stimulating calcium release from the sarcoplasmic reticulum with subsequent increases in inotropy. This therapy may also benefit patients poisoned with β-blockers; however, additional caution against acute hypoglycemia must be exercised as those patients lack the hyperglycemia seen from calcium channel blockade.

9. **How does intravenous lipid emulsion (ILE) therapy work?**

ILE therapy uses intravenous administration of a 20% lipid emulsion as a polyvalent antidote to poisoning by lipophilic drugs. The emulsion, originally developed for parenteral nutrition, may act as a "sink" within the plasma for lipophilic drugs. In various animal models and human case reports, it appears that the drugs are sequestered within this lipid phase and thus prevented from acting at potential target organs, such as the brain and the heart. Other theoretical mechanisms of action include the provision of free fatty acid fuel to starving cardiac mitochondria and increasing cardiac myocyte calcium influx. A large and growing body of data demonstrates benefit of ILE for several types of cardiotoxic drugs, including sodium channel blockers, calcium channel blockers, and some β-blockers. Consider giving lipid emulsion to any poisoned patient who has ingested a highly lipid-soluble drug and has significant hemodynamic instability.

10. **What else can be done for the patient with cardiovascular collapse in whom other medical therapies are failing?**
Several heroic options are described for patients in whom maximal medical therapies are failing, though none have been validated prospectively. Potential therapies include intraaortic balloon counterpulsation, left ventricular assist, cardiopulmonary bypass, and extracorporeal membrane oxygenation.

KEY POINTS: POISONING BY CARDIOVASCULAR DRUGS

1. Distinguishing among digoxin, β-blocker, and calcium channel blocker toxicity may be difficult, but digoxin toxicity is often associated with other systemic symptoms, such as nausea, weakness, and visual changes.

2. If digitalis toxicity is suspected, prompt administration of digoxin immune Fab is indicated.

3. Glucagon remains a first-line treatment for β-blocker toxicity.

4. The treatments of choice for calcium channel blocker toxicity include high-dose, direct-acting vasopressors and hyperinsulinemia-euglycemia therapy.

5. ILE has shown benefit in treatment of poisonings for several types of cardiotoxic drugs and should be considered for any poisoned patient who has ingested a highly lipid-soluble drug with significant hemodynamic instability.

BIBLIOGRAPHY

1. Bauman JL, Didomenico RJ, Galanter WL: Mechanisms, manifestations, and management of digoxin toxicity in the modern era. Am J Cardiovasc Drugs 6:77-86, 2006.

2. Cave G, Harvey M: Intravenous lipid emulsion as antidote beyond local anesthetic toxicity: a systematic review. Acad Emerg Med 16:815-824, 2009.

3. Engebretsen KM, Kaczmarek KM, Morgan J, et al: High-dose insulin therapy in beta-blocker and calcium channel-blocker poisoning. Clin Toxicol (Phila) 49:277-283, 2011.

4. Levine M, Nikkanen H, Pallin DJ: The effects of intravenous calcium in patients with digoxin toxicity. J Emerg Med 40:41-46, 2011.

5. Manini AF, Nelson LS, Hoffman RS: Prognostic utility of serum potassium in chronic digoxin toxicity: a case–control study. Am J Cardiovasc Drugs 11:173-178, 2011.

6. Page C, Hacket LP, Isbister GK: The use of high-dose insulin-glucose euglycemia in beta-blocker overdose: a case report. J Med Toxicol 5:139-143, 2009.

7. Patel NP, Pugh ME, Goldberg S, et al: Hyperinsulinemic euglycemia therapy for verapamil poisoning: a review. Am J Crit Care 16:498-503, 2007.

8. Rothschild L, Bern S, Oswald S, et al: Intravenous lipid emulsion in clinical toxicology. Scand J Trauma Resusc Emerg Med 5:51, 2010.

9. Vivo RP, Krim SR, Perez J, et al: Digoxin: current use and approach to toxicity. Am J Med Sci 336:423-428, 2008.

CHAPTER 82

NEUROLEPTIC MALIGNANT SYNDROME

Jennifer M. Hall, DO, and James L. Jacobson, MD

1. **What is neuroleptic malignant syndrome (NMS)?**
   NMS is a rare, potentially fatal, idiosyncratic complication of antipsychotic medications. The usual presentation consists of four primary features:

   - Hyperthermia
   - Extreme generalized muscular rigidity
   - Autonomic instability
   - Altered mental status

   These features generally appear 24 to 72 hours after the administration of an antipsychotic; however, NMS can also occur with chronic use. Altered mental status is the first presenting symptom in 80% of NMS cases. Mean recovery time after antipsychotic discontinuation is 7 to 10 days but may be prolonged when long-acting depot antipsychotics are implicated. For other common features of NMS, see Box 82-1.

   BOX 82-1. SIGNS AND SYMPTOMS OF NEUROLEPTIC MALIGNANT SYNDROME

   Primary Features
   Hyperthermia
   Altered mental status
   Autonomic instability
   Extreme generalized rigidity (often called lead pipe rigidity)

   Other Common Features
   Laboratory evidence of muscle injury (elevated creatine kinase muscle fraction)
   Tremor
   Mutism
   Leukocytosis
   Labile hypertension (less often hypotension)
   Tachycardia
   Tachypnea
   Dysphagia
   Diaphoresis
   Sialorrhea
   Incontinence

   ---

2. **How common is NMS?**
   Recent data suggest that the incidence of NMS in patients treated with antipsychotics ranges between 0.01% and 0.02%. Previous estimates were as high as 3%; however, because of increased awareness, judicious antipsychotic use, and rapid recognition and treatment the incidence of NMS has declined.

3. **What is the mortality rate for NMS?**
   Despite the declining incidence of NMS, it remains a significant source of morbidity and mortality among patients receiving antipsychotics. The original description of NMS in 1968 estimated

a mortality rate as high as 75%, which subsequently declined to 20% to 30% in the 1980s. More recently, the U.S. Agency for Healthcare Research and Quality reports that, of an estimated 2000 cases diagnosed annually in hospitals, mortality rates approximate 10%. Cause of death in NMS is usually a result of cardiac or respiratory arrest (cardiac failure, infarction, arrhythmia, aspiration pneumonia, or pulmonary emboli), myoglobinuric renal failure, or disseminated intravascular coagulation.

4. **What is the pathogenesis of NMS?**
Although the pathophysiology of NMS is poorly understood, dopamine receptor antagonism in the basal ganglia, hypothalamus, and postganglionic sympathetic neurons is hypothesized to be the primary culprit. Given the complexity of NMS, it is also hypothesized that other neurotransmitter systems involving γ-aminobutyric acid (GABA), serotonin, and glutamate have a contributing role in initiation and progression of NMS.

5. **What are the diagnostic criteria for NMS?**
The diagnosis of NMS is a clinical diagnosis of exclusion in which the administration of an antipsychotic medication has occurred (usually 24-72 hours) before the onset of the syndrome.
    Research criteria in the American Psychiatric Association's *Diagnostic and Statistical Manual,* fourth edition (DSM-IV-TR), include the following:
    A. The development of severe muscle rigidity and elevated temperature associated with the use of neuroleptic medication.
    B. Two or more of the following: diaphoresis, dysphagia, tremor, incontinence, changes in level of consciousness ranging from confusion to coma, mutism, tachycardia, elevated or labile blood pressure, leukocytosis, and laboratory evidence of muscle injury.
    C. The symptoms in criteria A and B are not due to another substance or a neurologic or other general medical condition.
    D. The symptoms in criteria A and B are not better accounted for by a mental disorder.

6. **What is the differential diagnosis of NMS?**
NMS is a clinical diagnosis of exclusion; therefore central, systemic, and toxic causes of hyperthermia, rigidity, rhabdomyolysis, and altered mental status must be excluded. See Box 82-2.

7. **Are there specific laboratory findings for NMS?**
No laboratory findings are pathognomonic for NMS, but findings may support or confirm the diagnosis of NMS while excluding other systemic illnesses. Common laboratory abnormalities include the following:
- Elevated serum creatine kinase level of 1000 to 100,000 International Units/L
- Leukocytosis (10,000-40,000/mm^3)
- Elevated lactate dehydrogenase, alkaline phosphatase, and liver transaminase levels
- Electrolyte disturbances: hypernatremia, hyponatremia, hyperkalemia, hypocalcemia, hypomagnesemia, and hypophosphatemia
- Metabolic acidosis
- Myoglobinuric acute renal failure: proteinuria, elevated blood urea nitrogen and creatinine levels
- Low serum iron concentration

8. **Are special diagnostic tests or imaging studies useful?**
Cerebrospinal fluid values are usually normal, but nonspecific elevations in protein have been reported in 37% of cases. Electroencephalogram may show diffuse slowing without focal abnormalities. Magnetic resonance imaging and computed tomography results are typically normal, but cerebral edema has been reported in the setting of severe metabolic imbalances.

BOX 82-2. DIFFERENTIAL DIAGNOSIS OF NEUROLEPTIC MALIGNANT SYNDROME

Infectious
Meningitis or encephalitis
Postinfectious encephalomyelitis syndrome
Brain abscess
Sepsis

Psychiatric or Neurologic
Idiopathic malignant catatonia
Agitated delirium
Benign extrapyramidal side effects
Nonconvulsive status epilepticus
Structural lesions, particularly involving the midbrain

Toxic or Pharmacologic
Anticholinergic delirium
Salicyl poisoning
MH (inhalational anesthetics, succinylcholine)
Serotonin syndrome (monoamine oxidase inhibitors, triptans, linezolid)
Substances of abuse (amphetamines, hallucinogens)
Withdrawal from dopamine agonists, baclofen, sedative-hypnotics, and alcohol

Endocrine
Thyrotoxicosis
Pheochromocytoma

Environmental
Heat stroke

9. **Which agents have been implicated in the development of NMS?**
   First- and second-generation antipsychotic medications have been reported to
   cause NMS:
   - First-generation antipsychotics include chlorpromazine, fluphenazine, haloperidol,
     paliperidone, perphenazine, and thioridazine.
   - Second-generation antipsychotics include aripiprazole, clozapine, olanzapine, quetiapine,
     risperidone, and ziprasidone.
     NMS also has been reported with antiemetic medications such as domperidone,
   droperidol, metoclopramide, prochlorperazine, promethazine, and trimethobenzamide, as a
   result of their dopamine antagonism. Abrupt withdrawal of dopaminergic medications
   (amantadine or L-dopa) and GABA-ergic medications has been reported to precipitate an
   NMS-like reaction.

10. **What are risk factors for development of NMS?**
    Several clinical, systemic, and metabolic risk factors have been associated with NMS. Suggested
    risk factors include history of NMS, baseline electrolyte disturbances, preexisting abnormalities
    in CNS dopamine activity or receptor function, iron deficiency, acute medical or neurologic
    illness, dehydration, primary diagnosis of an affective disorder (particularly bipolar disorder and
    psychotic depression), comorbid substance use disorder, acute catatonia, psychomotor
    agitation, use of restraints, delirium, dementia, concurrent use of other psychotropic
    medications, high doses of antipsychotics, rapid dose escalation, and parenteral administration
    or depot formulations of antipsychotics.

Recent evidence also suggests genetic vulnerability as a potential risk factor for the development of NMS. Age and sex alone are not considered independent risk factors; however, younger male patients may be more likely to receive higher doses of antipsychotics to control combative behavioral symptoms, which results in their overrepresentation in NMS case studies. Although the variables listed above correlate with the risk of NMS, they are not practical in predicting the development of NMS.

11. **Does NMS have a genetic predisposition?**
Some evidence has suggested a familial predisposition in the development of NMS. The human dopamine D2 receptors gene (*DRD2*) contains a TaqI A restriction fragment polymorphism containing A1 and A2 alleles. Subjects with one or two A1 alleles have lower dopamine D2 receptor density and also have diminished dopaminergic activity and glucose metabolism in brain regions abundant with dopamine receptors. Previous studies have shown that the proportion of subjects with the A1/A1 or A1/A2 genotype was significantly higher in patients with NMS than in those without NMS. This polymorphism is not regarded as a specific marker as 60% of patients without NMS also have the A1 allele.

12. **What is the suggested management for NMS?**
Early recognition and diagnosis of NMS is crucial to provide appropriate and prompt treatment. The mainstay of management is to:
- **Stop the offending agent** and other psychotropic agents.
- **Provide the necessary supportive care.**

Volume resuscitation should be aggressive as most patients are severely dehydrated in the acute phase of the illness. Serial monitoring and correction of electrolyte and metabolic abnormalities are critical, and using alkalinized fluids or bicarbonate loading may be helpful in preventing renal failure. Hyperthermia should be addressed by using physiologic cooling measures because peak and duration of temperature elevation are predictive of morbidity and mortality. Markedly elevated blood pressures should be lowered pharmacologically, and heparin or low-molecular-weight heparin should be administered to prevent deep venous thrombosis. Patients should be closely monitored in the intensive care unit for complications including cardiorespiratory failure, acute renal failure, aspiration pneumonia, and coagulopathies that may require prompt intervention or additional supportive measures.

13. **What pharmacologic treatments are useful?**
In most cases, cessation of antipsychotic medications and supportive medical management are sufficient to reverse the symptoms of NMS. Several empirical off-label treatment approaches can be used in a case-by-case basis:
- Recent clinical reports suggest that benzodiazepines (oral or parenteral) may ameliorate symptoms of agitation or catatonia and hasten recovery of NMS. A trial of lorazepam 1 to 2 mg parenterally is a reasonable first-line intervention for patients with acute NMS.
- Dopamine agonists, such as amantadine and bromocriptine, have been reported to reverse Parkinsonian symptoms, hasten recovery, and decrease mortality rates when used alone or in combination with other pharmacologic agents. Amantadine is generally initiated at 200 to 400 mg/day orally in divided doses. Bromocriptine can be started at 2.5 mg two to three times a day orally with a maximum daily dose of 45 mg. Be advised that bromocriptine can worsen psychosis and hypotension, as well as precipitate vomiting, and must be used with caution. Abrupt discontinuation of bromocriptine can also precipitate rebound symptoms.
- Dantrolene may be useful in cases of extreme hyperthermia, rigidity, and hypermetabolism. Typical dosing is 1 to 2.5 mg/kg intravenously initially and may be increased to 1 mg/kg every 6 hours. Side effects include respiratory impairment and hepatic toxicity.
- Electroconvulsive therapy (ECT) has been shown to be effective when NMS symptoms are refractory to supportive care and pharmacologic treatment. The typical ECT course was six to 10 bilateral treatments with initial response expected in the first few treatments. During ECT

succinylcholine should be avoided in patients with rhabdomyolysis to prevent acute hyperkalemia and cardiovascular complications.

14. **Will NMS recur with subsequent use of neuroleptic medications?**
The likelihood of development of NMS after restarting antipsychotic medications once the original episode of NMS has resolved is approximately 30%. To reduce risk of recurrence allow at least 2 weeks of recovery before restarting any antipsychotic medications. It is best to choose a low-dose or low-potency antipsychotic and titrate gradually while closely monitoring for subtle signs or symptoms of NMS.

15. **Is there any way to prevent NMS?**
No. When clinically indicated, reducing antipsychotic dose, avoiding parenteral or depot antipsychotic formulation, avoiding rapid dose escalation, and minimizing other risk factors (e.g., dehydration) may decrease the overall risk for development of NMS. Given that catatonia may be a strong risk factor for the development of NMS, antipsychotics should be avoided in patients with catatonia, if possible, for whom benzodiazepines may be effective treatment.

16. **Are there alternatives to antipsychotic medications for acutely psychotic patients?**
A number of alternative treatment options exist for acutely psychotic patients. Benzodiazepines may help reduce agitation in a hyperactive psychotic patient and may potentially lower the absolute dose of antipsychotic needed to manage symptoms. When the primary diagnosis is an affective disorder, aggressive treatment with mood stabilizers or antidepressants is indicated. However, if psychotic symptoms are present in the context of an affective disorder, antipsychotic medications are usually necessary. ECT is also a viable nonpharmacologic alternative for treatment of manic psychosis, depressive psychosis, and catatonia.

17. **Are there alternatives to antipsychotic medications for patients with chronic psychotic illnesses?**
In chronic psychotic disorders (e.g., schizophrenia, schizoaffective disorder, delusional disorder) there may be no alternative treatment to antipsychotic medications that adequately manages symptoms. Hence, if NMS has occurred caution is advised on rechallenging with a different class of antipsychotics. Special attention must be paid to second-generation antipsychotics and treatment of reversible risk factors. Efforts must also be made to minimize polypharmacy when clinically indicated.

18. **Are malignant hyperthermia (MH) and NMS related?**
MH and NMS have similar clinical presentations but different pathophysiologies. MH develops after exposure to inhalation anesthetics, such as halothane, and depolarizing muscle relaxants, such as succinylcholine. MH is characterized by diffuse muscle rigidity, fever, hypermetabolism, elevated serum creatine kinase level, hyperkalemia, tachycardia, hypoxemia, metabolic acidosis, and myoglobinuria. MH is caused by a genetic defect in a sarcoplasmic reticulum calcium channel protein, which results in excessive calcium release into skeletal muscle after exposure to triggering medications. Susceptibility to MH is diagnosed by the muscle contracture test. In susceptible people, excessive contractions occur in muscle strips exposed to varying concentrations of halothane and caffeine. Family studies and muscle contracture testing indicate that patients with one of the disorders do not appear to be at increased risk for the other.

19. **What is serotonin syndrome?**
Serotonin syndrome is a rare but potentially fatal syndrome characterized by the triad of altered mental status, autonomic dysfunction, and neuromuscular abnormalities, which is thought to result from central and peripheral hyperserotonergic activity. The similarity between serotonin syndrome and NMS often leads to misdiagnosis. Serotonin syndrome can develop after the addition of a serotonergic medication (e.g., monoamine oxidase inhibitor, tricyclic antidepressant, selective

serotonin reuptake inhibitor) to a regimen that already includes serotonin-enhancing drugs or after overdoses of serotonergic drugs. The presentation is heterogeneous, but common clinical features include confusion, agitation, restlessness, myoclonus, hyperreflexia, diaphoresis, tachycardia, blood pressure fluctuation, shivering, tremor, diarrhea, incoordination, and fever.

20. **How is serotonin syndrome differentiated from NMS?**
Serotonin syndrome follows a history of exposure to serotonergic medications, not antipsychotic medications. Compared with NMS, the observed tremor and myoclonus in serotonin syndrome are more prominent than muscle rigidity. Fever is present less often and the laboratory abnormalities seen in NMS (e.g., elevated creatine phosphokinase level) are usually absent in serotonin syndrome. Discontinuation of serotonergic medications and supportive measures are most important during treatment of serotonin syndrome. As with NMS, the role of pharmacologic treatment in serotonin syndrome is unclear. Lorazepam, propranolol, and cyproheptadine may be effective in symptomatic management.

Acknowledgments

The authors gratefully acknowledge the contribution of Ryan Peirson, MD, and Erin Fellner, MD, for revisions to a previous edition.

KEY POINTS: NEUROLEPTIC MALIGNANT SYNDROME

1. NMS can develop with exposure to any antipsychotic medication—acute or chronic use.

2. When considering the differential diagnosis, the physician should pay particular attention to recent changes in doses and psychotropic polypharmacy.

3. Other agents, such as antiemetic agents, can also cause NMS.

4. Treatment is primarily supportive.

5. In most cases, the most important factors that distinguish NMS from serotonin syndrome are hyperthermia and rigidity.

BIBLIOGRAPHY

1. Addonizio G, Susman VL: Neuroleptic Malignant Syndrome: A Clinical Approach, St. Louis, Mosby, 1991.

2. Boyer EW, Shannon M: The serotonin syndrome. N Engl J Med 352:1112-1120, 2005.

3. Brown T, Frian S, Mareth T: Pathophysiology and management of the serotonin syndrome. Ann Pharmacother 30:527, 1996.

4. Pope HG Jr, Keck JR, McElroy SL: Frequency and presentation of neuroleptic malignant syndrome in a large psychiatric hospital. Am J Psychiatry 143:1227-1232, 1986.

5. Rosebush P, Stewart T: A prospective analysis of 24 episodes of neuroleptic malignant syndrome. Am J Psychiatry 146:717-725, 1989.

6. Shalev A, Heresh H, Munitz H: Mortality from neuroleptic malignant syndrome. Clin Psychiatry 50:18-22, 1989.

7. Strawn J, Keck P, Caroff S: Neuroleptic malignant syndrome. Am J Psychiatry 164:870-876, 2007.

8. Suzuki A, Kondo T, Otani K, et al: Association of the TaqI A polymorphism of the dopamine D(2) receptor gene with predisposition to neuroleptic malignant syndrome. Am J Psychiatry 158:1714-1746, 2001.

9. Velamoo V: Neuroleptic malignant syndrome: recognition, prevention and management. Drug Safety Concept 1:73-82, 1998.

CARE OF THE CRITICALLY ILL PREGNANT PATIENT

CHAPTER 83

Stephen E. Lapinsky, MBBCh, MSc, FRCPC

1. **What are normal arterial blood gas findings in pregnancy?**

   Pregnancy results in increased ventilation because of elevated carbon dioxide production, as well as an increase in respiratory drive mediated largely by progesterone. These changes cause a low arterial partial pressure of carbon dioxide, at about 30 mm Hg by term. Plasma bicarbonate is decreased to 18 to 21 mEq/L, maintaining the arterial pH in the range of 7.40 to 7.45. Alveolar to arterial oxygen tension difference is usually unchanged, and the mean arterial PO_2 is generally about 100 mm Hg.

2. **How does pregnancy affect hemodynamics?**

   Cardiovascular physiology changes significantly during pregnancy, characterized by an increase in blood volume, an elevation in cardiac output, and a small decrease in blood pressure, resulting in a number of changes in the normal hemodynamic values in the third trimester (Table 83-1). In the supine position, the gravid uterus may produce significant mechanical obstruction of the inferior vena cava, reducing venous return and resulting in a decrease in cardiac output and hypotension. Maternal syncope or fetal distress may result. Supine hypotension syndrome may be avoided by positioning the patient on her left side, or at least with the right hip slightly elevated.

TABLE 83-1. EFFECT OF LATE PREGNANCY ON PULMONARY ARTERY CATHETER MEASUREMENTS

PARAMETER	CHANGE FROM NONPREGNANT VALUE
Central venous pressure	No change
Pulmonary capillary wedge pressure	No change
Cardiac output	30%-50% increase
Systemic vascular resistance	20%-30% decrease
Pulmonary vascular resistance	20%-30% decrease
Oxygen consumption	20%-40% increase
Oxygen extraction ratio	No change

3. **What factors affect oxygen delivery to the fetus?**

   Oxygen delivery to the fetus is determined by the maternal arterial oxygen content, uterine blood flow, and placental function. A number of factors may adversely affect blood flow to the uteroplacental vasculature, which is normally maximally vasodilated. A decrease in maternal cardiac output reduces fetal oxygenation. The maternal response to hypotension does not favor the uterus, and catecholamines (endogenous or exogenous) may aggravate fetal hypoxia by producing uterine vasoconstriction. Uterine blood flow may also be reduced by maternal alkalosis and during uterine contractions.

4. **Are there any special concerns to be considered when inserting an endotracheal tube in a critically ill pregnant patient?**

The upper airway in pregnancy may be edematous and friable because of the effects of estrogen and aggravated in the presence of preeclampsia because of excessive edema. The nasal route should be avoided, and a smaller endotracheal tube may be necessary. Because of the reduced functional residual capacity and increased oxygen consumption, hypoxemia will develop in a pregnant woman more rapidly than in nonpregnant, critically ill patients during intubation. Intubation should be carried out by the most skilled person available.

Note: The incidence of failed intubation is eight times higher in the obstetric population than in nonobstetric patients.

5. **Describe the principles of management of severe preeclampsia.**

The most important aspect of management is the well-timed delivery of the fetus. Supportive treatment involves fluid management, control of hypertension, and prevention of seizures:

- Patients with preeclampsia usually have volume depletion and require volume expansion, but excessive fluid administration may result in pulmonary or cerebral edema.
- Hypertension is managed to prevent maternal vascular damage and does not alter the pathologic process of preeclampsia. Commonly used regimens include small boluses of hydralazine (5–10 mg intravenous [IV]), boluses or infusion of labetalol, or oral calcium antagonists.
- Seizure prophylaxis should be undertaken with magnesium sulfate, with use of a loading IV bolus of 4 g over a 20-minute period followed by an infusion of 2 to 3 g/hour. Toxic levels (usually >5 mmol/L) can cause respiratory muscle weakness and cardiac conduction defects and are usually seen in a patient with associated renal failure. Hypocalcemia is common and should not be treated unless symptomatic. The effects of magnesium sulfate (toxic as well as therapeutic) can be reversed with IV calcium.

6. **What are the clinical features of the HELLP syndrome?**

The HELLP syndrome (i.e., **h**emolysis, **e**levated **l**iver enzyme levels, and **l**ow **p**latelet count) is a complication of preeclampsia characterized by multiorgan dysfunction. The diagnostic features are the presence of thrombocytopenia, elevated liver enzymes, and a microangiopathic hemolytic anemia. The patient may present with epigastric or right upper quadrant pain, nausea, and vomiting, with or without other features of preeclampsia. Significant hemorrhage may result from the thrombocytopenia. A rare but catastrophic consequence of HELLP syndrome is hepatic hemorrhage, manifesting with sudden shock or acute abdominal pain.

7. **What is acute fatty liver of pregnancy?**

This is an uncommon complication of pregnancy manifesting with acute fulminant hepatic failure during the third trimester. Increased awareness of this condition has resulted in earlier diagnosis, with milder liver disease and an improved outcome. The clinical presentation is with malaise, anorexia, and vomiting, followed by abdominal pain and jaundice. The patient deteriorates rapidly with acute liver failure manifested by coagulopathy, hemorrhage, renal failure, and encephalopathy. Management requires urgent delivery of the fetus and supportive therapy for fulminant hepatic failure.

8. **How does amniotic fluid embolism present?**

Amniotic fluid embolism is a rare but catastrophic obstetric complication usually associated with labor, delivery, or other uterine manipulations. The typical presentation is a sudden onset of severe dyspnea, hypoxemia, and cardiovascular collapse, which may be accompanied by seizures. The maternal presentation is accompanied or preceded by sudden fetal distress. A significant portion of patients die acutely within the first hour. Survivors commonly have a disseminated intravascular coagulopathy and acute respiratory distress syndrome. Management is supportive, and the prognosis for mother and fetus is poor.

9. **What are the causes of acute respiratory failure in pregnancy?**
The pregnancy-specific diseases (Box 83-1) include amniotic fluid embolism, pulmonary edema resulting from the use of tocolytic therapy or related to preeclampsia, or peripartum cardiomyopathy. Although pregnant patients may have diseases similar to those in nonpregnant patients, pregnancy may increase the risk for venous thromboembolism, acute asthmatic attacks, and gastric aspiration. Changes in immune function in pregnancy predispose to increased severity of influenza pneumonitis (particularly H1N1), varicella pneumonia, as well as coccidioidomycosis infections. Of interest is an association between the presence of pyelonephritis and the development of acute respiratory distress syndrome in pregnancy.

BOX 83-1. CAUSES OF RESPIRATORY FAILURE IN PREGNANCY

Pregnancy-Specific Factors
Amniotic fluid embolism
Tocolytic pulmonary edema
Preeclampsia complicated by
  pulmonary edema
Pulmonary edema due to peripartum
  cardiomyopathy
Obstetric sepsis with ARDS
Trophoblastic embolism

Risk Increased by Pregnancy
Venous thromboembolism
Asthma
Pulmonary edema due to preexisting heart
  disease
Aspiration
ARDS associated with pyelonephritis
Pneumonia (e.g., varicella, influenza)

ARDS, Acute respiratory distress syndrome.

---

10. **Does the management of pulmonary embolism differ in pregnant patients?**
Investigation of suspected pulmonary embolism is similar to that in nonpregnant patients, beginning with duplex ultrasound. False-positive results may occur because of venous occlusion by the enlarged uterus. Ventilation-perfusion scanning and chest computed tomography angiogram can be carried out with a low risk for fetal radiation exposure. Unfractionated heparin and low-molecular-weight heparin are safe and effective in pregnancy. Warfarin is usually avoided because of the risk for embryopathy with first-trimester use and central nervous system abnormalities and bleeding risk with second- and third-trimester use. Thrombolysis has been used successfully during pregnancy and the postpartum period but should be limited to life-threatening situations.

11. **What are the risks of radiologic procedures in pregnancy?**
Estimated fetal radiation exposure varies from <0.01 rad (0.1 mGy) for a chest radiograph to about 2 to 5 rad (20-50 mGy) for pelvic computed tomography (Table 83-2). Abdominal shielding with lead and use of a well-collimated x-ray beam can effectively reduce exposure. The potential adverse effects of fetal exposure to radiation are oncogenicity, teratogenicity, and neurologic compromise. A twofold increased risk for childhood leukemia may occur with relatively low-dose radiation (2-5 rad). Teratogenicity is thought to require greater than 10 rad exposure; microcephaly and hydrocephaly have been described after exposure of 10 to 150 rad. Although radiation exposure in pregnancy carries definite risks, the likelihood of any adverse effect is about 0.1% per rad. The perception of risk by patients, family members, and physicians is often vastly higher than the actual risk.

12. **How do the manifestations of severe trauma differ in pregnant patients?**
Trauma is a common cause of morbidity and mortality in pregnancy. The increased blood volume allows the mother to tolerate moderate blood loss, but this higher volume of hemorrhage necessitates more rapid IV fluid replacement. Fetal or amniotic injury may cause

TABLE 83-2. ESTIMATED FETAL RADIATION EXPOSURE DURING RADIOGRAPHIC STUDIES WITH APPROPRIATE SHIELDING

RADIOGRAPHIC STUDY	ESTIMATED FETAL DOSE (RAD)
Chest radiograph	0.001
Ventilation-perfusion scan	0.012-0.050
CT scan of head	0.001
CT scan of chest	0.05-0.1
CT scan of abdomen or pelvis	2-5

CT, Computed tomography.

maternal coagulopathy, which can exacerbate hemorrhage. Occult uterine or retroperitoneal hemorrhage always should be considered. Deceleration injuries may precipitate placental abruption, after 20 weeks gestation. In the third trimester, abdominal trauma usually involves the uterus. Other intraabdominal organs may be compressed in the upper abdomen, and injury in this area may cause significant organ damage. Physical signs of peritonism may be reduced because of stretching of the peritoneum. The bladder is at increased risk for injury as it extends above the pubis, and it should be remembered that some degree of ureteric dilation is normal in pregnancy. The fetus is at risk for morbidity resulting from maternal hypotension, direct injury, fetomaternal hemorrhage, or placental abruption.

13. **Is management of cardiac arrest different for pregnant patients?**
Management of cardiac arrest in pregnancy follows usual protocols with some modifications. Because cardiopulmonary resuscitation in the supine position may cause impaired venous return, the uterus should be manually displaced to the left, or alternatively a left lateral tilt position should be achieved with a firm wedge. IV access should be established above the diaphragm, and a difficult airway should be anticipated. No change in pharmacologic therapy is necessary, and drugs should not be withheld when clinically indicated. Consider calcium administration if the mother was receiving a magnesium sulfate infusion. Electrical defibrillation may be performed in pregnancy after removal of any fetal monitoring device. When initial attempts at resuscitation have failed, perimortem cesarean section should be considered if the fetus is at a viable gestation and no return of spontaneous circulation has occurred within 4 minutes. Ideally, delivery should occur within 5 minutes of cardiac arrest for optimal fetal outcome. Cesarean section has been reported to reverse aortocaval compression and allow successful resuscitation of both the mother and infant.

14. **How is massive obstetric hemorrhage managed?**
Supportive measures include adequate venous access, rapid volume replacement, and blood product support. A dilutional coagulopathy should be anticipated. Ultrasound allows assessment of the uterine cavity for retained placental fragments that necessitate uterine curettage. Uterine massage and intramuscular methylergonovine (which should be avoided in the presence of hypertension) are used for uterine atony. Oxytocin infusion is administered in a dose higher than that used for augmentation of labor (e.g., 20-40 units in 1000 mL normal saline solution at a rate up to 0.1 units/minute). Prostaglandin analogs are effective; carboprost

tromethamine is given by intramuscular or intramyometrial injection in a dose of 0.25 mg, which may be repeated. Intrauterine balloon tamponade is increasingly being used as an early adjunctive intervention. Prohemostatic drugs such as tranexamic acid and recombinant factor VIIa may be used, but good evidence is lacking. If bleeding remains uncontrolled, more invasive approaches may be required. These include radiologic arterial embolization and surgical exploration to repair lacerations, to reduce blood flow by arterial ligation, or, if necessary, to remove the uterus.

15. **Which cardiac lesions present problems in pregnancy?**
The changes in cardiovascular physiology in pregnancy may result in decompensation in a patient with preexisting heart disease, because of the rise in cardiac output reaching a peak at about 28 weeks, 40% to 50% above baseline levels. Cardiac lesions limiting cardiac output (e.g., mitral stenosis, aortic stenosis) therefore present a significant risk for precipitating pulmonary edema or hypotension in the third trimester. This risk is particularly high during labor because of the tachycardia and volume shifts associated with delivery. Pulmonary hypertension is associated with significant morbidity and mortality because of the limitation of cardiac output and the inability to respond to postpartum fluid shifts. Congenital heart abnormalities are generally better tolerated in pregnancy unless complicated by pulmonary hypertension. Pregnancy may also predispose the patient to the development of cardiomyopathy.

16. **Does termination of pregnancy improve the outcome of a critically ill mother?**
An understanding of the physiologic effects of late pregnancy may suggest that delivery of the pregnant patient with respiratory failure will improve the mother's condition. However, this has not been found to be correct; some improvement in oxygenation may occur, but without improvement in positive end-expiratory pressure requirements or compliance. If the fetus is at a viable gestation and is at risk because of severe maternal hypoxia, there may be a benefit from removing the fetus from the intrauterine environment. However, delivery is usually not appropriate solely in an attempt to improve maternal oxygenation or ventilation. Consultation by a neonatologist is essential to evaluate fetal risks or benefits, and obstetric indications should determine the mode of delivery. Although cesarean section allows more rapid delivery, the increased physiologic stress may be associated with a higher mortality in critically ill patients.

KEY POINTS: CAUSES OF ADMISSION TO THE INTENSIVE CARE UNIT BECAUSE OF PREGNANCY-SPECIFIC CONDITIONS

1. Respiratory failure can result from amniotic fluid embolism, tocolytic pulmonary edema, preeclampsia, or peripartum cardiomyopathy.

2. Hepatic dysfunction may occur, including acute fatty liver of pregnancy or HELLP syndrome.

3. Renal failure (e.g., preeclampsia or HELLP syndrome, idiopathic postpartum renal failure) may prompt admission to the ICU.

4. Hypertensive complications in the form of preeclampsia may occur.

5. Pregnant patients might require intensive care because of hemodynamic compromise, such as obstetric hemorrhage or obstetric sepsis.

BIBLIOGRAPHY

1. ANZIC Influenza Investigators and Australasian Maternity Outcomes Surveillance System : Critical illness due to 2009 A/H1N1 influenza in pregnant and postpartum women: population based cohort study. BMJ 340:c1279, 2010.

2. Clark SL, Cotton DB, Lee W, et al: Central hemodynamic assessment of normal term pregnancy. Am J Obstet Gynecol 161(6 Pt 1):1439-1442, 1989.

3. Conde-Agudelo A, Romero R: Amniotic fluid embolism: an evidence-based review. Am J Obstet Gynecol 201:445.e1-e13, 2009.

4. Georgiou C: Balloon tamponade in the management of postpartum haemorrhage: a review. BJOG 116:748-757, 2009.

5. Lapinsky SE: Cardiopulmonary complications of pregnancy. Crit Care Med 33:1616-1622, 2005.

6. Lapinsky SE, Kruczynski K, Slutsky AS: State of the art: critical care in the pregnant patient. Am J Resp Crit Care Med 152:427-455, 1995.

7. Lowe SA: Diagnostic radiography in pregnancy: risks and reality. Aust N Z J Obstet Gynaecol 44:191-196, 2004.

8. Marik PE, Plante LA: Venous thromboembolic disease and pregnancy. N Engl J Med 359:2025-2033, 2008.

9. Mercier FJ, Bonnet MP: Use of clotting factors and other prohemostatic drugs for obstetric hemorrhage. Curr Opin Anaesthesiol 23:310-316, 2010.

10. Munnur U, de Boisblanc B, Suresh MS: Airway problems in pregnancy. Crit Care Med 33(10 Suppl):S259-S268, 2005.

11. Oxford CM, Ludmir J: Trauma in pregnancy. Clin Obstet Gynecol 52:611-629, 2009.

12. Ratnapalan S, Bentur Y, Koren G: "Doctor, will that x-ray harm my unborn child?" CMAJ 179:1293-1296, 2008.

13. Siu SC, Colman JM: Heart disease and pregnancy. Heart 85:710-715, 2001.

14. te Raa GD, Ribbert LS, Snijder RJ, et al: Treatment options in massive pulmonary embolism during pregnancy: a case-report and review of literature. Thromb Res 124:1-5, 2009.

15. Tomlinson MW, Caruthers TJ, Whitty JE, et al: Does delivery improve maternal condition in the respiratory-compromised gravida? Obstet Gynecol 91:108-111, 1998.

16. Vanden Hoek TL, Morrison LJ, Shuster M, et al: Part 12: cardiac arrest in special situations: 2010 American Heart Association Guidelines for Cardiopulmonary Resuscitation and Emergency Cardiovascular Care. Circulation 122 (18 Suppl 3):S829-S861, 2010.

ETHICS

Alexandra F.M. Cist, MD

1. **Where is the locus of decision-making authority in the intensive care unit (ICU) regarding end-of-life care?**
   The process of *shared decision making* locates the responsibility between the patient or surrogate and the caregivers, thus aiming to respect the autonomy of the patient or surrogate, as well as the beneficent and nonmaleficent intentions of clinicians. The surrogate's responsibility is to express a substituted judgment, that is, to convey an understanding of *what the patient would want*. If the patient's preferences are unknown, the best interests standard is used—a presumed understanding of *what a reasonable person would want*. The attending physician has the ultimate responsibility in deciding on a reasonable plan.

2. **Describe the *shared decision-making* paradigm.**
   The key to the paradigm is communication. The process includes meetings to allow the caregivers to learn about the patient's values and goals, as well as to allow the patient or surrogates to learn about the patient's condition and about the interventions that might be reasonable to use, in light of the patient's values and prognosis. The dynamic process allows for reassessment and readjustment of plans, befitting the patient's changing condition and goals.

3. **What if clinicians disagree with the patient or surrogate?**
   After additional clarification of values, goals, prognosis, and treatment options, both parties can try to persuade the other and/or seek common ground. A time-limited trial of continued therapy, followed by reassessment, may bring about resolution. Consider additional informational or supportive services from other persons and clinicians who know the patient well, second-opinion consultations, social services, chaplaincy, ethics consultation, psychiatry, and/or palliative care.

4. **What if the clinical team believes some interventions are futile?**
   There is no agreement on a precise definition of *futility*, yet clinicians clearly recognize when they are in a futility quagmire. The term comes up when "the team" thinks some interventions are ineffective, overburdensome, wasteful, and harmful, but they are faced with a family that demands that "everything be done" to prolong the patient's life. Tensions increase, and people get edgy, cagey, defensive, or elusive in reaction to conflict, mistrust, and power struggles. If the procedures described in answers 2 and 3 have been tried and are unsuccessful, then the clinicians might:
   - Attempt to transfer the patient to another caregiver
   - Seek adjudication (possibly to replace the surrogate)
   - Override the patient or surrogate and decide to withhold or withdraw life-sustaining treatment (LST), with institutional support plus forewarning to the surrogate so that she or he has the opportunity to seek legal action.

   Some institutions have developed a procedural "Futility Policy" or "Conflict Resolution Policy" that outlines a stepwise process for a committee to review the perspectives of the team and family before making a recommendation regarding the LSTs in question.

5. **What if there is no surrogate decision maker for the patient?**
Gather as much information as possible about the person to best understand the patient's story, lifestyle, functional status, and values. Consider contacting neighbors, work colleagues, clergy, community members, primary care providers, and other outside health care providers. Use the information gained to approximate a *substituted judgment* to supplement the "best interests" standard to make decisions. Ethics consultation and advice from hospital legal counsel may be required to complement the plans devised by the attending physician and ICU team.

6. **How prevalent is conflict in ICUs, and what are some of the sources and consequences of conflict?**
The prevalence of conflict in ICUs is high, up to 70%, and most conflicts are rated as "severe," "dangerous," and/or "harmful." Yet 70% of conflicts are perceived to be preventable. Conflicts occur among staff members and between staff and families. Sources of conflict include personal animosity, mistrust, poor communication, and troublesome end-of-life care. Concerns about end-of-life care include lack of psychological support, suboptimal decision making, suboptimal symptom control, treatment futility, and disregard for family and patient preferences. The perception that *futile* care is being rendered is strongly associated with moral distress, especially among nurses. Conflict contributes to moral distress, burnout, and job turnover. A high level of burnout has been measured in intensivists. This is disturbing, because burnout is characterized by a detached or dehumanizing attitude and a lack of concern for others.

7. **List means to lessen or resolve moral distress and intrateam or team-family conflicts.**
Proactive family meetings, open visitation, family presence on rounds, respect of cultural norms, routine unit-level meetings, staff debriefings, collaborative care, spiritual support, relieving patients' distressing symptoms, ethics consultation, and integration of palliative care principles and practices into the ICU.

8. **What will an ethics consultant want to know when a consultation is requested?**
An ethics consultant will want to know:
- Who is this person?
- What are the issues that led to the consultation?
- What is the diagnosis?
- What is the prognosis (likelihood of best case and worst case scenarios)?
- Use of LSTs
- Code status and patient's decision-making capacity or identification of surrogate
- Understanding of patient's values and advance directives
- Identification of others who know the patient well
- Involvement of social worker and pastoral care
- Current goals of care (and areas of agreement and disagreement regarding these)
  Equipped with this information, the consultant may then help:
- Clarify areas that need elucidation
- Identify the ethical issues
- Help discern a good process for arriving at decisions
- Identify relevant guidance from clinical policy, literature, and/or case precedent
- Help formulate justifications for courses of action
- Help caregivers address moral distress

9. **Have *ethics interventions* been shown to reduce ICU length of stay or improve other ICU quality indicators?**
Yes. A large multicenter randomized controlled trial of ethics consultation in the ICU showed mitigation of treatment conflicts and, for nonsurvivors, reduced ICU length of stay by 1.44 days, days of ventilator use by 1.7 days, hospital length of stay by 2.95 days, and costs (range of

savings: $3000 to $40,000). These reductions were achieved without altering mortality between the intervention and control groups. Proactive multidisciplinary family meetings and palliative care interventions reduce length of stay and improve communication, symptom control, and quality of dying in the ICU.

10. **What are overlapping common concerns of critical care and palliative care?**
Optimizing the care of critically ill patients, whether living or dying, requires competencies shared by critical care and palliative care clinicians. These competencies include symptom management, communication and relational skills, interdisciplinary collaboration, prognostication, shared decision making, defining goals of care and setting plans, and providing psychosocial and spiritual assessment and support. Given high ICU mortality rates, the provision of excellent end-of-life care, including managing withholding and withdrawing LSTs, is a critical care priority.

11. **What is the difference between acceptable end-of-life care in the ICU and active euthanasia?**
Good end-of-life care in an ICU involves focusing on comfort (physical, psychosocial, and spiritual) while withholding or withdrawing LST from a patient who is expected to die in the near term of his or her underlying condition. The focus—the intent—is on achieving relief of distressing symptoms and on forgoing burdensome therapies. Occasionally, patients with life-threatening conditions survive treatment withdrawal (11%).
   On the other hand, the goal of active euthanasia is the death of the patient. Direct euthanasia is illegal in the United States and in most other countries. Practitioners of active euthanasia usually also intend the comfort of the patient, but one of the means they use to achieve that goal is by killing the patient. Many persons note an ethical difference between "letting die" and "killing."

12. **Why is the administration of narcotics and sedatives during the terminal withdrawal of LSTs not considered active euthanasia?**
It is not considered active euthanasia when doses are titrated "to effect," with the intent being the relief of particular distressing symptoms. The foreseen but unintended consequences of lowering blood pressure or slowing respirations are ethically acceptable if it is clear, from the titrating of doses, that the intention is palliation. Such dosing is justifiable under the "doctrine of double effect." However, if doses are given with the intent of causing death, then that would be considered active euthanasia (killing).

13. **My patient has a "Do Not Attempt Resuscitation" status yet needs surgery. Do we need to make him or her "full code" for the operating room?**
No or maybe. It depends on what the patient's goals of care are, what he or she hopes to achieve from the surgery, and what the patient has delineated as unacceptable outcomes. Thus a discussion must occur before the surgery in the context of discussing the expected benefits and risks of the procedure in light of the patient's condition, values, hopes, fears, and reasonable goals.

14. **Are there acceptable *crisis standards of care* under conditions of true scarcity, such as during an influenza pandemic or a major disaster?**
Crisis standards of care or *altered* standards of care have been proposed by various state organizations to address possibilities of severe medical shortages. Yet such altered standards, and clinical guidelines based on them, have not been widely promulgated or accepted for several reasons:
- The relative newness of attention to the problem
- Denial that shortages could reach crisis proportions
- Lack of consensus regarding prognostic scoring systems
- Concerns about legal liability
- Uneasiness about shifting from a focus on individual patients to a focus on populations of patients

Though a utilitarian goal of "the greatest good for the greatest number" makes intuitive sense to many (and already influences our allocation of organs for transplantation), clinicians accustomed to usual standards of care may find it difficult to withhold a treatment from a person in front of them for that treatment to be allocated to another person. Furthermore, the public will not easily accept being deprived of treatments to which it previously felt entitled.

CONTROVERSIES

15. **Should physicians be able to withhold cardiopulmonary resuscitation (CPR) from patients against the wishes of patients and surrogates?**

    Pro: Physicians should be able to refrain from attempting CPR when they think CPR would not be beneficial—even against the express demands of the patient/surrogate—because it is an affront to human dignity and professional integrity to perform such an aggressive brutal intervention under conditions when it is deemed to be inappropriate. Not only would the attempt be ineffective, but it is likely to be wasteful and harmful too.

    Con: Given that (1) medical decision making is rooted in respecting the autonomous choices of patients, (2) prognostication is an inexact science, and (3) physicians frequently underestimate the value patients might place on seemingly undesirable states of being, physicians should not be allowed to override the stated preferences of patients or surrogates regarding something so crucial as attempting resuscitation. Providers should respect a family's belief that one should fight for life. A family's convictions and psychological aftereffects take priority over the providers' transitory interest in the patient's welfare.

16. **Do *universal* or *bundled* consent forms for commonly performed procedures in the ICU improve patient-centered decision making?**

    Yes: The need to perform invasive and possibly life-saving procedures can arise suddenly in the course of routine intensive care. Yet it is often difficult to find someone quickly who can give consent to these procedures (such as intubation, mechanical ventilation, placement of arterial and venous lines, blood transfusions, bronchoscopy, chest tube placement). Therefore it is efficient and respectful of patient-centered care to discuss a whole *bundle* of procedures at the time of patient arrival in the ICU and then to request voluntary consent, allowing the patient or surrogate to learn about and decide about the whole *big picture* that comprises the complexities of critical care.

    No: The tenets of good informed consent include the patient's or surrogate's capacity to understand information, giving and receiving adequate information, and the opportunity for the patient or surrogate to voluntarily consent or refuse the treatment being proposed. These are nearly impossible to achieve in a one-time orientation discussion to the ICU when a patient or surrogate may be under a great deal of undue influence to agree with whatever is being offered. The value of autonomous well-informed consent should not be sacrificed for the sake of efficiency. Clinicians should engage in the informed consent process for each invasive procedure. If they cannot locate a surrogate and if they believe performing the procedure would be consistent with the patient's values and goals and in the patient's best interests, the "emergency exception" to informed consent allows clinicians to proceed with that procedure.

17. **Once family consent has been given to proceed with organ donation, using donation after cardiac death (DCD) guidelines, may interventions be done before death to improve organ viability?**

    Pro: Patients and families who consent to organ donation want to optimize the outcome of that gift. If the patient is bound to die anyway, the viability of his or her precious organs becomes paramount. It is respectful to the patient *as a donor* to optimize the value of his or her gift by intervening before death is declared to preserve the organs for transplantation.

Con: The preceding argument suggests that organs could be taken from persons before it is really known whether they would die of treatment withdrawal. Adhering strictly to the "dead donor rule" is respectful of patients *as persons*, upholds the integrity of clinicians as healers and patient advocates, and upholds the public's trust in the medical profession. DCD guidelines make it clear that the critical care team is caring for the dying person. Not until the person dies does the transplant team begin to care for the dead donor.

KEY POINTS: INTRATEAM OR TEAM-FAMILY CONFLICTS

ICU communication tasks are like procedures and require training to gain expertise in:
1. Eliciting patients' values and goals

2. Listening and expressing empathy

3. Framing recommendations regarding care plans

4. Translating goals of care into treatment plans and code status orders

5. Disclosing errors to patients and/or surrogates

BIBLIOGRAPHY

1. Arbour R: Clinical management of the organ donor. AACN Clin Issues 16:551-580, 2005.

2. Azoulay E, Timsit JF, Sprung CL, et al: Prevalence and factors of intensive care unit conflicts: the Conflicus Study. Am J Respir Crit Care Med 180:853-860, 2009.

3. Curtis JR: Point: the ethics of unilateral "Do Not Resuscitate" orders: the role of informed assent. Burt RA: Counterpoint: is it ethical to order "Do Not Resuscitate" without patient consent? Chest 132:748-751, 2007.

4. Curtis JR, Treece PD, Nielson EL, et al: Integrating palliative and critical care: evaluation of a quality improvement intervention. Am J Resp Crit Care Med 178:269-275, 2008.

5. Davidson JE, Powers K, Hedayat KM, et al: Clinical practice guidelines for support of the family in the patient-centered intensive care unit: American College of Critical Care Medicine Task Force 2004-2005. Crit Care Med 35:605-622, 2007.

6. Fine RL: Point: the Texas Advance Directives Act effectively and ethically resolves disputes about medical futility. Truog RD: Counterpoint: the Texas Advance Directives Act is ethically flawed. Rebuttals from Drs Fine and Truog. Chest 136:963-973, 2009.

7. Institute of Medicine: Consensus Report. Guidance for Establishing Crisis Standards of Care for Use in Disaster Situations. Washington, D.C., National Academies Press, 2009.

8. Jonsen AR, Siegler M, Winslade WJ: Clinical Ethics: A Practical Approach to Ethical Decisions in Clinical Medicine, 4th ed. McGraw-Hill, New York, 1998.

9. Lanken PN, Terry PB, DeLisser HM, et al, on behalf of the ATS End-of-Life Care Task Force: An official American Thoracic Society clinical policy statement: palliative care for patients with respiratory diseases and critical illnesses. Am J Respir Crit Care Med 177:912-927, 2008.

10. Luce JM: End-of-life decision making in the intensive care unit. Am J Respir Crit Care Med 182:6-11, 2010.

11. Schneiderman LJ, Gilmer T, Teetzel HD, et al: Effect of ethics consultations on nonbeneficial life-sustaining treatments in the intensive care setting: a randomized controlled trial. JAMA 290:1166-1172, 2003.

12. Thompson BT, Cox PN, Thijs LG, et al: Challenges in end-of-life care in the ICU: statement of the 5th International Consensus Conference in Critical Care: Brussels, Belgium, April 2003: executive summary. Crit Care Med 32:1781-1784, 2004.

13. Truog RD, Campbell ML, Curtis JR, et al: Recommendations for end-of-life care in the intensive care unit: a consensus statement by the American Academy of Critical Care Medicine. Crit Care Med 36:953-963, 2008.

14. White D, Curtis JR, Wolf LE, et al: Life support for patients without a decision maker: who decides? Ann Intern Med 147:34-40, 2007.

CHAPTER 85

PALLIATIVE CARE

Ursula McVeigh, MD, and Allan Ramsay, MD

1. **What are the elements of palliative care that are important in the care of critically ill patients?**
   Palliative care is support provided by an interdisciplinary team that focuses on relief of suffering in the physical, emotional, and spiritual domains of health. In the intensive care unit (ICU), coincident with aggressive disease-directed therapies, a multidisciplinary team provides this support to patients and families as they face what can be an emotional and tumultuous journey. This care is provided by physicians, nurses, social workers, and chaplains.
   Specific elements of palliative care in the ICU:
   - **Communication skills** including running a family meeting, delivering bad news, empathetic communication, eliciting patient preferences, and discussing goals of care
   - **Decisional support** for patients or surrogates
   - **Prognostication**
   - **Symptom management**
   - **Psychosocial and spiritual support** for patients, family, and staff
   - **Decisions to withhold or withdraw** life-supporting therapies based on goals of care
   - **End-of-life care**

2. **What are the goals of the ICU family conference?**
   - Exchange medical information between the patient and family and the medical team
   - Engage in complicated medical decision making, frequently with surrogate decision makers
   - Provide emotional support to families

3. **What are the steps of a family meeting?**
   - Preparation
     □ Invite invested participants; plan agenda, time, and space.
   - Premeeting
     □ Discuss among team members to reach consensus on goals of the meeting, medical condition, prognosis, and treatment options.
   - Introductions
     □ Identify family, team members, roles, and goals of the meeting.
   - Perceptions
     □ Ask family members what they hope to have addressed in the meeting.
     □ Ask what the family members know about the illness and what they expect or hope for.
   - Information
     □ Provide medical information about condition, prognosis, and treatment options.
     □ Explain aspects of surrogate decision making.
   - Exploration
     □ Elicit questions, concerns, and values, and explore how these influence decisions.
   - Recommendation
     □ Provide medical guidance and recommendations based on stated goals and values and the clinician's professional knowledge and experience.
   - Summary
     □ Review medical plan, next steps, and follow-up.
     □ Document.

4. **What components of the family meeting are associated with better outcomes?**
    Research has identified specific elements of family meetings that are associated with increased quality of care, decreased negative psychological symptoms during bereavement, and improved family satisfaction with communication. See Box 85-1.

BOX 85-1. IMPORTANT COMPONENTS OF INTENSIVE CARE UNIT FAMILY CONFERENCE

- Hold family meeting within 72 hours of ICU admission.
- Listen more, speak less.
  - A higher proportion of time providers spend listening to families rather than speaking is associated with increased family satisfaction with the meeting.
- Make empathetic statements acknowledging the difficulty of:
  - Having an ill loved one
  - Surrogate decision making
  - Impending loss of loved one
- Make statements of nonabandonment and support for the decisions made.
- Explore patient values and treatment preferences.
- Explain principle of surrogate decision making.
- Reassure that the patient will be comfortable and not suffer.

Modified from Curtis J, White D: Practical guidance for evidence-based ICU family conferences. Chest 134:835–843, 2008.

---

5. **What communication tool has been shown to be beneficial in improving communication in the ICU family meeting?**
    Incorporating the **VALUE** mnemonic has been shown to significantly reduce family symptoms of anxiety, posttraumatic stress disorder, and depression measured 3 months after the patient's death:
    - **V**alue what the family says.
    - **A**cknowledge expressed emotions.
    - **L**isten.
    - **U**nderstand the patient as a person; ask questions that elicit this information.
    - **E**licit family questions.

6. **What is empathetic communication?**
    There are two elements of communication: one involves primarily sharing cognitive or informational content, and the other involves statements that refer or respond to emotional states. Expressing clinical empathy is an essential part of therapeutic communication and has been shown to strengthen the physician-patient relationship, improve patient satisfaction, and enhance treatment adherence. For example:
    - Family member: *John was just mowing his lawn last week. How can this be happening?*
    - Cognitive-informational response: *Unfortunately, John's underlying lung disease makes him susceptible to infections, and pneumonia can come on very fast and severe.*
    - Empathetic response: *I can't imagine how hard it is for you to see John so sick and for this to happen so fast.*
      The **NURSE** mnemonic can be used to express clinical empathy:
    - **N**ame the emotion
      - *A lot of people in your situation would feel angry.*
      - *It sounds like this has been frustrating.*
    - **U**nderstand
      - *I can't begin to understand how hard this is.*
      - *It is hard to be in a situation like this.*

- ☐ *It sounds like you are weighing wanting to be sure everything that can help has been tried against wanting to be sure that if she is at the end of her life she does not suffer.*
- ■ Respect
  - ☐ *We have a lot of respect for how you are so present and supportive of your loved one.*
  - ☐ *I can tell you have been taking very good care of your mother.*
- ■ Support
  - ☐ *You will not be going through this alone; we are here to help you.*
  - ☐ *Based on what you have told us, we think you are making the right decision for your loved one.*
- ■ Explore
  - ☐ *What is the most difficult part of this for you?*
  - ☐ *Can you help me understand...?*

7. **What is a goals-of-care discussion?**
   The patient or surrogate decision maker and the medical team need to have a shared understanding of the patient's goals of medical therapy. This involves the physician providing a medical prognosis and possible outcomes. With this information the patient or surrogate can provide information on his or her treatment preferences. The patient values can then be the primary driver of the goals of medical care, weighing burdens of treatments with likelihood of positive benefits or outcomes. Goals are fluid and can change on the basis of the medical condition and prognosis. Initial ICU goals of care have a curative or restorative intent. As survival becomes unlikely goals may transition to comfort and allowing a peaceful death. It is essential to establish the goals of treatment before discussing new treatment options.

8. **What are the steps in a goals-of-care discussion?**
   - ■ Elicit patient and family understanding of the illness and prognosis.
   - ■ Provide information about prognosis and likely outcomes, including best case scenarios and worst possibilities.
   - ■ Explore what constitutes quality of life, what is most important to the patient.
   - ■ Explore what one is hoping for.
   - ■ Explore situations or outcomes that would not be desired or acceptable.
   - ■ Summarize values and goals, and advise on a medical plan to best achieve these goals:
     - ☐ *I hear you say these are your values and goals, ... these elements of quality of life are important to you, ... this is what you are hoping for, ... and these are the situations where quality of life would not be acceptable. Based on this, the medical plan I think would best achieve these goals is. ...*

9. **What questions can be asked of a surrogate decision maker to help elicit patient values and goals?**
   - ■ *Help me understand how things were for your father before he got this sick. What did he enjoy doing? What things are most important to the quality of his life? Is there an outcome or quality of life that would not be acceptable to him?*
   - ■ *If your loved one were here listening to this conversation, what would she be thinking or saying?*
   - ■ *Did your loved one ever talk about his wishes if he were to get sicker and were nearing the end of his life?*
   - ■ *Has your father ever known anyone in this situation? Did he express what he would want for himself after seeing that?*

10. **How can dying and end-of-life planning be discussed?**
    When recovery is not possible, it can be hard to find the words to convey this in a clear, supportive, and empathetic manner. This involves delivering bad news and reframing hope for what goals can be accomplished.

- When prognosis is ambiguous but concerning:
  - □ *If despite our best efforts Jane's illness continues to worsen, I am concerned that her life may come to an end. While we hope and work for the best, we should also have a plan in place to provide the best care possible if she is at the end of her life.*
  - □ *Unfortunately we do know that at some point your life will come to an end from this illness. As hard as it is to discuss, putting a plan in place for the care that you want at the end of your life is very important for both you and your family. It is part of getting your affairs in order so if you are unable to speak for yourself at the end of your life, your family can feel comfortable that they know your wishes.*
- When further disease-directed therapies are not helpful and death is expected:
  - □ *I wish we had better treatments for your condition. . . .*
  - □ *Although it is not in our control that your life will come to an end from this illness, what we do have control over is what happens between now and then.*
  - □ *Although we can't control the disease, we can treat the symptoms of the disease and help you feel as comfortable as possible with the time that you have. And when you are at the end of your life, we can assure that you pass peacefully, comfortably, and on your own terms.*

11. **How should the clinician discuss stopping or withholding life-supporting treatments when recovery is not possible?**
When goals transition to providing comfort at end of life and the decision is made to stop life-prolonging treatments, family members can feel burdened that decisions they make are the cause of death. They also may worry that stopping or withholding treatments may cause suffering. It is important for providers to be clear that it is the underlying disease that causes death. Clinicians must be ready to provide support for the decisions made and take time to explain in detail how comfort is assessed and maintained.

Unfortunately we have reached the point where John cannot recover, and his life is coming to an end no matter what decisions we make today. Would it be helpful for you to know how we would care for John if the goals of his medical care shifted to focus on comfort and allowing a peaceful death? That would mean that we would aggressively treat pain, anxiety, and shortness of breath with medications like morphine, that once we were sure he was comfortable we would remove the breathing machine, and that we would allow his life to come to an end from his lung disease as peacefully as possible.

12. **What is spirituality?**
The 2009 Consensus Conference on Quality of Spiritual Care defined spirituality as *"the aspect of humanity that refers to the way individuals seek and express meaning and purpose and the way they experience their connectedness to the moment, to self, to others, to nature, and to the significant or sacred." (p. 887).*

13. **How should the clinician discuss spiritual and religious issues?**
Spiritual support is a fundamental pillar of palliative care. Most patients want their physicians to ask about their religious and spiritual beliefs, though many practitioners feel uncomfortable doing so. Some patients and families may base their preferences for starting or stopping treatment on their religious or spiritual beliefs.

The **FICA** tool has been shown to be an effective and feasible framework for a clinical spiritual assessment:
- **F**aith, belief, meaning
  - □ *Is spirituality, faith, or religion an important part of your life?*
  - □ *Do you have spiritual beliefs that help you cope with stress?*
  - □ *What gives your life meaning?*
- **I**mportance and influence
  - □ *What role do your beliefs play in your health care decisions?*

- **C**ommunity
  - ▫ *Are you part of a religious or spiritual community?*
  - ▫ *Is this helpful to you and how?*
- **A**ddress in care
  - ▫ *How would you like your health care providers to use this understanding of your beliefs as they care for you?*

14. **What are indicators of spiritual or existential distress?**
    When facing a life-threatening illness, individuals can experience great distress in psychological, spiritual, and existential domains. Indicators of existential or spiritual suffering include statements of meaninglessness, hopelessness, and guilt (see Box 85-2). Helpful responses to spiritual or existential distress are statements that acknowledge the pain, provide a nonjudgmental supportive presence, and bear witness to the patient and family. Hospital chaplains are specially trained to provide this type of therapeutic support irrespective of specific faith or belief system of the patient or family member.

BOX 85-2. MOST COMMON ELEMENTS OF SPIRITUAL SUFFERING AT THE END OF LIFE

Sense of disconnection from self, others, phenomenal world, ultimate meaning
Crisis of meaning; an existential vacuum; inability to find solace or peace
Preoccupation with future or past
Sense of victimization
A need to be in control

Modified from Mount B, Boston P, Cohen S: Healing connections: on moving from suffering to a sense of well-being. J Pain Symptom Manage 33:372–388, 2007.

---

15. **What is the role of the social worker in the ICU?**
    Social workers play a critical role in supporting patients and families in the ICU by providing communication, counseling, and assisting with practical needs. When coordinating a family meeting, they can help families anticipate what will be discussed, help clarify their questions for the medical team, and provide emotional support during and after the meeting.

KEY POINTS: PALLIATIVE CARE

1. Quality critical care requires highly coordinated team collaboration to attend to the physical, psychosocial, and spiritual needs of patients and families facing a life-threatening illness.

2. Only discuss treatment choices after the goals of medical care have been established.

3. Most patients and families want their physician to ask about their faith and support systems.

4. Statements expressing meaninglessness, hopelessness, remorse, regret, abandonment, or loss of control can signify spiritual or existential suffering. When these statements are present, the clinician should consider referral to a chaplain or pastoral care professional.

BIBLIOGRAPHY

1. Back A, Arnold R, Tulsky J, et al: Medical Oncology Communication Skills Training Learning Module 2: Giving Bad News, 2002: http://depts.washington.edu/oncotalk/learn/modules/Modules_02.pdf. Accessed May18, 2012.

2. Borneman T, Ferrell B, Puchalski CM: Evaluation of the FICA tool for spiritual assessment. J Pain Symptom Manage 40:163-173, 2010.

3. Curtis J, White D: Practical guidance for evidence-based ICU family conferences. Chest 134:835-843, 2008.

4. End of Life/Palliative Education Resource Center (EPERC) at the Medical College of Wisconsin: www.eperc.mcw.edu/EPERC. Accessed May18, 2012.

5. Hudson P, Quinn K, O'Hanlon B, et al: Family meetings in palliative care: multidisciplinary clinical practice guidelines. BMC Palliat Care 7:12, 2008.

6. Lautrette A, Darmon M, Megarbane B, et al: : A communication strategy and brochure for relatives of patients dying in the ICU. N Engl J Med 356:469-478, 2007.

7. McCormick AJ, Engelberg R, Curtis JR: Social workers in palliative care: assessing activities and barriers in the intensive care unit. J Palliat Med 10:929-937, 2007.

8. Palliative care and end of life care: www.fletcherallen.org/palliative. Accessed May18, 2012.

9. Puchalski C, Ferrell B, Virani R, et al: Improving the quality of spiritual care as a dimension of palliative care: the report of the Consensus Conference. J Palliat Med 12:885-904, 2009.

CHAPTER 86

ORGAN DONATION

Benjamin T. Suratt, MD, and Kapil Patel, MD

1. **Who governs the rules and regulations for organ donation?**
   - The Organ Procurement and Transplantation Network (OPTN) is a system for operating and monitoring the unbiased allocation, through established medical criteria, of organs donated for transplantation and maintaining a recipients' waiting list (including the listing and delisting of recipients).
   - The United Network for Organ Sharing (UNOS) is a nonprofit organization awarded the contract by the Department of Health and Human Services in 1986 to implement the OPTN.
   - Organ Procurement Organizations (OPO) serve specific regions in the country for clinical services including working with hospital staff to maintain donor-organ function, working with UNOS to match donor organs with recipients, coordinating organ recovery surgery, and giving compassionate and professional support to donors' families.

2. **Who can be a potential organ donor?**
   Potential for organ or tissue donation has few absolute contraindications: human immunodeficiency virus infection, active hepatitis B virus infection, active visceral or hematologic neoplasm, or active bacterial infection, with no age limitation. Appropriateness for donation is assessed when the occasion arises. The majority of cases that are considered for organ donation occur within the intensive care unit (ICU). Despite severe organ shortage, no set universal protocol exists for organ donation. It is at the discretion of the intensivist to consider cases for organ donation. If a case is considered, then the next step is to notify the local OPO, which will then gather data and discuss the critical care management with the regional organ donation specialist, usually an intensivist.

   The general rule for the possibility for organ donation is that there should be no evidence of end-organ damage (e.g., acute tubular necrosis, myocardial depression, or pneumonia), with the final decision per the accepting transplant center.

3. **Which organs can be donated?**
   - Organs: kidney, heart, lung, liver, pancreas, and the intestines. Of note, combined organ transplantations (kidney-pancreas, heart-lung, other transplant) can be performed.
   - Tissue: corneas, the middle ear, skin, heart valves, bones, veins, cartilage, tendons and ligaments.

4. **What is the current standard for organ donation?**
   Organ donation is possible in patients who are declared brain dead. New brain death guidelines have been published (see Box 86-1). Despite efforts to promote organ donation, an enormous shortage of available organs for transplant continues to exist. As a result, efforts have been undertaken to expand the settings in which organs may become available (i.e., donation after cardiac death (DCD); see later). See Boxes 86-2, 86-3, and 86-4 and Tables 86-1 and 86-2.

5. **What is organ DCD?**
   DCD is considered in patients who have expressed a wish to donate organs and who sustain severe, irreversible brain injury short of meeting criteria for brain death (see earlier), but in whom withdrawal of life support is planned. In this case, organ procurement occurs immediately

---

BOX 86-1. BRAIN DEATH CRITERIA

- Unresponsiveness or coma
- Core body temperature ($\geq 32°$ C)
- Absence of cerebral motor responses to pain in all extremities
- Absence of brainstem reflexes, that is, pupillary, oculocephalic (*doll's eyes*), vestibuloocular (cold calorics), corneal, gag, and cough reflexes
- Apnea test (see Boxes 86–2, 86–3, and 86–4)
- Exclusion of conditions that may confound clinical assessment of brain death, that is, metabolic or endocrine abnormality or drug intoxication

---

BOX 86-2. PREREQUISITES FOR PERFORMING THE APNEA TEST

Core body temperature $\geq 36.5°$ C
Systolic blood pressure ≥ 90 mm Hg (may use intravenous fluids or dopamine to achieve)
Eucapnia ($PaCO_2$ approximately 40 mm Hg) if possible
Normoxemia ($PaO_2 \geq 200$ mm Hg) if possible (typically 10 minutes at an FiO_2 of 1.0 will achieve)
FiO_2, Fraction of inspired oxygen.

BOX 86-3. APNEA TEST

1. Patient is disconnected from the ventilator.
2. Oxygen cannula is placed at the level of carina, and 100% oxygen is delivered at a rate of 6 L/min.
3. Patient is observed for respiratory movements (e.g., chest or abdominal excursions).
4. Arterial PaO_2, $PaCO_2$, and pH are measured after approximately 8 minutes.
5. Patient is reconnected to the ventilator.

BOX 86-4. INTERPRETATION OF APNEA TEST RESULTS

Confirmatory results: No respiratory movements witnessed with resultant arterial PCO_2 ≥ 60 mm Hg (or 20 mm Hg increase in PCO_2 over pretest baseline)
Contradictory results: Any evidence of respiratory movements (regardless of PCO_2 level)
Inconclusive results: No respiratory movements and $PCO_2 \leq 60$ mm Hg. Apnea test may be repeated within 10 minutes.
If cardiovascular or pulmonary instability occurs during the test (i.e., systolic blood pressure ≤ 90 mm Hg, dysrhythmia, or arterial oxygen desaturation), arterial blood gas value is immediately obtained, and the patient is reconnected to the ventilator. Alternative confirmatory testing to determine brain death (see Table 86–1) is then performed at the discretion of physician.

---

after death as declared by cardiopulmonary criteria. For organs to be successfully recovered for transplantation, death must occur between 60 and 120 minutes (depending on the institution) of withdrawal of life support. If death does not occur within the preset time frame, the patient is brought back to the ICU and provided comfort care measures without organ procurement.

TABLE 86-1. CONFIRMATORY BRAIN DEATH TESTING

ELECTROENCEPHALOGRAPHY	NO ELECTRICAL ACTIVITY FOR A PERIOD OF 30 MINUTES
Cerebral angiography	No intracerebral filling at the level of the carotid bifurcation or circle of Willis Patent external carotid circulation
Transcranial Doppler sonography	No diastolic or reverberating flow Systolic-only or retrograde diastolic flow Small systolic peaks in early systole
Somatosensory evoked potential	Bilateral absence of response to medial nerve stimulation
Cerebral scintigraphy (technetium Tc 99m brain scan)	No uptake of radionuclide in brain parenchyma (*hollow skull phenomenon*)
Magnetic resonance imaging	Not yet determined

TABLE 86-2. COMPARISON OF DONATION AFTER BRAIN DEATH AND DONATION AFTER CARDIAC DEATH

	DONATION AFTER BRAIN DEATH	DONATION AFTER CARDIAC DEATH
Cause of illness (e.g., anoxic, trauma, stroke)	Severe irreversible brain injury Does meet criteria of brain death	Severe irreversible brain injury Does not meet criteria of brain death
Organ procurement process	Physician (non–transplant team) declares brain death	Family elects withdrawal of life support
	Referral to OPO	Referral to OPO
	Await OR time for organ procurement	Withdrawal of life support in the OR or ICU
	Transplant team retrieves organs	Physician (non–transplant team) declares cardiac death
	Heart, lungs, kidneys, liver, pancreas, and/or intestines are transplantable	Transplant team waits 5 minutes after cardiac death is declared before procuring organs
		Transplant team retrieves organs
		Kidney, pancreas, and liver are generally transplantable

Modified from Organ Donation After Cardiac Death. Madison, Wis., University of Wisconsin Organ Procurement Organization, 2009.
OR, Operating room.

The most commonly procured organs in DCD are kidney, liver, and pancreas. The time period required between cardiac arrest and the initiation of organ retrieval is 5 minutes. This time frame leaves other organs susceptible to ischemia. Currently very limited data support the procurement of lungs after cardiac death. However, recent data on DCD lung transplantation from the Toronto Lung Transplant Program have demonstrated acceptable outcomes.

6. **Is donation after cardiac death ethically appropriate?**
A national conference on donation after cardiac death in 2005 concluded that it is "an ethically acceptable practice of end-of-life care, capable of increasing the number of deceased-donor organs available for transplantation." This national conference affirmed the ethical propriety of DCD as not violating the "dead donor rule."

7. **What is the dead donor rule?**
"Organ transplantation has been guided by the overarching ethical requirement known as the 'dead donor rule,' which simply states that patients must be declared dead before the removal of any vital organs for transplantation."

8. **What are some of the statistics for organ donation and transplantation?**
   - Every 11 minutes, a patient is added to the transplant waiting list (e.g., lung, kidney, heart).
   - Every day, approximately 75 patients receive an organ transplant. Yet every day approximately 20 patients die waiting for a transplant.
   - As of May 4, 2009, the percentage of recipients who were still living 5 years after solid organ transplantation was as follows:
     - Kidney: 69.3%
     - Heart: 74.9%
     - Liver: 73.8%
     - Lung: 54.4%
   - In 2008, 60% of living donors were women. Sixty percent of deceased donors were men.
   - In 2008, 67% of all deceased donors were white, 16% were black, 14% Hispanic, and 2.5% Asian.
   - As of November 2010, patients on the national waiting list were 45% white, 29% black, 18% Hispanic, and 6% Asian.
   - In 2007 (the most recent data), nearly 2.5 million people died in the United States. Yet only 8085 of these people donated their organs.
   - OPTN data show a progressive increase in the rate of organ recovery from DCD donors (844 DCD donors in 2008 compared with 268 in 2003).
   - Currently, more than 86 million people in the United States have indicated a wish to become a donor. Although impressive at first, this still will not be nearly enough to address the growing demand (see Fig. 86-1).

KEY POINTS: ORGAN DONATION

1. All patients with impending brain death or withdrawal of care should be screened for the possibility of organ donation.

2. To diagnose brain death all confounding factors must be excluded.

3. DCD is an ethically acceptable manner in which terminally ill patients can be considered for organ donation.

4. The gap between those patients awaiting transplants and those donating organs is widening exponentially—the vast majority of those on the transplant list will die waiting.

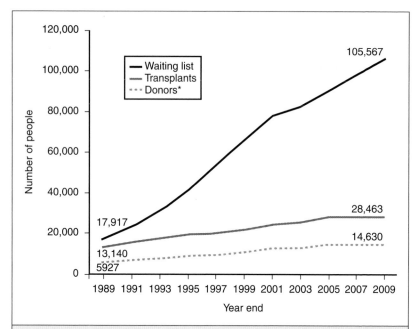

Figure 86-1. Over the past two decades, the gap between the number of patients waiting for a transplant and the number receiving a transplant has continued to widen. The substantial difference between the number of donors and the number of patients waiting for a transplant is one factor that contributes to waiting time from listing to transplantation. *Data include deceased and living donors. (From the University of Wisconsin Organ Procurement Organization: organdonor.gov/aboutStatsFacts.asp.)

WEBSITES

Association of Organ Procurement Organizations: aopo.org
Organ Procurement and Transplantation Network: optn.transplant.hrsa.gov
United Network for Organ Sharing: unos.org
U.S. Government Information on Organ and Tissue Donation and Transplantation: organdonor.gov

BIBLIOGRAPHY

1. Bernat JL, D'Alessandro AM, Port FK, et al: Report of a national conference on donation after cardiac death. Am J Transplant 6:281-291, 2006.
2. Cypel M, Sato M, Yildirim E, et al: Initial experience with lung donation after cardiocirculatory death in Canada. J Heart Lung Transplant 28:753-758, 2009.
3. Truog RD, Miller FG: The dead donor rule and organ transplantation. N Engl J Med 359:674-675, 2008.
4. Wijdicks EF, Varelas PN, Gronseth GS, et al: Evidence-based guideline update: determining brain death in adults. Neurology 74:1911-1918, 2010.

INTENSIVE CARE UNIT ORGANIZATION, MANAGEMENT, AND VALUE

Daniel Yagoda, MPH, Ulrich H. Schmidt, MD, PhD, and J. Perren Cobb, MD

CHAPTER 87

1. **How should intensive care units (ICUs) be organized?**

   Patient outcomes are best in units that provide care by multidisciplinary teams, including intensivists (physician ICU experts), nurses, respiratory and physical therapists, and clinical pharmacists and nutritionists. Our experience is that optimal team performance is critically dependent on open communication across disciplines, demonstrating respect and a willingness to listen to all. Experienced team leaders (typically provided by an intensivist director partnering with a nursing director) are required to create and maintain this environment while optimizing resource utilization. Important aspects of medical director involvement include bed triage, monitoring the system to ensure patient safety, and creation of a safety culture that promotes best practice. Several studies have shown decreased rates of complications and death and better resource utilization in units where patient care is managed primarily by ICU teams (*closed* ICUs). This may be due to better care for the critically ill provided by intensivist-led multidisciplinary teams and better coordination and fewer communication errors in closed units. Critical care educational programs should incorporate a management training component that addresses each of these issues.

   Hospitals with more than one ICU typically create an infrastructure that promotes better communication, usually in the form of a critical care committee. These committees are composed of ICU medical directors, nursing directors, and representatives from hospital administration, clinical pharmacy, respiratory therapy, physical therapy, and clinical nutrition, all of whom participate in the care of critically ill patients. The critical care committee often provides the necessary venue for multidisciplinary, open dialog to identify threats to patient safety and quality care. The committee also creates a mechanism to improve operations, including creation of guidelines and protocols to decrease unwanted variation in ICU clinical practice. The authority and responsibilities of these committees varies significantly across hospitals: many simply provide a convenient monthly venue to improve communication, whereas others are authorized and funded to plan strategically on behalf of the hospital.

   In our largest hospitals with multiple ICUs (e.g., academic medical centers), efficiency and cost pressures motivate evolution of the critical care committee to a hospital-based, center-type infrastructure. Center status within the hospital organization provides the opportunity to support a more robust and mission-specific governance across all ICUs, including standing committees for critical care clinical operations, patient safety, education, research, and outreach. The operational assumption for center leadership is that the center, on behalf of the hospital, has the authority to override directors of individual ICUs when the consensus is that patient safety and quality are at risk. A center without the appropriate level of authority may be ineffective at strategic planning and leading change that best serve the community (for example, lack of ICU care coordination and patient flow can increase waiting times in the emergency department and postanesthesia care units). In addition, resources are typically allocated better with this model, as it is much more efficient to redesign care and patient flow, establish informatics platforms, adhere to care protocols, and buy equipment working collaboratively across ICUs.

2. **What is the Leapfrog Group, and how has it affected ICU models of care?**

   The Leapfrog Group was created in 1998 by a large group of employers to leverage purchasing power to improve the quality and affordability of health care. The initial focus was on reducing preventable medical errors in hospitals. On the basis of available evidence, the group concluded that the quality of ICU care is particularly important in avoiding errors and improving outcomes in hospitalized patients. Subsequent Leapfrog Group recommendations included an ICU physician staffing standard:

- Intensivists are present during daytime hours and provide clinical care exclusively in the ICU.
- When not present on site or via telemedicine, intensivists return pages within 5 minutes and arrange for a qualified practitioner to reach ICU patients within 5 minutes.

The relative mortality reductions of 15% to 60% seen with this model are substantial. The mechanism for better outcomes is not well understood but appears to be related to multidisciplinary, team-based care led by intensivists. These recommendations motivated significant changes in intensivist staffing, because Leapfrog purchasers (businesses) collectively exert considerable influence over hospitals and their payers to staff ICUs appropriately. Nevertheless, in 2010, only 34% of hospitals responding to the national Leapfrog survey were fully compliant with this standard. Widespread adoption of the intensivist model is constrained by the limited number of intensivists, higher personnel costs, and perceived threats to physician autonomy.

3. **What can be done to address the shortage of intensivists and critical care nurses in the United States: Regionalization and telemedicine?**
Despite the overwhelming evidence that intensivist-led, team-based ICU care improves outcomes and decreases costs, only 50% of critically ill or injured patients, at most, have access to high-intensity intensivist staffing in the United States. This supply–demand inequity will continue, especially in underresourced areas, because of the high costs of intensivist staffing and a growing, nationwide shortage of intensivists.

Similarly, a nationwide shortage of critical care nurses threatens optimal outcomes. The traditional ratio of nurse to patients in an ICU for adults is 1:2 or 1:1 depending on disease severity. Excess mortality has been noted with nurse-to-patient ratios of 1:3 or greater. According to 2010 data from the American Association of Critical Care Nurses, approximately 40% of critical care nurses are aged 50 years or above. As this older cohort retires from practice, the available supply of ICU nurses will be insufficient. These staffing problems will be exacerbated by the aging of the baby boomers and the associated increased demand for intensive care. Therefore other organizational approaches will be required to optimize outcomes, in addition to efforts to grow the clinical workforce.

Increasing the availability of advanced nurse educational programs, such as those that train acute care nurse practitioners, is one solution. Regionalization of ICU care is another option, matching ICU patient needs to available resources, classifying providing institutions as level 1, 2, or 3 on the basis of the availability of procedural expertise and the intensity of ICU physician staffing.

A second, complementary approach leverages advances in telemedicine and systems engineering, using real-time data exchange, advanced informatics, and videoconferencing to optimize interactions among patients, caregivers, and families across the street or across great distances. Engineering health by optimizing use of regionalization and telemedicine promises to effectively extend the positive impact of intensivist-led, team-based care, the limits of which have not been established.

4. **What can be done to improve the value of intensive care: Checklists, process improvement, and automated decision support?**
Nationally, with the average daily costs of an ICU bed now over $3500, critical care costs account for approximately $81.7 billion or 0.66% of the gross domestic product. Not surprisingly, in light of these high costs, hospitals have increased the pressure on administrators and clinician leaders to document the value that ICUs provide to consumers and to the health care system. Value, in this instance, is defined as quality divided by cost, with use of whatever metrics are deemed appropriate by the system. One commonly used metric in the ICU setting is quality-adjusted life years or QALY, which accounts for both the quality and quantity of a patient's life after the ICU. This metric tries to account for the fact that 1 year of high-quality life after hospitalization is worth more to society than a year of low-quality life. If we then factor in the costs of care, we can begin to

make crude estimates of cost-effectiveness by computing the value of interventions as the cost per QALY saved. For instance, these types of analyses have been performed for elderly survivors of critical illness and injury to compare outcome variance dependent on diagnosis and intervention (for example, higher QALY after surgical vs. nonsurgical causes of critical illness).

Because value is defined as quality over cost, value can be improved by either increasing the quality of ICU care (the numerator) and/or decreasing the cost of that care (the denominator). One strategy successful at doing both (increasing quality while decreasing costs) leverages the simple but powerful checklist approach. An effective checklist accomplishes two tasks simultaneously: it ensures that every patient every day receives care that is best practice, and it decreases variance in practice that is deleterious to system efficiency. As one example, checklists as part of a multifaceted approach to system improvement have decreased dramatically the incidence of central line–associated bloodstream infections and their associated costs in the United States over the last decade. This success, coupled with the Institute of Medicine's report on the impact of preventable hospital errors, has fueled the mushrooming of an industry for quality assurance and performance improvement in medicine. To guide teams in critical care settings, a Society of Critical Care Medicine task force recently reported a how-to guide for quality improvement.

Improving on the pen-and-paper checklist model will require advances in information systems and automated decision analysis. Decision support tools are electronic systems designed to improve clinical decision making by matching individual patients' characteristics to a computerized knowledge base that generates patient-specific recommendations. When fully implemented, decision support tools can reduce unwanted practice variation and assist with a variety of tasks, including prevention reminders, a list of differential diagnoses, protocolized therapy, and notification of pharmaceutical dosing and drug incompatibilities. Examples in which decision support tools have improved ICU outcomes are antibiotic prescribing in the ICU, compliance with low tidal volume strategies, and glucose control. When selecting electronic decision support tools, it is important to consider a variety of issues, including workflow integration, compatibility with legacy applications, system maturity, and upgrade availability. Effective decision support tools have not supplanted the need for attentive on-site clinicians nor have they proved to undermine clinician education.

5. **What is patient- and family-centered care, and how has it changed the approach in the ICU?**
The benefits of patient- and family-centered care are widely appreciated. Historically, ICUs have been slow to accommodate the needs of patients' families, out of either convenience for ICU staff or fear of family-initiated disruptions. Happily, a growing literature strongly supports the patient- and family-centered approach to ICU care, as it improves communication and patient outcomes, including higher patient and family satisfaction. This has motivated a shift in ICU culture. State-of-the-art hospital renovations now include spacious and comfortable waiting areas accompanied by overnight accommodations for immediate family. Family participation on rounds and unrestricted visiting policies improve family satisfaction and may secondarily improve patient outcomes. As part of the quality assurance and process improvement imperative, several validated tools are available to assess family satisfaction: the Critical Care Family Satisfaction Survey (CCFS), Family Satisfaction in the Intensive Care Unit Questionnaire (FS-ICU), and the Critical Care Family Needs Inventory (CCFNI), among others.

6. **What is an "ICU without walls," and how does it affect care before and after ICU admission?**
Outcomes are strongly influenced by the care provided before arrival in the ICU, with patients typically being transferred from the emergency department, elsewhere in the hospital (the ward or the operating room), or even another institution. Therefore hospital intensive care operations have been redesigned to provide the "right care, right now," regardless of where a patient might physically be located. One component of this hospital-wide safety net is the rapid-response team (RRT), which (like the code team) is capable of providing intensive care "outside the walls of the ICU." RRTs have been widely adopted in the United States and elsewhere

to identify patients outside of the ICU at risk for acute organ dysfunction and physiologic deterioration. These activations in turn facilitate escalation of care at the bedside and evaluation for transfer potential to a higher acuity setting, such as an ICU. The U.S. Agency for Healthcare Research and Quality has endorsed the use of rapid-response systems, and the Joint Commission included as a 2008 National Patient Safety Goal the need for systems of care that allow "healthcare staff members to directly request additional assistance from a specially trained individual(s) when the patient's condition appears to be worsening." In addition, several studies have addressed the impact of RRTs, yet their benefit in the literature remains controversial. A large, prospective, cluster-randomized trial of RRTs in Australia failed to demonstrate changes in the incidence of cardiac arrest, unplanned ICU admissions, or unexpected deaths. Similarly, a recent meta-analysis examining the effectiveness of rapid-response systems on reducing major adverse events was inconclusive. Nevertheless, ongoing support for rapid-response systems is provided at the national and local levels by the rationale that early intervention is both effective in preventing emergencies and beneficial in limiting adverse consequences. The recent creation of the U.S. Critical Illness and Injury Trials Group provides the framework for testing these and other hypotheses at the national level.

KEY POINTS: INTENSIVE CARE UNIT ORGANIZATION, MANAGEMENT, AND VALUE

1. Patient outcomes are best in ICUs that are managed by multidisciplinary teams led by an intensivist. For hospitals with multiple ICUs, the Critical Care Center model provides the necessary vision and authority to realize economies of scale, optimized operational efficiencies, and infrastructure to maximize quality care and patient safety.

2. ICU staffing models have a significant impact on both the quality and cost of care. Staffing models shown to improve quality include multidisciplinary teams, intensivist coverage during daytime hours (and perhaps nighttime hours as well), and low patient-to-nurse ratios.

3. Because the demand for critical care clinicians significantly exceeds supply, several approaches are worth exploring to expand the available skill sets, including acute care nurse practitioners, RRTs, telemedicine, and regionalization of intensive care.

4. Health care value is defined as the quality of care divided by its cost. As the cost of ICU care continues to escalate faster than general economic indicators, increased emphasis has been placed on improving value through increased quality and decreased costs. To these ends, systematic approaches to improve performance provide significant benefit.

5. Patient- and family-centered care has been reported to improve outcomes. ICU structure should be evaluated to optimize communication and minimize stress with use of critical care–specific survey tools that measure patient and family satisfaction.

BIBLIOGRAPHY

1. Berenholtz SM, Pronovost PJ, Lipsett PA, et al: Eliminating catheter-related bloodstream infections in the intensive care unit. Crit Care Med 32:2014-2020, 2004.

2. Cobb JP: Engineering health in the intensive care unit. Arch Intern Med 170:319-320, 2010.

3. Cobb JP, Ognibene FP, Ingbar DH, et al: Forging a critical alliance: addressing the research needs of the United States critical illness and injury community. Crit Care Med 37:3158-3160, 2009.

4. Curtis JR, Cook DJ, Wall RJ, et al: Intensive care unit quality improvement: a "how-to" guide for the interdisciplinary team. Crit Care Med 34:211-218, 2006.

5. Dorman T, Paulding R: Is the time right for 24-hr/7-day coverage? Crit Care Med 39:1544-1545, 2011.

6. Garg AX, Adhikari NK, McDonald H, et al: Effects of computerized clinical decision support systems on practitioner performance and patient outcomes: a systematic review. JAMA 293:1223-1238, 2005.

7. Halpern NA, Pastores SM: Critical care medicine in the United States 2000–2005: an analysis of bed numbers, occupancy rates, payer mix, and costs. Crit Care Med 38:65-71, 2010.

8. Jones DA, DeVita MA, Bellomo R: Rapid-response teams. N Engl J Med 365:139-146, 2011.

9. Kaarlola A, Tallgren M, Pettilä V: Long-term survival, quality of life, and quality-adjusted life-years among critically ill elderly patients. Crit Care Med 34:2120-2126, 2006.

10. Kim MM, Barnato AE, Angus DC, et al: The effect of multidisciplinary care teams on intensive care unit mortality. Arch Intern Med 170:369-376, 2010.

11. Lee TH: Putting the value framework to work. N Engl J Med 363:2481-2483, 2010.

12. Lilly CM, Cody S, Zhao H, et al: for the University of Massachusetts Memorial Critical Care Operations Group: Hospital mortality, length of stay, and preventable complications among critically ill patients before and after tele-ICU reengineering of critical care processes. JAMA 305:2175-2183, 2011.

13. Nguyen YL, Kahn JM, Angus DC: Reorganizing adult critical care delivery, the role of regionalization, telemedicine, and community outreach. Crit Care Med 181:1164-1169, 2010.

14. Pronovost PJ, Angus DC, Dorman T, et al: Physician staffing patterns and clinical outcomes in critically ill patients: a systematic review. JAMA 288:2151-2162, 2002.

15. Tarnow-Mordi WO, Hau C, Warden A, et al: Hospital mortality in relation to staff workload: a 4-year study in an adult intensive-care unit. Lancet 356:185-189, 2000.

QUALITY ASSURANCE AND PATIENT SAFETY IN THE INTENSIVE CARE UNIT

Nitin Puri, MD, FACP, Antoinette Spevetz, MD, FCCM, FACP, and Carolyn E. Bekes, MD, MHA, FCCM

1. **How is quality assessed?**

   The definition of *quality* encompasses many things but clearly involves meeting the expectations of the consumer. In health care, this standard usually involves the satisfaction of patients, physicians, and payers, as well as good clinical outcomes, appropriate resource use, cost containment, and attention to patient safety.

2. **What is benchmarking?**

   To *benchmark* means to compare one's own performance-related data with similar data from another institution. The Joint Commission requires that hospitals benchmark with other hospitals. This process has grown tremendously, and numerous quality indicators are now reported and available to the public. The Surgical Care Improvement Project was a benchmarking process with a goal to reduce the incidence of surgical complications by 25% by 2010. The appropriate use of deep vein thrombosis prophylaxis is an example of a quality indicator that when compared among different hospitals gave insight into the quality of care they provided.

3. **What is the relationship between the intensive care unit (ICU) organization and quality of care?**

   Evidence indicates that the structure and organization of an ICU can influence outcome. A collaborative relationship among members of the health care team is critical. A multidisciplinary approach with the addition of a full-time intensivist greatly improves the quality of patient care in the ICU, as does the presence of critical care nurses with appropriate staffing ratios and clinical pharmacists on the unit. The use of clinical protocols continues to expand, with reliable data about their use leading to an improvement of care in critically ill patients. The use of spontaneous breathing trials has been validated in multiple studies, but worldwide its use remains stagnant at best. Not using a protocolized weaning system is an example of the need for organizational improvement in an ICU to improve care. Resistance to protocol use has come in many forms, but one of the primary arguments has been the unwillingness of physicians to reduce medicine to a *cookbook* profession and the need for individual tailored care for each patient. An inherent mistake in this argument is a lack of recognition of the individualized clinical data from each patient that is analyzed and used to treat the patient in a logical manner.

   Resistance to change in the practice of critical care medicine is reflective of a broader problem in medicine in which studies suggest that 30% to 40% of patients do not receive care consistent with current medical knowledge.

4. **List the uses to which severity of illness scoring systems are commonly applied.**

   - **Stratification:** Multiple scoring systems exist to stratify the severity or acuity of illness of critically ill patients. Examples of such classification systems are the:
     - □ Acute Physiology and Chronic Health Evaluation (APACHE)
     - □ Simplified Acute Physiology Score (SAPS)
     - □ Sequential Organ Failure Assessment (SOFA)
     - □ Multiple Organ Dysfunction Score (MODS)
   - These systems allow comparison of outcomes related to differing therapeutic approaches and attempt to match patients for severity of illness. The multiple scoring systems have not been

compared in a prospective manner. Scoring systems for specific disease processes in critically ill patients exist, such as the risk, injury, failure, loss (complete loss of kidney function × 4 weeks) and end-stage kidney disease (complete loss of kidney function × 3 months) (RIFLE) criteria for kidney injury. Disease-specific scoring systems allow for standardized assessment enabling uniformity for research.

- **Efficiency of care delivery:** Efficiency can be measured only if objective measures of resources are used together with models that define a population's acuity of illness. It is important that the stratification of illness models have some validity in predicting outcome. These may be provided by the APACHE system and the Therapeutic Intervention Scoring System, among others.
- **Decision making in clinical management:** Decision making may be aided by considering the information provided by scoring systems as these models allow physicians to stratify patients into cohorts. However, clinicians must be cognizant that scoring systems provide population illness overview, not specific patient prognosis. Individual patient data must be used when providing prognostic information for patients and their families.
- **Economics:** Scoring of patients can assist in appropriate billing and reimbursement code application.

5. **How is performance improvement carried out in the ICU?**
The unit director in collaboration with the nurse manager and other members of the health care team should identify areas for improvements in care delivery. Performance improvement committees exist for monitoring performance indicators in ICUs and noting deficiencies. A formal process to address problems should exist. Common systems used are the **PDSA** process (**p**lan, **d**o, **s**tudy, **a**ct) or **PDCA** process (**p**lan, **d**o, **c**heck, **a**ct). One proposed method for creating solutions for quality improvement in ICU is the barrier identification and creating solutions tool. It involves the creation of an interdisciplinary team that is given the authority to observe, interview, and simulate process in the ICU. The team is responsible for compiling the data and developing an action plan to create solutions to barriers to improvement in critically ill patients. This process is an example of a performance improvement method that can be generalized to solve many quality deficiencies in ICUs.

6. **List a number of observations on which to base assessment of outcome.**
Although a variety of indicators can be used to assess outcome, the following usually provide a reasonable database and can be used for benchmarking when similar data are available from other institutions:
- **Patient satisfaction:** This should include not only the patient's subjective opinions but also some objective observations of outcome such as activities of daily living scores. A significantly understudied aspect of this parameter is the posthospital status of the patient.
- **Length of stay:** The length of stay both in the hospital and in the ICU for patients who have been stratified by diagnosis, acuity, and comorbidities on admission provides valuable insight into outcomes and an excellent database for benchmarking, if studied consistently over a reasonable period.
- **Mortality indexed to severity of illness:** Although this information can provide a simple benchmarking tool, the data should be critically reviewed because death cannot always be equated with a bad outcome.
- **Incidence of unanticipated returns to the ICU during the same hospital stay:** This indicator may yield important information if examined in some detail. In addition to the actual incidence (which can be used for benchmarking), the individual cases should be reviewed. This may reveal a need to review the criteria for transferring patients from the unit or the compliance with the same. Alternatively, it may stimulate consideration of

the adequacy of the care capabilities of the environments receiving the patients on discharge from the unit.
- **Incidence of complications:** Complications may be linked to procedures (e.g., line placement, endotracheal intubation) or to general management (e.g., nosocomial infection, medication errors). Of major importance are those that have a clear impact on patient welfare. The criteria for identifying these and the methodology for data collection and analysis should be defined and consistently applied.

7. **How applicable to the ICU is the clinical or critical pathway approach to the maintenance of cost-effective care delivery?**
Although the development of so-called clinical pathways has had considerable success in reducing costs while maintaining or improving standards of care and clinical outcomes, this methodology appears to be applicable mainly to patients with diagnoses wherein there is a fairly homogeneous group of patients who run broadly similar courses. Good examples of these diagnoses are acute coronary syndromes and hip fractures. In the case of the patient population in a mixed adult medical-surgical ICU, however, there is no such homogeneity, and it is often virtually impossible to describe an average course for a given diagnosis. Such a diversity of progression exists that relates primarily to the individual patient circumstances that it is of little value to compare the course of an individual patient with the clinical pathway. A much better approach in the ICU is to write treatment algorithms applicable to discrete segments of the patient's care within the continuum of the entire illness (e.g., weaning with use of therapist-driven protocols or use of the ventilator bundle, Centers for Disease Control and Prevention line insertion bundle, or sepsis bundle) (Box 88-1). The use of this approach maintains all the advantages of getting groups together to discuss and agree on a unified approach toward aspects of care (thus reducing expensive diversity) without wasting time and energy on trying to define nonexistent average courses of these illnesses.

BOX 88-1. SURGICAL TIME-OUT CHECKLIST

- All team members have been introduced by name and role.
- Confirmation of the patient's identity, surgical site, and procedure.
- Review of anticipated critical events.
- Confirmation that prophylactic antibiotics have been administered ≤ 60 minutes before incision is made or antibiotics not indicated.
- Confirmation that all essential imaging results for the correct patient are displayed in the operating room.

---

8. **Is patient safety a concern in ICUs?**
Medical errors occur frequently in ICUs and can adversely affect outcome in critically ill patients. Errors occur more frequently in patients with more organ failures and in larger ICUs. Although individual mistakes may lead to errors in patient care, the solution to improving practice may be found in organizational changes.

9. **How can patient safety be improved?**
Health care providers can commit to a culture of safety to improve patient care. The Institute for Healthcare Improvement's 100,000 Lives Campaign and its later 5 Million Lives Campaign helped health care organizations set specific goals and targets to improve patient safety. These goals forced health care providers to reexamine the acceptance of previously tolerated errors that increased morbidity and mortality. A zero tolerance for errors and innovative strategies from other high-risk professions have helped physicians understand that safety can be improved. For example, although significant differences exist between the airline industry and the delivery of critical care medicine, one glaring similarity exists. Mistakes can have horrendous

consequences. The use of checklists in aviation has led to increased safety, and the similar use of checklists has dramatically decreased surgical complications (see Box 88-2).

BOX 88-2. FIVE COMPONENTS OF THE VENTILATOR BUNDLE

- Elevation of the head of the bed to at least 30 degrees
- Daily sedation vacation
- Daily assessments of readiness to extubate
- Peptic ulcer disease prophylaxis
- Deep vein thrombosis prophylaxis

---

10. **Can you give an example of a patient safety project that dramatically improved patient care in critically ill patients?**

   Multiple examples exist in the medical literature, but among the most dramatic was the Michigan Health & Hospital Association Keystone ICU project, which addressed central line–associated bloodstream infections (CLABSI). Catheter-related bloodstream infections cause close to 30,000 deaths in ICUs annually, and each infection leads to accrued cost over $40,000. The safety project used five proven techniques to reduce CLABSI (see Box 88-3). After 18 months of intervention, CLABSI decreased by 60%, and in a follow-up study the results were sustained at 36 months.

BOX 88-3. FIVE COMPONENTS OF THE KEYSTONE SAFETY PROJECT

- Hand hygiene.
- Maximal barrier precautions.
- Chlorhexidine skin antisepsis.
- Avoid femoral site when possible.
- Remove unnecessary catheters.

---

11. **What are common barriers to improvements in patient safety?**

   Introducing change into health care organizations is often fraught with difficulty. Common barriers to change include an unwillingness to abandon cultural and historical precedents that constrain a culture of safety. Health care providers must consider the partial loss of autonomy to promote patient care, such as the use of protocols in the critically ill. Education about safety deficits and also an improvement in communication among interdisciplinary team members remain important goals. Finally, resources must be invested into creating a culture of patient safety even when immediate benefits are not apparent.

KEY POINTS: QUALITY ASSURANCE AND PATIENT SAFETY IN THE INTENSIVE CARE UNIT

1. Quality assurance in the ICU means meeting the expectations of patients with the appropriate use of resources.

2. The use of multidisciplinary teams to provide care in ICUs has been validated.

3. Performance improvement projects are necessary to evaluate and improve care for the critically ill.

4. Patient safety is a major concern for critically ill patients.

5. Health care providers can improve patient safety in ICUs with a willingness to reexamine their own professional practices.

BIBLIOGRAPHY

1. Amalberti R, Auroy Y, Berwick D, et al: Five system barriers to achieving ultrasafe healthcare. Ann Intern Med 142:756-764, 2005.

2. Bota PD, Melot C, Ferreira FL, et al: The Multiple Organ Dysfunction Score versus the Sequential Organ Failure Assessment (SOFA) score in outcome prediction. Intensive Care Med 28:1619-1624, 2002.

3. Brilli RJ, Spevetz A, Branson RD, et al: Critical care delivery in the intensive care unit: defining clinical roles and the best practice model. Crit Care Med 25:2007-2019, 2001.

4. Curtis JR, Cook DJ, Wall RJ, et al: Intensive care unit quality improvement: a "how-to" guide for the interdisciplinary team. Crit Care Med 34:211-218, 2006.

5. Girard TD, Ely EW: Protocol-driven ventilator weaning: reviewing the evidence. Clin Chest Med 29:241-252, 2008.

6. Grol R, Grimshaw J: From best evidence to best practice: effective implementation of change in patients' care. Lancet 362:1225-1230, 2003.

7. Gurses AP, Marsteller JA, Ozok AA, et al: Using an interdisciplinary approach to identify factors that affect clinicians' compliance with evidence-based guidelines. Crit Care Med 38:S282-S291, 2010.

8. Haynes AB, Weiser TG, Berry WR, et al: Safety checklist to reduce morbidity and mortality in a global population. N Engl J Med 360:491-499, 2009.

9. Institute for Healthcare Improvement: www.ihi.org/IHI/Programs/Campaign/Campaign.htm?TabId=6. Accessed March 10, 2011.

10. The Joint Commission: www.jointcommission.org/. Accessed March 10, 2011.

11. Kane SL, Weber RJ, Dasta JF: The impact of critical care pharmacists on enhancing patient outcomes. Intensive Care Med 29:691-698, 2003.

12. Le Gall JR, Lemeshow S, Saulnier F: A new simplified acute physiology score (SAPS II) based on a European/North American multicenter study. JAMA 270:2957-2963, 1993.

13. Marshall JC, Cook DJ, Christou NV: Multiple organ dysfunction score: a reliable descriptor of a complex clinical outcome. Crit Care Med 23:1638-1652, 1995.

14. Moreno RP, Rhodes A, Donchin Y: for the European Society of Intensive Care: Patient safety in intensive care medicine: the Declaration of Vienna. Intensive Care Med 35:1667-1672, 2009.

15. Plost G, Nelson DP: Empowering critical care nurses to improve compliance with protocols in the intensive care unit. Am J Crit Care 16:153-157, 2007.

16. Pronovost P, Angus DC, Dorman T, et al: Physician staffing patterns and clinical outcomes in critically ill patients: a systematic review. JAMA 288:2151-2162, 2002.

17. Pronovost PJ, Dang D, Dorman T, et al: Intensive care unit nurse staffing and the risk of complications after abdominal aortic surgery. Eff Clin Pract 4:199-206, 2001.

18. Pronovost PJ, Goeschel CA, Colantuoni E, et al: Sustaining reductions in catheter related bloodstream infections in Michigan intensive care units: observational study. BMJ 340:c309, 2010.

19. Valentin A, Capuzzo M, Guidet B, et al: Patient safety in intensive care: results from the multinational Sentinel Events Evaluation (SEE) study. Intensive Care Med 32:1591-1598, 2006.

20. Valentin A, Capuzzo M, Guidet B, et al: Research group on Quality Improvement of the European Society of Intensive Care Medicine (ESICM); Sentinel Events Evaluation (SEE) Study Investigators: Errors in the administration of parenteral drugs in intensive care units: multinational prospective study. BMJ 338:b814, 2009.

CHAPTER 89

SCORING SYSTEMS FOR COMPARISON OF DISEASE SEVERITY IN INTENSIVE CARE UNIT PATIENTS

Benoit Misset, MD, and Islem Ouanes, MD

1. **What are severity scores?**

   Scoring systems have been developed to compare the severity of disease among patients in intensive care units (ICUs). These scores are established at admission or during the ICU stay, and they are widely used in the ICU; other scores were recently developed to be used at ICU discharge to predict worse outcome after discharge (early death or ICU readmission). The scores include the assessment of several physiologic parameters that have been documented to play an independent role in predicting hospital death. The scores presented in this chapter are only those used to assess general disease severity. Other scoring systems are used to assess particular organ function (i.e., Acute Lung Injury Score for evaluation of acute respiratory distress syndrome and Sequential Organ Failure Assessment [SOFA] or to assess resource and workload use (i.e., Therapeutic Intervention Scoring System [TISS]).

SCORES AT ICU ADMISSION

2. **Which scores are used for assessing the general severity of disease at ICU admission?**

   The three most frequently used systems are the:
   - Acute Physiology and Chronic Health Evaluation (APACHE)
   - Simplified Acute Physiology Score (SAPS)
   - Mortality Predictive Model (MPM)

   The most recent versions of each system are the APACHE IV (2006), the SAPS III (2005), and the MPM III (2007).

3. **Why were scores to assess general disease severity at ICU admission developed?**

   - **To assess performance of the ICU.** The ICU patient is a medical or a surgical patient who has either acute failure of one major vital function or a high risk for development of such failure. Because the mortality rate of ICU populations is usually high and varies widely depending on patient admission policies, an objective assessment of the patients' general disease severity is necessary to ensure that the mortality rate in an ICU is consistent with the overall severity of its patient population at admission. The ratio between observed and predicted mortality, called the standardized mortality ratio, is the simplest way to assess the performance of an ICU. It allows comparisons among mortality rates of various ICUs or the mortality rates documented in one ICU over time.
   - **To assess the patient's risk for death.** The scores give an objective evaluation that helps the clinician confirm the severity of the patient's illness. However, these scores cannot be used to make decisions about individual patients (e.g., withdrawal of support).
   - **To compare or match populations in clinical studies.** In randomized, controlled studies the scores have been used to confirm that the populations obtained by randomization had a

similar disease severity at admission to the ICU. In case-control studies, the scores have been used to match the control to the case patients.

4. **How were scores assessing general severity at ICU admission constructed?**
   Scores were constructed in large, multicenter, prospective populations. The variables were selected and weighed by consensus of panels of experts (first version of SAPS in 1984, first version of APACHE in 1981, and APACHE II in 1985) or through multiple logistic regression analyses used for most recently developed scores (SAPS II and III, APACHE III and IV, and MPM II and III) to determine whether the parameters were independent predictors of hospital death. The tested variables include age, worst values over the first 24 hours of ICU admission for certain acute physiologic abnormalities (e.g., sodium, potassium, partial arterial oxygen tension, urine output, Glasgow Coma Scale), category at admission (medical or surgical patient), and several underlying diseases (e.g., metastatic cancer, acquired immunodeficiency syndrome). The MPM system also includes several therapeutic measures (e.g., number of venous lines).

   The SAPS III is based on a more complex methodology. It has the advantage of being based on a worldwide population and of giving a larger place to prior health status and to circumstances of admission in addition to the physiologic imbalance at ICU admission. MPM0, MPM III, and SAPS III are collected entirely at admission to the ICU (i.e., within 1 hour), which reduces potential suboptimal care in the first day of the ICU in the assessment of severity.

   The most recent version of APACHE score is the APACHE IV developed in 2006 with use of a database of more than 100,000 patients admitted to 104 ICUs in 45 hospitals in the United States in 2002-2003, and remodeling the APACHE III score.

   MPM III is a recent update of MPM0 (2007) with use of a database of 124,885 patients from 135 ICUs. This recent score uses 16 variables including three physiologic parameters obtained within 1 hour of ICU admission to estimate mortality probability at hospital discharge.

5. **How were scores assessing general disease severity at ICU admission validated?**
   All of these models were validated in the initial studies in a subset of patients that was not used for construction of the scoring system. The performance of the scoring systems was considered adequate if they showed good discrimination in predicting hospital mortality and had a good calibration for the entire population under investigation. **Discrimination** in predicting hospital mortality is assessed with receiver operating characteristics (ROCs): the higher the area under the ROC curve, the more discriminative the test. The **calibration** in the entire population is measured with the goodness-of-fit test: the observed mortality must not be statistically different from the expected mortality in population deciles of equal probability intervals. The lower the Hosmer-Lemeshow H statistic value and the higher the corresponding p value, the better the calibration.

6. **Which scores have been validated adequately?**
   The APACHE I and II, SAPS I, and MPM I have not been constructed or validated with the current accepted methodologic standards. The SAPS II, MPM II, and APACHE III scores have been shown to have good discrimination and calibration in large multicenter studies.
   - The **SAPS II** is well validated. The score needs to be updated with more recent ICU populations.
   - The **MPM II** is well validated and has the advantage of being the only score available at ICU admission rather than at 24 hours after admission. This advantage is made possible because the score includes some therapeutic items (e.g., venous lines, drainage systems). The MPM II score also needs to be updated with more recent ICU populations.
   - The **APACHE III** is well validated and updated regularly, but its use is limited by the fact that clinicians must pay to know and use its equation for calculating death probability.
   - The **APACHE IV** and the **MPM III** are well calibrated, and they have a good discrimination; they were validated in a multicentered study of 11,300 ICU patients from California showing that APACHE IV had better discrimination and longer data extraction time than MPM III.

MPM III was also validated in 55,459 patients from 103 ICUs, 25 of which did not participate in the original development.

■ The **SAPS III** is well validated and updated as it was published in 2005, that is, 12 years after the most recent among the other ones. Unlike the APACHE III, its construction details were diffused to the entire scientific community. It appears to be a good candidate for an international benchmark, and its use is free of charge.

See Box 89-1.

BOX 89-1. STRUCTURE OF THE RECENT SIMPLIFIED ACUTE PHYSIOLOGY SCORE III

Box I
Age
Comorbidities
Length of stay before ICU admission
Intrahospital location before ICU admission
Use of major therapeutic options before ICU admission

Box II
ICU admission: planned or unplanned
Reason(s) for ICU admission (nine categories)
Surgical status at ICU admission (none, scheduled, emergency)
Anatomic site of surgery (six categories)
Acute infection at ICU admission (nosocomial, respiratory)

Box III
Glasgow Coma Scale score
Total bilirubin
Body temperature
Serum creatinine level
Heart rate
White blood cell count
Serum pH
Platelet count
Systolic blood pressure
Blood oxygenation

See also www.saps3.org.

SCORES OVER THE ICU STAY

7. **Why were scores assessing disease severity over the ICU stay developed?**
The scores measuring daily severity were developed to improve the prediction of an individual patient's death (already provided by scores at admission), to assess the activity and the performance of ICUs, and to match patients in clinical investigations. These scores are particularly useful as inclusion criteria in randomized studies in which patients are entered into the investigation several days after admission. These scores are also used as matching criteria in case-control studies addressing the attributable morbidity of ICU-acquired events, such as nosocomial infections.

8. **Which scores have been developed for assessing severity over the ICU stay?**
Various scores have been developed on ICU samples of various sizes. The scores developed on the largest ICU populations include the:
■ Organ System Failure score (OSF)
■ Organ Dysfunction and Infection score (ODIN)

- Logistic Organ Dysfunction Score (LODS)
- Sequential Organ Failure Assessment score (SOFA)
- Multiple Organ Dysfunction Score (MODS)

9. **How were the scores assessing severity over the ICU stay constructed?**
Sequential scores measure the number and/or the intensity of organ dysfunction. By contrast with the SAPS, MPM, and APACHE scores, they do not take age, category of admission, or underlying diseases into account, because these items do not change over the ICU stay.

The OSF, ODIN, SOFA, and MODS scores were constructed empirically. The OSF and ODIN scores assess the number of organ dysfunctions, and the SOFA and MODS scores also assess the intensity of organ dysfunction. The MODS construction included testing of its validity, reproducibility, and sensitivity of each test item between observers.

The choice and the weight of each LODS item are derived from a multiple logistic regression model, with use of hospital mortality as the dependent variable. The construction was made from the data collected during the first day in the ICU.

10. **How were they validated?**
Discrimination for predicting mortality is better in multivariate models when the evolution of the score account and its initial values are taken into account. This principle was demonstrated with the LODS score.

11. **What did these scores add to the description of ICU patients?**
    - The use of the OSF score initially showed that a 100% prediction of death could be made in the most severely afflicted patients after several days. However, the same score was eventually used to demonstrate that care in the ICU had improved over the years, so that published results were no longer valid 10 years later. These investigations documented that such scores are a method to assess ICU performance.
    - The mean time of occurrence of each organ failure is not the same. The peak of dysfunction for the neurologic system occurs usually before the second day; for the respiratory, cardiovascular, renal, and coagulation systems, around the third day; and for hepatic dysfunction, around the fifth day.
    - The weight of each organ failure in predicting death is not the same: hematologic and hepatic failures have less effect on mortality than respiratory, cardiovascular, renal, and neurologic failures.
    - The weight of each organ failure in predicting death is not the same over time. The same increase in respiratory dysfunction has a worse prognosis after 1 week of ICU stay. Hepatic dysfunction has an effect on mortality only after 3 weeks of ICU stay.

SCORES AT ICU DISCHARGE

12. **At what time of the ICU stay should either of these scores be used? (See Fig. 89-1.)**
Among critically ill patients, many experience clinical deterioration or death shortly after discharge from the ICU. These adverse outcomes might be ascribable to premature ICU discharge. Therefore determining the optimal time for ICU discharge is crucial. Moreover, ICU readmission is associated with a fivefold increase in hospital mortality compared with the initial prediction. Recently, scoring systems at ICU discharge are developed to predict prognosis after ICU discharge and to determine the optimal time of discharge to prevent unplanned ICU readmission or death. The Stability and Workload Index for Transfer (SWIFT) is a score for predicting unplanned ICU readmission that was developed in three ICUs. This score, which is determined at ICU discharge, is based on ICU length of stay, location before ICU admission, and neurologic and respiratory impairment on the discharge day. In two validation cohorts, the SWIFT value predicted ICU readmission but exhibited poor calibration.

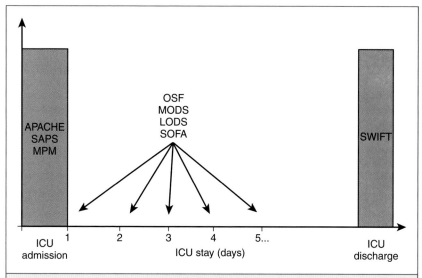

Figure 89-1. When should we measure the severity scores?

KEY POINTS: SCORING SYSTEMS FOR COMPARISON OF DISEASE SEVERITY IN INTENSIVE CARE UNIT PATIENTS

1. Most common items of the severity scores measured at ICU admission

   a. Age

   b. Previous health status

   c. Acute physiologic imbalance at ICU admission

   d. Reason for admission

   e. Mode of admission

2. Usual goals of measuring a severity score at ICU admission

   a. Prediction of death

   b. ICU populations comparison in scientific studies

   c. Performance and benchmarking, when linked to observed mortality

3. Common utilization of the organ dysfunction scores

   a. Match the patients in case-control or exposed-unexposed studies

   b. Adjust the cohorts in risk-factor multivariate analyses

BIBLIOGRAPHY

1. Cook R, Cook D, Tilley J, et al: Multiple organ dysfunction: baseline and serial component scores. Crit Care Med 29:2046-2050, 2001.

2. Fagon J-Y, Chastre J, Novara A, et al: Characterization of intensive care unit patients using a model based on the presence or absence of organ dysfunctions and/or infection: the ODIN model. Intensive Care Med 19:137-144, 1993.

3. Gajic O, Malinchoc M, Comfere TB, et al: The Stability and Workload Index for Transfer score predicts unplanned intensive care unit patient readmission: initial development and validation. Crit Care Med 36:676-682, 2008.

4. Higgins TL, Kramer AA, Nathanson BH, et al: Prospective validation of the intensive care unit admission Mortality Probability Model (MPM0-III). Crit Care Med 37:1619-1623, 2009.

5. Higgins TL, Teres D, Copes WS, et al: Assessing contemporary intensive care unit outcome: an updated Mortality Probability Admission Model (MPM0-III). Crit Care Med 35:827-835, 2007.

6. Knaus WA, Draper EA, Wagner DP, et al: APACHE II: a severity of disease classification system. Crit Care Med 13:818-829, 1985.

7. Knaus WA, Draper EA, Wagner DP, et al: Prognosis in acute organ-system failure. Ann Surg 202:685, 1985.

8. Knaus WA, Wagner DP, Draper EA, et al: The APACHE III prognostic system: risk prediction of hospital mortality for critically ill hospitalized adults. Chest 100:1619-1636, 1991.

9. Kuzniewicz MW, Vasilevskis EE, Lane R, et al: Variation in ICU risk-adjusted mortality: impact of methods of assessment and potential confounders. Chest 133:1319-1327, 2008.

10. Le Gall JR, Klar J, Lemeshow S, et al: The Logistic Organ Dysfunction system: a new way to assess organ dysfunction in the intensive care unit. JAMA 276:802-810, 1996.

11. Le Gall JR, Lemeshow S, Saulnier F: A new Simplified Acute Physiology Score (SAPS II) based on a European/North American multicenter study. JAMA 270:2957-2963, 1993.

12. Lemeshow S, Teres D, Klar J, et al: Mortality Probability Models (MPM II) based on an international cohort of intensive care unit patients. JAMA 270:2478-2486, 1993.

13. Marshall JC, Cook DJ, Christou NV, et al: Multiple organ dysfunction score: a reliable descriptor of a complex clinical outcome. Crit Care Med 23:1638-1652, 1995.

14. Metnitz PG, Lang T, Valentin A, et al: Evaluation of the logistic organ dysfunction system for the assessment of organ dysfunction and mortality in critically ill patients. Intensive Care Med 27:992-998, 2001.

15. Moreno RP, Metnitz PG, Almeida E, et al: SAPS 3—from evaluation of the patient to evaluation of the intensive care unit. Part 2. Development of a prognostic model for hospital mortality at ICU admission. Intensive Care Med 31:1345-1355, 2005.

16. Moreno R, Vincent JL, Matos A, et al: The use of maximum SOFA score to quantify organ failure/dysfunction in intensive care: result of a prospective multicenter study. Intensive Care Med 25:686-696, 1999.

17. Vincent JL, de Mendonca A, Cantraine F, et al: Use of the SOFA score to assess the incidence of organ dysfunction/failure in intensive care units: results of a multicenter, prospective study. Crit Care Med 26:1793-1800, 1998.

18. Zimmerman JE, Kramer AA, McNair DS, et al: Acute Physiology and Chronic Health Evaluation (APACHE) IV: hospital mortality assessment for today's critically ill patients. Crit Care Med 34:1297-1310, 2006.

INDEX

Page numbers followed by *f* indicate figures; *b*, boxes; *t*, tables.

A

A waves, 40
AAA. *See* Abdominal aortic aneurysm (AAA).
AAN. *See* American Academy of Neurology (AAN).
ABCDE bundle, 516
ABCDs of CPR. *See* Compressions, airway, and
 breathing (CAB) of CPR.
Abdomen
 acute, 352, 353, 356*b*
  causes of, 352-354
  in immunocompromised hosts, 356
  intraabdominal hypertension and, 354
  intraabdominal infections and, 355
  mesenteric ischemia and, 355
  Ogilvie syndrome and, 354-355
 examination of, 11-12
 pain in
  diabetic ketoacidosis-related, 361
  evaluation of, 352
  peritonitis-related, 353
  thoracic conditions and, 352
Abdominal aortic aneurysm (AAA), 356
Abdominal compartment syndrome, 4, 16-17, 354, 356
Abdominal reflexes, brain death and, 429
ABG analysis. *See* Arterial blood gas (ABG) analysis.
Abscesses
 abdominal, 355
 cutaneous, 266
 perivalvular, 226
Absolute hypovolemia, 24
Absolute insulin deficiency, 359, 360*f*
Abuse, definition of, 456
ACA. *See* Anterior cerebral arteries (ACA).
Acalculous cholecystitis, 355
Accessory muscle use, definition of, 9
ACE inhibitors. *See* Angiotensin-converting enzyme
 (ACE) inhibitors.
Acetaminophen, 509*t*
 overdose of, 6
 poisoning, 553, 554, 554*f*, 556
 side effects of, 508
 for thyroid storm, 380*t*
Acetazolamide, hypokalemia and, 316
Acetylcholine (ACh), 498
Acetylcholinesterase inhibitors for myasthenia
 gravis, 454

Acid-base abnormalities, 4, 11, 314*b*
 compensation for, 312*t*
 differential diagnoses of, 312-314, 312*b*
Acid-base status, 310-314, 501
Acidosis
 acute renal failure and, 302*t*
 anion-gap, 6
 cardiac arrest and, 24
 definition of, 310
 lactic, cancer and, 404
 metabolic
  abdominal pain and, 353
  anion gap, 312*b*, 359-360
  treatment of, 312*t*
 respiratory
  differential diagnosis of, 313
  treatment of, 312*t*
Acinetobacter sp.
 cellulitis and, 264
 multidrug-resistant, 137, 250
 sepsis and, 218
ACP. *See* American College of Physicians (ACP).
ACR. *See* Active core rewarming (ACR).
ACS. *See* Acute chest syndrome (ACS).
ACTH test. *See* Adrenocorticotropic hormone (ACTH)
 test.
Actinobacillus actinomycetemcomitans, 225
Activated charcoal, 547, 547*b*
 multiple-dose, 547-548
Activated protein C for heat stroke, 543
Active core rewarming (ACR), 537-538
Active external rewarming (AER), 537-538
Acute abdomen, 352, 353, 356*b*
 causes of, 352, 353-354
 in immunocompromised hosts, 356
 intraabdominal hypertension and, 354
 intraabdominal infections and, 355
 mesenteric ischemia and, 355
 Ogilvie syndrome and, 354-355
Acute adrenal crisis/insufficiency, 374
Acute asthma. *See* Severe asthma.
Acute bacterial pneumonia, 131-141
 See also Community-acquired pneumonia (CAP);
  Ventilator-associated pneumonia (VAP).
 health care–associated pneumonia, 136-140,
  138*t*, 139*f*

Acute bacterial pneumonia (*Continued*)
hospital-acquired pneumonia, 136-140, 138*t*, 139*f*
noninfectious, 136
nonresolving, 135-136
treatment failure in, 135
Acute chest syndrome (ACS), 169-170
Acute decompensated heart failure, 186-187, 186*t*, 191
Acute fatty liver of pregnancy, 572
Acute hepatic necrosis, 489
Acute illness
delirium and, 513*t*
hyperglycemia and, 369, 370*f*
steroids and, 419
Acute ischemic stroke, 11, 441, 446
blood pressure management in, 443-445, 446
IV recombinant tissue plasminogen activator for, 441, 442, 442*b*
Acute kidney injury (AKI), 55, 308
Acute lobar atelectasis, 112
Acute lung injury (ALI), 2, 167, 170
feeding formulas in, 55
sepsis-induced, 220-221
Acute meningitis, 232, 233*t*
Acute muscle paralysis, coma and, 424
Acute myocardial infarction (AMI), 3, 11, 192-196
cooling or hypothermia after, 195-196
diagnosis of, 192, 192*t*, 193
mortality and, 195
out-of-hospital cardiac arrest and, 193
treatment of, 193-196
unstable angina and, 194, 194*t*
Acute normovolemic intraoperative hemodilution (ANH), 387
Acute pancreatitis, 4, 336-342
antibiotics and, 339
biliary, 341
causes of, 336, 341*b*
diagnosis of, 336-337
nutritional therapy in, 55
severity and prognosis of, 337, 338*t*, 339*t*, 340*t*
signs and symptoms of, 336
treatment of, 338, 340-341, 356
Acute pericarditis, 212, 213
Acute Physiology and Chronic Health Evaluation (APACHE), 246, 598, 603-606
Acute renal failure (ARF), 4, 299-305
chronic vs., 299
classification of, 299*t*
diagnosis of, 299
differential diagnosis of, 299*t*, 300-301, 300*f*
electrolyte disorders and, 302, 302*t*
in neuroleptic malignant syndrome, 566
prevention of, 301
treatment of, 301-305, 304*b*
Acute respiratory distress syndrome (ARDS), 2, 167, 170
bronchoalveolar lavage performance in, 111
late, steroid use for, 375*f*

Acute respiratory distress syndrome (ARDS) (*Continued*)
low tidal volume in, 1, 60, 62
mechanical ventilation and, 1, 220-221
mortality with, 168
pneumothorax and, 470-471
pulmonary contusions and, 477
risk factors for, 167
sequelae in survivors of, 169
treatment of, 168
Acute respiratory failure (ARF), 166, 167, 170
in chronic obstructive pulmonary disease, 154
endotracheal intubation and mechanical ventilation for, 167
hypercapnic, 166
hypoxemic, 166
noninvasive ventilation for, 59
in pregnancy, 573, 573*b*, 575
types of, 166
Acute tubular necrosis (ATN), 300, 301
Addiction, definition of, 456
Addison disease, 374
Adenosine, 200, 200*f*, 201
Adenovirus, 290
ADH. *See* Antidiuretic hormone (ADH).
Adrenal insufficiency, 374-378
diagnosis of, 374-376, 375*f*
head trauma and, 377
risk factors for, 376
septic shock and, 377-378
steroids and, 376-378
types of, 374
Adrenocorticotropic hormone (ACTH) test, 374, 375*f*, 376
AEIOU mnemonic, 306
AER. *See* Active external rewarming (AER).
Aeromonas hydrophila, 264
AHA. *See* American Heart Association (AHA).
AIH. *See* Autoimmune hepatitis (AIH).
Airway
artificial, removal of, 65-66
definition of, 87
difficult, 90, 91
emergency nonsurgical, 91
evaluation of, 13
tracheotomy-related hemorrhage in, 2
Airway management, 87-92
in burns, 462
during CPR, 21
definition of, 87
in myasthenia gravis, 453-454
in trauma patients, 13, 14*f*, 18
Airway obstruction
evaluation of, 9
upper
after decannulation of tracheostomy tube, 98
emergency tracheotomy for, 94
endotracheal intubation for, 87, 92
Airway protection as indication for endotracheal intubation, 88

AKI. *See* Acute kidney injury (AKI).
Albumin
  as nutritional status indicator, 50
  as resuscitation solution component, 49
Alcohol abuse, 456
Alcohol addiction, definition of, 456
Alcohol dependence, definition of, 456
Alcohol poisoning, toxic, 6, 558-561
  diagnosis of, 559-560
  ethylene glycol, 558, 560
  isopropanol, 558, 561
  methanol, 558
  signs and symptoms of, 559
  treatment of, 560-561
Alcohol use
  immune function and, 456
  pathophysiology of, 457
Alcohol use disorders (AUDs), 456
Alcohol withdrawal, 5, 456-459
  clinical states of, 457
  criteria for, 456-457
  pathophysiology of, 457
  treatment of, 457-459
Alcoholic hepatitis, 4, 346
Aldosterone-producing adenoma (APA), 297-298
ALI. *See* Acute lung injury (ALI).
Alkalosis
  definition of, 310
  metabolic
    differential diagnosis of, 313
    treatment of, 312*t*
  respiratory
    differential diagnosis of, 313
    treatment of, 312*t*
Allen's test, modified, 70
Allergies, 529. *See also* Anaphylaxis.
Allograft rejection, 493
Allopurinol, 310
α_1-Antitrypsin replacement in chronic obstructive
    pulmonary disease, 152
ALS. *See* Amyotrophic lateral sclerosis (ALS).
Altered mental status
  evaluation of, 11
Alveolar gas equation, 1, 28-30, 36-37
Alveolar-arterial PO$_2$ difference (A − aO$_2$ gradient), 29-30
Amantadine
  for influenza, 272
  for neuroleptic malignant syndrome, 568
American Academy of Neurology (AAN), 428
American Association of Clinical Endocrinologists, 371*t*
American Association of Critical-Care Nurses, 594
American College of Cardiology, 207
American College of Physicians (ACP)
  glycemic target for critically ill patients, 371*t*
  web-based resource on bioterrorism, 259*t*
American Diabetes Association, 371*t*
American Heart Association (AHA)
  cardiopulmonary resuscitation guidelines, 20
  thoracic aortic disease guidelines, 207

American Society of Anesthesiologists, 113
American Thoracic Society, 371*t*
American-European Consensus Conference, 167
AMI. *See* Acute myocardial infarction (AMI).
Amino acids, acute kidney injury and, 308
Aminoglycoside
  for necrotizing skin and soft tissue infections, 266
  nondepolarizing neuromuscular blocking agents
      and, 501*t*
  for severe community-acquired pneumonia, 133*b*
Aminophylline for severe asthma attacks, 144
Aminosalicylic acid, acute pancreatitis and, 336
Aminosteroidal agents, 499, 499*t*
Amniotic fluid embolism, 572
Amoxicillin for anthrax exposure, 258*t*
Amoxicillin-clavulanate for cat or dog bites, 267
AmpC cephalosporinases, 248
Amphotericin B, 243-244
Amphotericin bladder irrigation, 241
Ampicillin-sulbactam
  for cat or dog bites, 267
  for endocarditis, 229
  for necrotizing skin and soft tissue infections, 266
  for severe community-acquired pneumonia, 133*b*
Amylase
  in abdominal pain, 353
  as pancreatitis indicator, 336-337
Amyotrophic lateral sclerosis (ALS), 452
ANA test. *See* Antinuclear antibody (ANA) test.
Anaerobes, 133
Analgesia
  in critically ill patients, 504, 510*b*
  during endotracheal intubation
  epidural, 510
  inadequate, 504
  during mechanical ventilation, 65
  nonopioid, 508-509, 509*t*
  opioid. *See* Opioids.
  patient-controlled, 507
  poisoning with, 552-553, 556
Anaphylaxis, 527-533
  antibiotics and, 529
  classification of immunologic reactions in, 527, 528*t*
  diagnosis of, 530-532
  heparin and, 530
  management of, 531*b*, 532
  neuromuscular blocking agents and, 528-529
  propofol and, 529-530
  to skin and oral disinfectants, 530
ANCA-associated vasculitis. *See* Antineutrophil
    cytoplasmic antibody (ANCA)-associated vasculitis.
Anemia, 5, 207
Anesthesia
  in bronchoscopy, 107-108, 110*t*
  general, in patients with cuffed tracheotomy tubes, 96
  Guillain-Barré syndrome and, 449
  inhaled, for severe asthma attacks, 144
  nondepolarizing neuromuscular blocking agents
      and, 501*t*

Aneurysms, intracranial mycotic, 230-231
Angina
  persistent refractory, 2
  unstable, 194, 194*t*, 196
Angiography
  as brain death confirmatory test, 431, 590*t*
  of gastrointestinal bleeding, 334
Angiotensin-converting enzyme (ACE) inhibitors
  acute pancreatitis and, 336
  hyperkalemia and, 319
  for hypertension, 294
ANH. *See* Acute normovolemic intraoperative
      hemodilution (ANH).
Animal bites, infections after, 267, 267*t*
Anion gap
  acid-base status and, 311, 314
  in diabetic ketoacidosis, 359-360, 363-364
  metabolic acidosis and, 312*b*
Anion gap acidosis, 6
Anorexia nervosa, chest tubes placement in, 103
Anterior cerebral arteries (ACA), 444
Anthrax, 252-254, 253*t*, 256*t*, 257, 258*t*
Antiarrhythmic drugs, 202, 501*t*
Antibiotic resistance, 262
Antibiotics
  for acute pancreatitis, 339
  after human bites, 268
  anaphylaxis and, 529
  for chest trauma, 480-481
  before chest tube placement, 103
  for chronic obstructive pulmonary disease
      exacerbations, 153
  for endocarditis, 229
  for febrile neutropenia patients allergic to penicillin,
      284
  for HAP, HCAP, or VAP, 136-140,
      138*t*, 139*f*
  for influenza, 273
  for intraabdominal infections, 355
  for neutropenic fever, 408
  for severe asthma attacks, 145
  thrombocytopenia and, 392
  for tularemia, 257
  for typhlitis, 290*b*
  for variceal bleeding, 349
Anticholinergic toxidromes, 546*t*
Anticholinergics
  for chronic obstructive pulmonary disease, 152
  for severe asthma attacks, 143, 144*t*
Anticholinesterases, side effects of, 502
Anticoagulation, 201, 202*t*
  for acute myocardial infarction, 195
  for continuous renal replacement therapy, 308
  for cor pulmonale, 162
  intraaortic balloon pumps and, 123
  for pulmonary embolism, 180-181
  reversal of, in warfarin-associated intracerebral
      hemorrhage, 446
  for stroke, 445

Anticoagulation (*Continued*)
  for superior vena cava syndrome, 407
Anticonvulsants
  for alcohol withdrawal, 458-459
  for brain metastasis, 406
Antidepressants
  for delirium, 517*t*
  tricyclic
    cardiac arrest and, 24
    hyponatremia and, 325
    poisoning, 555-556, 555*t*
Antidiuretic hormone (ADH), 322
Antifibrinolytic agents, 388
Antifungal agents, 242, 243
Antigens, anaphylaxis and, 531
Antihypertensive therapy
  for aortic dissection, 209
  for malignant hypertension or hypertensive crisis, 294
Anti-IgE therapy in acute anaphylaxis, 532
Antimicrobial therapy
  lack of response to, 135
  for necrotizing skin and soft tissue infections,
      266-267
  nondepolarizing neuromuscular blocking agents and,
      501*t*
  for severe community-acquired pneumonia, 132-133,
      133*b*
  for surgical site infections, 268, 269*t*
  topical, for burns, 465-466, 466*t*
Antineutrophil cytoplasmic antibody (ANCA)-associated
      vasculitis, 416*b*, 417
Antinuclear antibody (ANA) test, 414
Antioxidants as pharmaconutrients, 55
Antiphospholipid syndrome (APS), 415*t*, 416
Antiplatelet therapy for STEMI, 193, 196
Antipsychotic drugs
  alternatives to, in neuroleptic malignant syndrome
      treatment, 569
  for delirium, 516-518, 517*t*
  neuroleptic malignant syndrome and, 6
Antirejection medications, 291
Antithrombotic therapy for STEMI, 193, 196
Anti-TNF, 279*t*
Aortic dissection, 3, 204-211
  classification of, 204, 205*f*, 208, 210
  clinical findings with, 206-207
  definition of, 204
  diagnosis of, 207-208, 210
  differential diagnosis of, 208
  epidemiology of, 204-205
  hypertension and, 294
  risk factors for, 205-206
  signs and symptoms of, 206
  treatment of, 208-210
Aortic regurgitation, 189-190, 189*t*
  aortic dissection-related, 206
Aortic stenosis, 187-188, 188*t*, 191
Aortic valvuloplasty, 188
APA. *See* Aldosterone-producing adenoma (APA).

APACHE. *See* Acute Physiology and Chronic Health Evaluation (APACHE).
Apnea, emergency tracheotomy and, 94
Apnea testing, 430, 430*b*, 589*b*
APS. *See* Antiphospholipid syndrome (APS).
ARDS. *See* Acute respiratory distress syndrome (ARDS).
ARF. *See* Acute respiratory failure (ARF).
Argatroban, 393
Arginine, 55
Arginine vasopressin. *See* Antidiuretic hormone (ADH).
Arrhythmias, 3
   cardiopulmonary arrests and, 23
   in heart transplant patients, 493
   in hypothermic patients, 536
Arterial blood gas (ABG) analysis, 1, 28-32, 36-38, 36*f*
   in altered mental status, 11
   in cor pulmonale, 160
   indications for, 28
   oximetry versus, 30-31
   point-of-care, 30
   in pregnancy, 571
   in respiratory system evaluation, 10
Arterial catheters
   complications of, 69, 70, 72
   indications for, 69, 72
   ultrasound guidance for, 77
Arterial lines, 39-40, 43
Arterial pressure tracing, 123, 124*f*
Arterial pressure waveform, 69
Arterial tracings, 40
Arterial-end-tidal carbon dioxide gradient, 35
Artery infarction syndromes, 444*b*
Arthritis
   rheumatoid
      intubation and, 412-413, 413*f*
      shortness of breath and, 418
   septic, 411, 421
Ascites, cirrhotic, 347-348
Aseptic meningitis, 236-237, 237*b*
Aspergillus spp., 240
Aspiration, transbronchial needle, 109
Aspirin
   for acute myocardial infarction, 193
   for NSTEMI, 194-195
   platelets and, 395
   poisoning, 552-553
Assist control ventilation, 59, 62
Association for Professionals in Infection Control and Epidemiology, 259*t*
Asthma
   fatal/near-fatal, 143
   severe, 2, 131
      attacks
         indicators of, 142
         treatment of, 143-145, 144*t*
      discharge of emergency department patients with, 145

Asthma (*Continued*)
   endotracheal intubation and, 145-148, 148*b*
   helium admixtures and, 146
   history of patients with, 142, 142*b*
   mechanical ventilation and, 148, 148*b*
   new pharmacologic strategies for, 148-149
   noninvasive positive-pressure ventilation in, 146
   risk factors for, 149
   serum potassium and, 317
Asymptomatic candiduria, 241
Asystole, 25-26
Atelectasis
   acute lobar, 112
   treatment of, 2
ATN. *See* Acute tubular necrosis (ATN).
Atracurium, 499*t*
Atrial fibrillation, 200
   hypotension and, 201
   in hypothermia, 536
   treatment of, 201
Atrial tachycardias, 201
Atrioventricular (AV) block, 202-203
Atrioventricular nodal reentrant tachycardia (AVNRT), 199
Atrioventricular reentrant tachycardia (AVRT), 199
AUDs. *See* Alcohol use disorders (AUDs).
Autoimmune hepatitis (AIH), 346
Autologous blood transfusions, 387
Auto-positive end-expiratory pressure (auto-PEEP), 147, 468-469
AV block. *See* Atrioventricular (AV) block.
AVNRT. *See* Atrioventricular nodal reentrant tachycardia (AVNRT).
AVRT. *See* Atrioventricular reentrant tachycardia (AVRT).
Azathioprine
   for myasthenia gravis, 454
   nondepolarizing neuromuscular blocking agents and, 501*t*
Azithromycin, 133*b*
Aztreonam
   for cat or dog bites, 267
   immunocompromised hosts and, 284
   for severe community-acquired pneumonia, 133*b*

B

Bacillus anthracis, 252
Bacitracin, complications of, 466*t*
Back pain
   serious causes of, 419-420
   spinal cord compression-related, 405
Bacteria, multidrug-resistant, 3, 246-251
   causes of, 246-250, 247*f*
   risk factors for, 246
   treatment of, 249-251
Bacterial enteritis, community-acquired, 290
Bacterial pneumonia, acute. *See* Acute bacterial pneumonia.
BAL. *See* Bronchoalveolar lavage (BAL).
Balthazar score, 337, 339*t*

Barotrauma
  asthma-related, 147
  ventilator-related, 61
Basic life support (BLS), 20
Basilar artery, 444
BCI. *See* Blunt cardiac injury (BCI).
Beck triad, 213
Bedside index of severity in acute pancreatitis (BISAP)
  score, 337, 340*t*
Benchmarking, 598
Benzodiazepines
  for alcohol withdrawal, 5, 457-459
  for cocaine-induced hypertensive crisis, 294
  delirium and, 515, 517*t*, 518
  for poisoning, 549*t*
  for status epilepticus, 437
Benzylisoquinolinium agents, 499, 499*t*
β-Agonists for severe asthma attacks, 143, 144*t*
β$_2$-Adrenergic agents, 152
β-Blockers
  for cocaine-induced hypertensive crisis, 294
  heart transplantation and, 494
  hyperkalemia and, 319
  for hypertension, 294
  for mitral stenosis, 189
  poisoning, 563
  for thyroid storm, 380*t*
β-Lactam, 133*b*
Bicarbonate, 28
  for diabetic ketoacidosis, 365
  in salicylate poisoning treatment, 552-553
  for severe sepsis syndrome, 220
Bile, fluid loss from, 48
Biomarkers in diagnosing acute myocardial infarction,
  192, 192*t*
Biopsy
  lung, 285*f*
  for *Pneumocystis carinii* pneumonia, 288
  in spinal cord compression, 406
  transbronchial, 109
Bioterrorism, 252-261
  definition of, 252
  infection control in intensive care units, 255-257,
    256*t*
  possible agents in, 252-254, 253*t*, 522
  signs of, 252, 254-255, 260*b*
  treatment of victims of, 255, 257-258, 258*t*
  web-based resources on, 259*t*
Bird flu, 274
BISAP score. *See* Bedside index of severity in acute
  pancreatitis (BISAP) score.
Bisphosphonate therapy for hypercalcemia, 404
Bivalirudin for NSTEMI, 194-195
Blast injuries, 523
Blast lung, 523
Bleeding
  in arterial catheterization, 69
  gastrointestinal, 329-335
  variceal, 348-350

Blood cross-matching, 386
Blood cultures
  in endocarditis, 227
  for immunocompromised hosts, 281
Blood flow during closed-chest compressions, 22
Blood loss
  in hemorrhagic shock, 48*t*
  minimizing, 388
Blood pressure. *See also* Hypertension; Hypotension.
  after acute intracerebral hemorrhage, 445-446
  hemodynamic determinants of, 293
  in hemorrhagic shock, 48*t*
  during ischemic stroke, 443-446
Blood pressure measurement
  with arterial catheterization, 69
  arterial lines in, 39-40
  manual vs. automatic cuffs in, 39
Blood products, 385-391
  damage control resuscitation and, 15-16
  for disseminated intravascular coagulation, 400,
    401*f*
  fresh frozen plasma, 385, 388, 389, 389*t*
  packed red blood cells, 385
  red blood cell surface antigen systems and,
    385, 385*t*
  for sepsis, 220
Blood screening, 386
Blood transfusions
  autologous, 387
  infectious risks of, 387
  minimizing, 388
  packed red blood cells for, 385
  potential hazards in, 386-387
Blood typing, 386
Blood urea nitrogen (BUN), 299
Bloodstream infections, catheter-related, 1,
  70-72
BLS. *See* Basic life support (BLS).
Blunt cardiac injury (BCI), 482-487
  clinical features of, 482
  diagnosis of, 483, 484
  pattern of injury in, 482, 483*f*
Blunt chest trauma, 475
  adverse outcomes after, risk factors for, 475
  antibiotics and, 480-481
  fluid therapy for, 478
  management of, 484
  pain management in, 477-478
  penetrating cardiac injuries, 484-486
  positive end-expiratory pressure in, 479
  respiratory therapy for, 478
B-lymphocyte depletion, 279*t*
BMT. *See* Bone marrow transplantation (BMT).
Body, water distribution in, 47, 49
Bone marrow transplantation (BMT), 278
Botulism
  as bioterrorism agent, 253, 253*t*, 256*t*, 257, 258*t*
  bulbar weakness and, 452
Bowel. *See* Intestines.

Bradycardias, 202, 203
Bradykinin, 528
Brain
    blood supply to, 442
    hypertensive crisis and, 293
    injuries, coma and, 423-424
    metastasis, 406
Brain death, 5, 7, 428-433
    definition of, 428, 432
    examination and diagnosis of, 428, 429b,
        430-432, 430b
    movements in, 429, 430, 432
    organ donation and, 589b, 590t, 591
Brainstem function in coma, 425
Breathing
    during CPR, 21
    elevated work of, 1, 88
    normal, 9-10
    post-tracheotomy shortness of breath, 96-97
Bridge to bridge therapy, 128
Bromocriptine for neuroleptic malignant syndrome,
    568
Bronchial artery embolization, 2, 174-176
Bronchoalveolar lavage (BAL), 108, 111, 112, 285f
Bronchodilators for chronic obstructive pulmonary
    disease, 152
Bronchopleural fistula (BPF), 471, 471b
Bronchoscopy, 2, 106-112
    community-acquired pneumonia and, 109
    complications of, 109, 110t, 112
    contraindications for, 109
    definition of, 106
    fiberoptic, 107-108, 173, 175-176
    flexible, 106, 106f, 107f, 109, 111, 112
    in hemoptysis evaluation, 111, 173, 174
    in immunosuppression and pulmonary infiltrates,
        109-110
    indications for, 108, 108t, 112
    intubation prior to, 107
    in lung donors, 111
    mechanical ventilation and, 111
    rigid, 107
    during tracheotomy, 112
    ventilator-associated pneumonia and, 110, 111
BSP. See Bronchopleural fistula (BPF).
Bubonic plague, 253t, 254, 255, 256t, 257, 258t
Bulbar weakness, differential diagnosis of, 452
BUN. See Blood urea nitrogen (BUN).
Bundled consent forms in end-of-life care, 580
Burn centers, 463-464
Burn shock, 462, 466
Burns, 461-467
    chemical, 465
    electrical, 465
    thermal
        classification of, 461, 466
        hypermetabolism and, 464, 466
        ocular involvement after, 464
        treatment of, 461-466, 466t

C
C waves, 40, 45
CAB of CPR. See Compressions, airway, and breathing
    (CAB) of CPR.
Calcineurin inhibitors, 279t
Calcitonin, 404
Calcium channel blockers
    for cor pulmonale, 163
    heart transplantation and, 494
    for hypertension, 294
    nondepolarizing neuromuscular blocking agents
        and, 501t
    poisoning, 6, 563, 564
Caloric requirements of critically ill patients,
    51, 51t
CAM-ICU. See Confusion assessment method
    (CAM-ICU).
Campylobacter jejuni, 448
CA-MRSA. See Community-acquired methicillin-
    resistant Staphylococcus aureus (CA-MRSA).
Cancer. See Oncologic emergencies and specific types
    of cancer.
Candida sp.
    central venous catheter-related bloodstream
        infection, 71
    disseminated fungal infections. See Disseminated
        fungal infections.
    fluconazole-resistant, 243
    sepsis and, 218
Candidemia, 241, 242, 242t
Candiduria, asymptomatic, 241
CAP. See Community-acquired pneumonia (CAP).
Capnocytophaga canimorsus, 264
Capnography, 34-36, 35f, 38
Carbamazepine
    for alcohol withdrawal, 458
    nondepolarizing neuromuscular blocking agents
        and, 501t
Carbapenemases, 248, 250
Carbon dioxide, exhaled, 28, 34-36, 35f
Carbon monoxide poisoning, 24, 31
Carboprost tromethamine for obstetric hemorrhage,
    574-575
Carboxyhemoglobin (CoHb), 34
Cardiac arrest, 1
    out-of-hospital, acute myocardial infarction
        and, 193
    in pregnant patients, 574
    sodium bicarbonate and, 23
    therapeutic hypothermia and, 6
Cardiac conduction
    adenosine and, 200, 200f
    endocarditis-related abnormalities of, 228
Cardiac death, donation after, 580-581, 588-591,
    590t
Cardiac enzymes, 10, 483
Cardiac imaging, 74, 75f
Cardiac injury, blunt. See Blunt cardiac injury (BCI).
Cardiac lesions in pregnancy, 575

Cardiac output
    arterial lines and, 43
    as blood pressure determinant, 10
    impedance, 44
    measurement of, 44
    during pregnancy, 571*t*
    pulmonary artery catheters and, 42-43
Cardiac pump model, 22
Cardiac resynchronization therapy (CRT), 114
Cardiac tamponade
    aortic dissection-related, 207
    cardiac arrest and, 24
Cardiac trauma, 482-487
Cardiobacterium hominis, 225
Cardiogenic shock, 14, 193, 195
    treatment of, 195
Cardiomyopathy
    dilated, 492
    hypertrophic, 185
    restrictive, 185, 492
    stress-induced, 185*t*
Cardiopulmonary arrest
    arrhythmias associated with, 23
    iatrogenic, 20, 26
    reversible causes of, 24-26
Cardiopulmonary bypass
    extracorporeal membrane oxygenation vs., 79, 79*t*,
        85
    hypothermia and, 535, 538
Cardiopulmonary resuscitation (CPR), 1, 20-27
    capnography during, 36
    compressions, airway, and breathing (CAB) of,
        21-22, 26
    drug administration routes in, 26
    in hypothermic patients, 535, 539
    in-hospital outcomes, 26
    pharmacologic therapy during, 22-23
    pulse oximetry during, 33-34
    successful outcome of, factors in, 22
    withholding, 580
Cardiopulmonary Resuscitation and Emergency
        Cardiovascular Care (CPR & ECC), 20
Cardiovascular collapse, 4
Cardiovascular drug poisoning, 562-564
    β-Blockers and calcium channel blockers in,
        563
    digoxins in, 562
    treatment of, 563-564
Cardiovascular implantable electronic device (CIED)
    cardioversion or defibrillation in patients with, 119
    management of, 113
Cardiovascular system
    evaluation of, 10
    liver transplantation and, 490
    mechanical ventilation and, 61
Carotid arteries
    anatomy of, 442
    occlusion of, 444
Cat bites, infections after, 267, 267*t*

Catheters
    arterial
        complications of, 69, 70, 72
        indications and common sites for, 69, 72
        ultrasound guidance for, 77
    central venous, 70
        candidemia and, 241, 242*t*
        complications of, 70
        indications for, 70, 72, 536
        as infection cause, 1, 71, 72
        ultrasound guidance for, 70-71
    pulmonary artery, 40-43, 42*f*, 219-221, 536
CCFNI. *See* Critical Care Family Needs Inventory
        (CCFNI).
CCFS. *See* Critical Care Family Satisfaction Survey
        (CCFS).
CD4 cell count in HIV patients, 278
CDC. *See* Centers for Disease Control and Prevention
        (CDC).
Cefazolin
    for MSSA, 264*t*
    for necrotizing skin and soft tissue infections, 267
    for surgical site infections, 268
Cefepime, 133*b*
Cefotaxime, 133*b*
Ceftaroline fosamil, 249
Ceftriaxone
    for influenza, 273
    for severe community-acquired pneumonia, 133*b*
Cellulitis, 262-265
    impetigo vs., 262
    risk factors for, 264, 269
    treatment of, 264*t*
Centers for Disease Control and Prevention (CDC)
    definition of bioterrorism, 252
    web-based resource on bioterrorism, 259*t*
Central line placement, 40, 45
Central line-associated bloodstream infections
        (CLABSI), 601, 601*b*
Central nervous system
    evaluation of, 11
    in hemorrhagic shock, 48*t*
    infection, immunocompromised hosts and, 282,
        282*t*, 283
    liver transplantation and, 490
    metastasis, 406
    perfusion assessment of, 10
    vasculitis, 420
Central pontine myelinolysis, 326
Central venous catheter-related bloodstream infection
        (CRBSI), 1, 71, 72
Central venous catheters, 70
    candidemia and, 241, 242*t*
    complications of, 70
    indications for, 70, 72, 536
    as infection cause, 1, 71, 72
    ultrasound guidance for, 70-71
Central venous pressure monitoring, 40, 41*f*, 42
Cephalexin, 264*t*

Cephalosporins
  immunocompromised hosts and, 284
  for necrotizing skin and soft tissue infections, 266
Cerebellar artery, 444
Cerebral angiography, 431, 590*t*
Cerebral arteries
  anatomy of, 442
  anterior, occlusion of, 444
  middle
    ischemia of, 441
    occlusion of, 444
  posterior, 442, 444
Cerebral scintigraphy, 431, 590*t*
Cerebrospinal fluid analysis. *See also* Lumbar puncture.
  for delirium, 515
  for encephalitis diagnosis, 238
  for Guillain-Barré syndrome, 448-449
  for meningitis diagnosis, 235-236, 235*t*
  for neuroleptic malignant syndrome, 566
Cerebrovascular accidents (CVA), 293, 295.
    See also Stroke
Cervical spine
  rheumatoid arthritis of, 412-413
  of trauma patients, 17
Charcoal, activated, 547, 547*b*
  multiple-dose, 547-548
Checklists in intensive care units, 595
Chemical burns, 465
Chemotherapy
  cytotoxic, 288-289
  side effects of, 408-409
  spinal cord compression and, 406
  for superior vena cava syndrome, 407
Chemotherapy-induced neutropenia, 286*t*
Chest, blunt trauma to, 475
  adverse outcomes after, risk factors for, 475
  antibiotics and, 480-481
  fluid therapy for, 478
  pain management in, 477-478
  positive end-expiratory pressure in, 479
  respiratory therapy for, 478
Chest roentgenogram, 173
Chest tubes, 100-105. *See also* Thoracostomy, tube.
  complications of, 101*b*
  in hemothorax, 100, 100*b*
  indications for, 101*t*
  pigtails vs., 102*t*
  placement of, 101-104
  positive pressure ventilation and, 2
  PPV and, 104
  removal of, 102, 104
Cheyne-Stokes breathing, 425
Children
  diabetic ketoacidosis treatment in, 366
  fluid maintenance requirements for, 47
Chlorhexidine, anaphylaxis to, 530
Cholecystitis, acalculous, 355
Cholestatic cirrhosis, 489
Cholestyramine, 380*t*

Cholinergic toxidromes, 546*t*
CHR. *See* Corticotropin-releasing hormone (CHR)
  stimulation.
Chronic adrenal insufficiency, 374
Chronic cor pulmonale, 157
Chronic kidney disease, 319
Chronic obstructive pulmonary disease (COPD),
  151-156
  acute respiratory failure in, 154
  cor pulmonale and, 158-159
  exacerbations in, treatment of, 153-155,
    154*b*, 155*b*
  mortality prediction in, 153
  noninvasive ventilation in, 2, 66
  prevalence of, 151, 155
  severity grading of, 151, 152*t*, 155
  smoking cessation and, 151
  treatment of, 152-153
Ciaglia technique, 93
CIED. *See* Cardiovascular implantable electronic device
  (CIED).
CINM. *See* Critical illness neuromyopathy (CINM).
Ciprofloxacin
  for anthrax exposure, 258*t*
  immunocompromised hosts and, 284
  for necrotizing skin and soft tissue infections, 266
  for severe community-acquired pneumonia, 133*b*
Circadian rhythms and aortic dissection, 206
Circle of Willis, 442
Circulatory assist devices, 121. *See also* Intraaortic
  balloon pumps (IABPs); Ventricular assist devices
  (VADs).
Cirrhosis, 346, 350*b*
  causes of, 347
  cholestatic, 489
  complications of, 347
  diagnosis of, 347
  gastrointestinal bleeding and, 349
  liver transplantation and, 349-350
  noncholestatic, 489
Cirrhotic ascites, 347-348
Cisatracurium, 499*t*
CLABSI. *See* Central line-associated bloodstream
  infections (CLABSI).
Clindamycin, 249
  immunocompromised hosts and, 284
  for methicillin-resistant *Staphylococcus aureus*,
    264*t*
  for necrotizing skin and soft tissue infections, 266
  nondepolarizing neuromuscular blocking agents and,
    501*t*
  for surgical site infections, 268
Clinical/critical pathways approach, 600, 600*b*
Clonazepam, 437
Closed intensive care units, 593
Closed-chest compressions, blood flow during, 22
Closed-head injuries, 17
Clostridial gas gangrene, 266
Clostridium botulinum, 255

Clostridium difficile colitis, 352-354, 356
Clostridium perfringens, 266
CMV. *See* Cytomegalovirus (CMV).
Coagulation
    blood products and, 385-391
    in cor pulmonale, 160
    in sepsis, 218
Coagulopathies in pregnant patients, 574-575
Cocaine-induced hypertensive crisis, 294
Codeine, 507
Coffee-ground emesis, 329
CoHb. *See* Carboxyhemoglobin (CoHb).
Colestipol, 380*t*
Colistin, 250
Colitis
    Clostridium difficile, 352-354, 356
    ischemic, 334-335
Colloid therapy
    for blunt chest trauma, 478
    differentiated from crystalloid therapy, 1,
        48, 49
    for resuscitation, 49
Colon, fluid loss and, 48
Colorimetric detectors, 34-35
Coma, 5, 423-427
    causes of, 423-424, 426, 427
    definition of, 423
    diagnostic approach to, 425, 427
    hypoxic, 426-427
    managing patients with, 424-427
    myxedema, 379-382, 381*t*
    natural history and prognosis of, 426
    toxin-induced, 424
Communication
    in family meetings, 582-584, 583*b*
    goals-of-care discussion, 584
Community-acquired bacterial enteritis, 290
Community-acquired bacterial meningitis, 3,
    232, 234*t*
Community-acquired methicillin-resistant
    Staphylococcus aureus (CA-MRSA), 133, 134
Community-acquired pneumonia (CAP)
    diagnosis of, 109, 132
    in immunocompromised hosts, 284
    recent development in, 134-135
    severe, 131, 132
        antimicrobial therapy for, 132-133, 133*b*
        criteria for, 131*b*
    treatment of, 133, 134*b*
Compartment syndrome
    abdominal, 4, 16-17
    extremity, 13
Complete blood cell count
    in abdominal pain, 353
    in diabetic ketoacidosis and hyperosmolar
        hyperglycemic state, 363
Complications, incidence of, 600
Compressions, airway, and breathing (CAB) of CPR,
    21-22, 26

Computed tomography (CT)
    of acute pancreatitis, 337
    of aortic dissection, 208
    of cor pulmonale, 161
    of encephalitis, 238
    enhanced, for abdominal pain evaluation, 353
    hypotension and, 14-15
    intracranial mycotic aneurysms and, 230-231
    before lumbar puncture, 235
    prior to lumbar puncture, 3
    of pulmonary embolism, 179
Computed tomography angiography (CTA), 179
Conduction, cardiac. *See* Cardiac conduction.
Conflict Resolution Policy, 577
Confocal microscopes, 45
Confusion assessment method (CAM-ICU), 11, 513
Connective tissue diseases, 415*t*
Constrictive pericarditis, 213
Continuous positive airway pressure (CPAP), 5, 479
Continuous renal replacement therapy (CRRT),
    303-308, 314*b*
Contusions
    myocardial, 482-484
    pulmonary, 475-477, 480*b*
        acute respiratory distress syndrome and, 477
        flail chest associated with, 5, 476-477
        mechanical ventilation and, 479
        treatment of, 477
        radiographs of, 476, 477*f*
Convulsive status epilepticus, 434, 435
Cooling
    acute myocardial infarction and, 195-196
    heat stroke and, 542-543
Cor pulmonale, 157-165
    causes of, 157-158, 159*t*
    diagnosis of, 160-162
    epidemiology of, COPD and, 158-159
    left ventricle function in, 163-164
    mechanical ventilation and, 164
    signs and symptoms of, 160
    subtypes of, 157
    treatment of, 162-163
Core temperature afterdrop, 535
Coronary arteries, thrombosis of, 25
Corticosteroids
    acute pancreatitis and, 336
    immunosuppressive risks of, 279*t*
    inhaled, for chronic obstructive pulmonary disease,
        152
    for myasthenia gravis, 454
    for severe asthma attacks, 143, 144*t*
Corticotropin-releasing hormone (CHR) stimulation,
    376
Cough, post-tracheotomy, 96-97
Coumadin. *See* Warfarin.
Coxiella burnetii, 225
CPAP. *See* Continuous positive airway pressure
    (CPAP).
CPR. *See* Cardiopulmonary resuscitation (CPR).

CPR & ECC. *See* Cardiopulmonary Resuscitation and Emergency Cardiovascular Care (CPR & ECC).
CRBSI. *See* Central venous catheter-related bloodstream infection (CRBSI).
Creatine kinase, differentials of elevated levels of, 420-421
Cricothyroidotomy, 93, 94
Crisis standards of care, 579-580
Critical care committees, 593
Critical Care Family Needs Inventory (CCFNI), 595
Critical Care Family Satisfaction Survey (CCFS), 595
Critical care vs. palliative care, 579
Critical illness neuromyopathy (CINM), 500
Critically ill patients, general approach to, 9-12
CRRT. *See* Continuous renal replacement therapy (CRRT).
CRT. *See* Cardiac resynchronization therapy (CRT).
Cryoprecipitate
    definition of, 389
    indications for, 389
Cryptococcus neoformans, 264
Crystalloid therapy
    after blood loss, 48
    composition of, 48, 49*t*
    differentiated from colloid therapy, 1, 48, 49
    for rhabdomyolysis, 310
CTA. *See* Computed tomography angiography (CTA).
Culture-negative endocarditis, 227-228
Curling ulcers, 333
Cushing ulcers, 334
Cutaneous abscesses, 266
CVA. *See* Cerebrovascular accidents (CVA).
Cyanide poisoning, 24
Cyclosporine
    heart transplantation and, 494*t*
    hyperkalemia and, 319
    immunosuppressive risks of, 279*t*
    for myasthenia gravis, 454
Cytology brush, 109
Cytomegalovirus (CMV), 277
Cytotoxic chemotherapy, esophageal disease and, 288-289

D
Dabigatran, 390
DAI. *See* Diffuse axonal injury (DAI).
Damage control resuscitation, 15-16, 390
Damage control surgery, 16
Damping, 39
Danaparoid, 393
Dantrolene
    for heat stroke, 543
    for neuroleptic malignant syndrome, 568
    nondepolarizing neuromuscular blocking agents and, 501*t*
Daptomycin, 249
    for methicillin-resistant *Staphylococcus aureus*, 264*t*
    for streptococcal infections, 266

DCD. *See* Donation after cardiac death (DCD).
Dead donor rule, 591
Death. *See* Brain death; Mortality.
DeBakey classification of aortic dissection, 204, 205*f*
Decision-making
    in clinical management, 599
    in end-of-life care, shared, 577, 578
Deep tissue infections, 4
Deep venous thrombosis (DVT), 3
    chemical prophylaxis against, in trauma patients, 18
    diagnosis of, 177-178
    prevention of, 182, 510
    risk factors for, 177, 177*b*
    treatment of, 180-182
    ultrasound in screening for, 77, 78
Deep-tendon reflexes, brain death and, 429
Deferoxamine, 549*t*
Defibrillation/defibrillators, 22, 119*b*
    cardiovascular implantable electronic devices and, 119
    implantable cardioverter, 2, 113, 117
        central line placement and, 118-119
        differentiating pacemakers from, 113, 113*f*, 114*f*
        electrocautery affects on, 119-120
        magnets and, 117, 118*t*, 119
        pacemaker placement and, 119
    as ventricular fibrillation treatment, 1
Delayed hemolytic reactions, 386
Delirium, 6, 512-519
    causes of, 514-515
    clinical features of, 512-513
    definition of, 512
    diagnosis of, 512-515, 518
    differentiated from dementia, 515
    evaluation of, 11
    risk factors for, 513, 513*t*, 514*t*
    subtypes of, 513
    treatment of, 516-518, 517*t*
Delirium tremens (DTs), 457, 459
Dementia differentiated from delirium, 515
Department of Health and Human Services (HHS), 521
Department of Homeland Security (DHS), 521
Dependence, definition of, 456
Depolarizing neuromuscular blocking agents, 499*t*
Desmopressin, 388
Dexamethasone
    for myxedema coma, 381*t*
    for thyroid storm, 380*t*
Dexmedetomidine, 509
Dextrose for hyperkalemia, 302
DHS. *See* Department of Homeland Security (DHS).
Diabetes insipidus, 326
Diabetes mellitus
    in intensive care units, oral medications and, 369
    type 1, 360
    type 2, 360
Diabetic ketoacidosis (DKA), 4, 359-368
    complications in, 367-368

Diabetic ketoacidosis (DKA) (*Continued*)
definition of, 359
hyperosmolar hyperglycemic state versus, 361
hyponatremia and, 324
laboratory tests for, 362-364
pathogenesis of, 359, 360*f*
signs and symptoms of, 361
treatment of, 364-365
in children, 366
in pregnant women, 366
type 2 diabetes mellitus and, 360
Diagnostic and Statistical Manual of Mental Disorders
(DSM-IV), 512
Diagnostic maneuvers vs. therapeutic maneuvers, 9
Dialysis, 548. *See also* Hemodialysis; Peritoneal
dialysis
Diarrhea after abdominal aortic aneurysm repair,
bloody, 356
DIC. *See* Disseminated intravascular coagulation
(DIC).
Diclofenac, 509*t*
Dicloxacillin, 264*t*
Diffuse alveolar damage (DAH), 167, 417
Diffuse axonal injury (DAI), 426
Digoxin immune Fab, 562
Digoxin poisoning, 562
Dilated cardiomyopathy, 492
Diltiazem, 189
Disaster medicine, 521-526. *See also* Bioterrorism.
crisis standards of care in, 579-580
injury categories in, 522
phases of disaster response, 522-523, 522*t*
planning and response, 524-526
public health sector plan and, 521, 521*b*
triage, 523-524
Disinfectants, anaphylaxis to, 530
Disseminated fungal infections, 3, 240-245
diagnosis of, 241
mortality and, 242
prevention of, 244
treatment of, 242-244
Disseminated intravascular coagulation (DIC), 5,
397-403, 397*f*
acute, 398, 400, 401*f*
chronic, pathophysiology of, 398
clinical presentation of, 398, 399*f*
definition of, 403
diagnosis of, 398, 399, 400*f*, 403
hemolytic transfusion reaction-related, 386
treatment of, 400-403, 401*f*
Diuretics
for aortic regurgitation, 190
for cor pulmonale, 162
hypokalemia and, 316
hyponatremia and, 325
loop
acute renal failure and, 301-302
hypokalemia and, 318
for rhabdomyolysis, 310

Diuretics (*Continued*)
for mitral stenosis, 189
nondepolarizing neuromuscular blocking agents and,
501*t*
DKA. *See* Diabetic ketoacidosis (DKA).
DNR orders. *See* Do-not-resuscitate (DNR) orders.
Dobutamine, 163
Dog bites, infections after, 267, 267*t*
Donation, organ. *See* Organ donation.
Donation after cardiac death (DCD), 580-581, 588-591,
590*t*
Do-not-resuscitate (DNR) orders, 579
Dopamine agonists for neuroleptic malignant
syndrome, 568
Dopamine for acute renal failure, 301-302
Doppler echocardiography
of aortic stenosis, 188*t*
of cor pulmonale, 161
of mitral stenosis, 189*t*
Doxycycline, 249, 264*t*
DRSP. *See* Drug-resistant *S. pneumoniae* (DRSP).
Drug overdose, 24
Drug-resistant *S. pneumoniae* (DRSP), 133, 133*b*
Drugs. *See also specific drugs.*
delirium and, 515
in Emergency Mass Critical Care, 525
heat stroke and, 541
hyperkalemia and, 319
hypokalemia and, 316
hyponatremia and, 325
QT prolongation from, 199*b*
thrombocytopenia and, 392
DSM-IV. *See Diagnostic and Statistical Manual of
Mental Disorders* (DSM-IV).
DTs. *See* Delirium tremens (DTs).
Duke criteria for endocarditis diagnosis, 224-225, 224*b*,
230
DVT. *See* Deep venous thrombosis (DVT).
Dyshemoglobinemia and pulse oximetry, 34
Dyspnea, superior vena cava syndrome-related, 406

E
EBU. *See* Endobronchial ultrasound examination
(EBU).
EBV. *See* Epstein-Barr virus (EBV).
ECG. *See* Electrocardiography (ECG).
Echinocandins, 243
Echocardiography
of acute pericarditis, 213
of aortic stenosis, 188*t*
of cor pulmonale, 161, 162
of endocarditis, 224-226
focused transthoracic, 74-75, 76*f*, 78
of mitral stenosis, 189*t*
of pericardial tamponade, 214-215
of pulmonary embolism, 179
severe hypovolemia and, 75
transesophageal. *See* Transesophageal
echocardiography (TEE).

Echocardiography (*Continued*)
  transthoracic. *See* Transthoracic echocardiography (TTE).
ECMO. *See* Extracorporeal membrane oxygenation (ECMO).
ECR. *See* Extracorporeal rewarming (ECR).
ECT. *See* Electroconvulsive therapy (ECT).
Edema
  airway, 463
  cerebral, 4
  pulmonary, 103, 471, 472
Edrophonium, 452, 502*t*
EEG. *See* Electroencephalography (EEG).
EGD. *See* Esophagogastroduodenoscopy (EGD).
Eikenella corrodens, 225
Elderly patients
  cardiogenic shock in, 193
  endocarditis in, 223
Electrical burns, 465
Electrocardiography (ECG), 10
  of aortic pericarditis, 213
  of endocarditis, 228
  of myocardial contusions, 483
  of pericardial tamponade, 214-215
  in poisoning, 547
  of pulmonary embolism, 178
  of right ventricular hypertrophy, 160
  of tachycardias, 197
  of tricyclic antidepressant poisoning, 555-556
Electroconvulsive therapy (ECT), 568
Electroencephalography (EEG)
  in brain death, 431, 590*t*
  for coma evaluation, 425
  in delirium, 515
  for neuroleptic malignant syndrome, 565
  for nonconvulsive status epilepticus, 434-435
Electrolarynx, 95
Electrolyte disorders, 11
  acute renal failure and, 302, 302*t*
  in neuroleptic malignant syndrome, 566
Electrolytes
  liver transplantation and, 491
  serum, neuromuscular blocking agents and, 501
  urinary, in acute renal failure, 300-301, 300*f*
Electromyography (EMG), 453
ELISA. *See* Enzyme-linked immunosorbent assay (ELISA).
Embolism
  amniotic fluid, 572
  fat, 182-183, 183*b*
  pulmonary, 3, 177, 183*b*
    acute, signs and symptoms of, 178, 178*b*
    diagnosis of, 178-180
    in pregnancy, 573
    prevention of, 182
    risk factors for, 177, 177*b*
    treatment of, 180-182, 181*b*
EMCC. *See* Emergency Mass Critical Care (EMCC).
Emergency department, discharge of asthma patients from, 145

Emergency Mass Critical Care (EMCC), 525
Emergency nonsurgical airway, 91
Emergency tracheotomy, 94
Emesis, coffee-ground, 329
EMG. *See* Electromyography (EMG).
Empathetic communication, 583-584
Empiric replacement fluids for fluid loss, 48
EN. *See* Enteral nutrition (EN).
Encephalitis, 237-239
Encephalopathy
  hepatic, 349
  hypertensive, 293, 295
Endobronchial ultrasound examination (EBU), 109
Endocarditis, 3, 223-231
  blood cultures and, 227
  clinical manifestations of, 223
  conduction abnormalities and, 228
  culture-negative, 227-228
  diagnosis of, 226
  Duke diagnostic criteria for, 224-225, 224*b*, 230
  in elderly patients, 223
  etiologic agents of, 225
  health care-associated, 226
  intracranial mycotic aneurysms and, 230-231
  neurologic manifestations of, 229-230
  nonbacterial thrombotic, 227
  perivalvular abscesses and, 226
  prosthetic valve, 228
  right-sided vs. left-sided, 228-230
  treatment of, 226, 229
End-of-life care
  active euthanasia vs., 579
  cardiopulmonary resuscitation and, 580
  conflicts in, 578, 581*b*
  crisis standards of care and, 579-580
  critical care vs. palliative care concerns, 579
  discussion of, during palliative care, 584-585
  DNR orders in, 579
  organ donation and, 580-581
  shared decision-making in, 577, 578
  universal or bundled consent forms in, 580
Endoscopic retrograde cholangiopancreatography (ERCP), 336, 341
Endoscopic variceal ligation (EVL), 348
Endoscopy
  for lower gastrointestinal bleeding, 334, 335
  for upper gastrointestinal bleeding, 332-333, 333*t*, 335
Endothelin receptor antagonists, 163
Endotracheal intubation, 2, 87
  in acute respiratory failure, 167
  after liver transplantation, 491
  in asthma patients, 145-148, 148*b*
  complications of, 91-92
  confirmation of, 91, 92
  difficult, 90-91, 90*f*
  drugs to facilitate, 89
  in Guillain-Barré syndrome, 449
  in hypothermia, 536, 539

Endotracheal intubation (*Continued*)
  indications for, 87, 88, 92
  noninvasive positive pressure ventilation vs., 58-59, 58*f*
  nonsurgical techniques for, 88
  in pregnant patients, 572
  surgical techniques for, 88
  for upper airway obstruction, 87
End-tidal carbon dioxide, 28
Enteral nutrition (EN), 1, 50, 54-55, 56*b*
  in acute kidney injury, 55
  in acute pancreatitis, 55
  complications of, 53-54
  composition of, 52
  continuous vs. in boluses, 52
  contraindications to, 53
  gastric vs. small-bowel, 52
  indications for, 51
  initiation of, 51
  monitoring of tolerance to, 52-53
  in pancreatitis, 339
  positioning during, 53
Enteritis
  bacterial, community-acquired, 290
  viral enteritis, 290
Enterobacter sp., sepsis and, 218
Enterobacteriaceae, 249
Enterocolitis, neutropenic. *See* Typhlitis.
Enterovirus, 290
Enzyme-linked immunosorbent assay (ELISA), 531
Enzymes, cardiac, 10
Epidemics, influenza, 273
Epidural analgesia, 510
Epinephrine
  for anaphylaxis, 531*b*
  in cardiopulmonary resuscitation, 22
  inhaled, for severe asthma attacks, 144
Epoprostenol for cor pulmonale, 163
Epstein-Barr virus (EBV), 277
ERCP. *See* Endoscopic retrograde
    cholangiopancreatography (ERCP).
Ertapenem, 267
Erysipelothrix rhusiopathiae, 264
Erythromycin resistance, 262
Erythropoietin, recombinant, 388
ESBL. *See* Extended-spectrum β-lactamases
    (ESBL).
Escherichia coli
  central venous catheter-related bloodstream infection
      and, 71
  infected pancreatic necrosis and, 340
  sepsis and, 218
Esmolol, 380*t*
Esophageal disease, cytotoxic chemotherapy and,
    288-289
Esophageal intubation, 2
Esophagitis, candidal, 289
Esophagogastroduodenoscopy (EGD), 348
Ethanol in alcohol poisoning, 560

Ethics consultants, 578
Ethics in end-of-life care, 577-581
  cardiopulmonary resuscitation, 580
  conflicts in, 578, 581*b*
  crisis standards of care, 579-580
  critical care vs. palliative care concerns, 579
  DNR orders and, 579
  euthanasia, 579
  organ donation and, 580-581
  shared decision-making, 577, 578
  universal or bundled consent forms, 580
Ethics interventions, 578-579
Ethylene glycol poisoning, 558, 560
Euthanasia, 579
Euthyroid sick syndrome. *See* Nonthyroidal illness
    syndrome (NTIS).
Evaluation of critically ill patients, 9-12
EVL. *See* Endoscopic variceal ligation (EVL).
Exertional heat stroke, 541
Extended-spectrum β-lactamases (ESBL), 246
Extracorporeal membrane oxygenation (ECMO), 2,
    79-86
  cardiopulmonary bypass vs., 79, 79*t*, 85
  circuit components, 81-82, 81*f*, 82*f*, 85
  common problems during, 83-84
  complications of, 84, 85
  contraindications to, 81
  goals for management during, 82, 83*t*
  indications for, 80, 80*b*, 85
  transferring of patients receiving, 85
  vascular access for, 82, 83*t*
  ventilation management during, 82-83
  ventricular assist devices vs., 125-126
  weaning from, 84, 84*t*
Extracorporeal rewarming (ECR), 538
Extremity compartment syndrome, 13
Eyes
  after burns, 464
  hypertensive crisis and, 293

F

Family meeting, 582-584, 583*b*
Family Satisfaction in the Intensive Care Unit
    Questionnaire (FS-ICU), 595
Family-centered care in intensive care units, 595,
    596
Fasciitis, necrotizing, 4
FAST. *See* Focused assessment with sonography in
    trauma (FAST).
Fat embolism syndrome (FES), 182-183, 183*b*
Fatal asthma, 143
Febrile neutropenia, 284
Febrile nonhemolytic reaction, 386
Federal Bureau of Investigation, 259*t*
Femur fractures, 15
FENa test, 300-301
Fenestrated endografts, 209-210
Fentanyl, 505, 506*t*
FES. *See* Fat embolism syndrome (FES).

Fetus
    oxygen delivery to, 571
    radiation exposure in, 6, 573, 574*t*
Fever
    in endocarditis, 224
    in immunocompromised hosts with pulmonary
        infiltrates and, 284-285, 285*b*, 286*t*
    neutropenic, 5, 407, 408
    in sepsis, 219
FFP. *See* Fresh frozen plasma (FFP).
FHF. *See* Fulminant hepatic failure (FHF).
Fiberoptic bronchoscopy, 107-108, 173, 175-176
Fibrinogen concentrate, 388
Fibrinolytic inhibitors, 402
Fibroproliferative phase, 167
FICA tool, 585-586
Fick's principle, 44
Finder needles, 70
First-degree burns, 461
First-degree heart block, 202
Fistula
    bronchopleural, 471, 471*b*
    tracheoarterial, 2, 174
    tracheoesophageal, 96-97
Flail chest, 475, 476*f*, 477, 480*b*
    diagnosis of, 475
    long-term morbidity in, 480
    mechanical ventilation and, 479
    pulmonary contusions associated with, 5, 476-477
    surgical stabilization of, 479
    treatment of, 477
Flatbush diabetes, 360
Flexible bronchoscopy, 106, 106*f*, 107*f*, 109, 111, 112
Fluconazole, 243, 244
Flucytosine, 243
Fluid loss
    categories of, 47
    empiric replacement fluids for, 48
Fluid responsiveness in critically ill patients, 43, 45
Fluid therapy, 47-49
    3:1 rule in, 48
    4:2:1 rule in, 47
    for acute pancreatitis, 4
    for adrenal insufficiency, 377
    for blunt chest trauma, 478
    for burn patients, 462-463
    for children, 47
    for diabetic ketoacidosis patients, 4
    for hyperosmolar hyperglycemic state, 366-367
    for hypotension, 11
    for myxedema coma, 381*t*
    for rhabdomyolysis, 310
    for thyroid storm, 380*t*
    for trauma patients, 16
Flumazenil, 549*t*
Fluoroquinolone
    for necrotizing skin and soft tissue infections, 266
    for severe community-acquired pneumonia, 133*b*
Fluoroscopy, 52

Fluticasone, inhaled, 148-149
Focal status epilepticus, 434
Focused assessment with sonography in trauma
    (FAST), 15, 76-77
Focused transthoracic echocardiography, 74-75,
    76*f*, 78
Fomepizole, 559-561
Food and Drug Administration, 259*t*
Fosphenytoin, 436, 438*t*
Fourth-degree burns, 461
Fractures
    femur, 15
    pelvic, 15, 17-18
    rib, 475-478
Francisella tularensis, 254
Frank hemoptysis, 171
Frank-Starling curve, 43
Fresh frozen plasma (FFP), 385, 388, 389, 389*t*
Frostbite, 465, 466
FS-ICU. *See* Family Satisfaction in the Intensive Care
    Unit Questionnaire (FS-ICU).
Fulminant hepatic failure (FHF), 343, 346, 350
Fungal infections
    disseminated, 3, 240-245
        diagnosis of, 241
        mortality of, 242
        prevention of, 244
        treatment of, 242-244
    as sepsis cause, 218
Furosemide, 336, 404
Futility Policy, 577

G

GAD-65 antibody testing. *See* Glutamic acid
    decarboxylase-65 (GAD-65) antibody testing.
Gas gangrene, 4, 266
Gastric enteral nutrition, 52
Gastric lavage as poisoning treatment, 6, 547, 550
Gastric tonometry, 45
Gastrointestinal (GI) bleeding, 329-335
    acute, 330, 331*f*, 332*f*
    causes of, 330
    cirrhosis and, 349
    lower, 329, 330, 330*t*, 334, 335
    management of, 331-334
    ulcer appearance and, 333*t*
    upper, 329, 329*t*, 330, 332-333, 335
Gastrointestinal system, liver transplantation and, 490
Gastrointestinal tract
    evaluation of, 11-12
    fluid loss from, 49
GCA. *See* Giant cell arteritis (GCA).
Gell and Coombs classification, 527, 528*t*
Gemifloxacin, 133*b*
General anesthesia in patients with cuffed tracheotomy
    tubes, 96
General approaches
    to critically ill patients, 9-12
    to trauma patients, 13-19

Gentamicin
  for endocarditis, 229
  for plague or tularemia exposure, 258t
GFR. See Glomerular filtration rate (GFR).
Giant cell arteritis (GCA), 418
Global Registry of Acute Coronary Events (GRACE), 194
Glomerular filtration rate (GFR)
  in acute renal failure, 299
  in severe hypertension, 296, 297f
Gloves, 255, 257, 275
Glucagon, 563, 564
Glucocorticoids
  adverse effects of, 419b
  in chronic obstructive pulmonary disease, 155
  for myxedema coma, 381t
  for thyroid storm, 380t
Glucose
  insulin and, 321
  liver transplantation and, 491
  poisoning and, 549t
  sepsis and, 220
Glutamic acid decarboxylase-65 (GAD-65) antibody
      testing, 360
Glutamine, 54, 55
Glycemic targets and hyperglycemia, 370-372, 371t
Glycoprotein, 392
GNRs. See Gram-negative rods (GNRs).
Goals-of-care discussion, 584
Gout, 411
Gowns, 255, 257, 275
GRACE. See Global Registry of Acute Coronary Events
      (GRACE).
Graft-versus-host disease (GVHD), 278
Gram stain of sputum for pneumonia diagnosis, 132
Gram-negative rods (GNRs), 132
Grey Turner sign, 336
Guidewire dilating forceps. See GWDF technique.
Guillain-Barré syndrome, 5, 448-451
  autonomic dysfunction and, 449
  diagnosis of, 448-450
  management of, 449, 450
  Miller Fisher variant, 452
GVHD. See Graft-versus-host disease (GVHD).
GWDF technique, 93

H
HAART therapy, 290-291
HACEK organisms, 225, 230
Haemophilus influenzae, 132
  cellulitis and, 264
  chronic obstructive pulmonary disease and, 154
  convulsive status epilepticus and, 435
  endocarditis and, 225
  meningitis and, 234t
Haloperidol, 517, 518
Hand hygiene, 12
HAP. See Hospital-acquired pneumonia (HAP).
Harris-Benedict equation, 51t

HAV. See Hepatitis A virus (HAV).
HBV. See Hepatitis B virus (HBV).
HCAP. See Health care–associated pneumonia (HCAP).
HCV. See Hepatitis C virus (HCV).
HDV. See Hepatitis D virus (HDV).
Head trauma
  adrenal insufficiency and, 377
  closed, in trauma patients, 17
  intensive care unit and, 13
Health care–associated endocarditis, 226
Health care–associated pneumonia (HCAP), 136-140,
      138t, 139f
Heart
  hypertensive crisis and, 293
  perfusion assessment of, 10
Heart block, degrees of, 202-203
Heart failure
  acute decompensated, 186-187, 186t, 191
  causes of, 185, 191
  classification of, 186t
  diagnosis of, 186, 187
  reduced ejection fraction, 185, 185t
  treatment of, 3
Heart failure reduced ejection fraction (HFREF), 185,
      185t
Heart Rhythm Society (HRS), 113
Heart transplantation, 492-495, 591
  complications of, 493
  contraindications to, 492
  extracorporeal membrane oxygenation and, 80b
  indications for, 492
  postoperative management, 493-495, 494t
Heat loss, modes of, 534
Heat stroke, 6, 541-544
  complications of, 542
  diagnostic criteria for, 543, 543b
  prevention of, 542, 543
  treatment of, 542-543
  types of, 541
Helium admixtures in asthma treatment, 146
HELLP (hemolysis, elevated liver function, low platelet)
      syndrome, 400, 572
Hemagglutinin, 273
Hematemesis, 329
Hematochezia, 329
Hematologic system, 490
Hematopoietic stem cell transplant recipients, 278
Hemicraniectomy, 445
Hemodiafiltration, 307
Hemodialysis
  for acute renal failure, 303, 304
  definition of, 307
  for poisoning, 548, 550, 556
  for salicylate poisoning, 553
  for toxic alcohol ingestion, 6
  for toxic alcohol poisoning, 560
Hemodynamic monitoring, 1, 39-46, 215
Hemodynamically stable tachycardias, 200
Hemofiltration, 307

Hemoglobin
  abnormal or variant, 31
  blood oxygen content and, 10
  fetal, 34
Hemoglobin-based oxygen carriers, 388
Hemolytic reaction, 386-387
Hemolytic uremic syndrome (HUS), 395
Hemoptysis, 171-176
  bronchial artery embolization for, 2, 174-176
  bronchoscopy-based evaluation of, 111, 173, 174
  differential diagnosis of, 171, 172*b*
  evaluation of, 173
  massive, 2, 3, 171, 173-176
Hemorrhage
  of airway, tracheotomy-related, 96
  damage control resuscitation and, 15-16
  damage control surgery and, 16
  gastrointestinal, 4, 330, 331*f*, 332*f*
  hypotensive resuscitation and, 16
  intracerebral, 295-296, 445-446
  massive, in pregnant patients, 574-575
  subarachnoid, 295
Hemorrhagic shock
  classes of, 48, 48*t*
  in trauma patients, 13-15
Hemostasis, role of platelets in, 392
Hemothorax
  definition of, 100
  tension, 103*b*
  treatment of, 100, 104
  on ultrasound, 76
Heparin
  action mechanism of, 390
  anaphylaxis to, 530
  for deep venous thromboembolism, 182
  disseminated intravascular coagulation and, 402
  hyperkalemia and, 320
  intraaortic balloon pumps and, 123
  low-molecular-weight, 390
    hyperkalemia and, 319
    for pulmonary embolism or deep venous
      thrombosis, 180, 182
    standard heparin vs., 390
  thrombocytopenia and, 392-394, 394*t*
Heparin-induced thrombocytopenia (HIT), 392-394,
  394*t*, 396
Hepatic encephalopathy, 349
Hepatitis, 350*b*. *See also specific types of hepatitis*
  acute, 345
  alcoholic, 4, 346
  autoimmune, 346
  chronic, 345
  definition of, 343
  nonviral causes of, 346
  severe alcoholic, 4
  types of, 343
Hepatitis A virus (HAV), 343
Hepatitis B virus (HBV), 344
  blood transfusions and, 387

Hepatitis B virus (HBV) (*Continued*)
  concurrent infection with, 277
  diagnosis of, 344
Hepatitis C virus (HCV), 344, 345
  concurrent infection with, 277
  diagnosis of, 345
  genotypes of, 345
  screening for, 345
Hepatitis D virus (HDV), 345
Hepatitis E virus (HEV), 343-344
Hepatopulmonary syndrome, 349
Hepatorenal syndrome, 348
Hepatotoxicity, acetaminophen-induced, 553
Herpes simplex virus 2 (HSV-2), 237
HEV. *See* Hepatitis E virus (HEV).
HFOV. *See* High-frequency oscillatory ventilation
  (HFOV).
HFREF. *See* Heart failure reduced ejection fraction
  (HFREF).
HHS. *See* Department of Health and Human Services
  (HHS); Hyperosmolar hyperglycemic state (HHS).
HHV-6. *See* Human herpes virus 6 (HHV-6).
High-frequency oscillatory ventilation (HFOV), 168
Hirudin, recombinant, 393
Histamine, anaphylaxis and, 530
Histamine 2, 392
HIT. *See* Heparin-induced thrombocytopenia (HIT).
HIV. *See* Human immunodeficiency virus (HIV).
H1N1, 274
H5N1, 274
Hofmann elimination, 499
Hospital disaster preparedness, 524
Hospital surge operations, 525, 526
Hospital-acquired pneumonia (HAP), 136-140,
  138*t*, 139*f*
HRS. *See* Heart Rhythm Society (HRS).
HSV-2. *See* Herpes simplex virus 2 (HSV-2).
Human bites, infections after, 268, 270
Human herpes virus 6 (HHV-6), 277
Human immunodeficiency virus (HIV)
  CD4 cell count and, 278
  chest tubes placement in, 104
  concurrent infection with, 277
  HAART therapy for, 290-291
  radiographic patterns of pulmonary disease in, 286*t*
HUS. *See* Hemolytic uremic syndrome (HUS).
Hydralazine, 294
Hydrocortisone
  for myxedema coma, 381*t*
  for thyroid storm, 380*t*
Hydrofluoric acid exposure, 465
Hydromorphone, 506, 506*t*
Hydroxocobalamin, 549*t*
Hyperactive delirium, 513
Hyperbaric oxygen therapy, 24
Hypercalcemia, 404
Hypercapnia
  acute respiratory failure and, 166
  asthma and, 146

Hypercarbia, 30, 31, 61
Hyperglycemia, 5, 369-373
    acute illness and, 369, 370*f*
    glycemic targets and, 370-372, 371*t*
    in intensive care units, 369-370
    treatment of, 369-372, 372*b*
Hyperglycemic crisis, 368*b*
Hyperinsulinemia-euglycemia therapy, 6, 563, 564
Hyperkalemia, 11, 319-321
    acute renal failure and, 302, 302*t*, 305
    cardiac arrest and, 24
    causes of, 319
    clinical manifestations of, 319
    diagnosis of, 320
    drug-related, 319
    rhabdomyolysis and, 309-310
    treatment of, 302, 320-321
Hypermagnesemia, 302*t*
Hypermetabolism, burn-induced, 464, 466
Hypernatremia, 326-327
Hyperosmolar hyperglycemic state (HHS)
    complications in, 367
    diabetic ketoacidosis vs., 361
    laboratory tests for, 362-364
    pathogenesis of, 361-362
    signs and symptoms of, 362
    treatment of, 366-367
Hyperosmolar therapy for closed-head injuries, 17
Hyperphosphatemia, 302*t*
Hypertension, 293-298
    accelerated, 293
    aortic dissection and, 205, 207, 209
    cerebrovascular accidents and, 295
    intraabdominal, 354
    ischemic heart disease and, 296, 298
    malignant, 293, 298
    nonemergent, 293
    ongoing angina and, 296, 298
    portal, cirrhosis-related, 347
    preeclampsia and, 296
    pulmonary
        cor pulmonale and, 157-158, 159*t*
        pathophysiology of, 158
        during pregnancy, 572
    reactive, 296
    renal artery stenosis and, 293, 296
    secondary, 296, 297
    severe, 4, 296, 297*f*
    treatment of, 294-296, 298
Hypertensive crisis, 293, 294, 298
Hypertensive encephalopathy, 293, 295
Hypertensive urgency, 293
Hyperthermia, malignant, 569, 570
Hypertonic saline solutions, 49
Hypertrophic cardiomyopathy, 185
Hypoactive delirium, 513
Hypocalcemia
    acute renal failure and, 302*t*
    chemical burns and, 466

Hypoglycemia, 372
    clinical impact of, 371-372
    definition of, 371
    treatment of, 11
Hypokalemia, 4, 315-319
    cardiac arrest and, 24
    causes of, 316
    clinical manifestations of, 316
    diagnosis of, 316-317, 317*f*
    drug-related, 316
    treatment of, 318-319, 318*b*
Hyponatremia, 4, 322
    acute vs. chronic, 324
    diabetic ketoacidosis and, 324
    diagnosis of, 323*f*, 324, 327*b*
    drug-related, 325
    hypoosmolality vs., 322-323
    hypovolemia and, 323, 324
    signs and symptoms of, 324-325
    translocational, 322-323
    treatment of, 325-326
Hypoosmolality, 322-323
Hypoperfusion, tissue, 1, 11
Hypotension, 1
    aortic dissection-related, 207
    atrial fibrillation and, 201
    β-Blocker/calcium channel blocker poisoning and, 563
    diabetic ketoacidosis-related, 4
    hemorrhage-related, 14-15
    permissive, 16
    in trauma patients, 13-14, 18
    treatment of, 11, 12
Hypotensive resuscitation, 16
Hypothermia, 534-540
    acute myocardial infarction and, 195-196
    arrhythmias in, 536
    cardiac arrest and, 24
    cardiopulmonary resuscitation in, 535, 539
    definition of, 534
    J waves during, 534, 535*f*
    management of, 536-538, 537*f*
    therapeutic, 6, 538-540
Hypothyroidism, nonthyroidal illness syndrome versus, 382
Hypoventilation as indication for endotracheal intubation, 88
Hypovolemia
    absolute versus relative, 24
    hyponatremia and, 323, 324
    peritonitis and, 356
    severe, echocardiography and, 75
Hypoxemia, 1
    acute respiratory failure and, 166
    after blood component transfusions, 387
    altered mental status from, 11
    as an indication for endotracheal intubation, 88
    pulmonary hypertension and, 2
Hypoxia and cardiac arrest, 24
Hypoxic coma, 426-427

I

IABPs. *See* Intraaortic balloon pumps (IABPs).
IAH. *See* Intraabdominal hypertension (IAH).
Iatrogenic cardiopulmonary arrest, 20, 26
Iatrogenic pneumothorax, 468-469
Ibuprofen, 509*t*
ICDs. *See* Implantable cardioverter defibrillators (ICDs).
ICMAs. *See* Intracranial mycotic aneurysms (ICMAs).
ICS. *See* Incident Command System (ICS).
ICU-acquired weakness, 500, 501
IDSA. *See* Infectious Diseases Society of America (IDSA).
IgE. *See* Immunoglobulin E (IgE) antibodies.
ILE. *See* Intravenous lipid emulsion (ILE).
ILI. *See* Influenza-like illness (ILI).
Illness, severity of, scoring systems for, 2, 598-599, 603, 607*b*
    scores at ICU admission, 603-605, 605*b*
    scores at ICU discharge, 606-608, 607*f*
    scores during ICU stay, 605-606
Imipenem, 133*b*
Immune function
    alcohol ingestion and, 456
    in pregnancy, 573
Immune thrombocytopenic purpura (ITP), 394-395
Immunocompromised hosts, 277-292. *See also* Human immunodeficiency virus (HIV).
    acute abdomen in, 356
    central nervous system infection in, 282, 282*t*, 283
    community-acquired bacterial enteritis in, 290
    community-acquired pneumonia in, 284
    esophageal disease, cytotoxic chemotherapy, and BMT, 288-289
    evaluation of infections in, 278-281
    febrile neutropenia and, 284
    with fever and pulmonary infiltrates, differential diagnosis for, 284-285, 285*b*, 286*t*
    HAART therapy for HIV patients in the ICU, 290-291
    hematopoietic stem cell transplant recipients, 278
    immunosuppressive medications and, 279*t*
    infections after transplantation, timing of, 280*t*
    in intensive care units, 277
    meningitis in, 283-284
    patient without spleen, 281-282
    Pneumocystis carinii pneumonia in, 288, 289*t*
    pulmonary infiltrates in, 109-110
    solid organ transplant recipient with severe sepsis, 291
    typhlitis and, 289
Immunoglobulin E (IgE) antibodies, 527, 531
Immunosuppression
    assessment of, 277-278
    heart transplantation and, 494, 494*t*
    liver transplantation and, 492
    net state of, 277, 291
Immunosuppressive medications, 501*t*
Impedance cardiac output, 44
Impella, 128

Impetigo vs. cellulitis, 262
Implantable cardioverter defibrillators (ICDs), 2, 113, 117
    central line placement and, 118-119
    differentiating pacemakers from, 113, 113*f*, 114*f*
    electrocautery affects on, 119-120
    magnets and, 117, 118*t*, 119
    pacemaker placement and, 119
Incident Command System (ICS), 524-525
Infarction
    artery, 444*b*
    lacunar, 443, 443*b*
    venous sinus thrombosis and, 443
    watershed, 443
Infection control
    bioterrorism and, 255-257, 256*t*
    burns and, 464
    influenza and, 275
Infections. *See also specific types of infections.*
    after animal bites, 267, 267*t*
    after human bites, 268, 270
    after liver transplantation, 492
    after transplantation, 278, 280*t*
    catheter-related, 1, 70-72
    central nervous system, 282, 282*t*, 283
    deep tissue, 4
    in immunocompromised hosts, 278-281
    intraabdominal, 355
    surgical site, 268-270, 269*t*
Infectious Diseases Society of America (IDSA), 71, 131, 259*t*
Inferior vena cava (IVC) filters, 181-182
Infiltrates, pulmonary
    bronchoscopy and, 108*t*
    in immunocompromised patients, 109-110, 284-285, 285*b*, 286*t*
Inflammatory myopathy, 421
Influenza, 271-276
    complications from, 271-272
    diagnosis of, 272
    epidemics, 273
    intensive care unit and, 274-275
    pandemics, 273-274, 579-580
    prevention of, 275
    strains of, 271
    symptoms of, 271
    treatment of, 272
Influenza season, 4
Influenza vaccine, 275
Influenza-like illness (ILI), 272-273, 273*f*
INR. *See* International normalized ratio (INR).
Institute for Healthcare Improvement, 68, 600-601
Insulin deficiency, diabetic ketoacidosis and, 359, 360*f*
Insulin therapy
    for diabetic ketoacidosis, 4, 364-366
    for hyperglycemia, 369-372
    for hyperkalemia, 321
    for hyperosmolar hyperglycemic state, 367

Intensive care unit (ICU) patients
  adrenal insufficiency in, 374, 375f, 376, 377
  alcohol and, 456
  delirium in, 512
  delirium tremens in, 457
  diabetes mellitus in, oral medications and, 369
  diffuse alveolar damage in, 417
  gastrointestinal bleeding in, 329, 330, 331f, 332f
  Guillain-Barré syndrome in, 450
  hemoptysis in, 173
  HIV, HAART therapy for, 290-291
  hyperglycemia in, 369-370
  immunocompromised, 277
  influenza in, 274-275
  influenza season and, 4
  liver transplantation, 491
  platelet dysfunctions in, 395
  rheumatologic disease in, 411-422
  scoring systems for comparison of disease severity
      in, 603-608
    scores at admission, 603-605, 605b
    scores at ICU discharge, 606-608, 607f
    scores during ICU stay, 605-606
  septic shock in, 5
  tachycardias in, 197
  thrombocytopenia in, 392, 396
  thyroid conditions in, 379
  trauma, 13
Intensive care units (ICU), 593-597
  administration of, 593, 596b
  bioterrorism and, 255-257, 256t
  checklists in, 595
  closed, 593
  cost of, 594-595, 600, 600b
  end-of-life care in, ethics in. See Ethics in end-of-life
      care.
  family conference, 583, 583b
  improving value of, 594-595, 596b
  Leapfrog Group and models of care, 593-594
  multidrug-resistant bacteria in, 248-250
  neuromuscular blocking agents in, 497, 498, 499t
  organization of, 593, 596b, 598
  pain management in, 504-511
  patient- and family-centered care in, 595, 596
  patient safety in, 600-602, 601b
  quality assurance in, 598-600, 601b
  reducing patient morbidity in, 12
  shortage of intensivists and critical care nurses in,
      594
  social workers' role in, 586-587
  ultrasound in, 74-78
  volume status in, determining, 43
  "without walls," 595-596
Intensivists, 594
International normalized ratio (INR), 389
Intestines
  obstruction of, 11-12
    large, 355-357
    small, 355

Intestines (Continued)
  perforation of, 11-12
Intraabdominal hypertension (IAH), 354
Intraabdominal infections, 355
Intraabdominal pressure monitoring, 354
Intraaortic balloon pumps (IABPs), 2, 121, 123, 128b
  arterial pressure tracing and, 123, 124f
  complications of, 122
  contraindications for, 122
  failure to augment, 123-124, 125t
  indications for, 122, 122b
  removal of, 123
  weaning from, 123
Intraarterial thrombolysis, 442
Intracerebral hemorrhage, 295-296, 445-446
Intracranial mycotic aneurysms (ICMAs), 230-231
Intraoperative blood salvage, 387
Intravenous alcohol, 458
Intravenous drug abusers, 3
Intravenous lipid emulsion (ILE), 563-564
Intrinsic PEEP. See Auto-positive end-expiratory
      pressure (auto-PEEP).
Intubation. See also Endotracheal intubation;
      Nasogastric intubation.
  for chronic obstructive pulmonary disease
      exacerbations, 154, 155b
  esophageal, nonrecognition of, 2
  in myasthenia gravis, 453-454
  in pericardial tamponade, 215
  prior to bronchoscopy, 107
  rheumatologic disease and, 412-413, 413f
  translaryngeal, 2
Iodide for thyroid storm, 380t
Iohexol, 380t
Iopanoic acid, 380t
Ipecac, syrup of, 6, 548
Ireton-Jones equation for obesity, 51t
Ischemia, abdominal pain and, 355
Ischemic colitis, 334-335
Isopropanol poisoning, 558, 561
ITP. See Immune thrombocytopenic purpura (ITP).
Itraconazole, 243
IV recombinant tissue plasminogen activator (IVtPA),
      441, 442, 442b
IVC filters. See Inferior vena cava (IVC) filters.

J

J waves, 534, 535f
Johns Hopkins Center for Civilian Bio-Defense Studies,
      259t
Joints, septic, 411, 421

K

Ketamine, 509-510
Ketoacidosis, diabetic. See Diabetic ketoacidosis (DKA).
Ketones, 362
Ketorolac, 509t
Ketosis-prone type 2 diabetes, 360
Keystone Safety Project, 601, 601b

Kidneys
    hypertensive crisis and, 293
    perfusion assessment of, 10
    transplantation, 591
Klebsiella sp., 218
Korotkoff sound, 39
Kussmaul sign, 214

L

Labetalol, 294
Lactate levels, 1, 11
Lactated Ringer's solution, 48, 49, 49*t*
Lactic acidosis, cancer and, 404
Lacunar syndromes, 443, 443*b*
Lacune, 443
Lambert-Eaton myasthenic syndrome (LEMS), 452
Large bowel obstruction, 355-357
Laryngoscopy, 88-91, 89*f*
Lasix. *See* Furosemide.
Lateral medullary syndrome, 444
Latex allergies, 529
Lazarus sign, 429
Leapfrog Group, 593-594
Left ventricular assist devices (LVADs), 127-129
Left ventricular dysfunction, cor pulmonale-related, 163-164
Leg raise, passive, 43
Legionella sp., 132
Legionnaires disease, 284
LEMS. *See* Lambert-Eaton myasthenic syndrome (LEMS).
Leplace's law, 356
Leukocytosis
    aortic dissection-related, 207
    in neuroleptic malignant syndrome, 566
Leukopenia, 277
Leukostasis, 407
Leukotriene blockade for asthma, 148-149
Levetiracetam, 438*t*
Levofloxacin, 133*b*
Levothyroxine, 5, 381*t*
Lidocaine
    in bronchoscopy, 107-108
    nondepolarizing neuromuscular blocking agents and, 501*t*
    for tricyclic antidepressants poisoning, 556
Life-supporting treatment, termination of, 585
Limb posturing, brain death and, 429
Linezolid, 249
    for methicillin-resistant *Staphylococcus aureus*, 264*t*
    for streptococcal infections, 266
Liothyronine, 381*t*
Lipase
    in abdominal pain, 353
    as pancreatitis indicator, 336-337
Listeria monocytogenes, 232-234, 234*t*
Lithium carbonate, 501*t*
Lithium dilution, transpulmonary, 43-44

Liver disease
    disseminated intravascular coagulation and, 399
    pulmonary syndromes associated with, 349
    severity classification of, 6, 489
Liver function tests, 343
    in abdominal pain, 353
Liver transplantation, 489-492, 591
    cirrhosis and, 349-350
    complications of, 490-491, 494
    contraindications to, 489-490
    indications for, 489
    pathophysiology before, 490
    postoperative management, 491-492
LMWH. *See* Low-molecular-weight heparin (LMWH).
Locked-in syndrome, 423
LODS. *See* Logistic Organ Dysfunction Score (LODS).
Logistic Organ Dysfunction Score (LODS), 606
Loop diuretics
    for acute renal failure, 301-302
    hypokalemia and, 318
    for rhabdomyolysis, 310
Lorazepam
    for alcohol withdrawal, 458
    for delirium, 517*t*
    for status epilepticus, 434-435, 437, 438*t*
Low-molecular-weight heparin (LMWH), 390
    hyperkalemia and, 319
    for pulmonary embolism or deep venous thrombosis, 180, 182
    standard heparin vs., 390
Lumbar puncture
    computed tomography prior to, 3
    immunocompromised hosts and, 278
    for meningitis evaluation, 235, 236, 239
Lung donors, bronchoscopy in, 111
Lung injuries, ventilator-associated, 61, 63
Lung sliding, 1, 75, 78
Lung volume reduction surgery, 153
Lungs
    blast, 523
    fluid therapy and, 47
    function of, 9
    infiltrates of
        biopsy in, 285*f*
        in community-acquired pneumonia, 132
    perfusion assessment in, 10
    transplantation, 591
    ultrasound of, 75, 76, 78
LVADs. *See* Left ventricular assist devices (LVADs).

M

Macrophage activation syndrome (MAS), 420
Maddrey's discriminate score, 4
Mafenide, complications of, 466*t*
Magnesium and potassium, 315-316
Magnesium sulfate
    for status asthmaticus, 145
    for status epilepticus, 437

Magnetic resonance imaging (MRI)
for acute pancreatitis, 337
for aortic dissection, 208
for brain death, 590*t*
for cor pulmonale, 161
for encephalitis, 238
for intracranial mycotic aneurysms, 230-231
for neuroleptic malignant syndrome, 566
Magnets
ICDs and, 117, 118*t*, 119
pacemakers and, 115, 116*t*
Malignant pericardial effusion, 407
Malnutrition, critical illness-related, 50
Mannitol
for closed-head injuries, 17
for rhabdomyolysis, 310
MAS. *See* Macrophage activation syndrome (MAS).
Mask intolerance, 61-62
Masks, 275
Mass lesions in immunocompromised hosts, 284
Massive hemoptysis, 2, 3, 171, 173-176
Mast cells, anaphylaxis and, 527-528
MCA. *See* Middle cerebral arteries (MCA).
MCS. *See* Minimally conscious state (MCS).
MDAC. *See* Multiple-dose activated charcoal (MDAC).
Mechanical ventilation, 58-62. *See also* Noninvasive
ventilation (NIV).
in acute respiratory distress syndrome, 1, 220-221
in acute respiratory failure, 167
assist control, 59, 62
auto-PEEP in, 60
bronchopleural fistula and, 471, 471*b*
cardiovascular system and, 61
for chronic obstructive pulmonary disease
exacerbations, 154, 155, 155*b*
complications of, 61
cor pulmonale and, 164
discontinuation of, 63-68
assessment for, 63-65, 64*f*, 67
criteria in, 65-66
sedation/analgesia and, 65, 67
fiberoptic bronchoscopy in, 107-108
in flail chest, 479
indications for, 1, 58, 62
modes of, 59
optimal PEEP setting in, 60
peak and airway pressure in, 61
pneumothorax and, 469
pressure support, 59, 60, 62
prolonged, 67
in pulmonary contusion, 479
in respiratory failure, 10
in sepsis-induced acute lung injury, 220-221
setting adjustments in, 61
in severe asthma, 148, 148*b*
synchronized intermittent mandatory ventilation, 59,
60
tidal volume selection for, 60
tracheotomy and, 95-97

Mechanical ventilation (*Continued*)
transbronchial biopsies during, 111
types of, 58, 58*f*
ventilator settings in, 60, 148
weaning from, 1, 63-68
assessment for, 63-65, 64*f*, 67
effect of early tracheotomy on, 97
parameters for, 65
Medial medullary syndrome, 444
Medical errors in intensive care units, 600
MELD. *See* Model for end-stage liver disease (MELD).
Melena, 329
Meningitis, 232-237
acute, 232, 233*t*
aseptic, 236-237, 237*b*
bacterial, postexposure prophylaxis in documented
settings of, 236
chronic, 232
community-acquired bacterial, 3, 232, 234*t*
diagnosis of, 235, 239
in immunocompromised hosts, 283-284
treatment of, 232-235
viral causes of, 237
Mental status evaluation, 11
Meperidine, 506*t*, 507
delirium and, 515
Meropenem, 133*b*
Mestinon. *See* Pyridostigmine.
Metabolic acidosis
abdominal pain and, 353
anion gap, 312*b*, 359-360
treatment of, 312*t*
Metabolic alkalosis
differential diagnosis of, 313
treatment of, 312*t*
Metabolic emergencies, 404-405
Metabolic environment, evaluation of, 11
Metformin, 369
Methadone, 507
Methanol poisoning, 558
MetHb. *See* Methemoglobin (MetHb).
Methemoglobin (MetHb), 31, 34
Methicillin-resistant *Staphylococcus aureus* (MRSA),
248-249, 262
community-acquired, 133, 134
treatment for, 137, 264*t*
Methimazole, 380*t*
Methylergonovine, 574-575
Methylxanthines, 152
Metronidazole
acute pancreatitis and, 336
for necrotizing skin and soft tissue infections, 266
Microscopes, confocal, 45
Midazolam, 436, 438*t*
Middle cerebral arteries (MCA)
ischemia of, 441
occlusion of, 444
Mifflin equation, 51*t*
Migraines, complicated, 441

Miller Fisher variant Guillain-Barré syndrome, 452
Milrinone, 163
Minerals, 55, 308
Minimally conscious state (MCS), 423, 426
Minitracheotomy, 93
Minocycline, 264*t*
Minoxidil, 294
Minute ventilation, calculation of, 28
Mitral regurgitation, 2, 190-191
Mitral stenosis, 188-189, 189*t*
Mitral valve in endocarditis, 228
Mixed agonist-antagonist opioids, 507
Model for end-stage liver disease (MELD), 6
Modified Allen's test, 70
MODS. *See* Multiple Organ Dysfunction Score
    (MODS).
Monitoring, hemodynamic, 1, 39-46
Montelukast for asthma, 148-149
Moraxella catarrhalis, 154
Morphine, 505, 506*t*
Mortality
    in acute chest syndrome, 169-170
    in acute myocardial infarction, 195
    in acute respiratory distress syndrome, 168
    in aortic dissection, 204-205
    blunt trauma, 475
    in burns, 464
    in candidemia, 242
    of cirrhotic ascites, 348
    in cor pulmonale, 160
    delirium and, 512
    in delirium tremens, 457
    in diabetic ketoacidosis, 360
    in flail chest, 477
    in heat stroke, 542
    indexed to severity of illness, 599
    Leapfrog Group and, 594
    in neuroleptic malignant syndrome, 565-566
    in NSTEMI, 194
    in pulmonary contusions, 477
    of reexpansion pulmonary edema, 471
    in sepsis, 218, 221
    in unstable angina, 194
    in upper gastrointestinal bleeding, 330
Mortality Predictive Model (MPM), 603-606
Motility agents in critically ill patients, 53
Motor weakness, subacutely evolving,
    generalized, 448
Mouth opening, evaluation of, 90-91, 90*f*
Moxifloxacin, 133*b*
MPM. *See* Mortality Predictive Model (MPM).
MRI. *See* Magnetic resonance imaging (MRI).
MRSA. *See* Methicillin-resistant *Staphylococcus aureus*
    (MRSA).
MSSA, 264*t*
MUDPILERS acronym, 312-314, 312*b*
Multidrug resistant (MDR) pathogens in HAP, HCAP, or
    VAP, 136-137
    treatment and, 136-137, 138*t*

Multidrug-resistant bacteria, 3, 246-251
    causes of, 246-250, 247*f*
    risk factors for, 246
    treatment of, 249-251
Multiple Organ Dysfunction Score (MODS), 606
Multiple-dose activated charcoal (MDAC), 547-548
Multiple-organ dysfunction syndrome, 2, 168, 217
Muscle relaxants. *See* Neuromuscular blocking agents
    (NMBs).
Myasthenia gravis, 5, 452-455
    diagnosis of, 452-453
    pathophysiology of, 453
    treatment of, 454, 455
Myasthenic crisis, 453, 455
Mycophenolate mofetil
    heart transplantation and, 494*t*
    immunosuppressive risks of, 279*t*
Myelinolysis, central pontine, 326
Myocardial contusion, 482-484
Myocardial infarction
    acute. *See* Acute myocardial infarction (AMI).
    aortic dissection-related, 207
    intraaortic balloon pumps and, 2
    serum potassium and, 317
Myocardial ischemia, aortic dissection-related, 207
Myocarditis, 185*t*
Myoclonic status epilepticus, 434, 437
Myonecrosis, 266
Myopathy, inflammatory, 421
Myxedema coma, 379-382, 381*t*

N
N-Acetylcysteine, as acetaminophen overdose
    treatment, 6, 553, 554
Nafcillin
    for endocarditis, 229
    for MSSA, 264*t*
    for necrotizing skin and soft tissue infections, 267
Naloxone, 549*t*
Narcotics. *See* Opioids.
Nasogastric intubation, 329, 330
National Institute for Allergy and Infectious Diseases
    Biodefense Research, 259*t*
National Response Plans, 521, 521*b*
NBTE. *See* Nonbacterial thrombotic endocarditis
    (NBTE).
Near-fatal asthma, 143
Necrosis
    hepatic, 489
    pancreatic, 340
Necrotizing fasciitis, 4
Necrotizing skin and soft tissue infections, 266-267
Needle decompression, 103
Negative-pressure ventilation, 58
Neisseria meningitidis, 232-234, 234*t*, 236
Neostigmine, 502*t*
Net state of immunosuppression, 277, 291
Neuraminidase, 273

Neuroleptic malignant syndrome (NMS), 6, 546*t*, 565-570
  diagnosis of, 566
  differential diagnosis of, 566, 567*b*, 570
  malignant hyperthermia and, 569, 570
  prevention of, 569
  risk factors for, 567-568
  serotonin syndrome and, 570
  signs and symptoms of, 565*b*
  treatment of, 568-570
Neurologic evaluation, 11
Neuromuscular blocking agents (NMBs), 497-503. *See also specific neuromuscular blocking agents*
  active metabolites of, 501-502
  anaphylaxis and, 528-529
  classification of, 497
  depolarizing, 499*t*
  drug interactions of, 501*t*
  Guillain-Barré syndrome and, 449
  monitoring of, 500
  nondepolarizing, 498, 499, 499*t*, 500, 502, 502*t*
  prolonged, 502, 503*b*
  sedation and analgesia during, 500
  use during endotracheal intubation
Neuromuscular junction, 497
Neutropenia, 284
  central venous catheters and, 71
  chemotherapy-induced, 286*t*
Neutropenic enterocolitis. *See* Typhlitis.
Neutropenic fever, 5, 407, 408
Newborns, water weight in, 47
Nicardipine, 209
NICE-SUGAR study. *See* Normoglycemia in Intensive Care Evaluation-Survival Using Glucose Algorithm Regulation (NICE-SUGAR) study.
NIPPV. *See* Noninvasive positive-pressure ventilation (NIPPV).
Nitric oxide, inhaled, 163
Nitroglycerin for cocaine-induced hypertensive crisis, 294
Nitroprusside
  for aortic dissection, 209
  for aortic regurgitation, 190
  mitral regurgitation, 190
Nitrous oxide
  for in cor pulmonale, 163
  in patients with cuffed tracheotomy tubes, 96
NIV. *See* Noninvasive ventilation (NIV).
NMBs. *See* Neuromuscular blocking agents (NMBs).
NMS. *See* Neuroleptic malignant syndrome (NMS).
Nonbacterial thrombotic endocarditis (NBTE), 227
Noncholestatic cirrhosis, 489
Nonconvulsive status epilepticus (NSE), 434-435
Nondepolarizing neuromuscular blocking agents, 498, 499, 499*t*, 500, 502, 502*t*
Noninvasive positive-pressure ventilation (NIPPV), 58, 58*f*
  in asthma patients, 146

Noninvasive ventilation (NIV), 10, 58-62
  in acute respiratory failure, 59
  advantages of, 58-59
  in chronic obstructive pulmonary disease, 2, 154, 154*b*, 155
  complications of, 61-62
  for cor pulmonale, 162
  disadvantages and contraindications of, 59
  modes of, 59
  positive-pressure. *See* Noninvasive positive-pressure ventilation (NIPPV).
  in respiratory failure after extubation, 66
Nonpurposeful movements, brain death and, 429
Nonresolving pneumonia, 135-136
Nonsteroidal antiinflammatory drugs (NSAIDS)
  hyperkalemia and, 319
  side effects of, 508
Nonthyroidal illness syndrome (NTIS), 5, 379, 382-383
Normoglycemia in Intensive Care Evaluation-Survival Using Glucose Algorithm Regulation (NICE-SUGAR) study, 371-372
NSAIDS. *See* Nonsteroidal antiinflammatory drugs (NSAIDS).
NSE. *See* Nonconvulsive status epilepticus (NSE).
NSTEMI, 194-196
NTIS. *See* Nonthyroidal illness syndrome (NTIS).
Nuclear imaging of cor pulmonale, 161
NURSE mnemonic, 583-584
Nurses, critical care shortage of, 594
Nutritional status assessment, 50
Nutritional therapy. *See also* Enteral nutrition (EN); Parenteral nutrition (PN).
  in acute kidney injury, 55, 308
  in acute pancreatitis, 55
  in critically ill patients, 50-57
  propofol and, 55-56

O
Obesity
  heat stroke and, 541
  Ireton-Jones equation for, 51*t*
  morbid, chest tubes placement in, 103
Obstructive shock, 13-14
Occult pneumothorax, 100, 104
Octreotide, 331, 549*t*
ODIN. *See* Organ Dysfunction and Infection score (ODIN).
Ogilvie syndrome, 354-355
Olanzapine, 517*t*
Omalizumab, 532
Omega-3 fatty acids, 55
Oncologic emergencies, 404-409. *See also specific types of cancer.*
  definition of, 404
  hematologic, 407-408
  metabolic, 404-405
  side effects of chemotherapy, 408-409
  structural, 405-407
  types of, 404

Opioids, 505
  administration of, 507
  for aortic dissection, 209
  contraindicated, 507
  delirium and, 515
  for routine administration in ICU patients, 505-507, 506*t*
  side effects of, 508, 508*t*
  during terminal withdrawal of life support, 579
  toxidromes, 546*t*
OPO. *See* Organ Procurement Organizations (OPO).
OPSI. *See* Overwhelming postsplenectomy infection (OPSI).
OPTN. *See* Organ Procurement and Transplantation Network (OPTN).
Organ donation, 580-581, 588-591, 590*t*
  after cardiac death, 580-581, 588-591, 590*t*
  apnea test and, 589*b*
  brain death and, 589*b*, 590*t*, 591
  dead donor rule in, 591
  growing number of patients waiting for, 591, 592*f*
  potential donors for, 588
  rules and regulation on, 588
  statistics on, 591-592
  websites on, 592*b*
Organ Dysfunction and Infection score (ODIN), 605, 606
Organ Procurement and Transplantation Network (OPTN), 588
Organ Procurement Organizations (OPO), 588
Organ System Failure score (OSF), 605, 606
Orogastric lavage as poisoning treatment, 547
Osborn wave, 534
Oseltamivir, 272
OSF. *See* Organ System Failure score (OSF).
Osmolal gap, 559
Outcome assessment, 599-600
Overtriage, 524
Overwhelming postsplenectomy infection (OPSI), 281
Owen equation, 51*t*
Oxacillin
  for endocarditis, 229
  for MSSA, 264*t*
  for necrotizing skin and soft tissue infections, 267
Oxcarbazepine, 458
Oximetry, 30-31. *See also* Pulse oximetry
Oxygen carriers, 388
Oxygen consumption during pregnancy, 571*t*
Oxygen delivery to fetus, 571
Oxygen saturation, 10, 33-34, 37
Oxygen therapy
  in altered mental status from hypoxemia, 11
  for chronic obstructive pulmonary disease, 153
  for cor pulmonale, 162
  in Emergency Mass Critical Care, 525
  extracorporeal membrane, 2
  for myxedema coma, 381*t*
  for severe asthma attacks, 143, 144*t*
  for thyroid storm, 380*t*

Oxygenation, assessments of, 28-32. *See also* Pulse oximetry.
Oxyhemoglobin, 33
Oxytocin for obstetric hemorrhage, 574-575

P
PABD. *See* Preoperative autologous blood donation (PABD).
Pacemakers, 2, 113-120
  codes for, 114, 114*t*, 115
  differentiating ICDs from, 113, 113*f*, 114*f*
  electrocautery affects on, 119
  magnets and, 115, 116*t*
  modes of, 115, 116
  placement of, 118-119
  "R on T" phenomenon, 116-117
  websites on, 120*b*
Packed red blood cells (PRBCs) transfusions, 385
PACO₂. *See* Partial pressure of carbon dioxide in the alveolus (PACO₂).
PACs. *See* Pulmonary artery catheters (PACs).
Pain
  abdominal
    diabetic ketoacidosis-related, 361
    evaluation of, 352
    peritonitis-related, 353
    thoracic conditions and, 352
  adverse effects of, 505
  assessment of, 504, 504*f*
  back
    serious causes of, 419-420
    spinal cord compression-related, 405
  chest, aortic dissection-related, 206
Pain management, 504-511
  in blunt chest trauma, 477-478
  epidural analgesia in, 510
  inadequate, 504
  nonopioids in, 508-509, 509*t*
  opioids in, 505
    administration of, 507
    contraindicated, 507
    for routine administration in ICU patients, 505-507, 506*t*
    side effects of, 508, 508*t*
  patient-controlled analgesia in, 507
  in rib fractures, 478
Palliative care, 582-587
  discussion of end-of-life care, 584-585
  in end-of-life care, 579
  family's role in, 582-584, 583*b*
  goals-of-care discussion and, 584
  spirituality and, 585-586, 586*b*
Pancreas, fluid loss from, 48
Pancreatic pseudocysts, 341
Pancreatitis
  acute, 4, 336-342
    antibiotics and, 339
    biliary, 341
    causes of, 336, 341*b*

Pancreatitis (*Continued*)
    diagnosis of, 336-337
    nutritional therapy in, 55
    severity and prognosis of, 337, 338*t*,
        339*t*, 340*t*
    signs and symptoms of, 336
    treatment of, 338, 340-341, 356
   enteral nutrition in, 339
Pancuronium, 499, 499*t*
Pandemics, influenza, 273-274, 579-580
PaO$_2$. *See* Partial arterial oxygen tension (PaO$_2$).
PAOP. *See* Pulmonary artery occlusion pressure
    (PAOP).
Papilledema, 3
Paradoxic respirations, 9-10
Paralysis
   bioterrorism pathogens and, 255
   coma and, 424
Paralytic agents. *See* Neuromuscular blocking agents
    (NMBs).
Parenteral nutrition (PN), 50
   complications of, 54
   indications for, 54
Parkland Burn Center, 462
Partial arterial oxygen tension (PaO$_2$), 28-29, 111
Partial pressure of carbon dioxide in the alveolus
    (PACO$_2$), 35
Partial pressure of end-tidal carbon dioxide (PETCO$_2$),
    35, 35*f*, 36
Partial thromboplastin time (PTT), 389, 397
Passive leg raise, 43, 45
Pasteurella multocida, 264
Patient safety, 7, 600-602, 601*b*
Patient satisfaction, 599
Patient-centered care in intensive care units,
    595, 596
Patient-controlled analgesia (PCA), 507
PCA. *See* Patient-controlled analgesia (PCA).
PCI. *See* Penetrating cardiac injury (PCI).
PCP. *See* Pneumocystis carinii pneumonia (PCP).
PE. *See* Pulmonary embolism (PE).
PEA. *See* Pulseless electrical activity (PEA).
PEEP. *See* Positive end-expiratory pressure (PEEP).
Pelvic fractures, 15, 17-18
Pelvic immobilization, 18
Penetrating cardiac injury (PCI), 484-486
Penicillin
   anaphylaxis and, 529, 532
   hypokalemia and, 316
   for streptococcal infections, 266
Penicilloyl polylysine (Pre-Pen), 532
Pentobarbital, 436
PEP. *See* Postexposure prophylaxis (PEP).
Peptic ulcer disease (PUD), 333, 333*t*
Percutaneous mitral balloon valvotomy, 189
Percutaneous tracheotomy, 93
   dilational, 93
   with positive end-expiratory pressure, 94
   surgical vs., 93-94

Percutaneous valve implantation, 188
Perfluorocarbons, 388
Performance improvement in intensive care
    units, 599
Perfusion, assessment of, 10, 45
Pericardial disease, 204-211
   acute pericarditis, 212, 213
   constrictive pericarditis, 213
   pericardial tamponade, 13-14, 213-216, 216*b*
    acute, 214
Pericardial effusion, malignant, 407
Pericardial tamponade, 13-14, 213-216, 216*b*
   acute, 214
Pericardiocentesis, 213, 215
Pericarditis
   acute, 212
   constrictive, 213
Pericardium, 212
Peripheral blood smears, 398, 400*f*
Peritoneal dialysis, 303, 304
Peritonitis, 352-353, 356*b*
   clinical manifestations of, 353
   diagnosis of, 353
   spontaneous bacterial, 347, 348
Perivalvular abscesses, 226
Permissive hypercarbia, 61
Permissive hypotension, 16
Persistent vegetative state (PVS), 423, 426
PETCO$_2$. *See* Partial pressure of end-tidal carbon dioxide
    (PETCO$_2$).
Pharmaconutrients, 54-55
Pharyngeal space, evaluation of, 90-91, 90*f*
Phenobarbital, 438*t*
Phentolamine, 294
Phenytoin
   nondepolarizing neuromuscular blocking agents
    and, 501*t*
   for status epilepticus, 436, 438*t*
Pheochromocytoma, 294
Phlebotomy for cor pulmonale, 162
Phosphodiesterase-4 and chronic obstructive
    pulmonary disease, 153
Physostigmine, 549*t*
Pigtails, 102, 102*t*, 104
Piperacillin-tazobactam, 133*b*
PIRO score, 217
Pituitary dysfunction, nonthyroidal illness syndrome
    and, 382
Plague as bioterrorism agent, 253*t*, 254, 255, 256*t*,
    257, 258*t*
Platelet transfusions, 395, 396
Platelets
   aspirin and, 395
   dysfunctions of, 392, 395, 396
   role in hemostasis, 392
Pleural effusions
   aortic dissection-related, 207-208
   on ultrasound, 76
Pleural space on ultrasound, fluid in, 76

PMV. *See* Prolonged mechanical ventilatory support (PMV).
PN. *See* Parenteral nutrition (PN).
Pneumocystis carinii pneumonia (PCP), 288, 289*t*
Pneumonia
  acute bacterial, 131-141
    noninfectious, 136
    treatment failure in, 135
  community-acquired
    diagnosis of, 109, 132
    in immunocompromised hosts, 284
    recent development in, 134-135
    severe, 2, 131-133, 131*b*, 133*b*
    treatment of, 133, 134*b*
  health care–associated, 136-140, 138*t*, 139*f*
  hospital-acquired, 136-140, 138*t*, 139*f*
  multiple rib fractures and, 478
  nonresolving, 135-136
  Pneumocystis carinii, 288, 289*t*
  ventilator-associated, 61, 97, 136
    bronchoscopy-based diagnosis of, 110, 111
    diagnosis of, 2
    MDR pathogens and, 136-137
    prevention of, 137
    treatment of, 136-140, 138*t*, 139*f*
Pneumonic plague, 253*t*, 254, 256*t*
Pneumothorax, 468-474
  acute respiratory distress syndrome and, 470-471
  bronchopleural fistula and, 471, 471*b*
  causes of, 468, 468*b*
  chest tube treatment of, 101*t*, 102*t*
  clinical manifestations of, 469
  diagnosis of, 469-470
  iatrogenic, 468-469
  occult, 104
  pleural ultrasound for, 75, 78
  recurrent, 2
  reexpansion pulmonary edema and, 103, 471, 472
  spontaneous, 468
  tension, 5, 9, 103*b*, 472
    cardiac arrest and, 24
    clinical manifestations of, 473*b*
    diagnosis of, 13-14
    treatment of, 472
  traumatic, 468
  treatment of, 470, 472-473
Pneumothorax, tension, 5
Point-of-care ABGs, 30
Point-of-care ultrasound, 74
Poisoning, 545-551
  acetaminophen, 553, 554, 554*f*, 556
  cardiovascular drug, 562-564
    β-Blockers and calcium channel blockers in, 563
    digoxin in, 562
    treatment of, 563-564
  common toxidromes, 545, 546*t*
  diagnostic testing in, 545-547, 550
  salicylate, 552-553, 556

Poisoning (*Continued*)
  toxic alcohol, 559-560
    ethylene glycol, 558, 560
    isopropanol, 558, 561
    methanol, 558
    signs and symptoms of, 559
    treatment of, 560-561
  treatment of, 6, 547-548, 547*b*, 549*t*, 550
  tricyclic antidepressant, 555-556, 555*t*
Portal hypertension, cirrhosis-related, 347
Positioning
  in acute respiratory distress syndrome, 168
  during enteral nutrition, 53
Positive end-expiratory pressure (PEEP), 59
  in acute respiratory distress syndrome, 168
  in asthma patients, 148
  in blunt chest trauma, 479
  in chronic obstructive pulmonary disease, 155
  iatrogenic pneumothorax and, 468-469
  intrinsic. *See* Auto-positive end-expiratory pressure (auto-PEEP).
  optimal setting, 60
  percutaneous tracheotomy with, 94
Positive pressure ventilation (PPV), 2, 58
  chest tube removal and, 104
  iatrogenic pneumothorax and, 468-469, 472-473
  noninvasive, 58*f*
Postanoxic myoclonic status epilepticus, 437
Posterior cerebral arteries, 442, 444
Postexposure prophylaxis (PEP), 257-258
Postsplenectomy syndrome (PSS), 281
Potassium
  in digoxin overdose, 562
  magnesium and, 315-316
  serum
    in diabetic ketoacidosis and hyperosmolar hyperglycemic state, 363
    levels of, 315
    myocardial infarction or severe asthma and, 317
    regulation of, 315
  total body levels of, 315
Potassium replacement therapy, 318-319, 318*b*, 365
PPIs. *See* Proton pump inhibitors (PPIs).
PPV. *See* Positive pressure ventilation (PPV).
Prasugrel, 194-195
PRBCs transfusions. *See* Packed red blood cells (PRBCs) transfusions.
Prealbumin as nutritional status indicator, 50
Prednisone, heart transplantation and, 494*t*
Preeclampsia
  hypertension and, 296
  seizures and, 437
  severe, management of, 572
Pregabalin, 458-459
Pregnancy
  acute fatty liver of, 572
  acute respiratory failure during, 573, 573*b*, 575
  amniotic fluid embolism during, 572
  aortic dissection and, 206

Pregnancy (*Continued*)
arterial blood gas findings during, normal, 571
cardiac arrest during, 574
cardiac lesions and, 575
critical care during, 571-576
diabetic ketoacidosis treatment during, 366
endotracheal intubation during, 572
HELLP and, 572
hemodynamic values during, 571, 571*t*
massive hemorrhage during, 574-575
preeclampsia during
hypertension and, 296
seizures and, 437
severe, management of, 572
pulmonary embolism and, 573
severe trauma manifestations during, 573-574
termination of, 575-576
radiographs during, 573, 574*t*
Preoperative autologous blood donation (PABD), 387
Pre-Pen. *See* Penicilloyl polylysine (Pre-Pen).
Preperitoneal pelvic packing, 18
Pressure support ventilation, 59, 60, 62
Primary adrenal insufficiency. *See* Addison disease.
Primary aldosteronism, 297-298
Procainamide
acute pancreatitis and, 336
nondepolarizing neuromuscular blocking agents and,
501*t*
Prolonged mechanical ventilatory support (PMV), 67
Prone positioning in acute respiratory distress
syndrome, 168
Propofol
anaphylaxis to, 529-530
nutritional therapy and, 55-56
for postanoxic myoclonic status epilepticus, 437
for status epilepticus, 438*t*
Propranolol for thyroid storm, 380*t*
Propylthiouracil, 380*t*
Prostacyclins for cor pulmonale, 163
Prosthetic heart valves, endocarditis of, 228
Protein C, activated, 543
Prothrombin complex concentrate, 388
Prothrombin time
definition of, 389
in disseminated intravascular coagulation, 397
Proton pump inhibitors (PPIs), 331
Pseudocysts, pancreatic, 341
Pseudohemoptysis, 171
Pseudohyperkalemia, 320
Pseudomonas
multidrug resistant, treatment for, 137
as pneumonia cause, 132
Pseudomonas aeruginosa
chronic obstructive pulmonary disease and, 154
endocarditis and, 225
as meningitis cause, 234
multidrug-resistant, 249
as pneumonia cause, 132
sepsis and, 218

PSS. *See* Postsplenectomy syndrome (PSS).
PTT. *See* Partial thromboplastin time (PTT).
PUD. *See* Peptic ulcer disease (PUD).
Pulmonary artery, thrombosis of, 25
Pulmonary artery catheters (PACs), 40-43, 42*f*,
219-221, 536
Pulmonary artery occlusion pressure (PAOP), 41
Pulmonary capillary wedge pressure
liver transplantation and, 490
during pregnancy, 571*t*
Pulmonary contusions, 475-477, 480*b*
acute respiratory distress syndrome and, 477
flail chest associated with, 5, 476-477
mechanical ventilation and, 479
treatment of, 477
radiographs of, 476, 477*f*
Pulmonary edema, reexpansion, 103, 471, 472
Pulmonary embolism (PE), 3, 177, 183*b*
acute, signs and symptoms of, 178, 178*b*
diagnosis of, 178-180
in pregnancy, 573
prevention of, 182
risk factors for, 177, 177*b*
treatment of, 180-182, 181*b*
Pulmonary hypertension
cor pulmonale and, 157-158, 159*t*
pathophysiology of, 158
Pulmonary infiltrates
bronchoscopy and, 108*t*
in immunocompromised patients, 109-110, 284-285,
285*b*, 286*t*
Pulmonary reexpansion, rapid, 103
Pulmonary rehabilitation, 153
Pulmonary vascular resistance during pregnancy, 571*t*
Pulse oximetry, 1, 28, 33-34, 38*b*
in altered mental status, 11
cost effectiveness of, 37-38
definition of, 28, 33
double counting and, 40
in respiratory system evaluation, 10
in sickle cell disease, 169
Pulse rate in hemorrhagic shock, 48*t*
Pulseless electrical activity (PEA), 23
Pulseless idioventricular rhythm, 25
Pulsus paradoxus, 3, 214, 214*f*
PVS. *See* Persistent vegetative state (PVS).
Pyridostigmine, 454, 502*t*
Pyridostigmine toxicity, 454

Q
QALY. *See* Quality-adjusted life years (QALY).
QRS, very wide, 198, 198*f*
QRS complex, 116-117
QT prolongation, 199*b*
Quality assurance in intensive care units, 598, 601*b*
clinical/critical pathways approach and, 600, 600*b*
performance improvement and, 599
scoring systems for severity of illness and, 2,
598-599

Quality-adjusted life years (QALY), 594-595
Quetiapine, 517t
Quinupristin-dalfopristin, 249, 266

R

"R on T" phenomenon, 116-117
Rabies, 267
Radial artery, 40
Radial artery catheterization, permanent ischemic
    damage after, 69
Radiation, fetal exposure to, 6
Radiation therapy for superior vena cava
    syndrome, 407
Radioallergosorbent test (RAST), 531
Radiography. See radiographs.
Radiographs
    chest
        of cor pulmonale, 161
        of implantable cardioverter defibrillator, 113f
        of pacemaker, 114f
        for pneumothorax, 469
        in poisoning, 547
        of pulmonary contusions, 476, 477f
        of pulmonary disease in immunocompromised
            hosts, 286t
        of pulmonary embolism, 178
        for respiratory system evaluation, 10
        of rib fractures, 475
        in thoracic bleeding, 15
    in pregnant patients, 573, 574t
Randomized Evaluation of Mechanical Assistance for
    the Treatment of Congestive Heart Failure study.
    See REMATCH (Randomized Evaluation of
    Mechanical Assistance for the Treatment of
    Congestive Heart Failure) study.
Ranitidine
    acute pancreatitis and, 336
    nondepolarizing neuromuscular blocking agents and,
        501t
Ranson's criteria for acute pancreatitis,
    337, 338t
Rapid influenza diagnostic tests (RIDT), 272
Rapid regular narrow-complex tachycardias, 201
Rapid shallow breathing index (RSBI), 64
Rapid-response teams (RRTs), 595-596
RAS. See Renal artery stenosis (RAS).
RAST. See Radioallergosorbent test (RAST).
Recombinant human factor VIIa, 388
Rectal examination, 11-12
Red blood cell surface antigen systems,
    385, 385t
Red blood cell transfusions, 387
REE. See Resting energy expenditure (REE).
Reexpansion pulmonary edema, 103, 471, 472
Reflexes, brain death-associated, 429, 432
Relative adrenal insufficiency, 374
Relative hypovolemia, 24
Relative insulin deficiency, 359

REMATCH (Randomized Evaluation of Mechanical
    Assistance for the Treatment of Congestive Heart
    Failure) study, 128-129
Renal artery stenosis (RAS), 293, 296
Renal dysfunction in liver transplant patients, 491
Renal failure
    acute, 4, 299-305
        chronic vs., 299
        classification of, 299t
        diagnosis of, 299
        differential diagnosis of, 299t, 300-301, 300f
        electrolyte disorders and, 302, 302t
        in neuroleptic malignant syndrome, 566
        prevention of, 301
        treatment of, 301-305, 304b
    chronic, 299
    pregnancy and, 575
Renal replacement therapy, 306-308
    continuous, 303-308, 314b
    hybrid, 306
    indications for, 306
    modes of, 306
Renal system, liver transplantation and, 490
Respiration
    in hemorrhagic shock, 48t
    paradoxic, 9-10
Respiratory acidosis
    differential diagnosis of, 313
    treatment of, 312t
Respiratory alkalosis
    differential diagnosis of, 313
    treatment of, 312t
Respiratory failure
    acute. See Acute respiratory failure (ARF).
    chronic obstructive pulmonary disease-related, 2
    extracorporeal membrane oxygenation in, 2
    Guillain-Barre syndrome-related, 449
    postextubation, 66
    in pregnancy, 573, 573b, 575
    treatment of, 10
Respiratory system
    evaluation of, 9-10
    liver transplantation and, 490
Respiratory therapy for blunt chest trauma, 478
Resting energy expenditure (REE), 51, 51t
Restrictive cardiomyopathy, 185, 492
Resuscitation. See also Cardiopulmonary resuscitation
    (CPR).
    of burn victims, 462-464
    damage control, 15-16, 390
    hypotensive, 16
    of septic shock patients, 220
Resuscitation fluids, 48t, 49
Retina, hypertensive crisis and, 293
Retroperitoneal bleeding, evaluation of, 15
Rewarming of hypothermic patients, 536-538, 537f
Rhabdomyolysis, 309-310
    causes of, 309, 309b
    diagnosis of, 309

Rhabdomyolysis (*Continued*)
    signs and symptoms of, 309
    treatment of, 310, 313*b*
Rheumatoid arthritis
    intubation and, 412-413, 413*f*
    shortness of breath and, 418
Rheumatologic disease, 411-422
    ANCA-associated vasculitis, 416*b*, 417
    antiphospholipid syndrome, 415*t*, 416
    central nervous system vasculitis, 420
    inflammatory myopathy, 421
    macrophage activation syndrome, 420
    scleroderma renal crisis, 413, 414
    synovial fluid analysis and, 412*t*
Rib fractures, 475-477
    pain management in, 478
Richet, Charles, 527
RIDT. *See* Rapid influenza diagnostic tests (RIDT).
Right ventricular assist devices (RVADs), 124, 125, 127, 128
Right ventricular failure, 185
    in heart transplant patients, 493
    pathophysiology of, 157, 158*f*
Right-to-left shunt, 29
Rigid bronchoscopy, 107
Rimantadine, 272
Ringer's solution, lactated, 48, 49, 49*t*
Risperidone, 517*t*
Rocuronium, 499, 499*t*
Roentgenogram, chest
    in evaluation of hemoptysis, 173
    in evaluation of pneumothorax, 469
Roflumilast, 153
Rotavirus, 290
RRTs. *See* Rapid-response teams (RRTs).
RSBI. *See* Rapid shallow breathing index (RSBI).
Rumack-Matthew treatment nomogram, 553, 554*f*
RVADs. *See* Right ventricular assist devices (RVADs).

S

Safety, patient. *See* Patient safety.
Salicylate poisoning, 552-553, 556
Saline solutions
    composition of, 48, 49*t*
    hypertonic, 49
SAPS. *See* Simplified Acute Physiology Score (SAPS).
SBT. *See* Spontaneous breathing trial (SBT).
Scant hemoptysis, 171
SCh. *See* Succinylcholine (SCh).
Scleroderma renal crisis (SRC), 413, 414
Scoring systems for severity of illness, 2, 598-599, 603, 607*b*
    scores at ICU admission, 603-605, 605*b*
    scores at ICU discharge, 606-608, 607*f*
    scores during ICU stay, 605-606
SE. *See* Status epilepticus (SE).
Seasonal variation and aortic dissection, 206
Secondary adrenal insufficiency, 374

Secondary hypertension, 296, 297
Second-degree burns, 461
Second-degree heart block, 202-203
Second-hit phenomenon of disaster scenes, 524
Secrets, top 100, 1-8
Sedation
    in asthma patients, 148
    during endotracheal intubation
    during mechanical ventilation, 65, 67
    during neuromuscular blockade, 500
    during terminal withdrawal of life support, 579
Seizures
    prophylaxis during pregnancy, 572
    status epilepticus-related, 5, 434, 437-439
    stroke and, 441
Selective serotonin reuptake inhibitors, hyponatremia and, 325
Sepsis, 217-222
    definition of, 217, 221
    hypotension from, 11
    incidence of, 217-218
    microorganisms associated with, 218-219
    nomenclature of disorders related to, 217, 218
    pathogenesis of, 218
    in patient without spleen, 281-282
    severe. *See* Severe sepsis.
    signs and symptoms of, 219
Septic arthritis, 411, 421
Septic shock, 3, 217, 218
    adrenal insufficiency and, 377-378
    incidence of, 217-218
    pathogenesis of, 218
    steroid therapy for, 5, 377-378
Septicemic plague, 253*t*
Sequential Organ Failure Assessment (SOFA), 598, 606
Serotonin syndrome, 546*t*, 569-570
Serratia sp., 218
Serum electrolytes, neuromuscular blocking agents and, 501
Serum potassium, 315
    in diabetic ketoacidosis and hyperosmolar hyperglycemic state, 363
    myocardial infarction or severe asthma and, 317
    regulation of, 315
Serum sodium, 363
Severe asthma, 2, 131
    attacks
        indicators of, 142
        treatment of, 143-145, 144*t*
    discharge of emergency department patients with, 145
    endotracheal intubation and, 145-148, 148*b*
    helium admixtures and, 146
    history of patients with, 142, 142*b*
    mechanical ventilation and, 148, 148*b*
    new pharmacologic strategies for, 148-149
    risk factors for, 149
    serum potassium and, 317
Severe community-acquired pneumonia (CAP), 131, 131*b*

Severe sepsis, 3, 217, 221
  antirejection medications and, 291
Severity of illness, scoring systems for, 2, 598-599,
    603, 607*b*
  scores at ICU admission, 603-605, 605*b*
  scores at ICU discharge, 606-608, 607*f*
  scores during ICU stay, 605-606
Shared decision-making in end-of-life care, 577
Shivering
  postoperative, 507
  significance of, 534
  during therapeutic hypothermia, 539
Shock
  in bioterrorism, pathogens presenting with,
      254-255
  burn, 462, 466
  cardiogenic, 14, 193, 195
    aortic dissection-related, 207
    treatment of, 195
  hemorrhagic
    bleeding sources in, identifying, 14-15
    classes of, 48, 48*t*
  obstructive, 13-14
  septic, 3, 217, 218
    incidence of, 217-218
    pathogenesis of, 218
    steroid therapy for, 5
  spinal, 14
SIADH. *See* Syndrome of inappropriate secretion of
    antidiuretic hormone (SIADH).
Sickle cell disease/anemia, 169
Silver nitrate, complications of, 466*t*
Silver sulfadiazine, complications of, 466*t*
Simplified Acute Physiology Score (SAPS), 598,
    603-606, 605*b*
SIMV. *See* Synchronized intermittent mandatory
    ventilation (SIMV).
Sirolimus, 279*t*
SIRS. *See* Systemic inflammatory response syndrome
    (SIRS).
Skin
  fluid therapy and, 47
  perfusion assessment of, 10
Skin infections, 4, 269*b*
  after animal bites, 267, 267*t*
  after human bites, 268, 270
  cutaneous abscesses, 266
  diagnosis of, 262, 263*t*
  necrotizing, 266-267
  treatment of, 264*t*
Skin tests in anaphylaxis, 531, 532
SLE. *See* Systemic lupus erythematosus (SLE).
SLUDGE syndrome, 454
Small intestine
  fluid loss from, 48
  obstruction, 355
Small-bowel enteral nutrition, 52
Smallpox as bioterrorism weapon, 253*t*, 255, 256*t*,
    257, 258*t*

Smoking cessation and chronic obstructive pulmonary
    disease, 151
Social workers, 586-587
Society of Critical Care Medicine, 514
Sodium, serum, 363
Sodium balance and volume control, 322
Sodium bicarbonate
  cardiopulmonary resuscitation and, 23
  for poisoning, 549*t*, 556
Sodium nitroprusside for cocaine-induced hypertensive
    crisis, 294
Sodium valproate, 501*t*
SOFA. *See* Sequential Organ Failure Assessment
    (SOFA).
Soft tissue infections, 262-270
  after animal bites, 267, 267*t*
  after human bites, 268, 270
  cellulitis, 262-265, 264*t*, 269
  diagnosis of, 262, 263*t*
  necrotizing, 266-267
  signs of, 262
  surgical site, 268-270, 269*t*
Solid organ transplant patients,
  antirejection medications for, 291
  radiographic patterns of pulmonary disease in, 286*t*
Somatosensory evoked potential, 590*t*
Somatostatin analogs for gastrointestinal bleeding, 331
Speaking tracheostomy tube, 95
Spinal cord compression, oncologic, 405, 406
Spinal cord injuries, 17
Spinal shock, 14
Spirituality, 585-586, 586*b*
Spirometry in grading chronic obstructive pulmonary
    disease severity, 155
Splenectomy, 13
Spontaneous bacterial peritonitis (SBP), 347, 348
Spontaneous breathing trial (SBT), 63-65, 64*f*
  failure during, 65, 66*b*
Sputum Gram stain, 132
SRC. *See* Scleroderma renal crisis (SRC).
SSIs. *See* Surgical site infections (SSIs).
St. Louis encephalitis, 237
Stability and Workload Index for Transfer (SWIFT),
    606-608, 607*f*
Stanford classification of aortic dissection, 204, 205*f*,
    208, 209
Staphylococcus aureus
  antibiotic resistance and, 262
  as bacteremia cause, 227
  cellulitis and, 262
  central venous catheter-related bloodstream infection
    and, 71
  as endocarditis cause, 3, 225, 227, 230
  as meningitis cause, 234, 234*t*
  methicillin-resistant, community-acquired,
    133, 134
  as pneumonia cause, 132
  septic arthritis and, 411
Status asthmaticus, 145

Status epilepticus (SE), 5, 434-440
  classification and clinical presentation of, 434
  convulsive, 434, 435
  definition of, 439
  nonconvulsive, 434-435
  postanoxic myoclonic, 437
  treatment of, 435-439, 438*t*
ST-elevation MI (STEMI), 193, 196
Stem cell transplant recipients, 278
STEMI. *See* ST-elevation MI (STEMI).
Stenotrophomonas maltophilia, 250
Steroids. *See also* Corticosteroids.
  acute illness and, 419
  adrenal insufficiency and, 376, 377
  adverse effects of, 419*b*
  for anaphylaxis, 531*b*
  for brain metastasis, 406
  for chronic obstructive pulmonary disease
    exacerbations, 154
  inhaled for asthma, 148-149
  for meningitis, 234-235
  nondepolarizing neuromuscular blocking agents
    and, 501*t*
  for *Pneumocystis carinii* pneumonia, 288
  for sepsis, 221
  for septic shock treatment, 5, 375*f*
  for severe alcoholic hepatitis, 4
  spinal cord compression and, 405
  for spinal cord injuries, 17
  stress-dose, 377-378
  for superior vena cava syndrome, 407
StO$_2$. *See* Tissue oxygenation (StO$_2$).
Streptococcus agalactiae, 233*t*
Streptococcus bovis, 223, 224
Streptococcus iniae, 264
Streptococcus pneumoniae
  chronic obstructive pulmonary disease and, 154
  in convulsive status epilepticus, 435
  as meningitis cause, 3, 232-234, 234*t*
  as pneumonia cause, 132
Streptococcus pyogenes
  antibiotic resistance and, 262
  cellulitis and, 262
Stress ulcers, 333
Stroke, 441-447
  acute ischemic, 11, 441, 446
    blood pressure management in, 443-446
    IV recombinant tissue plasminogen activator for,
      441, 442, 442*b*
  anticoagulation and, 445
  arterial, infarcts from venous sinus thrombosis vs., 443
  artery infarction syndromes and, 444*b*
  definition of, 441
  differential diagnoses of, 441
  intracerebral hemorrhage and, 295-296, 445-446
  lacunar, 443, 443*b*
  large hemispheric, 445
  primary hemorrhagic, 445
  transient ischemic attack, 445

Structural brain injuries, coma and, 423, 424
Subarachnoid hemorrhage, 295
Succinylcholine (SCh)
  action mechanism of, 497-498
  contraindications to, 498, 499
  hyperkalemia and, 319
  indications for use of, 498
  rhabdomyolysis and, 310
Sufentanil, 506*t*, 507
Sugammadex, 502
Superior vena cava (SVC) syndrome, 404, 406, 407
Supraventricular tachycardia (SVT), 197
Surfactant replacement therapy, 168
Surge operations, hospital, 525, 526
Surgical site infections (SSIs), 268-270, 269*t*
Surgical time-out checklist, 600*b*
Surrogate decision maker, 584
Surviving Sepsis Campaign Guidelines, 219, 220*b*, 221
SVC syndrome. *See* Superior vena cava (SVC)
  syndrome.
SVT. *See* Supraventricular tachycardia (SVT).
Sweat, fluid loss from, 48
SWIFT. *See* Stability and Workload Index for Transfer
  (SWIFT).
Sympatholytic toxidromes, 546*t*
Sympathomimetic toxidromes, 546*t*
Synchronized intermittent mandatory ventilation
  (SIMV), 59, 60
Syncope, aortic dissection and, 206
Syndrome of inappropriate secretion of antidiuretic
  hormone (SIADH), 324
Synercid. *See* Quinupristin-dalfopristin.
Synovial fluid analysis, 412*t*
Syrup of ipecac, 6, 548
Systemic inflammatory response syndrome (SIRS), 5,
  218, 219
Systemic lupus erythematosus (SLE), 5, 414-415
Systemic vascular resistance during pregnancy, 571*t*
Systems engineering, 594

T

Tachycardias
  adenosine and, 200, 200*f*
  atrial, 201
  atrioventricular nodal reentrant, 199
  atrioventricular reentrant, 199
  hemodynamically stable, 200
  rapid regular narrow-complex, 201
  supraventricular, 197
  torsades de pointes, 198, 199*f*, 203
  treatment of, in intensive care units, 197
  ventricular, 197, 198, 198*f*, 203
  Wolff-Parkinson-While syndrome-related,
    198-199
Tachypnea, 5
Tacrolimus
  heart transplantation and, 494*t*
  immunosuppressive risks of, 279*t*
Tagged red blood cell scans, 334

Tamoxifen, 501*t*
Tamponade, cardiac. *See* Cardiac tamponade.
TandemHeart, 128
Tapazole. *See* Methimazole.
TBW. *See* Total body water (TBW).
TEE. *See* Transesophageal echocardiography (TEE).
Telemedicine, 594
Televancin, 249
Tensilon. *See* Edrophonium.
Tension pneumothorax, 5, 9, 103*b*, 472
    cardiac arrest and, 24
    clinical manifestations of, 473*b*
    diagnosis of, 13-14
    treatment of, 472
Tetanus, 267
Tetracycline
    acute pancreatitis and, 336
    nondepolarizing neuromuscular blocking agents
        and, 501*t*
Therapeutic hypothermia, 6, 538-540
Therapeutic maneuvers vs. diagnostic
    maneuvers, 9
Thermal injuries
    classification of, 461, 466
    hypermetabolism and, 464, 466
    ocular involvement after, 464
    treatment of, 461-466, 466*t*
Thermodilution, transpulmonary, 43-44
Thiamine, 435
Thiazide
    acute pancreatitis and, 336
    hypokalemia and, 316
    hyponatremia and, 325
    for rhabdomyolysis, 310
Thioureas, 380*t*
Third space, fluid loss from, 48
Third-degree burns, 461
Third-degree heart block, 202
Thoracic pump model, 22
Thoracostomy, tube
    antibiotics and, 480-481
    needle decompression vs., 103
    placement of, 102
    for pneumothorax, 5, 104, 470, 472-473
Thoracotomy, indications for, 100, 100*b*
Thrombocytopenia, 392-396
    definition of, 392
    disseminated intravascular coagulation-related,
        398
    drug-induced, 392
    heparin-induced, 392-394, 394*t*
    mechanisms of, 392
    prevalence of, 392
Thromboembolic cerebrovascular disease, 295
Thrombolysis, intraarterial, 442
Thrombolysis in Myocardial Infarction (TIMI), 194
Thrombolytic therapy
    for pulmonary embolism, 181, 181*b*
    for superior vena cava syndrome, 407

Thrombosis
    of coronary arteries, 25
    deep venous, 3
    of pulmonary arteries, 25
    venous sinus, 443
Thrombotic thrombocytopenic purpura (TTP), 395
Thymectomy, 454
Thyroid disease, 379-383
    myxedema coma, 379-382, 381*t*
    nonthyroidal illness syndrome, 5, 379, 382-383
    thyroid storm, 379, 380*t*, 382
Thyroid hormone replacement therapy, 381*t*
Thyroid storm, 379, 380*t*, 382
Thyromental distance, 91
Thyrotoxicosis, 452
TIA. *See* Transient ischemic attack (TIA).
Tidal volume selection in mechanical ventilation, 60
Tigecycline, 250
TIMI. *See* Thrombolysis in Myocardial Infarction
    (TIMI).
TIPS. *See* Transjugular intrahepatic portosystemic
    shunt (TIPS).
Tissue hypoperfusion, 1, 11
Tissue oxygenation (StO_2), 45
Tissue perfusion, assessment of, 10, 45
Tissue plasminogen activator, 11, 441
T-lymphocyte depletion, 279*t*
TMP-SMZ, 264*t*
TNF-α antagonists, 418-419
TNX-901, 532
Tobramycin, 229
Tonometry, gastric, 45
Top 100 secrets, 1-8
Torsades de pointes, 198, 199*f*, 203
Total body potassium, 315
    deficit in, 315
Total body water (TBW)
    in hypernatremia, 327
    in hyponatremia, 327
Total energy expenditure, 51
Toxic alcohol poisoning, 6, 558-561
    diagnosis of, 559-560
    ethylene glycol, 558, 560
    isopropanol, 558, 561
    methanol, 558
    signs and symptoms of, 559
    treatment of, 560-561
Toxicology. *See* Poisoning.
Toxidromes. *See* Poisoning.
Toxin-induced coma, 424
Toxins. *See also* Poisoning.
    cardiac arrest and, 24
    heart failure and, 185*t*
Trace minerals, acute kidney injury and,
    308
Tracheal buttons, 97, 98*f*
Tracheoarterial fistula, 2, 174
Tracheoesophageal fistula, 96-97
Tracheostomy. *See* Tracheotomy.

Tracheotomy, 2, 93-99
  airway hemorrhage and, 96
  aspiration after removal of tubes, 98
  bronchoscopy during, 112
  complications of, 2, 94, 95*b*
  cuff pressure of, 95, 96, 96*b*
  cuffed, precautions for general anesthesia, 96
  emergency, 94
  fenestrated, 97
  indications for, 93
  mechanical ventilation and, 95, 97
  mini, 93
  percutaneous, 93
    dilational, 93
      with positive end-expiratory pressure, 94
    surgical vs., 93-94
  tube sizes for, 95
  upper airway obstruction after decannulation of
      tracheostomy tube, 98
  ventilator weaning and, 97
TRALI, 387
Tranexamic acid, 402
Transbronchial biopsy, 109, 111
Transbronchial needle aspiration, 109
Transcranial Doppler, 431, 590*t*
Transcutaneous pacing pads, 203
Transducers, ultrasound, 74, 78
  for cardiac imaging, 74, 75*f*
  for vascular access, 77
Transesophageal aortic Doppler, 44
Transesophageal echocardiography (TEE), 80
  of aortic dissection, 208
  of blunt cardiac injury, 484
  of cor pulmonale, 161, 162
  of endocarditis, 225, 226
Transient ischemic attack (TIA), 445
Transjugular intrahepatic portosystemic shunt (TIPS),
      347, 348, 350
Translaryngeal intubation, 2
Translocational hyponatremia, 322-323
Transplantation, organ, 7. *See also* Heart
      transplantation; Liver transplantation.
  antirejection medications and, 291
  growing number of patients waiting for, 591, 592*f*
  immunosuppression after, 4
  risk of infection and time from, 278, 280*t*
  statistics on, 591-592
Transpulmonary lithium dilution, 43-44
Transpulmonary thermodilution, 43-44
Transthoracic echocardiography (TTE)
  of blunt cardiac injury, 484
  of cor pulmonale, 161
  of endocarditis, 226
  focused, 74-75, 76*f*, 78
Transtubular potassium gradient (TTKG), 320
Trauma patients. *See also* Blunt cardiac injury (BCI).
  abdominal compartment syndrome in, 16-17
  airway management in, 13, 14*f*, 18
  cervical spine of, 17

Trauma patients (*Continued*)
  chemical deep venous thrombosis prophylaxis in, 18
  closed-head injuries in, 17
  damage control surgery and, 16
  FAST examination of, 15
  general approach to, 13-19
  hemorrhagic shock in, 14-15
  hypotension in, 13-14, 18
  intensive care unit and, 13
  pelvic fractures in, massive bleeding from, 17-18
  pregnant, 573-574
  resuscitation of, 15-16
  spinal cord injuries in, 17
Trazodone, 517*t*
Triage in disaster medicine, 523-524
Triangle of safety in chest tube placement, 101
Tricuspid valve in endocarditis, 228
Tricyclic antidepressants
  cardiac arrest and, 24
  hyponatremia and, 325
  poisoning, 555-556, 555*t*
Trimethoprim-sulfamethoxazole (TMP-SMX), 249
Triple flexion response, brain death and, 429
Troponins, cardiac, 483
Tryptase, 531
TTE. *See* Transthoracic echocardiography (TTE).
TTKG. *See* Transtubular potassium gradient (TTKG).
TTP. *See* Thrombotic thrombocytopenic purpura (TTP).
Tuberculosis, 104
Tularemia, 253*t*, 254, 256*t*, 257, 258*t*
Tumor lysis syndrome, 405, 409*b*
Type 1 diabetes mellitus, 360
Type 2 diabetes mellitus, 360
Typhlitis, 289, 290*b*, 408-409

U
UDDA. *See* Uniform Determination of Death Act (UDDA).
Ulcers
  Curling, 333
  Cushing, 334
  gastrointestinal bleeding and appearance of, 333*t*
  stress, 333
Ultrasound
  abdominal, 353
  bedside, in monitoring hemodynamics in ICU, 44-45
  cardiac, 74, 75*f*
  for central venous access, 77
  for deep venous thrombosis, 77, 78
  endobronchial, 109
  guidance for central venous catheterization, 70-71
  in intensive care units, 74-78
  learning critical care techniques in, 77-78
  pleural, 75, 76, 78
  for pneumothorax, 469-470
  point-of-care, 74
  transcranial Doppler, 431, 590*t*
  transducers. *See* Transducers, ultrasound.
  for vascular access, 77
Uniform Determination of Death Act (UDDA), 428

United Network for Organ Sharing (UNOS), 588
Universal consent forms in end-of-life care, 580
UNOS. *See* United Network for Organ Sharing (UNOS).
Unstable angina, 194, 194*t*, 196
Upper airway obstruction
    after decannulation of tracheostomy tube, 98
    emergency tracheotomy for, 94
    endotracheal intubation for, 87, 92
Uremia, renal replacement therapy and, 306
Uremic syndrome, 303, 395
Urine
    acute renal failure and, 300
    fluid therapy and, 47
    in hemorrhagic shock, 48*t*
    potassium excretion in, 316
    sepsis and, 219
Urine toxicology screen, 545-547, 550

V
V waves, 40, 45
Vaccines
    chronic obstructive pulmonary disease, 153
    influenza, 275
VADs. *See* Ventricular assist devices (VADs).
Valproate for status epilepticus, 438*t*
VALUE mnemonic, 583
Valvotomy, percutaneous mitral balloon, 189
Valvuloplasty, aortic, 188
Vancomycin
    for endocarditis, 229
    immunocompromised hosts and, 284
    for influenza, 273
    for methicillin-resistant *Staphylococcus aureus*, 264*t*
    for multidrug-resistant bacteria, 249
    for necrotizing skin and soft tissue infections, 267
    for neutropenic fever, 408
    for severe community-acquired pneumonia, 133*b*
    for streptococcal infections, 266
    for surgical site infections, 268
Vancomycin-resistant enterococcus (VRE), 284
VAP. *See* Ventilator-associated pneumonia (VAP).
Variceal bleeding, 348-350
Varicella-zoster virus (VZV), 237
Vasculitis
    antineutrophil cytoplasmic antibody-associated,
        416*b*, 417
    aortic regurgitation and, 189*t*
    central nervous system, 420
    systemic lupus erythematosus-related, 5
Vasoconstrictors, heart transplantation and, 494
Vasodilators
    for aortic dissection, 209
    for cor pulmonale, 162, 163
    heart transplantation and, 494
    for hypertension, 294
Vasopressors
    for β-Blocker/calcium channel blocker poisoning, 563
    for cardiogenic shock, 195
    for gastrointestinal bleeding, 331

Vasopressors (*Continued*)
    for hypotension, 11
    intraarterial catheters and, 69
    as severe sepsis syndrome treatment, 5
Vecuronium, 499*t*
Venous sinus thrombosis (VST), 443
Venous thromboembolism, 177, 177*b*, 408
Ventilation. *See also* Mechanical ventilation.
    in acute respiratory distress syndrome, 168
    extracorporeal membrane oxygenation and, 79*t*
Ventilation-perfusion (V/Q) scan, 179
Ventilator-associated lung injuries, 61, 63
Ventilator-associated pneumonia (VAP), 136
    bronchoscopy-based diagnosis of, 110, 111
    MDR pathogens and, 136-137
    prevention of, 137
    treatment of, 136-140, 138*t*, 139*f*
Ventricular assist devices (VADs), 124, 125, 128*b*
    complications with, 127
    contraindications for, 127
    extracorporeal membrane oxygenators versus,
        125-126
    indications for, 127, 128
    left, 127-129
    percutaneous options for, 128
    pulsatile vs. continuous systems, 125
    right, 124, 125, 127, 128
    types of, 126*t*
    weaning from, 128
Ventricular fibrillation
    in hypothermia, 536, 539
    treatment of, 1, 25
Ventricular tachycardias, 197, 198, 198*f*, 203
Vertebral arteries, occlusion of, 444
VHF. *See* Viral hemorrhagic fever (VHF).
Vibrio vulnificus, 264
Viral enteritis, 290
Viral hemorrhagic fever (VHF), 252, 253*t*, 254, 255,
        256*t*, 257, 258*t*
Virchow's triad, 177
Vital organ perfusion, assessment of, 10
Vitamins, 55, 308
Volume deficit, 47, 49
Volume excess, 47
Von Willebrand disease, 392
Voriconazole, 243
V/Q scan. *See* Ventilation-perfusion (V/Q) scan.
VRE. *See* Vancomycin-resistant enterococcus (VRE).
VST. *See* Venous sinus thrombosis (VST).
VZV. *See* Varicella-zoster virus (VZV).

W
Wallenberg syndrome. *See* Lateral medullary syndrome.
Walmart, 524
Warfarin
    action mechanism of, 389
    argatroban administration with, 394
    for cor pulmonale, 162
    intracerebral hemorrhage and, 446

Water deficit in hyperosmolar hyperglycemic state, 367
Water distribution in the body, 47, 49
Watershed syndrome, 443
WBI. *See* Whole-bowel irrigation (WBI).
Weakness
    bulbar, 452
    ICU-acquired, 500, 501
Weaning
    from extracorporeal membrane oxygenation, 84, 84*t*
    from intraaortic balloon pumps, 123
    from mechanical ventilation, 1, 63-68
        assessment for, 63-65, 64*f*, 67
        parameters for, 65
    from ventricular assist devices, 128
West Nile virus (WNV), 237
White, Paul Dudley, 157
Whole-bowel irrigation (WBI), 548
Withdrawal of treatment, 579

WNV. *See* West Nile virus (WNV).
Wolff-Parkinson-White (WPW) syndrome, 198-199
World Health Organization
    on pandemic of 2009, 274
    web-based resource on bioterrorism, 259*t*
WPW syndrome. *See* Wolff-Parkinson-White (WPW)
    syndrome.

X
Xolair. *See* Omalizumab.

Y
Yersinia pestis, 254

Z
Zanamivir, 272
Zapol, Warren, 80
Ziprasidone, 517*t*